DALE M. SCHULZ

Systemic Pathology

Authors

C. W. M. Adams
B. S. Cardell
*J. B. Cavanagh
K. G. A. Clark
C. A. G. Cook
T. Crawford
A. R. Currie
*P. M. Daniel
W. M. Davidson
I. M. P. Dawson
I. Doniach
B. Fox
I. Friedmann
H. Haber
*D. G. F. Harriman
B. E. Heard
Kristin Henry
R. E. B. Hudson
P. E. Hughesdon

M. L. Lewis
R. B. Lucas
*W. H. McMenemey
J. A. Milne
G. Morgan
B. C. Morson
D. A. Osborn
K. A. Porter
*H. A. Sissons
J. C. Sloper
*W. Thomas Smith
*Sabina J. Strich
*W. St C. Symmers
A. C. Thackray
K. Weinbren
C. P. Wendell-Smith
E. D. Williams
G. Payling Wright
A. H. Wyllie

* Contributors to Volume 5

Editor
W. St C. Symmers

Systemic Pathology

SECOND EDITION

by THIRTY-EIGHT AUTHORS

VOLUME 5

Nervous System
Muscle
Bone
Joints

CHURCHILL LIVINGSTONE
Edinburgh London and New York 1979

CHURCHILL LIVINGSTONE
Medical Division of Longman Group Limited

Distributed in the United States of America by Longman
Inc., 19 West 44th Street, New York, N.Y. 10036, and by
associated companies, branches and representatives throughout the world.

First Edition (edited by G. Payling Wright and W. St Clair Symmers) 1966

Second Edition 1979

ISBN 0 443 01333 0

British Library Cataloguing in Publication Data

Systemic Pathology.
  Vol. 5: Nervous system, muscle, bone,
  joints. — 2nd ed.
  1. Pathology
  I. Symmers, William St Clair
  616.07   RB111   78-40903

Printed in Great Britain by
T. & A. Constable Ltd, Edinburgh

Contents

Volume 4

Volume 5

Volume 6

Authors of Volume 5

J. B. CAVANAGH, MD (London), FRCP (London)

Professor of Applied Neurobiology in the University of London at the Institute of Neurology; Honorary Consultant Pathologist, National Hospitals for Nervous Diseases, London.

P. M. DANIEL, MA (Oxford and Cambridge), DM (Oxford), DSc (London), MB, BChir (Cambridge), FRCP (London), FRCS (England), FRCPath, FRCPsych

Emeritus Professor of Neuropathology in the University of London; Senior Research Fellow in the Department of Applied Physiology, Royal College of Surgeons of England; formerly Honorary Consultant Pathologist, Bethlem Royal and Maudsley Hospitals, London, and Honorary Consultant in Neuropathology to the British Army at Home.

D. G. F. HARRIMAN, MD (Belfast), FRCP (London), FRCPath

Senior Lecturer in Neuropathology in the University of Leeds; Honorary Consultant Neuropathologist, Leeds Area Health Authority (Teaching); Honorary Director in Pathology, High Royds Hospital, Menston, Ilkley, West Yorkshire.

W. H. McMENEMEY, MA (Oxford), DM (Oxford), FRCPA (*Honorary*), FRCP (London), FRCPath, FRCPsych, DPM (England)

Emeritus Professor of Pathology in the University of London; Consulting Pathologist, National Hospitals for Nervous Diseases, London.

H. A. SISSONS, MD (Melbourne), FRCP (London), FRCS (England), FRCPath

Professor of Morbid Anatomy in the University of London at the Institute of Orthopaedics; Honorary Consultant Morbid Anatomist, Royal National Orthopaedic Hospital, London.

W. THOMAS SMITH, MD (Birmingham), FRCP (London), FRCPath

Professor of Neuropathology in the University of Birmingham; Honorary Consultant in Pathology, Birmingham Central Health District (Teaching); Honorary Consultant in Neuropathology to the West Midlands Regional Health Authority, Birmingham.

SABINA J. STRICH, MA (Oxford), DM (Oxford), MRCP (London), MRCPsych

Formerly Reader in Neuropathology in the University of London at the Institute of Psychiatry and Honorary Consultant Neuropathologist, Bethlem Royal and Maudsley Hospitals, London.

Editor

W. St C. SYMMERS, MD (Belfast), PhD (Birmingham), FRCP (London and Ireland), MRCP (Edinburgh), FRCPA

Professor of Histopathology in the University of London at Charing Cross Hospital Medical School; Honorary Consultant Pathologist, Charing Cross Hospital, London.

§

Acknowledgements for Illustrations

The caption of each illustration that requires an acknowledgement includes the symbol §, printed after the figure number (for example, Fig. 34.57.§). A footnote on the page on which the first such illustration in each chapter appears refers the reader to the page on which the acknowledgements are made. In the lists of acknowledgements, all the illustrations from each source are grouped together, in numerical sequence.

Some of the authors of the book and some of those who provided them with illustrations for the first volumes of this edition have found this method of acknowledgement to be inadequate. The § footnote, appearing only once in each chapter, is liable to be overlooked: this has led to a mistaken impression that acknowledgements have not been made in all instances requiring them.

The decision not to include acknowledgements in the captions of the illustrations but to collect them at the end of the chapter was made by the editor, who is responsible for the embarrassment caused to the authors and to those who helped to illustrate the book.

34: *The Central Nervous System*

by W. H. McMenemey

revised by THE AUTHOR *and* W. Thomas Smith

CONTENTS

1*

34: *The Central Nervous System*

by W. H. McMenemey *

* William Henry McMenemey: 16th May 1905–24th November 1977

revised by THE AUTHOR *and* W. THOMAS SMITH

Note: Except when stated otherwise, the histological preparations illustrated in this chapter are sections of tissues that were embedded in paraffin wax. See also footnote on page 2098.

THE CYTOLOGY OF THE CENTRAL NERVOUS SYSTEM

Introduction

The average weight of the brain is about 1400 g in men and 1250 g in women. In children, it rises steadily from its weight of 250 to 350 g at birth (see Table 34.1); at any age, the weight of a boy's brain is about 10 per cent greater than that of a girl.

The infolding of the brain during development and the resulting multiplicity of sulci accommodate a very large surface area of cortex. The two main divisions of the brain, the cerebrum and the cerebellum, are very different in structure. The two layers of the cortex of the cerebellum—the molecular

Table 34.1. *Mean Weight of the Brain of Children at Various Ages†*

Age	Weight (grams)	Age	Weight (grams)
6 months	660	5 years	1237
12 months	925	7 years	1263
2 years	964	9 years	1275
3 years	1141	12 years	1351

† Coppoletta, J. M., Wolbach, S. B., *Amer. J. Path.*, 1933, 9, 55.

and granular layers, with the cell bodies of the Purkyně cells‡ at the deep aspect of the former,

‡ Jan Evangelista Purkyně was born in 1787 in Libochovice, in Bohemia. He was professor of physiology in Breslau (Wrocław) from 1832 to 1850 and in Prague from 1850 until his death in 1869. The Czech spelling of his name is less familiar to the reader of English than the German transliteration, Purkinje, which was used in the paper in which he gave the first description, in 1837, of the cells of the cerebellar cortex that are now known as 'Purkyně cells' or 'Purkinje cells' (Purkinje, J. E., *Ber. Versamml. dtsch. Naturf. Aertz.* [Prag 1837], 1838, 179).

abutting on the latter—contrast with the more numerous layers of the cerebral cortex, which are still conventionally described as consisting of six laminae. Each cerebral lamina has a number of synonyms, including the following sequence—outer molecular, outer granular, outer pyramidal cell, inner granular, inner pyramidal cell, and fusiform cell layers. The distinctive lamination of the cerebral cortex is best appreciated in celloidin sections, about 30 μm thick and stained with cresyl violet by Nissl's method. The cells of the cerebral cortex reach their location in these layers during the period of migration of the neuroblasts from the centre of the fetal brain—the so-called 'mantle' (Fig. 34.1): this mainly occurs during the later months of intrauterine life. In children up to the age of 10 years, however, neurons are sometimes present in the white matter, especially of the occipital lobes; this misplacement has no significance. Occasionally, clusters of neuroblasts fail to reach their destination, but develop in abnormal sites (*heterotopia*).

The high metabolic activity of the brain requires a blood flow of about three-quarters of a litre a minute (roughly one-seventh of the cardiac output at rest).[1, 2] From studies on arteriovenous oxygen differences, it is estimated that the brain extracts rather more than 50 ml of oxygen from this volume of blood. This high oxygen requirement reflects the very large number of cells in the brain: the neurons alone are believed to number at least 26×10^9, and the glial cells are more numerous. In the cortex beneath every square millimetre of the surface of the cerebrum there lie some 50 000 nerve cells, a concentration of about 10 000 cells in each cubic millimetre.[3, 4] Cell density studies on the striate cortex of a young man showed $17 \cdot 5 \times 10^6$ neuronal

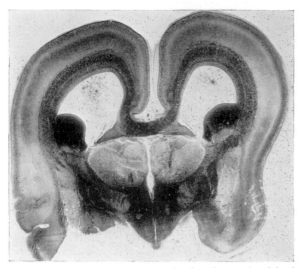

Fig. 34.1.§ The human brain at the fourth month of fetal development. The broad band surrounding most of the lateral ventricles is the mantle layer: a few of the migrating cells have already reached the rudimentary cortex, which at this stage is without gyral pattern. *Stern–Weil–Davenport stain.* × 3.

nuclei and 77×10^6 glial nuclei in each gram of fresh brain tissue; the figures are similar in the rhesus monkey and the rat.[5] It has been calculated that the neurons, although much outnumbered by the glial cells, utilize over half the oxygen supplied to the brain; nearly three-quarters of the oxygen is believed to be consumed in the grey matter and the rest in the white matter.[6]

The whole of the nervous system, with the exception of the blood vessels, their accompanying mesenchymal cells, the leptomeninges and the dura mater, is derived from the ectoderm. The medullary epithelium, which in early embryonic life lines the primitive neural canal, differentiates in two directions, forming the neurons (the excitable cells of the nervous system) and the neuroglia (the supporting and nutritive cells).

The Neuroglia[7–10]

The *neuroglia** is generally taken to comprise the astrocytes and the oligodendrocytes; it is usual to include also the ependymal cells, which retain a

---

* Virchow believed that the neuroglial cells, of which he could see only the nuclei, constituted the connective tissue or 'glue' (hence the name *glia*) of the brain (Virchow, R., *Virchows Arch. path. Anat.*, 1854, **6**, 135). There seems to be little doubt that he recognized that some of the cells also had a phagocytic function.

§ See *Acknowledgements*, page 2293.

---

closer resemblance to embryonic medullary epithelium than any other mature cells of the nervous system. The term glia is used in a general sense to refer to these cells; the tumours that originate from them are the gliomas. The term gliosis is generally used with the restricted meaning of proliferation of the fibrillary processes of the astrocytes.

The Astrocyte*

It is usual, with the light microscope, to distinguish two varieties of astrocyte, the *protoplasmic astrocyte*, found in the grey matter, and the *fibrous astrocyte*, found in the white matter throughout the brain and spinal cord, and less widely in the grey matter. Both varieties have a similar cell body; it is in their cytoplasmic processes that they differ. In paraffin wax sections stained with haematoxylin and eosin, the astrocyte can be identified by its round or ovoid, vesicular nucleus, some 8 to 10 μm in diameter (Fig. 34.2); unlike most neurons the normal astrocyte lacks a prominent nucleolus, and this is helpful in differentiating cells in the grey matter. Its cytoplasm, when visible at all in haematoxylin-eosin preparations, appears to be scanty, and its processes are seldom recognizable, and then only for a fraction of their length. When the processes are seen, they generally project in a radial pattern from the cell body: this arrangement led early neuro-histologists to name the cells 'spider cells' or, alternatively, 'stellate cells' ('astrocytes'). If stained by Holzer's crystal violet or Anderson's Victoria blue methods, the processes of the fibrous astrocytes become more distinct, especially in the white matter, and their tenuous prolongations can be followed for 300 μm or more. To demonstrate astrocytes in grey matter, Mallory's phosphotungstic acid haematoxylin is preferable; in white matter this method is less valuable, largely because

---

* Deiters in 1865 was the first to recognize the astrocyte (Deiters, O., *Untersuchungen über Gehirn und Rückenmark des Menschen und der Säugethiere*; Braunschweig, 1865), but it was not until the introduction of the carmine wash method that its manifold cytoplasmic processes could be identified with any certainty. The method of metallic impregnation, apparently first tried by Krause in 1844, helped to disclose the many ramifying processes possessed by these cells, and the early silver and gold techniques of Ranvier (Ranvier, L. A., *Leçons sur l'histologie du système nerveux*; Paris, 1878) and Golgi (reference 13a on page 2227) were later modified by Ford Robertson (Robertson, W. F., *Scot. med. J.*, 1899, **4**, 23), Ramón y Cajal (Ramón y Cajal, S., *Rev. Cienc. méd.* [*Madr.*], 1892, **18**, 457; and many subsequent publications) and del Río Hortega (reference 34 on page 2227).

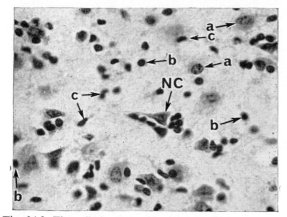

Fig. 34.2. The cells in diseased cerebral cortex. The nuclei of astrocytes (a) are of moderate size and roundish, with palely-stained contents: surrounding the nucleus a rim of pale cytoplasm can often be discerned together with the beginnings of the processes, but the cell outline is always indistinct, tending to fade imperceptibly into the background; the cytoplasm is more prominent and the nucleus often lies eccentrically when, as in the present instance, these cells are reacting. The nuclei of oligodendrocytes are small, round and pyknotic (b) and are usually surrounded by a fine unstained halo or, less often, by a thin rim of palely-stained cytoplasm. Intermediate in size and in their ability to hold the haematoxylin are the nuclei of Hortega cells (microglia): they are often reniform (c) but in cross section are round and so may resemble oligodendrocytes; they have to be distinguished from the endothelial cells of capillaries. The degenerating nerve cell in the centre (NC) is adjoined by Hortega cells, but the cluster of round cells to its right could be oligodendrocytes. *Celloidin. Haematoxylin–eosin.* × 300.

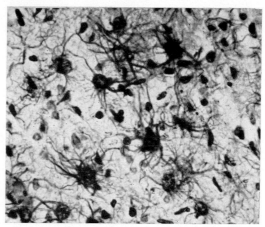

Fig. 34.3. Proliferating protoplasmic astrocytes in cerebral cortex. *Frozen section. Hortega silver method for astrocytes.* × 360.

the cell processes are obscured by the presence of myelin, which also takes up the haematoxylin.

While most of the astrocytes in the cerebral cortex are of the protoplasmic variety, fibrous astrocytes are present in the outer cellular layer and also round the penetrating arterioles. The distinction between protoplasmic and fibrous astrocytes can be shown microscopically by various methods of metallic impregnation of histological sections. The processes of the protoplasmic astrocytes are short and stout (Fig. 34.3), and they branch oftener than the long, fine, fibrillary processes of the fibrous astrocytes (Fig. 34.4); these differences in structure may reflect differences in the functions of the two varieties of cell. When the protoplasmic astrocytes react—for instance in lesions in which cortical neurons have been lost—their processes become fibrous, fibrils developing in them that are clearly revealed by the methods of Anderson and of Holzer. The glial fibrils were shown by del Río Hortega to be within the cytoplasmic processes and not extracellular structures,[11]

a finding that has since been confirmed with the electron microscope. In fact, on the evidence of electron microscopy, the distinction between protoplasmic and fibrous astrocytes is not always possible. The fibrils that are seen with the light microscope probably consist of compact bundles of the intracellular filaments that are disclosed by the electron microscope (Figs 34.5 and 34.6).

Electron microscopy shows that the cytoplasm of astrocytes contains—in addition to the filaments noted above—rough endoplasmic reticulum, Golgi complexes, mitochondria and lipid droplets (Fig. 34.5). The foot processes (see below) are also easily recognized in electron micrographs (Fig. 34.6); they are separated from the capillary endothelial cells by their basal lamina.

Protoplasmic astrocytes are present in the

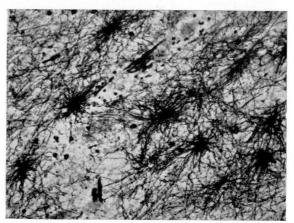

Fig. 34.4. Proliferating fibrous astrocytes in white matter. *Frozen section. Golgi–Cox stain.* × 200.

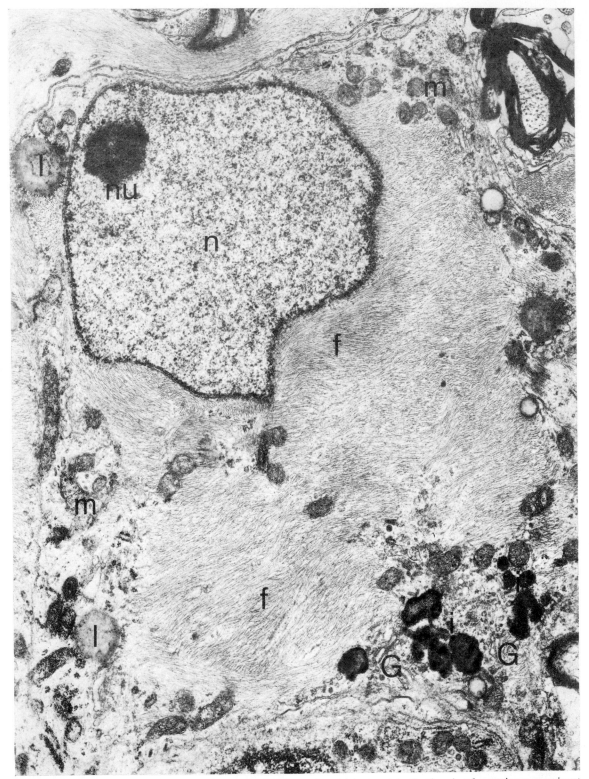

Fig. 34.5.§ Electron micrograph of a reacting astrocyte. The nucleus (n) is eccentrically placed and contains a prominent nucleolus (nu). The abundant cytoplasm contains large numbers of filaments (f); there are also Golgi complexes (G), mitochondria (m), lipid droplets (l) and electron-dense inclusions (i). × 16 400.

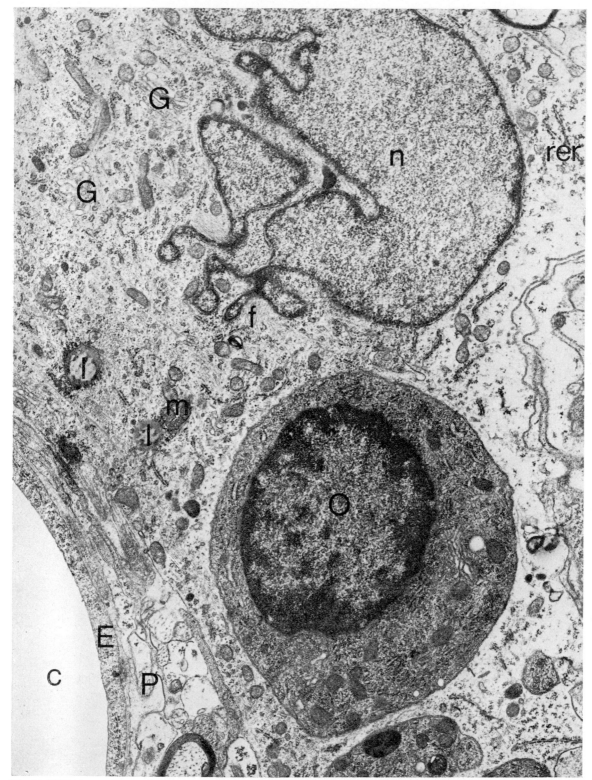

Fig. 34.6.§ Electron micrograph of a reacting astrocyte surrounding an oligodendrocyte (O). The nucleus of the oligodendrocyte has a regular outline; its electron-dense cytoplasm contains closely-packed ribosomes, rough endoplasmic reticulum and organelles. The outline of the nucleus of the astrocyte (n) is very irregular; its chromatin is evenly distributed. The abundant cytoplasm of the astrocyte contains cisternae of rough endoplasmic reticulum (rer), Golgi complexes (G), filaments (f), mitochondria (m) and lipid droplets (l). A capillary (c) is seen: its endothelial cells (E) are separated from the clear foot processes of the astrocytes (P) by a basal lamina. ×9200.

caudate nuclei and putamina, and in the granular layer of the cerebellum. Elsewhere in the central nervous system most astrocytes are of the fibrous type, although variations among them have been observed. Some, the *Bergmann cells*, found in the granular layer of the cerebellum near the Purkyně cells, have a well-developed fibrous process that extends to the pial surface, while others, the *Fañanás cells*,[11a] lying more superficially in the cerebellar cortex, have processes that are shorter and stouter than usual, somewhat resembling those of the protoplasmic astrocytes.

Astrocytes have been compared with the fibroblasts of other tissues of the body, for one of their functions is to close, by means of glial scar formation, any gaps caused by the destruction of neurons or of the myelin that surrounds the axons.[12] The analogy should not be carried too far, for fibroblasts are of mesodermal origin, and the collagen fibres that they produce are extracellular structures,[13] whereas astrocytes are of ectodermal origin and the glial fibres are part of their cytoplasm. Moreover, the astrocyte by no means completely replaces the fibroblast within the central nervous system, for under certain circumstances collagenous scars can develop, as, for instance, in the wall of abscesses, round foreign bodies, and in post-trau-matic meningocortical adhesions; these collagenous scars are stronger, and more rapidly produced, than astroglial scars. Nevertheless, the ability of astrocytes to form dense masses of glial fibrils is at times remarkable, notably in multiple sclerosis, in which an abundance of fibrils may soon obscure the cells that have produced them. When gliosis develops along the course of demyelinated axons, the fibrils assume a regular and parallel arrangement (*isomorphic gliosis*) (Fig. 34.7).

Gliosis is not always pathological. It may be found to some extent in the normal brain, for instance in the olivary nuclei, the floor of the fourth ventricle and round the aqueduct and the central canal of the spinal cord.

Astrocytes possess one or more terminal protoplasmic expansions that embrace the adjacent capillaries; these 'sucker feet', which were first noted by Golgi,[13a] are especially well seen in Cajal preparations of the white matter. They are so numerous that it has been suggested that they constitute an anatomical blood–brain barrier (Held's limiting membrane). Electron microscopy, however, has indicated that there may be gaps in this investment round some capillaries.[14] In addition to their attachment to blood vessels, astrocytes that are near the surface of the cortex—for instance,

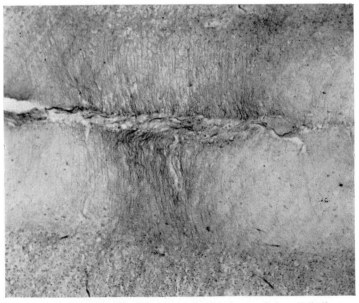

Fig. 34.7. Isomorphic gliosis in the molecular layer of the cerebellum, a not infrequent finding indicative of local ischaemia. These glial fibrils have developed in the processes of the Bergmann astrocytes (in the Purkyně cell layer) and extend to the pial surface. The distended venule near the right of the centre of the picture lies at the bottom of a sulcus. *Celloidin section. Holzer stain.* × 90.

the Fañanás cells—often have a process that is secured to the pial membrane. Studies on the ultrastructure of astrocytes indicate that their processes ramify very widely and are much more voluminous than other histological techniques suggest: within the substance of the central nervous system they are believed to fill all the available space between the other cells and their processes.[15-17]

In tissue culture, chick embryo astrocytes grow best when the oxygen tension is reduced to 2 per cent and the carbon dioxide tension is 4 per cent.[18] In human pathology, the stimulus to the proliferation of the cortical astrocytes appears to be death of nearby neurons. For example, within 48 hours of a hypoxic or hypoglycaemic episode in which neurons have been lost, the astrocytes in the vicinity of the dead cells swell and begin to proliferate. The nuclei of the dividing astrocytes can be seen lying in pairs, and the cytoplasmic processes become grouped into two sets, one associated with each nucleus. If many neurons have been destroyed, and the patient survives, further proliferation of astrocytes takes place, with the formation of cell clusters (*astrocytosis*) (Fig. 34.8). In grey matter, the presence of astrocytic nuclei paired or clustered in this way is presumptive evidence of neuronal loss. Sometimes nuclear division takes place without separation of the swollen cytoplasm, the formation of a multinucleate giant astrocyte resulting. Under other conditions, the cell body of the astrocyte swells considerably, its nucleus enlarges and assumes an eccentric position, and its cytoplasm and nucleolus usually become clearly visible, even in haematoxylin–eosin preparations. The German word *gemästet* ('fattened', 'plump') was applied to this type of cell, and has been 'anglicized' in the names *gemistocytic astrocyte* and *gemistocyte*. Such swollen forms are to be seen in oedematous white matter and near rapidly expanding inflammatory, ischaemic or neoplastic lesions. They may also be found in the white matter within as little as six hours after the onset of acute oedema.

Under normal circumstances astrocytes seldom, if ever, undergo division. There has been much debate whether astrocytes in pathological states divide by mitosis or in some other way: that they proliferate round focal lesions is not in doubt, for experimental studies, using perfusion fixation, mitotic inhibitors and autoradiography, have shown that division does occur.[19]

There is no evidence that astrocytes are capable of phagocytosis. Like other cells, they may undergo fatty degeneration, and, in old age, their cytoplasm, like that of neurons, may contain granules of lipochrome. Like other cells, too, they are susceptible to bacterial toxins and other poisons, undergoing a form of degeneration in which the cell and its processes swell (*'cloudy swelling'*); in the severer, irreversible forms of degeneration, the nucleus disappears (*karyolysis*), and the processes fragment (*clasmatodendrosis*) (Fig. 34.9) and are ingested by phagocytic cells (*dendrophagocytosis*).

The Oligodendrocyte

In sections stained with haematoxylin and eosin or by Nissl's method, the oligodendrocyte is recognized

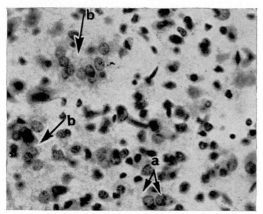

Fig. 34.8. Cerebral cortex showing an unusual degree of astrocytosis. The pale-staining nuclei of astrocytes can be seen in pairs (a) and in clusters (b), lying eccentrically in ill-defined cytoplasm. *Celloidin section. Haematoxylin–eosin.* × 360.

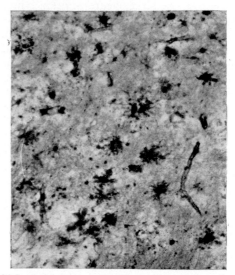

Fig. 34.9. Astrocytes, some in pairs, showing clasmatodendrosis: fragments of processes can be seen adjacent to the contracted proximal stumps. *Frozen section. Cajal's gold sublimate method.* × 120.

by its small, dense nucleus, which is about 7 μm in diameter (Fig. 34.2). The cytoplasm seldom takes these stains but is often recognizable in the form of a clear halo round the nucleus. In the immediate vicinity of a blood vessel it may prove impossible, with ordinary stains, to distinguish the oligodendrocyte from a lymphocyte, but with Golgi's rapid method the nucleus of the former stains selectively as an orange sphere some 6 to 9 μm in diameter.[20]

Oligodendrocytes possess processes, as del Río Hortega showed,[21] but these are difficult to demonstrate and few in number—hence the name of the cell. Although the nucleus of the oligodendrocyte appears round in haematoxylin–eosin preparations, giving an impression that the cell itself is round, the cytoplasm appears angulate when impregnated with silver; silver preparations show that most of the processes are long, and they tend to originate from four corners of the cell. In tissue cultures, the oligodendrocyte and the astrocyte are not dissimilar, and it has even been suggested that they are different forms of a single cell type,[22, 23] a view in keeping with Hortega's schema, which groups them together as the neuroglia. Although the nuclei of oligodendrocytes and astrocytes are generally easy to identify correctly, it may prove impossible at times to distinguish between them; in fact, in pathological states of the white matter, a gradation may sometimes be recognized between the typical forms of these two cells.

Oligodendrocytes outnumber all other cells in the central nervous system.* They are frequently seen in attendance on the larger neurons, often lying close to the cell body and wedged between dendrites. The accumulation of oligodendrocytes round a neuron is known as *satellitosis*, and the arrangement of the clustered nuclei led Spielmeyer to name the cells *Traubenzellen* ('bunch-of-grapes cells').† Satellitosis is specially noticeable round the large and medium-sized pyramidal cells of the frontal cortex and the large neurons of the basal ganglia. It is not so apparent round Betz cells of the motor cortex and cells of the anterior grey columns of the spinal cord. When white matter is sectioned in the long axis of the axons, oligodendrocytes are visible in

---

* As implied above, the word oligodendrocyte means—literally—cell with few dendrites. The increasing tendency to abbreviate the term to oligocyte ignores this derivation and is objectionable also as implying that these cells are few in number, which, as noted in the text, is the opposite of the case.

† The corresponding observation of perineuronal satellite cells in the ganglia of the dorsal roots of the spinal nerves is mentioned on page 2298. The satellite cells in these ganglia are modified neurolemmal cells.

long regular rows: these are the periaxonal or interfascicular oligodendrocytes, and they are particularly well seen in the corpus callosum. Oligodendrocytes are also to be found in close relation to small blood vessels (perivascular oligodendrocytes), and it has been suggested that they control the opening and closing of the vessels.[24]

It has been supposed that the flat, delicate processes of these cells are wrapped round the neuron, including its axon and dendrites.[25, 26] The views of electron microscopists on this matter are still divided, for some believe that the processes are numerous and extensive while others find them scanty. This difference of opinion may depend, in part, on the existence of more than one form of the oligodendrocyte.

The oligodendrocyte is a sensitive cell and there are many pathological conditions—among them hypoxia, ischaemia, acute infections and trauma—in which it undergoes acute swelling. The pathologist must recognize that some degree of acute swelling is inevitable in tissues fixed by immersion and in biopsy specimens obtained under anaesthesia. In experimental studies perfusion fixation is always desirable.

The cytoplasm of the normal oligodendrocyte is more electron-dense than that of the astrocyte (Fig. 34.6), because of the close packing of the ribosomes, which are often arranged in rosettes or associated with rough endoplasmic reticulum. The usual organelles are present. There are no cytoplasmic filaments in oligodendrocytes, in contrast to astrocytes, but microtubules have been recognized. Electron microscopy and histochemical and biochemical findings together indicate that there is considerable metabolic activity in oligodendrocytes: this may be concerned in maintenance of myelin, and possibly is related to a continuous need for synthesis of certain components of myelin. Interfascicular oligodendrocytes are often surrounded by the clearer cytoplasmic processes of fibrous astrocytes (Fig. 34.6).

There is firm evidence that oligodendrocytes are responsible for the synthesis of the myelin in the central nervous system.[27] The compacted layers of the myelin in the central nervous system are disposed in a spiral and have a cytoplasmic component that is derived from and continuous with the oligodendrocytic perikaryon. A single oligodendrocyte, by a connecting process that may be lengthy, may contribute to several internodes and to internodes of more than one axon.

Oligodendrocytes are morphologically heterogeneous, comprising four types, of which three occur in white matter and are concerned with myelin.[27] Whether the normal oligodendrocyte is 'dormant' throughout life, like its counterpart in the peripheral nerves, the Schwann cell, is still uncertain. There is also still no firm evidence that the oligodendrocyte is capable of mitotic division.

It has been suggested that the glia includes uncommitted cells that can mature into either oligodendrocytes or astrocytes. There is also some evidence that limited remyelination of axons of the central nervous system can occur under experimental conditions.[28, 29]

Nodes that correspond to the nodes of Ranvier of peripheral nerves are present in the central nervous system. The available data suggest that the ratio of internodal length to fibre diameter may be similar to that in the peripheral nerves.

It is possible that oligodendrocytes may assume a phagocytic role in the early stages of myelin breakdown.[30] This view has been disputed, for the presence of myelin breakdown products within the cytoplasm of these cells in such circumstances might equally result from passive transfer, in consequence of their intimate contact with the myelin.

Both Ford Robertson and Cajal failed to distinguish the oligodendrocyte from microglia (see page 2095). The former asserted that the small 'glial cells', which he recognized to be neither neurons nor astrocytes, were mesodermal in origin and phagocytic in character; he referred to them as mesoglia,[31, 32] a term that is now obsolete. Cajal called them the 'third element'.[33] It was Cajal's pupil, del Río Hortega, who first clearly distinguished these two types of cell.[34, 35] He classified the oligodendrocyte with the astrocytes as neuroglia: the microglial cell he regarded as the real 'third element', because it is neither a neuron nor a true neuroglial cell.

The Ependymal Cell[36]

The epithelium-like ependymal cells cover the choroid plexuses and line the ventricles, the aqueduct and the central canal of the spinal cord. They are ciliate. One or several fibrillate tapering processes may extend from the base of the cell into the subependymal layer of glial cells and fibres. In the developing brain the subependymal zone (subependymal plate) includes undifferentiated dividing cells that are an important source of mature neurons and neuroglia, which migrate into the surrounding brain.

At the base of the cilia of the ependymal cells are the small, round or rod-shaped bodies known as blepharoplasts. The blepharoplast stains with phosphotungstic-acid haematoxylin and corresponds to the basal corpuscle seen with the electron microscope. Ultrastructurally, the cilia consist of nine peripheral pairs of filaments that surround a central pair, an arrangement common to most cilia and flagella. The peripheral filaments continue into the basal corpuscle. Adjacent cells are bound together by complex lateral interdigitation. The cells differ in morphology in different areas: those covering white matter are usually flattened and have scant cilia and basal processes; those covering grey matter have many cilia and basal processes and a microvillous border. The presence of mitochondria, a Golgi complex, ergastoplasm and dense bodies is suggestive of metabolic activity. Thorium dioxide and other particulate material injected into the ventricular system is taken into ependymal cells by pinocytosis: this supports the view that there is transfer of substances between the cerebrospinal fluid and the brain by way of the ependyma. It is clear that these cells influence the formation and composition of the cerebrospinal fluid by a combination of active secretion, diffusion, absorption and exchange.

In most respects the covering cells of the choroid plexuses resemble the ependymal cells elsewhere, except that in man they rarely have cilia and blepharoplasts.

The ependymal cells are usually considered to have relatively little capacity to react to pathological conditions or to regenerate. In chronic inflammatory states, such as neurosyphilis, there is often a reactive proliferation of the subependymal astrocytes, which may break through the ependymal surface as 'granulations' and then grow over the adjacent ependyma by confluence: ependyma that is covered in this way may react and form rosettes or small clefts. Similar changes may be found in association with hydrocephalus.

'Corpora Amylacea'

Rounded bodies, about 10 to 15 μm in diameter, and sometimes laminate, are often found in elderly people in the white matter adjacent to the ventricles and to the pial surface of the spinal cord. They stain grey or greyish blue in haematoxylin–eosin and cresyl violet preparations, and they are periodic-acid/Schiff-positive. They receive the name corpora amylacea because of their supposed resemblance to starch granules. They have been thought to represent the end-stage in degeneration of either oligodendrocytes or astrocytes: electron microscopy indicates that the latter is the probable explanation.[37] These bodies provoke no glial reaction and they are thought not to have any pathological significance except in so far as they may be seen in the brain and spinal cord of younger people as a result of earlier disease, particularly poliomyelitis.

The Neuron[10, 38, 39]

Neurons differ widely in size, as judged by the dimensions of the cell body, the extremes being 80 μm (the greatest dimension of the cell body of the Betz cells) and 5 μm (the diameter of the cell body of the granule cells of the cerebellum). But the axon must also be taken into account when considering the size of a neuron: that of the Betz cell, for instance, has more than 1000 times the volume of the cell body (*perikaryon*) of which it is a process. Neurons vary in shape, some being round, others oval, fusiform or pyramidal. Each possesses a single axon; the number of its dendrites varies from one to as many as 80, according to the type of cell (Fig. 34.10). The dendrites branch freely and repeatedly to produce terminal twigs. Axons may branch, but they do so infrequently: the branches (collaterals) tend to leave the main trunk at a right angle.

Whatever their size or function, all neurons have certain features in common: they have a high metabolic rate, they are peculiarly sensitive to oxygen lack, and at about the time of birth they lose the ability to multiply. The well-known phenomena of ageing, with the intellectual deterioration that accompanies them, are generally believed to be associated with a progressive loss of neurons, or, perhaps, with a reduction in the number of those that remain capable of functioning. This gradual wastage of neurons through 'wear and tear' is probably accentuated under certain conditions, as, for instance, by insults inflicted by alcohol, the temporary hypoxia associated with nitrous oxide anaesthesia, and the excessive use of certain drugs. Any loss of neurons must be considerable, however, before it is recognizable in histological sections of the cortex, unless attention is drawn to it by the presence of a compensatory astrocytosis (see page 2083). Some progress is being made in the assessment of neuronal loss by applying quantitative morphometric methods with the aid of computers: unpublished recent evidence suggests that the degree of this loss in cases of senile dementia is not as great as was previously believed.[39a, 39b]

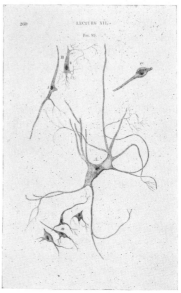

Fig. 34.10. Neurons. This illustration is from a preparation by Gerlach (1847) and is reproduced because of its historical interest. By a simple process of teasing fresh preparations the early microscopists learned a great deal about the axon and dendrites of nerve cells. In the centre can be seen a 'many-rayed' or multipolar motor cell from the anterior column of the spinal cord. Two 'sensory cells from the spinal cord' are shown at the top left, and bottom left is a group of small cells from the cerebral cortex. (Virchow, R., *Cellular Pathology as Based upon Physiological and Pathological Histology*, translated from the second German edition by F. Chance, Fig. 89, page 298; Philadelphia, 1863 [republished in New York, 1971].)

The specialized character of certain neurons is apparent from their size, shape, and cytoplasmic contents; they also differ in their neurohumoral transmitter agents. The relatively large size of the perikaryon of the Betz cells in the cerebral cortex and of the cells of the anterior grey columns of the spinal cord is clearly related to the great length of their axons. It is, in fact, because of the metabolic demands of the long axon that their content of Nissl substance (see below) is so abundant. In some metabolic deficiencies and intoxications that injure such neurons, it is the distal parts of the long fibres that are affected first, and most severely. The smaller neurons, in the middle lamina of the cerebral cortex, have shorter axons and much less Nissl substance.

The Nucleus of the Neuron

Because of their large size, the Betz cells of the precentral gyrus and the cells of the anterior grey columns of the spinal cord have been studied in particular detail. The round, centrally placed nucleus is characterized by a prominent nucleolus that contains ribonucleic acid (RNA) linked to a protein. It would seem that the RNA is synthetized in the nucleolus or at its periphery. As in all cells, the nuclear chromatin, which appears finely granular, is composed of deoxyribonucleic acid (DNA). The DNA, which has little if any metabolic turnover, except during mitosis, carries the genetical information of the cell, and thus determines the nature of the RNA, which is constantly being formed and utilized in cellular activities.[40]

The Cytoplasmic Constituents of Neurons

Nissl Substance.—In the cytoplasm of the neuron, certain polygonal, basiphile structures, known collectively as Nissl substance,[41] are present, often packed against the limiting membrane of the cell body. Because of a supposed likeness to the markings on the skin of the tiger, these bodies have sometimes been called the 'tigroid substance'. They consist of aggregates of complex, iron-containing, protein molecules linked to RNA, and in the unfixed cell they can be identified and estimated quantitatively by means of ultraviolet light of 257 nm wavelength.[42] With phase-contrast microscopy, they can be seen in neurons in tissue culture,[43] corresponding precisely to the structures found in the same cells when subsequently fixed and stained.[44] They are equated with the granular endoplasmic reticulum seen in electron micrographs. In conventional histological sections of fixed tissue, these bodies are shown best by methylene blue or cresyl violet stains, but they are readily visible in haematoxylin–eosin preparations. Nissl substance is not confined to the cytoplasm but is also present in the dendrites up to some distance from the perikaryon. It is absent, however, from the axon hillock (the origin of the axon), and also from the axon itself. The amount in any one perikaryon seems, in general, to be proportional to the length of its axon: it is particularly plentiful in the Betz cells and in the cells of the anterior grey columns of the spinal cord (the upper and lower motor neurons respectively).

Under conditions of stress the Nissl substance disappears, at first from that part of the perikaryon nearest to the nucleus, and later from the rest of the cytoplasm, with the exception of its periphery, where a thin rim usually remains identifiable.[45] This process of depletion, which occurs both under physiological conditions of heightened activity and in many pathological states, is known as *central chromatolysis* (or 'tigrolysis'). Under physiological

conditions, the Nissl substance is wholly restored after a resting period of a few days (seven days in the case of the anterior horn cells);[46] the newly formed substance appears first at the periphery of the perikaryon. It would seem that new RNA emerges from the vicinity of the nucleolus, travels to the periphery of the nucleus, traverses its membrane, and appears as Nissl substance in the cytoplasm.[47-49]

When the axon is severed, chromatolysis follows, and is accompanied by swelling of the perikaryon and, usually, by displacement of the nucleus from near the centre of the cell to its periphery. This is known as the *axonal reaction*, or *retrograde degeneration*; the change has frequently been used for identifying the cell groups that form the brainstem nuclei of certain cranial nerves. If the proximal end of the divided axon succeeds in sprouting and making contact with suitable dendrites, or with a muscle or other effector organ, some recovery of axonal function may follow, but it is not easy to ascertain how often this is achieved. In the central nervous system it probably happens rarely, for within the brain and spinal cord the newly growing axon, unlike that of a peripheral nerve, has no neurolemmal sheath to guide its progress. Many cells that are thus injured die; there is some evidence that a cell is likelier to survive if its afferent fibres still function.[50] Among cells that die when their axons have been cut, those of the thalami, the lateral geniculate bodies and the spiral ganglion of the organs of Corti are of particular neurosurgical importance.

The subject of central chromatolysis and the axonal reaction has recently been reappraised.[50a] The degree of chromatolysis may range from extensive to almost none, regardless of the outcome of the reaction. Electron microscopy may show a degree of disruption of the endoplasmic reticulum that varies appreciably although the chromatolytic cells look similar under the light microscope. Variation may be related to the type of injury, age, species, area affected and other factors. Regeneration of the axon appears to be accompanied by an increase in the synthesis of RNA and protein in the perikaryon.

In pathological states Nissl substance may disappear completely. The functional recovery of a neuron seems to be associated with restoration of this substance, which takes place more slowly after injury than after physiological exhaustion. If the injury has rendered the nucleolus incapable of forming RNA, Nissl substance is not replaced, and death of the cell probably follows soon.

Nissl substance appears to fill the whole cyto-plasm of the nerve cells of the anterior grey columns of the spinal cord: in contrast, it is present more sparsely in neurons of some other types. For instance, the cells of the nuclei dorsales of the spinal cord (Clarke's columns[51]) are oval, with an eccentric nucleus: the centre of the perikaryon is occupied by lipochrome, and Nissl substance is present only at the periphery of the cytoplasm. Unless familiar with this appearance—which is common to many neurons in the brainstem and elsewhere—it is easy to mistake this normal state for central chromatolysis.

Mitochondria.—The Nissl substance is not to be confused with the *mitochondria*, which are present in all cells of the body; in the neurons, mitochondria are to be found throughout the cytoplasm, including the axon hillock and the axon itself. Each mito-chondrion has an outer double membrane that encloses a series of transversely placed inner membranes, or cristae.[52, 53] Oxidative phosphoryla-tion and electron transport take place in these organelles, with the formation of substances such as adenosine triphosphate, which play an important part in the metabolism of the cell. The mitochondria carry enzyme systems: these remain unaffected when the Nissl substance is depleted physiologically but disappear when the cell is irrecoverably injured by, for example, toxins or viruses.

Neurofibrils.—In neurons fixed by the usual methods, delicate filaments known as neurofibrils can be seen by means of Bielschowsky's silver impregnation technique to traverse the cytoplasm from the dendrites to the axon. They lie between the Nissl bodies and tend to be packed closely together. Under certain circumstances neurofibrils become swollen and seemingly fused together: they can then be seen much more easily (see page 2275).

It has been much disputed whether neurofibrils are present as such in living cells, or whether they are formed from some previously invisible element during the coagulative process of fixation. The birefringence of the cytoplasm of neurons, and especially of their axons, makes it likely that there is, in fact, some organized system of molecular complexes arranged with a linear orientation throughout the cell and its processes. Two types of neurofilaments can be identified with the electron microscope (Fig. 34.11): some—known as neuro-tubules—are about 24 nm in diameter and have a lumen that is about 15 nm in diameter; others are about 10 nm in diameter and have a poorly-defined lumen. It has been suggested that these filaments, oriented longitudinally in the perikarya and axon, represent the fibrous protein that is synthetized in the Nissl complex.[54–57] They are too fine to be resolved by the light microscope, unless a fixation artefact results in their side-to-side aggregation, when they may become visible, especially in silver impregnation preparations.[58]

Melanin.—Some of the neurons in the brainstem contain melanin. These cells lie in two main groups, forming the substantia nigra in the midbrain and the substantia ferruginea in the pons; the heavy pigmentation of the latter makes it visible in the upper part of the floor of the fourth ventricle as the tiny locus caeruleus. Melanin is also found in small amounts in other brainstem nuclei, including the dorsal motor nucleus of the vagus.

The suggestion has been made that there are differences between neuronal melanin and melanin elsewhere.[59] The significance of the melanin in the brain remains controversial. The melanin in the substantia ferruginea appears at an early stage in fetal development; in contrast, none is found in the substantia nigra until the eighteenth month after birth.[60] Both these cell groups are characterized by an exceptionally high content of copper.[61] It is noteworthy that these are the neurons that seem to be particularly subject to degenerative changes in Parkinson's disease (see page 2267).

Melanin has been found in neurons of the sub-stantia nigra in species representing five mammalian orders:[62] the amount of pigment seems to parallel the phylogenetic increase in size and cellularity of this nucleus. The pigmentation is most marked in simians, particularly in apes closely related to man. In lower animals the amount of melanin is not great enough to be visible to the naked eye: microscopically visible amounts are present in the cat, dog, sheep and horse. Melanin has not been found in the pig, rabbit, guinea-pig, rat or mouse.

Melanophores are present in the meninges in man. Meningeal pigmentation with melanin occurs in many animals: it is most marked in sheep and cattle, greatly exceeding the amount found in man.

Lipochrome.[63]—The cytoplasm of some neurons contains fatty substances in the form of Sudanophile granules, many of them near the nuclear membrane. This material is known generically as *lipofuscin*, or *lipochrome*. In unstained preparations it is seen to have a yellowish colour, and it is not wholly removed from fixed cells by alcohol or xylene. It is

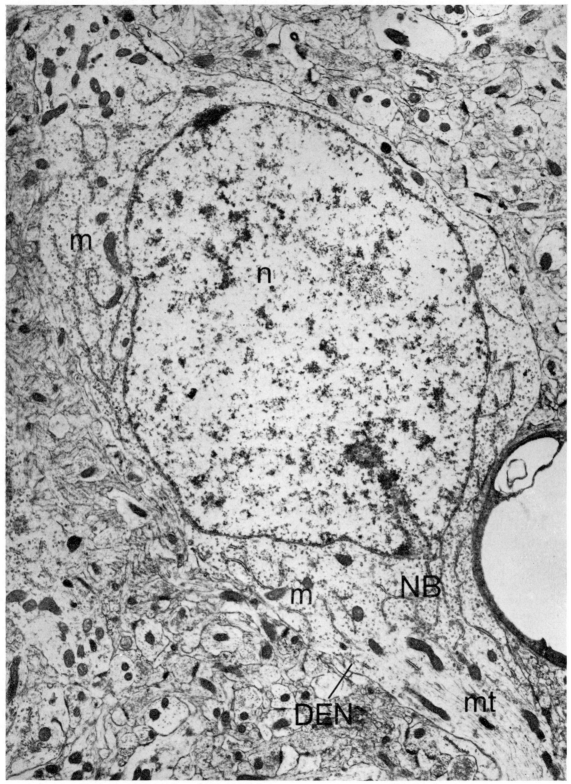

Fig. 34.11.§ Electron micrograph of a neuron from the caudate nucleus of a rat. The large, central, rounded nucleus (n) contains homogeneously dispersed karyoplasm. The apical dendrite (DEN) contains Nissl bodies (NB), mitochondria (m) and microtubules (mt). The neuron is surrounded by glial, axonal and dendritic processes. × 18 900.

believed to have a role in the normal metabolism of the neurons in which it occurs, namely those of the nuclei dorsales (Clarke's columns) of the spinal cord, the dorsal root ganglia, the colliculi and the thalami.

Lipofuscin is thought to be associated with peroxidative attack on cell systems, which many believe to be a major factor in the ageing of neurons. Many neurons of the brain and spinal cord of old people contain a quantity of lipochrome substance and this has long been regarded as a degenerative phenomenon. Antioxidant drugs are said to prevent deposition of this pigmented material in the course of ageing and in experimental encephalopathies.[64]

Lipofuscin and the related substance ceroid accumulate in the brain and autonomic ganglia in juvenile amaurotic family idiocy (Batten–Mayou disease—see page 2236 and Volume 6, Chapter 40).[65]

Secretion.—The neurons of the supraoptic and paraventricular nuclei are noteworthy for their ability to form a secretion that is carried along their axons to the neurohypophysis, particularly the posterior lobe of the pituitary, where normally it is stored before it is passed into the blood (see page 1875, Volume 4).[66] This neurosecretion contains vasopressin and oxytocin.

Axons, Dendrites and Synapses

From the behaviour of neuronal processes in tissue culture it seems likely that the outgrowing axon in the developing nervous system makes contact with adjacent dendrites of other cells. It is through these axonal connexions that nervous impulses are received by dendrites. These effective sites of cellular contact are the *synapses*. Cajal believed that the neuron is polarized in such a way that the impulse always passes from the dendrites to the perikaryon and thence down the axon to the synapse at its extremity: no serious objection to this view has been advanced.

The axoplasm has been shown to contain mitochondria, vesicles and longitudinal filaments similar to and continuous with those in the perikaryon. There is uncertainty about the precise relation between somal and axonal filaments and their functions. In addition to synapses with adjacent dendrites, many axonal twigs make close contact with the bodies of nerve cells by means of end bulbs (*boutons terminaux*).[67] The cellular territories subserving particular neurological activities remain functionally discrete, and it is only at the synapses with the second, or recipient, neurons that neuro-

humoral agents, such as acetylcholine, are released from synaptic vesicles and, by creating local ionic changes, propagate the nervous impulse.

The excitatory, cholinergic, presynaptic axon terminal in the central nervous system expands into a synaptic knob, filled with clear, acetylcholine-containing vesicles and mitochondria. The thickened membrane of the axon terminal is separated by a narrow space (the synaptic cleft) from the postsynaptic membrane; the latter is thick and is formed on the soma, dendrite or dendritic spine of the neuron that it is in contact with. Denser membrane-bound vesicles containing catecholamines have also been described in axon terminals. Axo-axonic terminals are also recognized: they are thought to be inhibitory in nature.

Myelin[68]

In man, the process of myelination extends over many months; some axons in the central nervous system, in the spinal cord particularly, are myelinated at birth, but the majority acquire their sheath only during the first year of life.

The myelin sheath is thin in comparison with the axon it surrounds: the histological appearances in post-mortem material fixed in formal saline are deceptive, for this form of fixation causes swelling of the myelin and substantial shrinkage of the axon.[69] X-ray diffraction studies and electron microscopy have shown that the sheath has a highly organized internal structure, consisting of many successive layers of protein and lipid wrapped round the axon.[70] There is still uncertainty as to how this wrapping process begins and how the successive layers are deposited. Geren, who studied peripheral nerves, suggested that a fine film of protoplasm from the enclosing Schwann cell gradually advances round the axon, surrounding it with a coil of myelin layers,[71] and this view has been supported by studies with tissue cultures.[72] On the other hand, Luse, who studied the process of myelination in the central nervous system, believed that the successive layers are laid down by what may be termed a 'plastering process', through the repeated deposition on the surface of the axon of film-like elements of proteolipid formed in the cytoplasm of the investing oligodendrocytes.[73] This view has not received general acceptance.[74]

Each layer of myelin is believed to be composed of alternating laminae of lipid and protein. The lipid element is made up of cholesterol, phospholipids and cerebrosides: the lipid molecules seem to be arranged with their long axes radially, while the much larger protein molecules lie circumferentially. Examination of human tissue suggests that the larger nerve fibres may be surrounded by up to 100 such layers: a current suggestion is that a process of a glial cell becomes applied to the axon and spirals round it.[75]

There is evidence that the myelin sheath has a structural stability comparable to that of collagen: its metabolic turnover is probably small, and may be negligible. When radioactive cholesterol is injected into young rabbits, it is at first widely distributed in all organs: after a few weeks, however, it is found virtually to have disappeared from the blood, heart, liver and kidneys, whereas it is retained in the white matter of the brain, in which it scarcely diminishes in amount over a period of many months.[76] The cerebroside component of myelin can be synthetized from radioactive serine: it, too, can then be shown to persist once it is laid down in the central nervous system of young rabbits.[77] Such findings agree with experimental observations that the turnover of cholesterol in the brain of adult rats is very slow.[78] More recently, evidence has been found that there is also a considerable turnover of components related to mature myelin.[79]

The possibility of a metabolic turnover of the components of myelin in the normal adult human brain is of special importance in relation to the pathogenesis of multiple sclerosis (see page 2257). In this disease, the loss of myelin might be regarded as due either to a failure in myelin maintenance or to the action of some myelinolytic agent. The latter now seems the more probable.

Chemical analysis of the myelin lipids, which began with the classic work of Thudichum at the end of the last century,[80] has shown that cholesterol, phospholipids (sphingomyelin and lecithin) and cerebrosides (glycosphingosides) are present in the proportions of 2 : 2 : 1. Analytical methods have not advanced sufficiently to state whether there are species differences in the constitution of myelin, or differences between families or between individuals. Such differences, should they exist, would probably be in the proteins (neurokeratin or proteolipids) rather than in the lipids themselves. In general, however, the laminate pattern of myelin structure appears to be the same in all the mammals, birds, reptiles and invertebrates that have been studied. Nevertheless, in molecular associations of such complexity there may be occasional deviations from the normal composition, and a consequent instability of the myelin structure might be a factor in the pathogenesis of some leucodystrophies (see page 2232).

By no means all the axons in the central nervous system are myelinated: indeed, the number without a discernible myelin sheath is considerable. In the anterior part of the corpus callosum, for instance, only about half the axons are myelinated.[81] The thickness of a myelin sheath seems to be related to the speed of conduction in the fibre. All long axons, both motor and sensory, are myelinated, the latter acquiring their sheaths before the former. Phylogenetically, as well as in human ontogenesis, the fibres subserving the highest functions, notably those in the frontal and parietal lobes, are the last to become myelinated; only when myelination is completed is full cerebral function possible. Physical agility in an infant in all probability does not become fully developed until myelin sheaths have appeared in the pyramidal system, and a child does not become fully educable until the fibres in the frontal and parietal lobes are myelinated.

Artefacts and Pathological Changes in Neurons

Before the pathologist can assess the state of normality or abnormality of a nerve cell in a section, he must be familiar with the changes in its appearance that may take place during the interval between death and the exposure of the tissue to histological fixatives. If a piece of cortex is removed and placed immediately in a 10 per cent solution of formalin, it will be found that the neurons near the surface of the sample are shrunken, that the nuclei of these cells stain deeply with basic dyes, and that their axons and dendrites are twisted in a corkscrew fashion. Deeper in the cortex, however, the neurons are seen to have very pale, distended nuclei, with an indistinct nucleolus; often a clear space can be seen in the cytoplasm, and sometimes in the nucleus as well ('water change'). The appearances of these cells, both those near the surface and those more deeply placed, are the result of artefact: the changes in the former are a shrinkage effect and probably due to the fixative while those in the latter appear to result from the imbibition of water. Both types of artefact may be seen in biopsy specimens, or in pieces of brain that have been fixed within a few hours of sudden death. The deeper-lying cells are not reached by the fixative as soon as the more superficial ones, and, therefore, they are able to take up a considerable amount of fluid consequent upon the osmotic changes that occur in dying tissues.

Most of the tissues studied by pathologists are

from patients who have died after an illness of at least some hours' duration. Such tissues have been modified by metabolic disturbances inseparable from the pre-mortal period. Moreover, there is usually a delay of many hours before the necropsy is performed, and fixation of much of the brain is certain to be delayed in the course of the usual procedure of immersion in formal saline. It is the average findings in such brains that are conventionally described as the 'normal' state with which the changes caused by disease must be contrasted (see also page 2099).

Central chromatolysis (see page 2087) may follow physiological exhaustion of the neuron or injury by toxins or viruses. When chromatolysis is pathological, other damage to the neuron is evident: the cytoplasm may be swollen and vacuolate, the neurofibrils may break up and eventually disappear, the nuclear membrane often becomes crinkled, the chromatin disappears and the nucleolus becomes enlarged and distorted. The electron microscope shows changes in the organelles.[50a]

A neuron that is shrunken and has an abnormally darkly staining, contracted and maybe crenated nucleus must be regarded as damaged, if the possibility of a fixation artefact can be excluded. It is not always possible to assess the state of the Nissl substance in the condensed cytoplasm of shrunken cells, but if Nissl substance can still be recognized in such cells, the shrinkage is almost certainly an artefact. Certain well-recognized patterns of pathological change in nerve cells are associated with the names of Nissl and Spielmeyer: they will be referred to later (see page 2098).

An aggregation of Hortega cells (see page 2095) on the surface of a nerve cell is presumptive evidence of its death; for instance, a neuron that has been killed by the virus of poliomyelitis will be found to be surrounded by these phagocytic cells (and also neutrophils) within two to three days of the onset of paralysis. This phenomenon is known as *neuronophagia* (Fig. 34.15) and it must not be confused with satellitosis (see page 2084). It is not by any means an invariable accompaniment of neuronal death, for neurons seem sometimes to die and disappear by lysis without leaving any trace.

Occasionally, at the edge of an old infarct, shrunken neurons are found that are more or less heavily impregnated with finely granular pigment (Fig. 34.12): the pigment gives Perls's Prussian blue reaction for iron and is presumably haemosiderin derived from the breakdown of red blood cells. These pigmented neurons can readily be mistaken

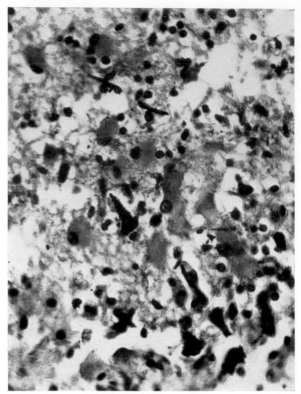

Fig. 34.12. In the centre there is a ferruginized nerve cell, encrusted with pigment. Above it are two elongated and darkly-stained bodies which are probably the rod form of microglia containing ingested pigment. The astrocytes are readily recognized in this preparation—which is taken from the edge of a small infarct—because of their copious and swollen cytoplasm. *Haematoxylin–eosin.* × 300.

for haemosiderin-containing phagocytes. This degeneration is known as *ferrugination of nerve cells*: such cells are probably not viable. Adjacent to contusions, however, neurons may be seen that contain a small amount of iron pigment in their cytoplasm, but otherwise appear normal or only slightly shrunken.

Although it is believed that neurons in the central nervous system are incapable of regeneration, binucleate nerve cells may, rarely, be found in some diseases and in tissues recovering from trauma. These cells give every appearance of being healthy, and presumably result from the division of a normal nucleus without subsequent separation of the cytoplasm.

As has already been mentioned, the severance of an axon is followed by central chromatolysis and swelling of its cell body (*axonal reaction*). Although the neuron may recover (see page 2087), the distal part of the severed axon undergoes dissolution.

Augustus Volney Waller, a cosmopolitan English physiologist, whose classic experiments were published in 1850,[82] noted that the myelin sheath, which was inevitably damaged when the axon was divided, disintegrated below the level of the cut, with conversion of the myelin into fatty globules (*Wallerian degeneration*—see also page 2305). These globules, which, unlike myelin, stain intensely with Sudan dyes, may be demonstrated in degenerating fibres within eight days after the experimental cutting of a nerve trunk. In such experiments on peripheral nerves it may take weeks before the degradation products of myelin disappear completely;[83, 83a] in the central nervous system they may persist for months.

The integrity of the myelin sheath depends on that of the axon but the reverse does not hold: in a primary demyelinating disease, such as multiple sclerosis, the axons may remain more or less intact, although their myelin sheath has disappeared. The disparity between the clinical disability and the extensive loss of myelin in multiple sclerosis is, in fact, often striking.

Other forms of neuronal degeneration will be described when dealing with various diseases in the later sections of this chapter. Some of them take the form of changes in the cytoplasm or in the neurofibrils; in others the nucleus is primarily affected.

The Neuron–Neuroglial System

From the earliest days of neurohistology, the nerve cell has been recognized as the executive cell and the neuroglia has been regarded as a supportive tissue; more recently, the neuroglia has also been credited with an important metabolic function. The neurons exhibit the greatest variety of morphological and, presumably, functional differentiation. The neuroglial cells, especially astrocytes, also vary considerably in the details of their appearance in different parts of the central nervous system. Both the neuron and the neuroglial cell have a common developmental origin, and it is not unreasonable to assume that their relationship is in some way complementary. In adult life, the neuron has little direct contact with the capillary bed of the brain, and its metabolic requirements are believed to be mediated by astrocytes, each of which has at least one attachment to a blood vessel (see Figs 34.3 and 34.4, page 2079).

Oligodendrocytes also have links with neurons in the form of small, ring-like attachments.[84] These neuron–oligodendrocyte contacts have attracted much attention, and it has been suggested that oligodendrocytes may receive some of the information that is transmitted to and from the neurons.[85] It may be that in addition to having a nutritive function, like the astrocytes, interfascicular oligodendrocytes are concerned in amplifying or facilitating the nervous impulse.[85a]

The astrocyte–neuron–oligodendrocyte system should be regarded as an integral unit. The respiratory activity of the neuron may seem to differ considerably from that of the glial cells, but the differences are found to be much reduced if the rate of respiration is correlated with the surface area of the three types of cell.[86] The least vulnerable is the astrocyte, which may survive degrees of injury that kill the neurons and oligodendrocytes. This vulnerability is well exemplified by the great susceptibility of neurons and oligodendrocytes to cyanide and other agents that inhibit cellular oxidation.[87]

'Ground Substance' in the Central Nervous System

Studies with the electron microscope have tended to support the view that there is no ground substance as such in the cerebral cortex. The distribution of oxidative enzymes suggests that much or all of what was formerly believed to be ground substance in fact consists of dendrites and collaterals. Material that gives a positive periodic-acid/Schiff reaction, and formerly thought to be ground substance,[88] is now known to consist partly of submicroscopical and ubiquitous constituents of astrocytes and oligodendrocytes and partly of myelin.[89, 90] The term *neuropil* is used to designate the dense complex of glial and neuronal processes that lies between the cell bodies of the cortex.

The question of the amount of intercellular fluid in the nervous system has been controversial.[91] Between the membranes of contiguous cells there is a potential space, which is estimated by electron microscopists to be 20 nm wide:[92] it is in this space that ionic movements are believed to occur. The dimensions of the intercellular space are fairly constant when studied in material fixed rapidly in osmium tetroxide; it has to be remembered, however, that such clefts might open up under pathological or even physiological conditions. One of the greatest difficulties in accepting the electron microscopists' low estimate of intercellular space in the brain is the high content of sodium and chloride ions in the central nervous system, for in other organs both these ions are almost wholly confined to the extracellular fluids. White matter differs from grey matter in being likelier under certain circumstances to contain intercellular fluid. Experimental evidence[93] supports this view and electron microscopy[94, 95] has confirmed it.

The Blood–Brain Barrier[96]*

The concept of a blood–brain barrier (to be distinguished from a blood–cerebrospinal-fluid barrier) originated from the work of Ehrlich in 1885 on the staining of tissues by vital dyes introduced into the circulation. The fact that the central nervous system is unstained by these dyes contrasts sharply with the staining of other organs. It has long been supposed, therefore, that the permeability of the lining cells of the small vessels of the brain must differ significantly from that of capillary endothelium elsewhere. It is only at sites of injury to the cerebral vasculature, such as might be associated with inflammation or hypoxia, that the vessels allow the dye to leak from the blood stream. More recently, with fuller knowledge of the relations of the various elements in the central nervous system, it has been suggested that the barrier may be formed not only by the endothelium but also by the attachment of glial cells to the capillary wall (see page 2082).[96, 97]

There are other possible explanations for this barrier effect. First, it is possible that many substances fail to escape from the smaller blood vessels because there is little—if any—extravascular fluid in the brain (see above). Fluid into which substances circulating in the blood could escape may collect in the brain only after its substance has been injured in some way. Second, even if tissue fluid is normally present in the central nervous system, the molecular size of a circulating substance, coupled perhaps with its molecular electrical charge, may be an important factor in determining whether or not it can escape from the blood into the brain. That size plays a part here, as elsewhere, is shown by the fact that proteins, identified by a radioactive label, are unable to pass across the endothelium of the cerebral capillaries.[98] On the other hand, small molecular size alone does not ensure the escape of substances from the blood: although some small molecules—among them volatile anaesthetics, barbiturates and glucose—enter the brain readily, others of equally small size, such as fructose, fail to do so.

* The so-called blood–spinal-ganglion barrier and blood–nerve barrier are referred to on page 2305.

It is this difference in the behaviour of certain small, diffusible molecules that has made it necessary to modify the idea of something comparable to a simple physical sieve as the explanation of the blood–brain barrier.[99] It has been suggested that some small molecular substances that are normally present in the blood (among them inorganic phosphates and most amino acids) fail to enter the tissues of the central nervous system because they do not participate in its metabolism, whereas others, notably glucose, on which neuronal activity almost wholly depends, pass readily.[100] To summarize this belief, large molecules are probably retained in the blood because of their size, while small molecules enter or fail to enter the brain according to whether or not they are utilized there in metabolic processes.

There are two sites where the blood–brain barrier seems to be relatively less effective: these are the *areae postremae* in the floor of the fourth ventricle[101] and the ganglia of the dorsal spinal roots.[102] It may be at these apparently more permeable sites that toxins and some neurotropic viruses gain access to the central nervous system.

The Mesodermal Elements of the Central Nervous System

The Dura Mater

The dura mater (pachymeninx) is a tough, fibrous membrane that surrounds and, by means of its extensions (the falx cerebri and the tentorium cerebelli), cradles the brain. It has a close attachment to the skull and, indeed, it forms the inner layer of the endocranial periosteum. In the spinal canal, however, there is a potential space (the epidural space) between the bone and the dura. The dura consists of two main layers of collagen fibres, among which there are few cells and few nutrient blood vessels; its inner aspect is covered by flat mesothelial cells. The intracranial venous sinuses are contained within the layers of the dura mater.

The Pia-Arachnoid

The pia mater and the arachnoid are delicate, vascular membranes and together constitute the leptomeninges or pia-arachnoid. The pia mater is closely in contact with the brain surface and is reflected over the blood vessels that enter and leave the brain. The arachnoid lies between the pia mater and the dura mater; it does not dip into the sulci but forms a roof over them and over the cisterns at the base of the brain. The space between the arachnoid and the pia contains cerebrospinal fluid (the *subarachnoid space*); there are extensions of this space between the wall of the blood vessels entering the brain and their pial sheath, and in this situation it is known as the circumvascular space (*Virchow–Robin space*). The diverticula of the subarachnoid space that are known as arachnoid villi are important as the pathway of drainage of the cerebrospinal fluid into the blood (see page 2106).

There is an important potential space between the dura mater and the arachnoid membrane, in which, under certain circumstances, blood, exudate or cerebrospinal fluid may collect (the *subdural space*).

The Hortega Cells (Microglia)[34]

The Hortega cell (microglial cell; cerebral histiocyte; brain phagocyte) is the representative in the central nervous system of the reticuloendothelial system and, like all reticuloendothelial cells, it takes up vital dyes and colloidal particles (see page 524, Volume 2).[103] It is a true phagocyte. The commonly used term 'microglia' is inappropiate, for, unlike the glial cells, the Hortega cell is not of ectodermal origin, it is mobile and not fixed, and it is small only during its resting phase. The term 'cerebral histiocyte' does not suffice because the Hortega cell is not confined to the cerebrum. In spite of its close relation to the macrophages in other parts of the body, it would seem to deserve a name of its own; it will generally be referred to here as the Hortega cell.

The quiescent Hortega cell has a bean-shaped nucleus, nearer in size to the nucleus of the astrocyte than to that of the oligodendrocyte but less vesicular than the former and less compact than the latter. The cytoplasm is scanty, and its branching is revealed by a special technique of silver impregnation devised by del Río Hortega; the processes are fewer than those of the astrocytes, but they are sometimes very elongated. Hortega cells are normally to be found near to small blood vessels and sometimes are wrapped round them: in such situations they are sometimes referred to as 'pericytes', a term fraught with confusion because of the variety of uses to which it has been put. When brain tissue is damaged these cells are mobilized, probably in response to chemotactic stimulation: they then move into the affected parts (Fig. 34.13).

The cytoplasm of the resting Hortega cell can

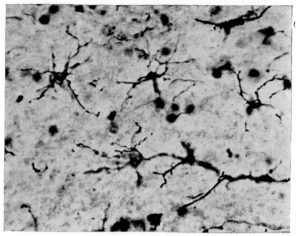

Fig. 34.13. Cerebral cortex. Reacting Hortega cells in pathological cerebral cortex. The cell bodies of some are swollen because they have already assimilated debris. One or two have adopted the rod form (see Fig. 34.16). *Marshall's silver impregnation method.* × 300.

be seen only with difficulty, but during phagocytosis it becomes conspicuous, and at the same time its processes become shorter, stouter, and fewer in number. In the actively phagocytic cell the nucleus tends to be eccentrically placed, and it may be close to the cell surface. As the cell body becomes more and more distended with ingested material, the processes continue to shrink: eventually, the Hortega cell appears as a large, round cell with an eccentric, spherical nucleus, and cytoplasm that is often turgid with droplets that, in frozen sections, are found to be Sudanophile. The finely reticulate pattern of the cytoplasm of the Hortega cell at this stage earned it the name *lattice cell* or, in its original German form, *Gitterzelle* (Fig. 34.14). It is also often known as the *compound granular corpuscle*, or *foam cell*. Once this metamorphosis has been completed, the cell migrates into the Virchow–Robin space and makes its way to the cerebrospinal fluid. The ingested material is believed to be absorbed through the arachnoid villi; however, it is also possible that some of the fat-laden Hortega cells become attached to the adventitia of the small blood vessels, and either pass through the vessel wall themselves or discharge their contents into the blood stream.

The Hortega cells reach the brain during embryonic development through the 'fountains of Hortega', which are subpial collections of amoeboid cells situated in the tela choroidea of the lateral and fourth ventricles and beneath the pia covering the

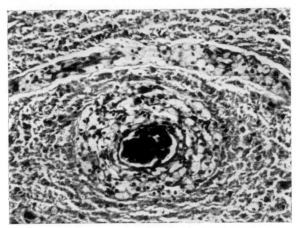

Fig. 34.14. Demyelination in a lateral funiculus of the spinal cord. A transversely-cut small venule is surrounded by rows of cells with pale-staining cytoplasm and small eccentric nuclei: these are macrophages containing ingested lipid. Above the venule there is a longitudinally-cut capillary, also surrounded by phagocytes. *Celloidin section. Haematoxylin–eosin.* ×150.

cerebral peduncles. In these situations, and in other places where the pia is in contact with white matter, subpial aggregations of amoeboid cells can be seen at the time of birth. After birth, the cells traverse the white matter; some remain in the vicinity of the blood vessels in the latter, but most pass into the cortex.

Under pathological conditions, Hortega cells may congregate in small clusters round capillaries, or round dead nerve cells (*neuronophagia*—see page 2146 and Figs 34.2, 34.15 and 34.59). Such appearances are suggestive of an infection, particularly a viral infection, and the focal collections of Hortega cells may be very numerous. Small aggregates of

these cells—the misnamed 'glial knots'—also occur in degenerating nerve tracts, for instance in cases of motor neuron disease or of anterior poliomyelitis, or in Wallerian degeneration from whatever cause. They may also be seen in the white matter in some cases in which there have been no clinical manifestations of neurological disease; in such instances they may represent a focal response to a terminal blood-borne infection or to agonal oligaemic hypoxia. It would seem that Hortega cells are sufficiently plentiful to meet the need for scavengers or 'fetch and carry' cells at all times except when a large focal lesion or a serious infection threatens the integrity of the nervous system. Under such circumstances the available Hortega cells may be reinforced by multipotential cells derived from the adventitia of blood vessels and from monocytes in the blood—not all fat-filled phagocytes in an area of softening are derived from Hortega cells.

As the nervous system has no direct lymphatic drainage it is likely that the Hortega cell also has an immunological function corresponding to that of the cells of the lymphoid tissue in other parts of the body.

In a few conditions—mostly chronic diseases of the cortex, and notably general paresis—Hortega cells become markedly attenuated in form, their processes being confined mainly to the two extremities. Such cells are often known as *rod cells*, or by the German equivalent, *Stäbchenzellen* (Fig. 34.16). Globules of fat may be detected within their scanty cytoplasm, and sometimes the cytoplasmic processes are encrusted with iron and calcium.

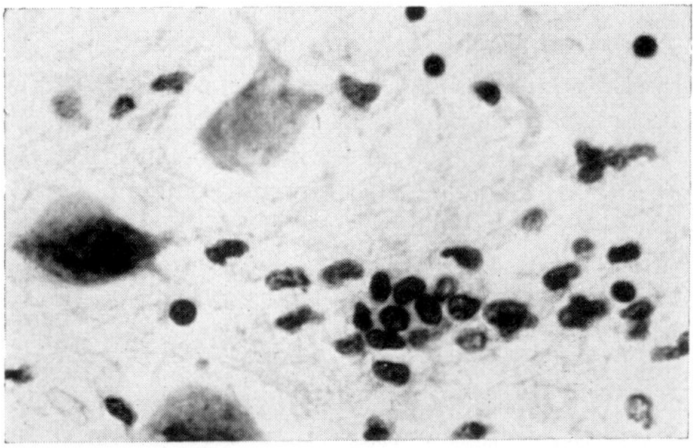

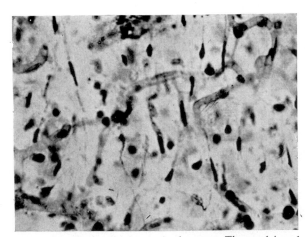

Fig. 34.15. Neurons in a dentate nucleus undergoing degeneration. Hortega cells are engaged in removing the remains of one of them. *Celloidin section. Nissl's stain.* ×400.

Fig. 34.16. 'Rod cells' in cerebral cortex. The nuclei and cytoplasm of these Hortega cells are elongated to a remarkable extent and have to be distinguished from the endothelial cells of capillaries. *Frozen section. Penfield's method.* ×350.

HYPOXIA[104-107]

INTRODUCTION

Neurons vary widely in their susceptibility to the effects of hypoxia. Our knowledge of this subject is founded upon both experimental and clinicopathological evidence. Weinberger and his colleagues[108] clamped the pulmonary artery of cats and found that when the period of circulatory arrest (as shown by lack of pulsation in the retinal vessels) lasted three and a half minutes the animals that survived had sustained permanent damage to the small pyramidal cells of the cortex. Very few animals lived for more than a few hours when the period of arrest exceeded seven and a half minutes. In dogs, permanent damage has been found in the cerebral cortex after two minutes of histamine-induced collapse.[109] Most sensitive to ischaemia are the small pyramidal cells of the frontal and occipital lobes and some cells of the hippocampal formation; the Purkyně cells of the cerebellum are next in order of sensitivity, and then the cells of the thalami and of the brainstem. The most resistant are the Betz cells of the motor cortex of the brain and the neurons of the anterior grey columns of the spinal cord; the latter, in fact, are able to survive 15 minutes of anoxia.

Observations following temporary cardiac arrest in man tend to support these findings. Unless the patient survives the period of anoxia for at least 12 hours, very few morphological changes will be observable in the neurons, even though at a biochemical level widespread damage may have taken place. When interpreting such observations, it has to be remembered that histological techniques are not adequate to allow us to observe the earliest departure from normality in man.

When the body temperature is normal, the longest period of cerebral anoxia that should be permitted during surgical operations on the cardio-vascular system is 90 seconds. Dementia has been known to follow three minutes of cardiac asystole at normal operating theatre temperature during an operation for ligation of a patent ductus arteriosus. In exceptional cases, it has been claimed that cardiac arrest lasting longer than four minutes at normal temperature has caused no damage to the brain: however, there has been neither direct observation of the heart nor continuous graphical registration of its activity in these cases, and complete suppression of the heart beat throughout the period of presumed arrest cannot be regarded as proved. Induced hypothermia, by reducing the

metabolic rate, prolongs the period during which the brain can safely be without oxygen.

Several factors may affect the neurological outcome of cardiac arrest during surgical operations: for instance, a young patient is better able to withstand the accompanying cerebral hypoxia than an older one, and anaemia, extensive lung disease, and premedication with drugs that have a central depressant action have an adverse effect on a patient's chances of survival without permanent injury. Important, too, are the efficiency and duration of cardiac massage, and of efforts to maintain arterial pressure. Following resumption of the natural heartbeat and the return of the arterial pressure to normal, the patient still faces the hazards of the recovery period, during which further cerebral injury can result from the hypoxia induced by retention of secretions in the air passages. The occurrence of hypoxia while a patient is in the sitting position, as in a dentist's chair, or with the head raised for other surgical or nursing purposes, is particularly dangerous.

There is some evidence, both clinical and experimental, that intravenous injections of substances of high osmotic value are helpful in reducing the cerebral swelling that may develop as a sequel of an ischaemic episode.[110]

Causes of Hypoxia[111]

Cerebral hypoxia may be defined as the state of the living brain when its supply of oxygen is insufficient to meet its requirements. There are many conditions that can give rise to cerebral hypoxia. Some of them, like cardiac arrest or sudden and sustained hypotension, act by depriving the brain cells of oxygen and glucose substrate (*ischaemic* or *oligaemic hypoxia*). Others, like anaemia, exposure to a high altitude, and carbon monoxide and nitrous oxide intoxication are the result of lowering of the oxygen content of the blood passing to the brain (*hypoxic* or *anoxic hypoxia*); cyanide poisoning proves fatal because the oxidative enzymes of the neurons are inhibited (*histotoxic hypoxia*). In general, whatever the nature of the hypoxic mechanism, the damage to the neurons is essentially the same.

The Vascular Effects of Hypoxia

The immediate effect of sudden hypoxia on the blood vessels of the brain is believed to be angiospasm, which is quickly followed by vasodilatation and stasis. The vasodilatation is usually evident even when death has occurred almost immediately; it is more marked if the patient has survived long enough for some of the nerve cells to disappear. Survival beyond three or four days may be associated with proliferation of cerebral capillaries.

Cell Changes in Hypoxia

Neurons.—Hypoxic injury to nerve cells may be shown in two ways—in the early period by alterations in their appearance, and later by their disappearance from the affected area. This is well illustrated by the behaviour of the Purkyně cells (Fig. 34.17) which, within as little as 24 hours of a hypoxic episode, may show cytoplasmic swelling and nuclear pyknosis. If the interval between the hypoxic episode and the patient's death is a few days, Hortega cells are usually found to have surrounded the dying neurons. If death is delayed for three to four weeks, the Purkyně cells and,

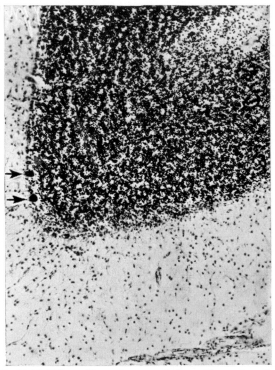

Fig. 34.17. Effect of hypoxia on cerebellum. The patient died four days after an episode of cardiac arrest (ischaemic hypoxia) lasting four minutes. Only two of the Purkyně cells have survived (arrows): the remainder have already disappeared and the Bergmann astrocytes of the Purkyně cell layer have proliferated. The more resistant nerve cells of the granular layer are unaltered. *Celloidin section. Nissl's stain.* × 120.

usually, the Hortega cells will have disappeared from the area. Purkyně cells are notably susceptible to hypoxia, and a deficiency in their number is suggestive of a previous hypoxic episode, such as perinatal asphyxia; it has to be remembered that they may be absent for reasons other than deprivation of oxygen—for instance, in primary cerebellar degeneration. Conversely, the presence of Purkyně cells does not exclude the possibility of a past hypoxic episode, for they are less susceptible to oxygen lack than the small ganglion cells of the cerebral cortex (Fig. 34.18), and they may survive an episode that is fatal to the latter.

Evidence of early neuronal damage is most easily seen in sections stained by Nissl's method.* In such preparations, many neurons show 'degenerative' changes, of which the commonest are swelling and pallor of the cytoplasm, loss of Nissl substance, swelling of the nucleus, and eccentricity of the nucleolus. These appearances were formerly known as *Nissl's acute cell change* or *Spielmeyer's acute cell swelling.* They are thought to be reversible. The designation *Nissl's severe cell change* was used when a nerve cell had swollen cytoplasm devoid of Nissl substance and a shrunken, darkly-staining nucleus. Some of these appearances are now recognized to be artefacts (see below).

Another type of degenerative change is characterized by contraction of the whole cell, and especially of the nucleus, which, instead of being round, with a well-defined nucleolus and scattered chromatin, becomes homogeneous and pyknotic, with a withered-looking nuclear membrane; the cytoplasm is acidophile. This change, in which the Nissl substance has been lost, is termed *ischaemic change* because it is commonly met with in ischaemic conditions. *Spielmeyer's homogenizing cell change,* originally described in Purkyně cells, is characterized by an appearance as if the nucleus were dissolving into the cell body. Occasionally, the cells appear wizened and have a darkly staining, angular nucleus (*Nissl's chronic cell change*). Generally,

* In general, paraffin wax embedding is perfectly suitable for the histological study of the brain. However, embedding in celloidin is often preferred, for three reasons: (1) the shrinkage of the tissues is more even; (2) celloidin preparations stained by Nissl methods are less liable to fade than paraffin wax sections; and (3) celloidin sections, which usually have to be cut about 30 μm thick, give a better picture than that seen in paraffin wax sections of equal thickness, and they are particularly well suited for the staining of myelin and for anatomical localization of lesions by means of the dissecting microscope. Many neuropathologists feel that the advantages justify the long wait (8 to 10 weeks) that celloidin processing entails.

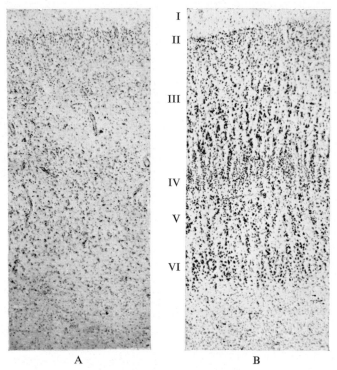

Fig. 34.18. Parastriate cortex (A) in the same case as Fig. 34.17: there is a considerable loss of cells, in all layers, on comparison with the control (B), although laminae II and IV are still identifiable. The Roman numerals indicate the cortical laminae. *Celloidin section. Nissl's stain.* × 30.

these severer alterations are regarded as irreversible, and indicate imminent death of the cell: indeed, it is likely that many cells that show such changes were already dead when the patient died.

These five named varieties of cell change have long been recognized and well illustrated,[112–114] yet recent experimental studies using perfusion fixation[115, 116] have shown that artefacts account for more than was realized (see page 2092). The recognition of significant acute ischaemic changes in human material can therefore be difficult in the absence of changes that unequivocally have occurred *in vivo*, such as secondary astrocytic and microglial reactions. The luxol-fast-blue/cresyl-fast-violet method is recommended for demonstrating ischaemic cell change:[117] it gives an intense mauve colour to the shrunken cytoplasm.

A combined study by light microscopy and electron microscopy of anoxic and ischaemic neuronal changes in the perfusion-fixed rat brain showed microvacuolation to be the earliest neuronal lesion and that this is followed within two hours by ischaemic cell change and surface 'incrusta-tion'.[105, 118] The microvacuoles correspond to swollen mitochondria and there is accompanying dilatation of the endoplasmic reticulum. Ischaemic cell change appears to result from condensation of cytoplasm and is sometimes associated with mitochondrial shrinkage. The incrustations result from irregularities of the neuronal surface, and from isolation of dense areas of the perikaryon between less dense areas. Swollen processes of astrocytes surround the affected neurons.

Some of the neurons in acutely damaged parts of the cortex may contain Sudanophile lipid which is more widely dispersed in the cell than the normal lipochrome material. Some of the fat in the cytoplasm in this form of degeneration is protein-bound and still demonstrable after treatment of the tissues with fat solvents.

The late stages of neuronal degeneration may not be easy to recognize. Neuronophagia, when present, is clear evidence that the cells are dying or dead, but it is an inconstant feature, and many neurons disappear with little or no sign of their former presence. Even the loss of as many as 30 per cent of the small nerve cells in the cerebral cortex may be difficult to detect; cell loss is most obvious when mainly confined to a particular lamina of the cortex.

Astrocytes.—Further evidence of nerve cell loss following hypoxia can be obtained from a study of the astrocytes. Within three days of the episode, proliferating astrocytes may be seen in haematoxylin–eosin preparations, in which they appear as oval, vesicular nuclei lying side by side in pairs (Fig. 34.19). After a period of three or four weeks, if the loss of neurons has been considerable, astrocytic nuclei are found in groups of eight or more, and stains for glial fibres will disclose an early stage in gliotic closure of the gaps resulting from death of the nerve cells. The deposition of glial fibres, which takes place as early as the sixth day, is most marked in three situations—at the surface of the cortex (Chaslin's *marginal gliosis*[118a]), deep to the ependyma, and round the transcortical arterioles.

Hortega Cells.—The Hortega cells begin to show signs of activity if the patient survives for 18 hours or more. The extent to which neuronophagia takes place varies in different parts of the brain: in the cerebral cortex it is by no means constant even when

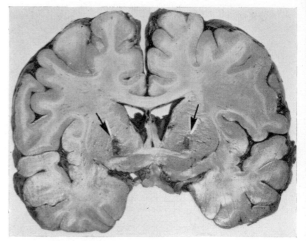

Fig. 34.20. Carbon monoxide poisoning ('hypoxic hypoxia'). The pallidum is vulnerable and reactive change in the damaged tissue may be expected after an interval of 24 hours or so. This patient survived for eight days, time enough for necrosis to develop and, where extensive, to be visible to the naked eye (arrows).

neuronal necrosis is widespread; it is found oftener in other situations, for example in the Purkyně layer of the cerebellar cortex, and in the dentate and olivary nuclei, the thalami and the corpora striata.

Neuronophagia may still be evident as late as 28 days after the hypoxic injury. Cells containing fat droplets are found in cases in which the white matter is involved, or when extensive cortical softening also implicates myelinated fibres; these fat-laden cells may be Hortega cells or, possibly, altered oligodendrocytes (see page 2085).

Distribution of the Lesions in Different Forms of Hypoxia

The different forms of hypoxia may be characterized by differences in the distribution of the lesions in the brain. Thus, in *carbon monoxide poisoning* (Fig. 34.20) the changes that occur in the cerebral cortex will almost certainly be accompanied by lesions in the pallidum and in the subthalamic nuclei. If the patient survives for two or more days, post-mortem examination may show that softening is already present; if he survives for weeks or months, there may be cavitation of the pallidum, and in such cases a Parkinsonian state may have developed. Each globus pallidus is supplied by a deep penetrating branch of the middle cerebral artery, which in older people is apt to become thickened, calcified, and encrusted with iron pigment (Fig. 34.21);[119, 120] this change may increase the liability to necrosis and cavitation.

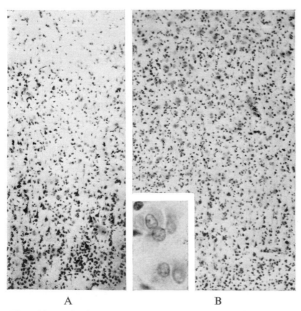

Fig. 34.19. Striate (A) and parastriate (B) cortex. The patient died one month after an episode of cardiac arrest lasting four minutes. Most of the small nerve cells in laminae III and V have been destroyed and replaced by astrocytes. The loss of cells in (A) is patchy. Proliferating astrocytes are particularly conspicuous in (B), some being shown inset; it is characteristic that the outline of the cytoplasm of these cells is blurred. *Celloidin section. Nissl's stain.* × 120 (inset × 450).

In *nitrous oxide poisoning* also the pallidum and the subthalamic nuclei are affected, and there may be extensive laminar necrosis of the cortex. Courville collected 30 fatalities due to this anaesthetic, three of them caused by the same faulty anaesthetic machine.[121] It should be pointed out that pallidal degeneration, although characteristic of carbon monoxide and nitrous oxide intoxication, may occur in other forms of 'hypoxic hypoxia'[122] and in hypoxia caused by cyanide and by carbon disulphide.[123]

Acute hypoxic hypoxia is the purest form of hypoxia, for it is initially uncomplicated by circulatory factors.[124, 125] In it the pallidum, the subthalamic nuclei and the dentate nuclei exhibit the greatest susceptibility to damage, whereas in cardiac arrest (*ischaemic hypoxia*) the cerebral and cerebellar cortex prove more sensitive; this may be because failure of the circulation deprives these parts of other essential substances as well as oxygen.[126] This distinction between hypoxic and ischaemic hypoxia is useful, although, in practice, it is by no means clear cut.

In all forms of hypoxia, the cortical cells of area h_1 (Sommer's sector*) of the hippocampus may undergo degeneration (Fig. 34.22). This is an

* Wilhelm Sommer, of Allenberg, in Bavaria, first drew attention to changes in this region in a study on epilepsy (*Arch. Psychiat. Nervenkr.*, 1880, **10**, 631).

important observation, for it provides a useful means of demonstrating that there has been damage to the central nervous system by hypoxia at some past time. However, care is needed in interpreting the histological appearances, for the cells of this area are normally disposed in an irregular manner: mere patchiness of their distribution, therefore, is not evidence of hypoxic damage. In practice, degeneration of this area is most easily recognized by studying Nissl-stained celloidin sections at a low magnification. In severe, but not immediately fatal, cases of hypoxia, the striking loss of cells in this area, which is the lasting mark of such an episode, is unmistakable. If the loss is recent there will be signs of neuronal degeneration, and there is likely to be activity of the phagocytes, amounting perhaps to neuronophagia. There may well be early astrocytic proliferation also; if this is of long standing, gliosis will be recognizable in suitably stained preparations, and this should always be looked for, as its presence is confirmation of neuronal loss.

The cortex in the depths of the cerebral sulci is more vulnerable to hypoxic damage than the convexity of the convolutions. The susceptibility of the cortex in the calcarine fissure is debatable; this part of the brain receives its blood supply from both the middle and the posterior cerebral arteries, and this dual supply, while tending to lessen the extent of the hypoxic damage should one

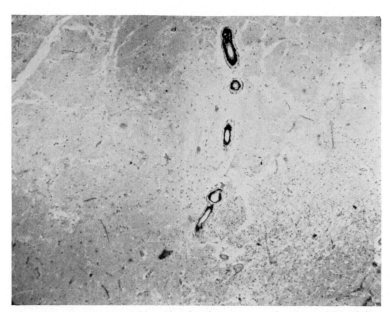

Fig. 34.21. Carbon monoxide poisoning (same case as in Fig. 34.20). Globus pallidus. The blood vessels show degenerative changes and thickening of their wall. The brain tissue is softened and breaking down. *Haematoxylin–eosin.* × 30.

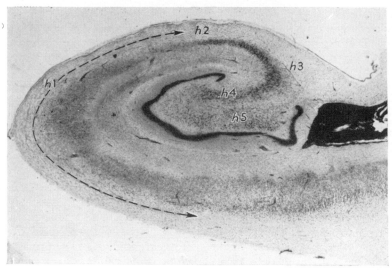

Fig. 34.22. The vulnerability of 'Sommer's sector'. That part of the pyramidal cell layer of the hippocampi known as area h_1 (Sommer's sector) is particularly vulnerable in hypoxia. The patient survived for six weeks after a period of cardiac arrest lasting 'something more than two minutes'. The dark staining nuclei of neurons so noticeable in sector h_3 disappear at the point marked h_2, the whole of sector h_1 being occupied by the proliferating astrocytes that take the place of the destroyed neurons and give the sector a blurred appearance. The nerve cell atrophy in such lesions tends to be followed by gliosis that, provided the patient has survived for more than a month, should be discernible with appropriate staining. In the bottom right-hand corner, beyond h_1, lies the subiculum, in which many neurons have survived and are well stained. Some of the cells of the end folium (end plate, or h_5) are intact. The most resistant part of all is sector h_2. *Celloidin section. Nissl's stain.* $\times 12$.

artery become occluded, does not protect the area from the effects of a general hypoxia and may, indeed, increase the liability to serious injury in the course of prolonged hypotensive episodes.

In some instances of hypoxia degeneration of the white matter may also occur, the destruction of myelin giving rise to a spongy state and later to fibrillary gliosis. This is especially apt to occur after carbon monoxide poisoning: it is believed to be caused by stasis and changes in capillary permeability, resulting from the local action on the white matter of carbon monoxide (and perhaps of other components of coal gas).[127, 128]

PERINATAL HYPOXIA

Under normal conditions there is an interval of less than a minute between the birth of a baby and its first cry; during this time a temporary state of hypoxia is developing. However, studies on animals suggest that at the time of birth the fetus is especially endowed to survive a period of hypoxia by reason of a high level of glycogen in the ventricles

of the heart that, provided the circulation is intact, ensures for the brain a supply of substrate for energy requirements.[129] Even so there are circumstances that favour the development of a pathological degree of perinatal hypoxia: these include the use of narcotic drugs during labour (these tend to depress the respiratory centre of both the mother and the baby), undue delay in the second stage of labour, strangulation by looping of the cord round the neck, and prematurity. A breech presentation carries a special risk, for breathing may begin while the head is still within the birth canal. Serious hypoxia is a feature of two clinical conditions in the neonatal period—white asphyxia and blue asphyxia. *White asphyxia* is, essentially, a form of shock; it is associated with a serious fall in blood pressure, and the hypoxia is therefore both oligaemic and hypoxic. *Blue asphyxia*, which has the better prognosis as regards both life and the liability to permanent cerebral damage, is accompanied by venous congestion and stasis, particularly of the head, and is predominantly a form of hypoxic hypoxia. Both types of neonatal asphyxia may be followed by fits in the early days of life; if there is permanent cerebral damage, mental retardation may become apparent.

Many of the pathological findings in cases of spastic palsy, or in backward children, have been attributed to neonatal asphyxia, sometimes without justification. It has to be remembered that there are other perinatal causes of mental retardation and spasticity: these include intracranial injuries and haemorrhage, which may be the result of using instruments during delivery, or of excessive moulding, or, in a breech delivery, of sudden release of the aftercoming head. Further, some cases of imbecility are due to causes that operate during the first or second year of life: some of these are vascular in origin, notably thrombosis of the venous sinuses, and others are infective or metabolic. Finally, the possibility of vascular and infective disorders of the fetus in utero must be remembered; these have to be distinguished not only from perinatal hypoxia but also from genetically determined anomalies of brain structure. Most of the credit for recognizing the importance of neonatal asphyxia in the aetiology of cerebral diplegia and mental deficiency is due to Little.[130]

The importance of venous congestion in the aetiology of damage to the brain at birth was recognized by Schwartz.[131] He showed that back pressure through the straight sinus and the great cerebral vein (vein of Galen) was responsible for the foci of softening so often found in the caudate, lenticular and subthalamic nuclei, with the accompanying loss of neurons, disordered myelination (erroneously called 'hypermyelination') and cystic cavitation in these nuclei. When the condition proves fatal within a few hours of birth, the venous distension may be recognizable from an examination of the great cerebral vein and, particularly, of the subependymal veins in the region of the caudate nuclei.

In contrast to blue asphyxia, the rare instances of survival after the prolonged hypotension of an episode of white asphyxia show most damage in the 'watershed' areas between the various arterial territories. For example, there may be ischaemic softening in the second frontal convolution, which is supplied by peripheral branches of both the anterior and middle cerebral arteries.[132]

In investigating any case in which there may have been an episode of cerebral hypoxia, the pathologist may be greatly helped by examining paired preparations stained to show neuroglial fibres and myelin respectively. These preparations of tissue from vulnerable areas, such as the cerebral cortex, the hippocampi, the basal ganglia and the inferior olivary bodies, will effectively supplement the Nissl picture, and will allow an assessment of the extent of the damage, particularly if celloidin sections are used.

Kernikterus[133-136]

The appearance of a yellow discoloration of parts of the basal ganglia, brainstem and cerebellum in cases of icterus gravis neonatorum was known long before 1903, when Schmorl recorded his classic studies and named the condition Kernikterus ('jaundice of the nuclei').[137] The most vulnerable areas are the pallidum, the subthalamic nuclei (of Luys) and the hippocampi, but the dentate nuclei, the inferior olivary bodies and some cranial nerve nuclei are often involved also. Phylogenetically, these are old parts of the brain; also, they are functional at the time of birth.[138] The corpus striatum and the neocortex, which are not functionally developed at birth, are seldom affected in this disease.

The yellow pigment is apparently unconjugated ('indirect') bilirubin, which circulates in loose association with the plasma proteins. It is lipid-soluble, and is deposited in the neurons that have succumbed to anaemic or histotoxic hypoxia. The unconjugated bilirubin is invariably present in excess in the plasma of the affected baby; this is, in part, because of a deficiency of glucuronyl transferase, the hepatic enzyme that is responsible for the conversion of the unconjugated lipid-soluble bilirubin to the water-soluble conjugated bilirubin. The critical concentration of the unconjugated bilirubin necessary for the development of Kernikterus is variable; a significant factor may be the occurrence of some of the bilirubin in a diffusible, non-protein-bound form.[139]

The abnormally high concentration of bile pigments in the blood of babies with Kernikterus is most commonly caused by haemolysis of their erythrocytes by maternal antibodies. The condition is then usually a manifestation of the form of haemolytic jaundice found in that proportion of the offspring of 'rhesus-negative' mothers in which erythroblastosis fetalis develops (see page 442, Volume 1). Theoretically, all the offspring should be affected if the father is homozygous 'rhesus-positive', and one in two if he is heterozygous. In practice, the incidence is less, because some 'rhesus-negative' mothers do not produce antibodies to rhesus antigens while some of those who do produce antibodies do so only in low titre. Even when the father is homozygous the first infant is usually unaffected. It is when the 'rhesus-negative' mother has developed antibodies (particularly anti-D antibodies) during a previous pregnancy, or after a transfusion of rhesus-positive blood, that a further pregnancy will result in a rapid rise in the titre of these antibodies in her serum. The infant may be stillborn and oedematous (hydrops fetalis), or may be born alive with severe haemolytic anaemia and jaundice. Once a rhesus-negative woman has given birth to a baby suffering from this disease it is inevitable—in the absence of appropriate preventive measures—that each subsequent child by a man who is rhesus-positive will present the condition in a severer form.

If the child is born alive with anaemia and jaundice, immediate exsanguination (aimed at ridding it of all the rhesus antibodies acquired from its mother) and transfusion of compatible blood may save its life. If an exchange transfusion is not given early, injury to neurons may be so severe that disorders of muscle tone and movement, and deafness, may result later in childhood.

Not all cases of *Kernikterus* are due to rhesus incompatibility. Other red-cell antigens, including those of the ABO system, may sometimes be concerned, or the abnormal haemolysis may be due to anomalies of the erythrocytes themselves, such as occur in congenital spherocytosis. It is now well-established that *Kernikterus* may also develop in the absence of demonstrable isoimmunization and of any congenital anomaly of the red cells; this is particularly liable to occur in premature infants.[140, 141] Further, in exceptional cases there may be a congenital (and probably hereditary) lack of the enzymes needed to convert unconjugated bilirubin into the conjugated form, as would appear to be the case in the Crigler–Najjar type of *Kernikterus* (see page 1273, Volume 3).[142]

The pigment in the brain in cases of *Kernikterus* is readily soluble in xylene, and so this solvent must not be applied to tissues that are to be examined for its presence; frozen sections in an aqueous mountant are suitable. The pigmentation is accompanied by degenerative changes in the neurons, loss of myelin, and gliosis; these changes are consistent with hypoxia, and indeed the disease has been reproduced experimentally in new-born monkeys that have been rendered hyperbilirubinaemic and hypoxic.[143] The pigmentation gradually disappears, and in older children who have shown the clinical after-effects of neonatal *Kernikterus* the typical discoloration of the brain cannot be found at necropsy.

EPILEPSY AND HYPOXIA

Recurrent attacks of major epilepsy may damage the brain if the episodes of hypoxia are severe. If fits are frequent, they may lead to hippocampal sclerosis, atrophy of the thalami and focal atrophy of the cerebellum. Other lesions have also been described, but it is always difficult to know whether a discovered abnormality in the brain of an epileptic has been the result of the seizures or their cause. Epilepsy may result from focal lesions, such as meningocortical scars, which may be the sequel of some past injury to the head (see page 2187), but as often as not no histological abnormality can be detected in the brain of an epileptic (no lesions were recognized in 37 per cent of a series of 294 cases[144]). No constant biochemical anomaly has ever been reported, and the cause of idiopathic epilepsy is still unknown. It would seem most likely that the attacks result from a functional disturbance of the neuron or of its associated glial cells.

Temporal Lobe Epilepsy.[145]—The risk that temporal lobe epilepsy will be established permanently is greatest when hypoxic damage occurs in a temporal lobe in early life, due either to ischaemia at the time of birth in the territory supplied by the anterior choroidal branches of the posterior cerebral artery[146] or to infantile convulsions. The clinical effects may be apparent from the time of such initial hypoxia or they may develop only later in life. In other cases a hamartoma of blood vessels or a slow-growing astrocytoma is found in the temporal lobe,[147] or there may be a focal anomaly of cortical architecture, with groups of giant neurons and other bizarre cells, probably of glial origin.[148]

HYPOGLYCAEMIA AND THE BRAIN

Metabolic investigations have shown that the energy requirements of the central nervous system are almost wholly derived from the oxidative metabolism of glucose; the functions of the nervous system are, therefore, adversely affected by hypoglycaemia as well as by hypoxia. From studies made on the oxygen and glucose content of arterial and jugular venous blood in normal people, it has been found that the brain has a respiratory quotient of almost unity, and that it utilizes about 100 g of glucose daily.[149] As long as the amount of glucose in the blood remains above 5·5 mmol/l (about 100 mg/dl) the carbohydrate requirements of the brain are met, but should the blood glucose level fall below about 3·0 mmol/l (about 55 mg/dl) a succession of symptoms indicative of disturbances in the functioning of the brain may appear: these symptoms of hypoglycaemia include inability to concentrate thought, irritability, hunger, and chilling of the skin. Should the blood glucose fall much below 3·0 mmol/l (55 mg/dl), memory becomes seriously impaired, disorientation increases, and finally consciousness is lost and convulsions develop. Inability of nervous tissue to use available oxygen in the absence or reduction of substrate glucose has been termed *oxyachrestia*.[150]

Should hypoglycaemia be very severe or prolonged, permanent injury to the brain may follow. The histological changes are said to differ from those of grave hypoxia only in the frequency with which the neurons are found to be swollen and their nuclei distorted into a triangular shape. This appearance and the 'homogenizing' change (see page 2098) are reputedly seen oftener as a result of hypoglycaemia than after ischaemic damage; however, reference in the literature to 'severe' and 'homogenizing' cell changes should be treated with caution as such change has not been a feature of the optimally fixed primate brain following controlled experimental hypoglycaemia.[151] Although, in general, it is the cells of laminae III and V of the cerebral cortex and hippocampi that are particularly implicated, the cells of the calcarine cortex are relatively lightly affected. The small cells of the caudate nuclei and putamina are sometimes involved, but the pallidum generally escapes damage. Recent experimental work on hypoglycaemia in primates and in the rat, including studies with the electron microscope, has confirmed the morphological similarities between the changes in hypoxia and those in hypoglycaemia.[152–154]

The varying effects of hypoxia and hypoglycaemia on different parts of the central nervous system seem not to be adequately explicable on the basis of differences in local vascular supply.[155] The inherent biochemical constitution of the cells is probably an important additional factor in determining whether they die or survive. This concept of cell specificity under adverse conditions has been referred to as *pathoclisis*.[156]

It has been claimed that neonatal hypoglycaemia can be recognized as a cause of cerebral damage,[157–159] marked neuronal degeneration being found in affected human neonates[159] and—under experimental conditions (including fixation by perfusion)—in newborn rats.[154]

BACTERIAL, RICKETTSIAL AND FUNGAL INFECTIONS, AND GRANULOMATOUS DISEASES OF UNCERTAIN CAUSE

PYOGENIC INFECTIONS

The cerebrospinal fluid circulates in the space between the arachnoid, or outer layer of the leptomeninges, and the pia mater, or inner layer. This subarachnoid space is maintained by the supporting arachnoid trabeculae and contains the arteries and veins, which, with their pial investment, enter the substance of the brain. The dissemination of microorganisms that gain access to this space from a focus of infection is, therefore, understandably rapid, and this, together with the fact that the cerebrospinal fluid with its glucose and other metabolites provides an excellent culture medium, accounts for the fulminating character of many forms of meningitis caused by bacteria capable of rapid growth: they include the meningococcus, the pneumococcus, *Streptococcus pyogenes* and *Staphylococcus aureus*. Various organisms may cause suppurative meningitis as a form of 'opportunistic infection' (see page 2109).

Changes in the Cerebrospinal Fluid in Meningitis

The great clinical importance of correct treatment requires that the diagnosis between pyogenic, tuberculous and viral meningitis be made quickly and reliably. The organism responsible must be sought by appropriate microbiological methods in every case. In cases of acute pyogenic bacterial infections the protein in the cerebrospinal fluid is usually above 1·0 g/l. The cells are predominantly neutrophils and their number usually exceeds $2 \times 10^9/l$ (2000/μl). The concentration of chloride in the cerebrospinal fluid is usually reduced but this has no diagnostic value (see page 2117). Glucose may be undetectable in cases of pyogenic infection.

In tuberculous meningitis (see page 2117) the amount of glucose in the fluid tends to be reduced to between 2·0 and 0·8 mmol/l (between 36 and about 15 mg/dl); the protein content is raised less than in cases of pyogenic infection and the cell count is usually of the order of 0·1 to $1·0 \times 10^9/l$

(100 to 1000/μl), lymphocytes predominating after the initial stages.

In cases of viral meningitis (see page 2151) the amount of glucose in the cerebrospinal fluid is usually normal. The cell count varies; most of the cells are lymphocytes.

Suppurative Leptomeningitis

Meningococcal Meningitis (Cerebrospinal Fever)

Although a small proportion of normal people harbour the meningococcus (*Neisseria meningitidis*) in the nasopharynx, sporadic cases of meningeal infection due to this organism are uncommon, and occur usually in infants. In 1970, there were 524 notified instances of meningococcal meningitis in England and Wales.[160] Other specified organisms were reported in 374 cases of acute meningitis; in 424 further cases the causal organism was not identified.[160] By 1974 the number of notified cases of meningococcal meningitis had risen to 1296 and there were 479 cases of acute meningitis due to other specified organisms and 447 due to unspecified organisms.[160] In the following year, 1975, the corresponding figures were 864, 881 and 892; in 1976 they had fallen to 718, 665 and 513.[160] This pattern of fluctuation in the annual incidence of meningococcal meningitis is characteristic:[160a] no serious outbreaks of the disease occurred in England and Wales during the period covered by these sets of figures, most of the notifications concerning single and apparently unrelated cases. The population at risk throughout this period numbered about 48 million.

The incidence of meningococcal meningitis characteristically rises, and outbreaks tend to occur, in conditions of overcrowding. The infection was formerly a notorious hazard for young soldiers in barracks; in such communities the carrier rate may rise to over 50 per cent, but even in an epidemic the case incidence is low. Augmentation of the virulence of the organism is a generally postulated but ill-understood reason for a periodical increase in the incidence of the infection. In time of war such factors as debility and malnutrition, mass movements of troops and of the civil population, and a deterioration of housing conditions contribute to the development of epidemics.

The organism enters the blood stream, probably by way of the lymphoid tissue of the pharynx. In its initial phases the disease is essentially a septicaemia, and in some cases the patient dies before there is time for meningeal involvement to show. Meningococcal septicaemia is the commonest infective cause of bilateral haemorrhage into the adrenal glands, with consequent acute adrenocortical failure (Waterhouse-Friderichsen syndrome—see page 1937, Volume 4): in these cases, too, death usually occurs before there is clinical evidence of infection of the meninges.

A high continuous fever, acute polyarthritis and an erythematous or petechial rash are frequent manifestations of the septicaemic illness. From the combination of rash and pyrexia the disease acquired the name '*spotted fever*', which it shared with typhoid fever and with typhus. In some cases, meningococcal endocarditis develops during the septicaemia. Usually, however, the bacteria show their remarkable affinity for the cerebrospinal fluid pathways. The main route of the infection is believed to be through the choroid plexuses, which become intensely inflamed: once in the cerebrospinal fluid the organisms multiply rapidly in the lateral ventricles,[161] whence they spread through the third and fourth ventricles and the apertures in the roof of the latter to reach the surface of the brain and spinal cord. They may also gain access to the meninges through the smaller meningeal vessels. It was formerly believed that the meningococcus might occasionally infect the leptomeninges by passing directly from the nose along the filaments of the olfactory nerves and the minute vessels that accompany them through the cribriform plate; this pathway is no longer regarded as having any part in the pathogenesis of this disease.

Meningococcal infection rapidly provokes a neutrophil leucocytosis in the affected tissues, and particularly in the subarachnoid space. It is in the cytoplasm of the neutrophils that the characteristic Gram-negative, bean-shaped diplococci are most frequently found. In favourable cases (which were uncommon before the days of specific antisera and chemotherapy) the number of neutrophils in the cerebrospinal fluid falls as the bacteria are destroyed: the neutrophils are replaced by increasing numbers of lymphocytes, and of macrophages containing bacteria (most of which are dead), fat and other debris. Some of these cells eventually return to the general circulation through the arachnoid villi; others die and disintegrate in the subarachnoid space.

Course

Some of the patients die of the fulminating toxaemia. In such cases the brain is greatly swollen and there is considerable inflammatory hyperaemia of the meninges, with many petechial haemorrhages and marked distension of the veins. Petechiae, from which the meningococcus can be recovered, are also numerous in the skin and mucous membranes, and in the serosal lining of the body cavities.

Within 48 hours of the onset of the disease, in typical cases, a thin layer of pus covers the brain, particularly its basal surface, and the ventricles are tensely distended with turbid fluid. In some untreated cases death may be delayed for several days, by which time the circulation of the cerebrospinal fluid is impeded by viscous exudate obstructing the median and lateral apertures in the roof of the fourth ventricle (foramina of Magendie and Luschka) and filling the pontine cistern. In treated cases, adhesions may develop if therapy has been delayed or inefficient (Fig. 34.23).

Although the disease is essentially a leptomenin-

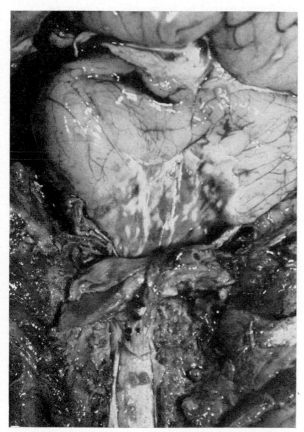

Fig. 34.23. Postmeningitic adhesions at necropsy in the case of a girl who died at the age of four years. When 10 days old she had developed meningococcal meningitis. Adhesions followed recovery from the infection and blocked the apertures of the fourth ventricle, necessitating several palliative operations for relief of the obstruction. The photograph shows the brain and spinal cord *in situ*, from behind: the markedly thickened leptomeninges over the distended fourth ventricle are well seen. The foramen magnum has not been opened when removing the occipital bone.

2*

gitis, there are other changes in the brain. The white matter swells and the downward expansion of the supratentorial part of the brain leads to compression of the brainstem at the tentorial opening, and to vascular engorgement of the pons and medulla; a consequent dysfunction of the reticular formation has been blamed for the early onset of unconsciousness. The nerve cells may show marked degenerative changes. Because of the accumulation of exudate, delay in treatment increases the risk of subsequent fibrosis of the leptomeninges, with resultant compression of the vestibulocochlear and other cranial nerves, dyspituitarism, and symptoms and signs of hydrocephalus.

'Post-Basic Meningitis'

A form of meningococcal meningitis that affects the meninges over the base of the brain predominantly, and particularly in the posterior fossa, occurs in young children. This so-called 'post-basic' form of meningitis, first described by Gee and Barlow,[162] is liable to be confused clinically with tuberculous meningitis.

Pneumococcal Meningitis

The pneumococcus (*Streptococcus pneumoniae*) usually gains access to the subarachnoid space from an infected air sinus, especially following a fracture of the base of the skull, but it may be blood-borne from the lungs, the pleural or peritoneal cavities, or, in cases of acute pneumococcal endocarditis, from the heart valves. The pneumococcus multiplies rapidly, and it is not surprising that within 48 hours of the commencement of the infection the surface of the brain is coated with pus (Fig. 34.24), which in this form of meningitis often has a distinctly greenish or greenish-yellow colour. If death occurs earlier, the presence of pus may be apparent only in the pontine, cerebellomedullary and interpeduncular cisterns, in the lateral sulci of the cerebral hemispheres, and over the spinal cord, particularly its posterior surface. In fulminating cases there may be no obvious pus, but the brain is swollen and tense, and the meningeal veins are grossly distended: if pus is present it is likeliest to be found as streaks of exudate alongside these veins. In the absence of treatment the patient may not survive beyond the third day, by which time the suppurative process has usually spread into the substance of the brain in the vicinity of the distended sulci. The pneumococci are even more readily found in the cerebrospinal fluid than are menin-

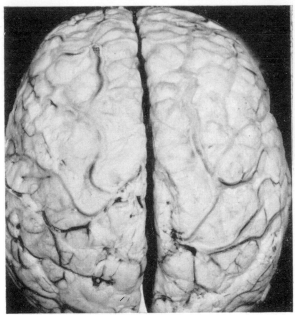

Fig. 34.24. Pneumococcal meningitis. A boy aged 10 months had been fretful for one week and had vomited on the day before he was admitted to hospital following a fit. He was found to have bilateral otitis media. He was treated with penicillin but died on the next day.

gococci in cases of meningococcal meningitis. Patients who, as a result of treatment, have survived the acute disease may develop fibrosis of the leptomeninges, and, consequently, obstructive hydrocephalus. Infarction of parts of the brain may result from secondary obliterative arteritis.[163]

Staphylococcal Meningitis

Meningitis caused by *Staphylococcus aureus* (Fig. 34.25) is commonly secondary to an infection elsewhere, such as a perinephric abscess, a boil or carbuncle, or acute osteomyelitis. To the naked eye, the appearances are, in general, indistinguishable from those of pneumococcal meningitis, except that the purulent exudate is yellowish, without any green tint. *Staphylococcus albus* has been known to cause meningitis as a complication of lumbar puncture.

Streptococcal Meningitis

Streptococcal meningitis, so named, is usually caused by *Streptococcus pyogenes*. The pathological picture is similar to that of pneumococcal and staphylococcal meningitis, but the exudate tends to be greyer and less viscous. The organisms gain access to the subarachnoid space from a source that may be local or distant. The commonest antecedent of

streptococcal meningitis is infection of the middle ear or nasal sinuses, which may be acute or chronic: in some instances, the meningitis develops as a complication of a fracture involving the wall of a sinus. Sometimes it accompanies a streptococcal infection of the skin of the upper lip or of the nose, or it may complicate erysipelas of the face: the bacteria in these cases may be conveyed to the leptomeninges as a result of a septic facial thrombophlebitis complicated by thrombosis of the cavernous sinus. In exceptional cases the infection has followed lumbar puncture: in such instances it is likely that the apparatus used in the operation has been contaminated by organisms carried in the throat of a member of the staff.

Meningitis caused by *Haemophilus influenzae*

Meningeal infection with *Haemophilus influenzae* occurs oftenest in the young, and it may be preceded by pneumonia; its maximum incidence is in the first year of life. It is rare over the age of 20 years: in this it contrasts with pneumococcal and staphylococcal meningitis, liability to which increases throughout childhood and into adult life. The changes in the brain do not differ appreciably from those in streptococcal meningitis, although cerebral phlebitis appears to be commoner.[164] In films of cerebrospinal fluid the organism is pleomorphic, ranging from coccoid forms to long filaments. It is less easily cultivated than the pathogenic cocci.

Other Forms of Acute Meningitis

Surprisingly many different types of organism may cause acute meningitis. It would appear, from the experience of neurosurgeons, that the exposed subarachnoid space has an unduly low resistance to bacterial infection, and even to infection by organisms that are usually regarded as no more than saprophytes. In effect, the wide variety of potential invaders of the subarachnoid space means that the accurate and complete diagnosis of meningitis is dependent upon laboratory studies. Every effort must be made to establish quickly the nature of the organism and its sensitivity to drugs: it is, therefore, essential to obtain a sample of cerebrospinal fluid before treatment is begun. In some cases it will be found that more than one species of organism is present.

Among the organisms that may cause acute meningitis are *Listeria monocytogenes*[165] and *Brucella melitensis. Pseudomonas aeruginosa (Pseu-*

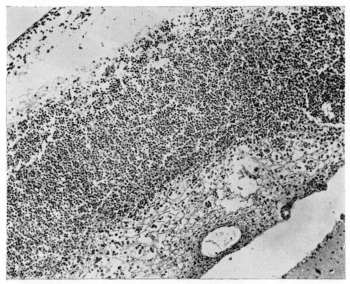

Fig. 34.25. Staphylococcal meningitis after four days of treatment. Most of the cells in the subarachnoid space are neutrophils, but there is already an attempt at organization: in a Gram-stained preparation organisms could no longer be found. *Haematoxylin–eosin.* × 60.

domonas *pyocyanea*), *Proteus vulgaris* and *Staphylococcus albus* are among the bacteria that are particularly liable to be the causes of infective complications after neurosurgical procedures. *Pseudomonas aeruginosa* has been known to infect solutions of spinal anaesthetics.[166] *Bacillus anthracis*, which has a distinct predilection for the meninges, may cause a fulminating, haemorrhagic meningitis (Fig. 34.26) as a complication of cutaneous or pulmonary anthrax.

Meningitis may occur in leptospirosis, particularly in cases of infection by *Leptospira icterohaemorrhagiae* (Weil's disease—see page 1226, Volume 3).[167] The meningeal involvement may be severe, or so trivial as to be virtually symptomless. The cellular response in the cerebrospinal fluid may be predominantly lymphocytic, and leptospirosis must, therefore, be considered in the differential diagnosis of benign lymphocytic choriomeningitis (see page 2151). Other species of leptospira may also invade the meninges, particularly *Leptospira canicola*, which typically is acquired from dogs: the organisms are passed in their urine—the infected animals are not necessarily ill.

Escherichia coli may give rise to acute meningitis during the early neonatal period in otherwise healthy babies, and the infection may even be well established before birth;[168] in other cases, *Escherichia coli* may gain access to the spinal meninges through the deficient covering of the

malformed parts at the site of a meningocele, meningomyelocele (see page 2201) or congenital occipital or lumbosacral sinus connecting the meninges and the skin.

Various serotypes of *Salmonella*, including the typhoid bacillus, may cause meningitis. This occurred in 1 per cent of a series of almost 8000 cases of salmonellosis in North America[168a] and in 6 per cent of a series of over 800 cases in West Africa.[168b]

The doctor in attendance on a patient with meningitis must always look for the portal of entry of the organisms: a failure to recognize a lesion that is the source of meningeal infection may result in repeated attacks of meningitis. An unsuspected fracture of the roof of an ethmoidal air cell may have this effect until such time as it is surgically repaired. Similarly, chronic infection of the middle ear may be the source of recurrent episodes of meningitis, and treatment of the latter will not eradicate the risk until the aural disease has been dealt with properly. Again, it has to be remembered that acute meningitis may be a complication of an unrecognized otitis media, and this possibility must always be considered when dealing with a delirious child with no localizing manifestations.

The possibility of a so-called 'opportunistic infection', caused by an unusual organism, may need consideration in patients whose immunolo-

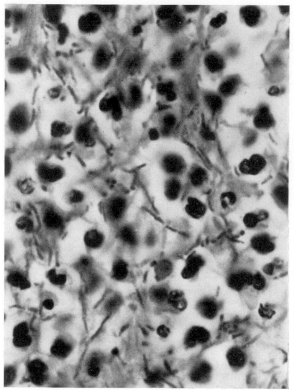

Fig. 34.26.§ Anthrax meningitis. Histological section showing chains of haematoxyphile anthrax bacilli in the meningeal exudate. Neutrophils are conspicuous in this field: often—as elsewhere in the specimen from which this preparation comes—leucocytes are sparse in the essentially haemorrhagic exudate that usually characterizes anthrax meningitis. Case of cutaneous and meningeal anthrax studied by R. B. Calwell and W. St. C. Symmers (Belfast, 1907). *Haematoxylin–eosin.* × 1000.

gical defences have been depressed by disease or therapy (see page 362, Volume 1).

Pachymeningitis

The tough and sparsely cellular dura mater is seldom, if ever, the seat of acute inflammation unless infected as an accompaniment of a fracture or of osteomyelitis of the skull or spine. An *extradural abscess* is a rare development in such cases. A *subdural abscess* may form if the dura has been penetrated by wounding or if infection spreads within the venous sinuses in cases of nasal sinusitis, otitis media or mastoiditis.

Extradural abscesses are less uncommon in the spinal canal, in which the dura is less firmly and less widely attached to the bones. In most instances, such abscesses are a haematogenous accompaniment

of cutaneous suppuration caused by *Staphylococcus aureus.*

Non-specific chronic granulomas of undetermined cause occasionally develop in the spinal extradural space and compress the cord. Histological examination of these lesions shows a variable degree of fibrosis and of accumulation of lymphocytes and plasma cells, and sometimes of eosinophils and multinucleate giant cells. The resemblance to some of the so-called 'pseudotumours' of the orbit (see Chapter 40, Volume 6) has attracted attention, but there is no evidence to link the two conditions.

Brain Abscess

An abscess in the brain may be the result either of direct spread of bacteria from a local source or of haematogenous spread from a distant infected focus. In the days before antibiotics, by far the commonest cause was otitis media and mastoiditis, complicating scarlet fever or an upper respiratory tract infection. Because of prompt, effective treatment of the primary infection, such abscesses are now much less common, although they still account for almost half the total number of brain abscesses. A brain abscess may also follow suppuration in the frontal sinus and, more rarely, in the ethmoidal or sphenoidal sinuses. Brain abscess may complicate cavernous sinus thrombosis, which itself may result from septic thrombophlebitis of the anterior facial vein. Infection may enter the brain as a result of a penetrating injury, or following a compound fracture of the skull or erosion of the bone by a malignant tumour.

Foci of suppuration in the lungs, especially in cases of bronchiectasis, and vegetations in infective endocarditis may be a source of haematogenous infection of the brain. Micro-organisms may, it is thought, sometimes find their way from the pelvis to the brain by way of the vertebral venous plexuses.

Because the pathological features of an abscess that results from extension of a nearby infected focus differ somewhat from those of a metastatic abscess, the two varieties will be considered separately. Otogenous abscess will be described as the type example of the former. The changes in the cerebrospinal fluid, which are common to both varieties, will be noted before the characteristics of the abscesses are described.

Changes in the Cerebrospinal Fluid.—The protein content of the cerebrospinal fluid in patients with a cerebral abscess is often within the normal range, and seldom exceeds 1·0 g/l. The cell count may be normal, but it may rise as high as $800 \times 10^6/l$, even in the absence of a complicating meningitis; usually it is of the order of 100 to $150 \times 10^6/l$.[169] A helpful point in diagnosis, when the cell count is low, is that both lymphocytes and neutrophils are generally present; the latter seldom reach 50 per cent of the total.

Otogenous Abscess

The source of otogenous brain abscess is suppuration in the middle ear (see Chapter 41, Volume 6). Most such abscesses develop in the temporal lobe (Fig. 34.27) but sometimes infection spreads by way of the mastoid air cells to the adjacent cerebellar hemisphere, giving rise to a cerebellar abscess.

Although in cases of acute suppurative otitis media the tympanic membrane may rupture spontaneously and thus allow pus to escape, such a mode of drainage is seldom as effective as that provided surgically. If free drainage is not established, the infection is likely to spread from the middle ear into the tegmen tympani, the thin plate of the petrous part of the temporal bone that forms the roof of the mastoid antrum and of the tympanic cavity.

This 'petrositis' is usually associated with localized pachymeningitis, but, surprisingly, the infection tends to cross the plane of the subarachnoid space without causing a spreading leptomeningitis; instead, it tracks through the cortex of the brain into the underlying white matter. It seems likely, therefore, that the bacteria traverse the pia-arachnoid and cortex in the blood vessels that penetrate from the pia, possibly in microscopical emboli originating as septic thrombi that form on the damaged endothelium of the vessels within the middle ear. At the junction of the grey and white matter, where each of the penetrating cortical branches of the cerebral arteries may divide into several branches, the emboli are arrested, and the bacteria multiply and invade the white matter which, relative to the grey matter, has a scanty blood supply. Sometimes, however, the abscess is superficial, and contiguous with the tegmen tympani.

Experimental work has suggested that the presence of bacteria in damaged brain parenchyma may bring about the release of a substance that is capable of promoting intravascular clotting,[170] and it is possible that consequent oligaemic changes in the area favour the establishment and eventual extension of the infection.

Very rarely, the frontal lobe is the site of an abscess that develops as a complication of middle ear disease. In these cases it is believed that the abscess is the result of retrograde carriage of infected emboli in the superior sagittal sinus.

The presence of multiplying bacteria stimulates the defence mechanisms of the tissues. Capillaries dilate and allow the prompt access of neutrophils and monocytes: the centre of the abscess soon consists of bacteria, pus and autolysing tissue debris. One of the earliest responses is shown by adventitial cells, which separate off as fibroblasts and lay down collagen fibres (Fig. 34.28). Lymphocytes, plasma cells and Hortega cells also collect: the last ingest the debris of myelin and cells. The astrocytes are also active, but their participation tends to be confined to the zone of brain tissue immediately abutting on the capsule produced by the fibroblasts. However, such astrocytes, especially those nearest to the abscess cavity, are liable to show evidence of toxic damage in the form of clasmatodendrosis (see page 2083). In the surrounding white matter, the blood vessels are often dilated, and many are cuffed by migrant cells. There is usually considerable swelling of the white matter of the affected lobe or hemisphere, with displacement of midline structures to the side opposite to the lesion. Sometimes the process of encapsulation is defective or is never initiated, and a spreading suppurative encephalitis extends through

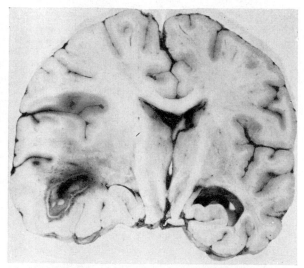

Fig. 34.27. Right temporal lobe abscess, with well-formed capsule. Note the marked swelling of the white matter that has obliterated the inferior horn of the lateral ventricle on the same side and displaced the midline structures to the opposite side. Swelling of the white matter tends, as in this instance, to lessen the depth of the sulci and widen the gyri, so making the brain surface flatter and smoother.

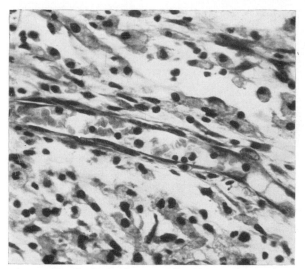

Fig. 34.28. Cerebral abscess. Fibroblasts migrate from the adventitial surface of a blood vessel to help form the fibrous wall (they are the cells with elongated nuclei, especially noticeable close above the vessel). *Haematoxylin–eosin.* × 260.

much of the white matter. The nerve cells near the abscess show degenerative changes.

When the contents of a brain abscess are aspirated in the course of treatment and replaced by a solution of an antibiotic, the opportunity may be taken to introduce a radio-opaque medium into the cavity to enable its position and extent to be defined radiologically. Following such an injection, phagocytes ingest the particles of the contrast medium and, as these laden cells collect among the proliferating fibroblasts, their presence can be demonstrated radiologically in the 'pyogenic membrane' that surrounds the abscess (Fig. 34.29). When the radio-opaque zone that thus delineates the cavity is seen to have become sharply defined, the surgeon knows that fibrosis is sufficiently advanced to justify drainage of the abscess: this is usually after about three weeks. It is appropriate to note here that the computer-assisted brain-scanner is likely to outmode conventional contrast radiography.

It is of practical importance to note that temporal lobe abscesses, although almost always solitary, may have an irregular outline, with pockets that lead out of the main cavity.

An abscess may eventually rupture into a ventricle or on to the surface of the brain, causing a terminal leptomeningitis. Rupture may be precipitated by a sudden lowering of intracranial pressure accompanying an injudicious lumbar puncture.

Most otogenous abscesses are caused by strepto-

cocci, some strains of which may prove difficult to cultivate. Somewhat less often a pneumococcus is found. In exceptional cases, diphtheroid bacilli, *Fusobacterium fusiforme* or *Bacillus anthracoides* may be responsible.

Abscesses secondary to infection in the nasal sinuses differ from otogenous abscesses only in their situation, which usually is in the subcortical white matter adjacent to the source of the infection. An abscess originating as a complication of frontal sinusitis, for instance, is likeliest to be found in the corresponding frontal lobe.

Elevation of the intracranial pressure is not usually a notable feature of a brain abscess complicating otitis or nasal sinusitis.

Metastatic Abscesses

Metastatic abscesses develop most frequently in the parts of the brain that are supplied by a middle cerebral artery. They usually appear—as do most embolic lesions in the brain—near the junction of the white and grey matter; however, when the route of infection is the central arteries supplying the

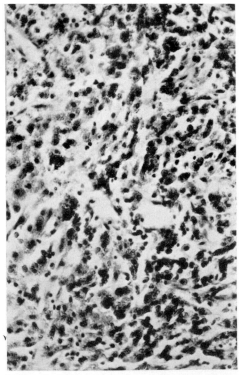

Fig. 34.29. Contents of abscess cavity three weeks after introduction of a radio-opaque material. The foreign substance has been taken up by histiocytes that by this stage tend to collect round the newly-formed blood vessels of the abscess wall. *Haematoxylin–eosin.* × 100.

interior of the brain, they are more deeply situated (for instance, in the basal ganglia). They are sometimes multiple. They differ from otogenous abscesses in being less well encapsulated: in consequence, diffuse suppurative encephalitis is less rare as a manifestation of haematogenous infection than as a complication of suppuration in the ear or in a nasal sinus. An infected embolus in a major branch of a cerebral artery gives rise to a large area of septic infarction. Considerable surrounding oedema may result, with a rise in intracranial pressure and the development of papilloedema, which is comparatively rare in cases of otogenous abscess.

Various organisms have been recovered from brain abscesses complicating disease of the lungs and bronchi; the commonest are streptococci, and, as in cases of streptococcal otogenous abscesses, they may be difficult to isolate in the laboratory. Spirochaetes are not infrequently found, especially in patients with bronchiectasis: *Borrelia vincentii* is the usual one, and is often accompanied by *Fusobacterium fusiforme*—these symbiotic organisms are common secondary invaders of bronchiectatic lesions and seem to find the milieu of a brain abscess equally suitable for their growth.

Acute bacterial endocarditis may give rise to metastatic brain abscesses. In contrast, embolism of the cerebral vasculature in cases of subacute bacterial endocarditis results in bland infarction, because the causative organisms do not ordinarily survive in the emboli; occasionally, however, a mycotic aneurysm results (see page 147, Volume 1).

Haematogenous brain abscess is a common complication of congenital cyanotic heart disease, observed in 3 to 11 per cent of cases in different series. It develops in the absence of bacterial endocarditis and its explanation is obscure.[171, 172] Such abscesses are usually solitary. They may develop after corrective cardiac surgery and it is possible that the presence of a central veno-atrial shunt is a predisposing factor, bypassing an as yet undefined pulmonary mechanism that in some way clears bacteria from the circulation.

Metastatic brain abscesses complicating peritonitis or suppurative infection of the pelvic organs are most commonly caused by streptococci, which in some instances are anaerobic.

TUBERCULOSIS OF THE CENTRAL NERVOUS SYSTEM

Tuberculous Meningitis

The condition that is familiar to us as tuberculous meningitis was first described as a clinicopatho-logical entity by Robert Whytt, of Edinburgh, in 1768.[173] Its association with tuberculosis of other organs was recognized some 50 years later by Antoine Laurent Jessé Bayle, in Paris.[174] The mortality from the disease has fallen dramatically since the second world war: the number of recorded deaths[174a, 174b] from tuberculous meningitis in England and Wales in 1946 was 1587, by 1962 it had declined to 67 and in 1976 it was 29. This is partly due to advances in treatment, and partly to the striking general decrease in the incidence of tuberculosis. However, it is important to recognize that even in countries, such as Britain, where there has been a very great reduction in the incidence of tuberculosis in the indigenous population, tuberculosis among particular sections of the community is still an important problem. In Europe this is specially true of various immigrant groups, particularly when living under inadequate conditions. It should also be remembered that the influence of ethnic, genetical and nutritional factors may determine unusual clinical syndromes in members of certain population groups, such as the range of atypical manifestations of tuberculosis of the central nervous system that has been recognized in India (see page 2118).[175]

In the days before streptomycin, tuberculous meningitis followed a downhill course of about three weeks. Death occurred nearly always because of interference with the circulation of the cerebrospinal fluid, the upward flow through the tentorial opening being obstructed by the inflammatory exudate in the pontine cistern, and the outflow from the ventricles being similarly hindered by blockage of the median and lateral apertures of the fourth ventricle (Fig. 34.30). Exudate at the base of the brain prevented the passage of the fluid through the foramen magnum into the spinal subarachnoid space. The fact that death occurs so much later in untreated cases of tuberculous meningitis than in cases of acute pyogenic meningitis is attributable to the slower progress of the inflammatory reaction. Chronic forms of meningeal tuberculosis were very rare before the introduction of modern treatment: they are now liable to be seen if treatment is delayed or inadequate (Fig. 34.31).

Aetiology and Pathogenesis

The disease is commonest in childhood, and in many instances it follows an acute respiratory tract infection, notably measles or whooping cough. Possibly for this reason, tuberculous meningitis is seen most frequently in the spring months. It is

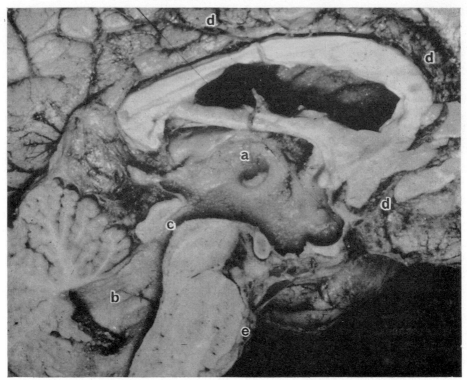

Fig. 34.30. Tuberculous meningitis. Untreated disease in a child dying on the 21st day of the illness. Note the dilatation of the ventricular system (a — interventricular foramen and third ventricle; b = fourth ventricle; c = aqueduct) and the tubercles on their ependymal lining and in the leptomeninges, especially along the course of the anterior cerebral artery (d) and in the interpeduncular fossa. The leptomeninges are characteristically thickened in the region of the pontine cistern (e).

usual to find that these children have a healing or healed Ghon focus in one lung with active hilar lymph node involvement (see page 331, Volume 1). If the interval between the primary pulmonary infection and the onset of meningitis is short, the Ghon focus also may still be advancing. Presumably, the superimposed acute infection of the respiratory tract lowers resistance to the tuberculous infection, with rapid exacerbation of the disease in the hilar lymph nodes, erosion of a vein, and discharge of bacilli into the blood stream. Sometimes the portal of entry of the infection is intestinal: in such cases an incompletely healed tuberculous lymphadenitis may be found in the mesentery. More rarely, meningitis is the result of invasion of the blood stream in the course of a tuberculous infection of bone or of cervical lymph nodes.

Tuberculous meningitis develops in between 70 and 85 per cent of cases of generalized miliary tuberculosis, and almost 90 per cent of cases of tuberculous meningitis are, in fact, a manifestation of the miliary disease. The belief that tuberculous meningitis is not an invariable accompaniment of miliary tuberculosis was confirmed when it was found that an intravenous or intra-arterial injection of virulent tubercle bacilli into rabbits caused miliary tuberculosis but not frank meningitis.[176, 177] Scattered miliary lesions developed in the brain and leptomeninges of the animals: they were clearly the result of chance haematogenous distribution to these situations, for they were no more frequent than the lesions in other parts of the body. In contrast, it was found that progressive meningitis regularly followed if the bacilli were introduced directly into the subarachnoid space.

For a long time it was not apparent why there was no associated miliary tuberculosis in some 10 per cent of children with tuberculous meningitis, or why, when the two conditions did coexist, the meningeal involvement was often so much more marked than the infection of other organs. Rich and McCordock,[177] working in Baltimore, took the view that, as a result of a minor tuberculous bac-

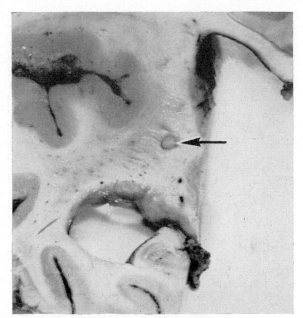

Fig. 34.31. Tuberculous meningitis, treated and chronic, showing marked ventricular dilatation. Tubercles can be seen in several parts of the leptomeninges (notably in the small sulcus crossing the centre of the bottom edge of the photograph). The arrow points to a small, deep-seated tuberculoma.

teriaemia, a metastatic tuberculous focus developed in the brain, and, in due course, enlarged until it ruptured into the subarachnoid space: this extension of the infection and the resulting dispersal of the bacilli in the cerebrospinal fluid they believed to account for the development of the meningitis. They observed such foci in over 90 per cent of a series of 82 cases of tuberculous meningitis.[177] The presence of these so-called Rich (or Rich–McCordock) foci was confirmed in a similar proportion of cases studied in Edinburgh;[178] it was also noted during the Scottish investigation that comparable foci were to be found in the brain in nearly half the cases of miliary tuberculosis in which there had been no clinical evidence of meningitis.

The *Rich focus* may be single or multiple: it is not always in the brain—in some instances it has been located in the spinal cord. It is usually only about 1 to 2 mm in diameter (Fig. 34.32), although sometimes considerably larger. It is not difficult to find, provided the fixed brain is cut coronally in thin slices (Rich recommended that the slices should be 3 mm thick and that they should be examined by transillumination). The foci are usually near the surface of the cortex (Fig. 34.32), although a not uncommon site is the junction of the grey and white

matter of the cortex, precisely where small emboli are prone to lodge (see page 2174).

Rich's view of the pathogenesis of tuberculous meningitis has been challenged. Some investigators have doubted that the meningeal infection spreads from the foci: they have been unable to find the relatively greater concentration of lesions in the adjacent meninges that they considered would have been evident if the focus had been the source of the meningeal infection.[179] They noted that in some cases the tubercles in the meninges were of different generations, indicating that there had been several showers of bacilli into the cerebrospinal fluid. Some investigators have commented on the considerable frequency with which tubercles are present in the choroid plexuses, although Rich and McCordock found foci in these structures in only a little more than 1 per cent of their cases (see above).[177] Others believe that the bacilli may enter the cerebrospinal fluid not only from the choroid plexuses but also by passage through the walls of the cerebral blood vessels elsewhere: certainly, tubercles are commonly present along the meningeal course of the major cerebral arteries. It seems likely, therefore, that there are several routes by which meningeal infection can take place, any or all of which may be concerned in particular cases. In fact, the pathogenesis of every case of tuberculous meningitis is an individual problem and must be studied in detail

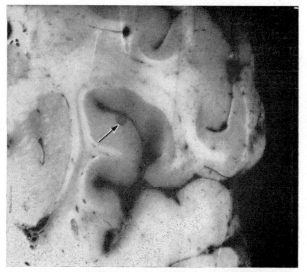

Fig. 34.32. Tuberculous meningitis. An inflammatory exudate occupies the recesses of the lateral sulcus. There is a small tuberculoma (arrow) impinging on the pial surface of the insula: expanding tuberculous lesions like this (Rich foci) are thought to give rise to meningitis when they rupture into the subarachnoid space.

accordingly. In particular, attention should be paid to the apparent age of the meningeal tubercles and to the possibility that they are of different generations, and their size and structure should be compared with those of tubercles present in other organs.

Structural Changes

Lesions that are typical of tuberculous meningitis may be greatly modified by treatment, which can prolong the course of the disease by many months, and often is curative.

In rapidly progressive cases, such as were formerly the rule, the tubercles were usually clearly visible in the leptomeninges. They have a predilection for the pontine cistern and the interpeduncular fossa, and they should also be sought on the upper surface of the cerebellum and along the course of the large blood vessels, especially the anterior and middle cerebral arteries. They are greyish and opaque, and, when viewed with a hand lens, they are seen to be slightly raised above their surroundings. They are best seen in direct light against a background of the blood contained in the thin-walled veins, but they have to be distinguished by digital pressure from the tiny air bubbles that collect in veins during the course of the necropsy (such bubbles can be moved by lightly stroking the vessel whereas tubercles are fixed, and firm to the touch). Tubercles may also be seen in the ependyma of the ventricles (Figs 34.30 and 34.33).

Sometimes tubercles are so few that they are easily overlooked. Indeed, evidence of tuberculous meningitis can be missed at necropsy, and this is

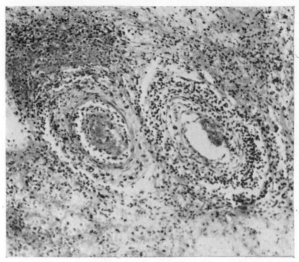

Fig. 34.34. Tuberculous meningitis. The inflammatory process is seen to involve all layers of the wall of the blood vessels in the subarachnoid space. Note the thrombi and the necrosis. Giant cells are scanty. *Haematoxylin–eosin.* ×90.

particularly so in cases that have been treated with antituberculous drugs. The diagnosis often depends on a particularly careful macroscopical examination of possibly affected structures. If necessary, selected pieces of the pia-arachnoid should be removed and studied with a hand lens by transillumination, for in this way the smallest tubercles are least liable to be overlooked. The brain is always swollen in cases of tuberculous meningitis, and the sulci therefore tend to become obscured; also, there is always some thickening of the leptomeninges covering the basal cisterns, and a characteristic gelatinous exudate collects in the interpeduncular fossa. Such findings should strongly suggest the possibility of tuberculosis.

When tuberculous meningitis occurs in infancy, before the anterior fontanelle has closed, there is no bony hindrance to expansion of the brain, and a marked degree of hydrocephalus may develop.

In cases treated with antituberculous drugs, the patient may survive for many months, and lesions of the local vasculature may develop. Tuberculous arteritis (Figs 34.34 and 34.35) is often accompanied by thrombosis, with infarction of the corresponding parts of the brain.[180] The arteries in the subarachnoid space at the base of the brain are most liable to be affected, but the branches over the cortex may also become involved. Vascular occlusion may develop even when treatment is far advanced (Fig. 34.36); the vessels affected are, particularly, the anterior and posterior cerebral arteries and the

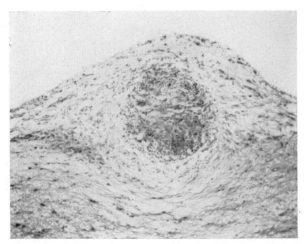

Fig. 34.33. Tuberculous meningitis. Small subependymal tubercle of the size seen in Fig. 34.30. *Haematoxylin–eosin.* ×30.

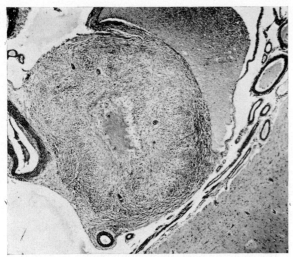

Fig. 34.35. Tuberculous meningitis. The wall of this small artery is completely replaced by tuberculous granulation tissue with well-formed giant cell systems. The lumen is blocked by a contracting thrombus. *Haematoxylin–Van Gieson.* × 30.

central arteries that supply the basal ganglia. An occasional complication of chronic tuberculous meningitis is thrombosis of the superior sagittal sinus.

Changes in the Cerebrospinal Fluid

Traditionally, it has been said that the feature most typical of the cerebrospinal fluid in tuberculous meningitis is its low chloride concentration. This is a dangerously misleading teaching, for if diagnosis and treatment are delayed until the chloride level has fallen significantly, the patient may be past any chance of recovery.[181] A low concentration of chloride in the cerebrospinal fluid simply means that there has been a heavy depletion of the chloride of the body as a whole: it can follow any sustained febrile state accompanied by vomiting, and it may, therefore, be found as an isolated change in the fluid in cases of acute pneumococcal pneumonia, or of miliary tuberculosis without meningeal involvement, or in other continued fevers. It is in no sense peculiar to tuberculous meningitis, and as a diagnostic feature it should be discarded. An earlier, and more significant, although also unspecific, change in the cerebrospinal fluid in cases of tuberculous meningitis is a reduction in the concentration of glucose. This is often attributed to a supposed avidity of the bacilli for glucose, but, in fact, it has no constant relation to the number of bacilli present: sometimes bacilli are plentiful when the

glucose content of the fluid is little reduced, and the reverse is occasionally found. It must be added, however, that bacilli may be few in the spinal fluid and yet plentiful in the subarachnoid cisterns.

In most cases of tuberculous meningitis the amount of protein in the cerebrospinal fluid is raised: the value is generally between 1·0 and 4·0 g/l. In unclotted fluid the cell count may lie between $0·1$ and $1·0 \times 10^9/l$ ($100/\mu l$ and $1000/\mu l$); neutrophils may be numerous at first but later are much outnumbered by lymphocytes.

It is imperative that the presence of tuberculous meningitis should be recognized at the earliest opportunity, for only prompt treatment holds out a reasonable hope of cure.[182] The longer the delay in starting effective therapy, the greater is the likelihood of death or residual disability. In fact, the aim should be to recognize the disease in the stage before generalized meningitis develops; sometimes this is possible, as, for instance, when a Rich focus that is about to break through at the surface of the brain presents with focal symptoms and a slight increase in the number of cells and in the amount of protein in the cerebrospinal fluid. With a past history of tuberculosis or, in the case of a child, a history of contact with a case of active tuberculosis, even slight neurological disturbances may be important as evidence of the pre-meningitic stage of tuberculous meningitis.

The only reliable way of making the diagnosis is to find the tubercle bacilli in the cerebrospinal

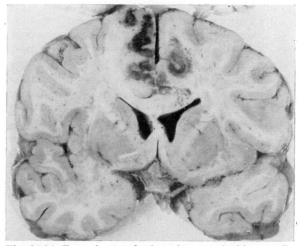

Fig. 34.36. Treated case of tuberculous meningitis complicated by occlusion of both anterior cerebral arteries. Note involvement of the left lateral part of the corpus callosum (on right of picture). The thickening of the leptomeninges is apparent round the optic chiasma and in the left lateral sulcus.

fluid, and every effort should be directed to this end. It is not always the fault of the laboratory if the bacilli are not found, for they are sometimes very scanty. They are most readily discovered by microscopical examination of the fine fibrin clot—the *'spider's web clot'*—that so constantly forms when a sample of the fluid from a case of this disease is allowed to stand, especially if kept at 37°C for a few hours. Attempts must always be made to cultivate the bacillus and so confirm the diagnosis, particularly in those cases in which treatment has had to be started on a presumption. It is also important to ascertain the in-vitro sensitivity of the organism to drugs: cultures are necessary for this purpose, and also for determining the specific identity of the mycobacterium. A working diagnosis, however, cannot await the results of these time-consuming procedures, and so, for this purpose, there is still no alternative to the diligent microscopical search for the causative organism in samples of cerebrospinal fluid.

Effects of Treatment

The main dangers in tuberculous meningitis are obstruction of the subarachnoid space by exudate and infarction of the brain due to thrombosis of involved cerebral arteries. It is logical, therefore, to treat the disease not only with antituberculous drugs, such as streptomycin, isoniazid and sodium aminosalicylate, but also with a corticosteroid, administered early enough to discourage the outpouring of cells and the formation of fibrin and granulation tissue.[183-185]

Both streptomycin and isoniazid act by killing the tubercle bacillus. If either drug is given alone, resistant variants of the organism may appear; when both are given together, there seems to be less liability for resistance to develop to either. Isoniazid has the potentially serious disadvantage that it encourages the growth of granulation tissue; to avoid the risks of such a development within the closed cavity of the skull, the combination of of streptomycin with sodium aminosalicylate is preferable.

Tuberculoma

Tuberculosis of the central nervous system may take the form of a single, large, caseous lesion. This possibility should always be considered when a patient with symptoms of a tumour in the brain or spinal cord comes from a country where tuberculosis is still rife (see below). Tuberculomas are found oftenest in the cerebellum, and less commonly in the cerebral hemispheres, brainstem (Fig. 34.37) or spinal cord. They may calcify. Their removal is attended with much risk of disseminating the bacilli throughout the subarachnoid space, and the prophylactic administration of antituberculous drugs is imperative during the preoperative and postoperative periods.

Surgical exploration is essential in all cases in which there is a possibility that spinal cord symptoms may be due to a tuberculoma. It is usually impossible to distinguish clinically or radiologically between intramedullary and extramedullary tuberculomas.[186] Unfortunately, the intramedullary tuberculoma is appreciably commoner than the extramedullary (subdural or extradural) lesion, which it may be possible to treat successfully by a combination of surgical measures and drugs.

It is an important observation, and in accordance with the role of diabetes mellitus in predisposing to tuberculosis, that some patients with intracranial tuberculomas prove to be unsuspected diabetics. The declining incidence of tuberculosis, and therefore of tuberculoma of the central nervous system, in Europe and North America since 1946 (see page 2113) contrasts with the situation in some parts of the world, such as India, where tuberculoma is the commonest form of intracranial mass to develop during childhood.[187]

SYPHILIS OF THE NERVOUS SYSTEM[188]

Syphilis is much less common than formerly, but it cannot yet be regarded as a disappearing disease. In England and Wales in 1946, 10 705 new cases were notified among men and 6970 among women.

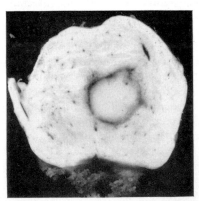

Fig. 34.37. Tuberculoma lying centrally in the pons. The patient was a middle-aged woman with a history of diplopia of sudden onset, followed by transient dysphagia. Her symptoms included failure of vision, giddiness, and dragging of the left leg, and her speech was difficult and thick. She died six months after the clinical onset of the disease.

In 1957, the numbers were down to 555 and 192 respectively, after which they rose to a combined peak of 2118 in 1965, falling again in 1970 to 1583.[189] By 1976, the latest year for which figures are available, the annual number—based on the figures for the first six months of that year—had risen to 3844 (2978 men and 866 women).[189a]

Since 1962, the number of cases of all forms of late syphilis in England and Wales has continued to decline. The figures for neurosyphilis was 349 in 1962 and 114 in 1974,[189b] which is the last year for which relevant records are at hand. In 1970 there were 27 recorded deaths from general paresis, 10 from tabes dorsalis and 11 from other forms of neurosyphilis. This trend was expected to change, a rise being forecast in the morbidity and mortality from late syphilis corresponding to the rise in the number of new cases of syphilis since the close of the 1950s. However, in 1976 there were still no more than 37 deaths in England and Wales from all forms of syphilis of the central nervous system (25 among men and 12 among women).[174b]

It has been established by studies of experimental infections in the higher apes that *Treponema pallidum* gains access to the blood stream almost immediately after it enters the body. In about 10 per cent of all cases of syphilis in the primary stage the cell count in the cerebrospinal fluid is found to be raised, although there are no meningeal symptoms. The treponemes have been identified in the fluid at this stage, even in the absence of any rise in the cell count.

In about a third of cases of syphilis in the secondary stage, changes in the cerebrospinal fluid indicate that the central nervous system has become involved, although neurological symptoms are absent or trivial. The Wassermann reaction in the cerebrospinal fluid is then often positive, and in many instances there is also an increase in the amount of gammaglobulin. It is often stated that no prognostic significance need be attached to these findings, in the belief that they are merely a transitory accompaniment of treponemal dissemination in the blood and do not necessarily indicate that the infection has become localized in the central nervous system. This is debatable, and the more widely held view is that abnormalities of the cerebrospinal fluid at any stage in the course of syphilis should be regarded as serious.

Meningeal Syphilis

Syphilitic meningitis commonly develops within a year of the initial infection; it may not occur until much later. The inflammation usually affects mainly the leptomeninges over the convexity of the cerebral hemispheres, and especially in the lateral sulci. Sometimes, however, it is the base of the brain that is involved: the cranial nerves are then liable to be affected by the exudate, and lower motor neuron paralysis, notably of the muscles supplied by the 9th, 11th and 12th cranial nerves, is a possible complication. Occasionally, the disease is more widespread, so that in addition to the meningitis there may be inflammation of the subependymal blood vessels and swelling of the ependymal cells of the ventricles and aqueduct, with a consequent liability to attacks of acute internal hydrocephalus from obstruction at the outlets of the fourth ventricle. Such cases of meningitis are essentially subacute in nature, although the symptoms, which include vomiting and headache, may be intermittent.

If a patient dies during this stage of neurosyphilis, the leptomeninges are found to be somewhat opaque. Histological examination shows an accumulation of lymphocytes, plasma cells and proliferating fibroblasts in the pia-arachnoid; this reaction is especially intense round the blood vessels. There is marked thickening of the intima of many of the vessels, and there may be lymphocytes and plasma cells in all the layers of the vessel wall. It is for this reason that syphilitic meningitis is more accurately designated *meningovascular syphilis*.

The Wassermann reaction in the cerebrospinal fluid in these cases is likelier to be negative than positive, although it is usually positive in the blood.

The dura mater may be involved in syphilis. The result is a *gummatous pachymeningitis*, and this is especially liable to occur over the cervical enlargement of the spinal cord, constricting the related nerve roots.

Syphilitic Cerebral Arteritis

The cerebral arteries are particularly prone to be affected by syphilis. In the later part of the secondary stage the treponemes may enter and pass through the vessel walls, causing proliferation of the intima and an accumulation of lymphocytes and plasma cells in the adventitia. The endarteritis becomes so marked that the lumen is considerably reduced, with a resulting liability to thrombosis, and therefore to infarction of the parts of the brain supplied by the affected vessels, most commonly the middle cerebral arteries.

Atherosclerosis may be present as well as syphilis: the yellowish patches of atheromatous material may then be the only macroscopical abnormality, apart from thickening of the wall of the vessels. Usually, there is no calcification, perhaps because syphilitic arteritis is commoner in younger people. In the advanced stages of syphilitic arteritis the elastic tissue in the vessel wall is replaced by fibrous tissue: this may lead to fusiform dilatation.

Changes in the Cerebrospinal Fluid.—The changes in the cerebrospinal fluid are a slight increase in the number of cells, and an increase in the protein content, which may exceed 2·0 g/l. There may be a relative increase in the amount of gammaglobulin. The Wassermann reaction in the fluid is positive in rather more than half the cases; the reaction in the blood is almost always positive.

Tabes Dorsalis (Locomotor Ataxia)

Tabes dorsalis was so named because there is macroscopically obvious atrophy of the dorsal aspects of the thoracic and lumbar segments of the spinal cord (the word *tabes* means wasting). The atrophy of the posterior funiculi produces a groove-like concavity along the cord. The overlying leptomeninges are thickened. The dorsal roots are noticeably thinner than the ventral roots, and, because of loss of myelin, may be grey instead of white. It has been claimed that the essential feature of tabes dorsalis is a degeneration of the dorsal roots central to the point where they pass through the leptomeninges. In this so-called 'root entry zone', or Obersteiner–Redlich space,[189c] the nerve fibres normally are surrounded by oligodendrocytes instead of Schwann cells: they are believed to be specially vulnerable to the treponemes because of this structural peculiarity. In time, the meninges become scarred and this results in constriction of the affected roots. The root entry zone of each successive spinal nerve in the lower segments of the spinal cord is longer than that of the nerve immediately above it: for this reason the lumbar and sacral roots are more vulnerable than those of the thoracic and cervical segments; impairment of the innervation of the legs is, therefore, the rule in tabes dorsalis. Consequently, in the cervical region of the spinal cord (Fig. 34.38), most atrophy is shown by the medially situated fasciculi graciles (columns of Goll), the fibres of which come from the lumbar enlargement. The fasciculi cuneati (columns of Burdach), which lie lateral to the fasciculi graciles, are not appreciably involved, because their fibres come from the upper limbs. In the lumbar and lower thoracic regions of the cord (Fig. 34.38), where the posterior funiculi consist only of the fasciculi graciles, their whole width tends to be atrophied.

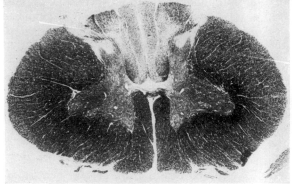

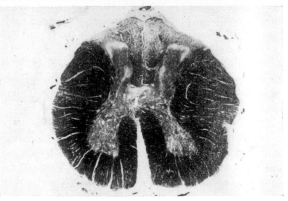

Fig. 34.38.§ Spinal cord in tabes dorsalis. *Celloidin sections. Heidenhain's stain.* ×6. A (8th cervical segment):§ The fasciculi graciles (medial in the posterior funiculi, and conveying axons from the lumbar region) have lost myelin; the fasciculi cuneati (lateral to the fasciculi graciles) show demyelination of their central part. B (2nd lumbar segment):§ The posterior funiculi consist only of the fasciculi graciles; myelin has been lost from their posterior half. Same specimen as Fig. 34.38A. See also Figs 35.30A and 35.30B, page 2334.

Tabes dorsalis is thus essentially the manifestation of low-grade inflammation localized to the root entry zone of the dorsal roots: this results in secondary degeneration of the afferent fibres of the spinal ganglia. The extent to which the dorsal root ganglia are directly involved in this inflammatory process is still uncertain. The characteristic atrophy of the posterior columns of the spinal cord and the clinical disability persist indefinitely after the inflammatory process has run its course and become completely inactive.

In view of the localized character of the lesions it may seem surprising that the cell count in the cerebrospinal fluid is so often raised in this condition. The total protein content of the fluid, including the gammaglobulin, may rise, but never so much as in general paresis. The typical second-zone curve ('tabetic curve') in the Lange colloidal gold reaction is found in about half the cases and a first-zone curve ('paretic curve') in roughly a quarter.* The Wassermann reaction in the fluid is positive in about 70 per cent of cases. Often the fluid presents no abnormality: this does not preclude the diagnosis of tabes dorsalis. In some cases the Wassermann reaction is negative in the blood also.

The optic atrophy common in this disease may also begin with a localized syphilitic leptomeningitis, although a chronic fibrosing interstitial neuritis of the optic nerve also develops. The anatomical lesion that gives rise to the Argyll Robertson pupil[190] has not been satisfactorily demonstrated but is believed to be the result of involvement of the ciliary ganglion or its afferent fibres in the inflammatory process.

Tabes dorsalis is commoner in men than in women. Its first symptoms have been known to appear more than 50 years after the infection was acquired.

General Paresis

This disease, which formerly was known as general paralysis of the insane, or dementia paralytica,

* Although comparatively little used nowadays, Lange's colloidal gold test had considerable diagnostic usefulness in its time. It was introduced in 1912 as an aid to the diagnosis of syphilis of the central nervous system (Lange, C., *Berl. klin. Wschr.*, 1912, **49**, 897; *Z. Chemother.*, 1913, **1**, 44). Changes in the total and relative quantities of albumin and of gammaglobulin in the cerebrospinal fluid produce changes in the colour of a colloidal gold sol, ranging from red through lilac and blue to colourless. The colours are represented numerically from 0 to 5 and are plotted as a graph that records the reading in each of 10 serial dilutions. The curve may take three distinct forms. A characteristic first-zone ('paretic') curve would be recorded as 5555542000, a mid-zone ('luetic', or 'tabetic') curve as 0133100000 and an end-zone ('meningitic') curve as 0001243200. The first-zone curve is typical of general paresis and, in less marked form, of active multiple sclerosis. The mid-zone curve is typical of tabes dorsalis and of many cases of active meningovascular syphilis. The end-zone curve is typical of suppurative meningitis; a 'weaker' curve—for example, 0001123100—is seen in cases of tuberculous meningitis and in some cases of tumour, especially a tumour obstructing the spinal canal, when the concentration of protein in the cerebrospinal fluid is substantially raised.

A first-zone curve is seen when the total concentration of protein in the cerebrospinal fluid is normal or no more than slightly increased although there is an increase in the concentration of gammaglobulin. A mid-zone curve is seen when the total protein content is raised, with a proportionately greater increase in the amount of gammaglobulin. An end-zone curve is seen when the total protein content is greatly raised due to a large increase in the amount of both albumin and gammaglobulin. *See*: Baron, D. N., *A Short Textbook of Chemical Pathology*, 3rd edn, page 209; London, 1973.

differs from the other forms of neurosyphilis in that the neurons themselves are heavily involved as well as the blood vessels and meninges. Although its syphilitic nature was long suspected, proof was not obtained until 1913, when Noguchi and Moore demonstrated the treponemes in the cerebral cortex.[190a]

At necropsy, the brain is shrunken and its weight is reduced (Fig. 34.39). The leptomeninges are thickened, pale bluish-white, and adherent to the underlying cortex. The cortical atrophy is much more apparent after the removal of the meninges. The frontal lobes are always affected early in the disease; the more advanced the condition, the more widespread is the cerebral involvement, until eventually the whole cerebrum, with the exception of the occipital lobes, may share in the shrinkage.

Occasionally, the atrophy is curiously local and it may even be confined to one side of the brain. This variety of general paresis, which is known as *Lissauer's atrophy*, or Lissauer's dementia, is, in most instances, a local accentuation of a generalized, but for the most part macroscopically inconspicuous, disease of the brain.[191, 191a] The area of overt atrophy is usually in the temporal lobe.

The lining of the fourth ventricle has a finely granular appearance, which is well seen if a good light is directed obliquely upon it. When this granularity is associated with the meningeal changes already described, the diagnosis of general paresis is in little doubt. The 'granular ependymitis' consists of subependymal collections of glial cells (Fig. 34.40), with lymphocytic cuffing of blood vessels: it is seldom absent, unless the disease is in an early stage or has been treated intensively. The whole ventricular system, particularly the lateral ventricles, is dilated, and often markedly so: this is usually the result of cerebral atrophy rather than of obstruction to the outflow of the cerebrospinal fluid.

Histological examination shows that there are lymphocytes and plasma cells in the pia-arachnoid. The blood vessels in the cortex are surrounded by cuffs of these cells, and their walls are so thickened, as a result of proliferation of the intima and adventitia, that they stand out prominently. Because there is so much general atrophy of the cortex, the blood vessels appear to be abnormally numerous, although it is unlikely that there is any real increase in their number (Fig. 34.41). The normal laminar disposition of the nerve cells is largely disrupted, and many of the neurons, especially in the third lamina, have disappeared (Fig. 34.42). Those that remain are often jumbled together in irregular fashion, and no longer lie in

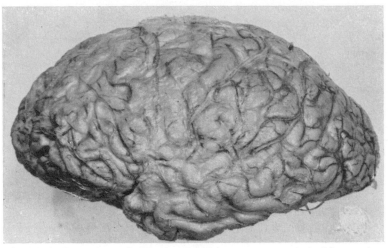

Fig. 34.39. General paresis. The leptomeninges are opaque and white, particularly over the frontal lobes and vertex and adjacent to the lateral sulcus. The frontal convolutions under the thickened pia-arachnoid are noticeably atrophied.

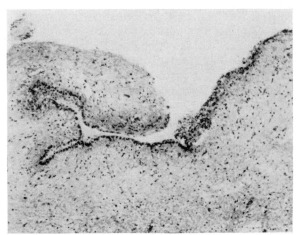

Fig. 34.40. General paresis. Ependymal granulations in the floor of the fourth ventricle. A nodule of glial proliferation appears to have sprouted through the ependymal lining. *Celloidin section. Haematoxylin–eosin.* × 100.

their neat, parallel rows. Individually, the cells may show 'acute swelling' or 'chronic cell change' (see page 2098). In severe cases, there is widespread atrophy of the Betz cells, and the pyramidal tracts in consequence lose many of their fibres. The cerebral cortex is not the only grey matter to be involved: the caudate nuclei and putamina, and other centrally placed nuclei, may also be affected.

The loss of neurons is accompanied by considerable proliferation of astrocytes (Fig. 34.43). This is manifest in the arrangement of the nuclei, which are frequently in pairs or small clusters: there is also an associated increase in the amount of neuroglial

fibre formation, especially in the outer two laminae of the cortex.

The Hortega cells are prominent (Fig. 34.44), characteristically appearing in the form of rod cells (see page 2096). Iron pigment is often present in their cytoplasm and free in the tissue spaces: its amount bears no relation to the severity of the disease. Treponemes may be found in Levaditi or

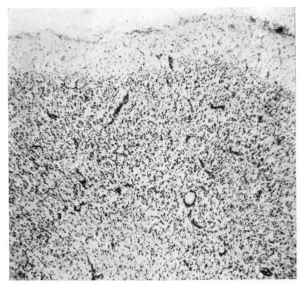

Fig. 34.41. General paresis. Frontal cortex. The blood vessels are conspicuous because of the circumvascular cuffing. There is disordered lamination, loss of nerve cells and an increased number of glial cells, especially astrocytes. *Celloidin section. Nissl's stain.* × 30.

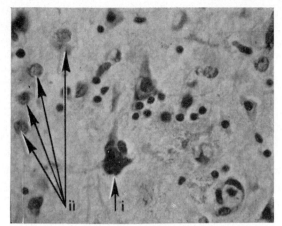

Fig. 34.42. General paresis. Frontal cortex, lamina III. Arrow 'i' points to a nerve cell showing chronic cell change: the nucleus is pyknotic and the cell outline is irregular. Arrows 'ii' point to proliferating astrocytes. *Haematoxylin–eosin.* × 260.

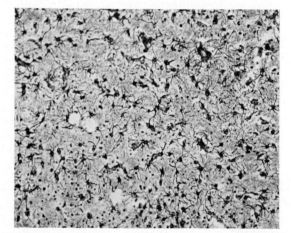

Fig. 34.43. General paresis. Frontal cortex, treated to show extent of astrocytic hyperplasia. *Frozen section. Cajal's method.* × 100.

other appropriate preparations, but usually are demonstrable in only very small numbers.

Changes in the Cerebrospinal Fluid.—The Wassermann reaction in the cerebrospinal fluid is almost always positive, even in those exceptional cases in which it is negative in the blood. If it is negative in the blood, other tests, such as the Meinicke and Venereal Disease Research Laboratory* (VDRL) flocculation tests, which tend to remain positive in old-standing and, sometimes, in treated cases of syphilis, may help in diagnosis. The *Treponema*

* Venereal Disease Research Laboratory, United States Public Health Service, Chamblee, Georgia.

pallidum immobilization test (TPI test) is even more specific: it is invariably positive in the blood in all varieties of neurosyphilis. For this reason, the VDRL and TPI tests tend to supplant the Wassermann reaction in neurological and psychiatric practice. The number of cells in the cerebrospinal fluid is increased in the untreated disease, and plasma cells and fibroblasts may be found among them. The protein content is usually of the order of 1·5 g/l, and there is a marked increase in the relative concentration of gammaglobulin. With adequate treatment, the cell count and the total protein and gammaglobulin content fall to normal, and the Wassermann and other serological reactions become negative.

Rarer Forms of Neurosyphilis

Other, less common, forms of syphilis of the nervous system may be briefly mentioned. *Gummas* of various sizes may be found in meningovascular syphilis, and occasionally one may be large enough to simulate an intracranial neoplasm. Such massive gummas are now rare: experience shows that a patient with signs of raised intracranial tension and a positive Wassermann reaction is likelier to have a neoplasm—or, a rarer alternative, syphilitic hydrocephalus—than a gumma.

Tabes dorsalis and general paresis can coexist as *taboparesis*; in such cases dementia is seldom marked, and the manifestations of both conditions are less severe than when they occur separately.

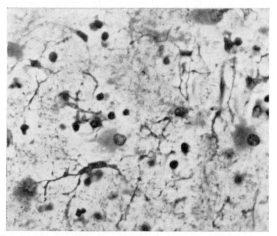

Fig. 34.44. General paresis. Frontal cortex. Hortega cells, the processes of which have been revealed by means of silver impregnation, are numerous and active: several, including one on the right, have adopted the 'rod cell' form. The cytoplasm of the reacting astrocytes is very obvious. *Frozen section. Penfield–Cone method.* × 260.

The cerebral lesions in cases of taboparesis are more akin to those of meningovascular syphilis than to the usual form of general paresis.[192]

Erb's spastic paraplegia[192a] is characterized by degeneration of the corticospinal tracts and, in a fair proportion of instances, of the posterior funiculi also. The blood vessels of the cord show periadventitial fibrosis, particularly in the subarachnoid space, where adhesive arachnoiditis and cuffing of blood vessels with lymphocytes and occasional plasma cells may result.

Comment

Although neurosyphilis has been described here under the successive headings of meningitis, arteritis, tabes dorsalis and general paresis, it must be stressed that these are not unrelated entities, but different, and sometimes coexisting, manifestations of a single disease. Syphilitic meningitis and arteritis are commonly classified together as *meningovascular syphilis*, and tabes dorsalis and general paresis as *parenchymatous neurosyphilis*. Meningovascular syphilis develops within the first few years after infection; tabes dorsalis and general paresis are, usually, later manifestations. The available evidence indicates that tabes dorsalis is not a form of 'parenchymatous' neurosyphilis comparable to general paresis but the end-stage of a localized, late form of meningovascular syphilis. Only general paresis differs from the others, being essentially a disease in which there is a pronounced loss of neurons: it is, in fact, a true syphilitic encephalitis. What determines whether meningovascular syphilis or general paresis will develop in the case of the individual patient is not known.

It has been suggested that general paresis may be the result of poisoning of the nerve cells by a toxin produced by the treponemes, but no such toxin has been demonstrated. It has also been suggested that death of nerve cells may be the result of chronic hypoxia, due to the functional inadequacy of the diseased blood vessels, but the histological findings do not support this view. An unexplained feature of the disease is the paucity of treponemes in the brain.

Why these late manifestations should develop in a small proportion of cases of syphilis is not known. It has been estimated that 10 per cent of patients with untreated syphilis die of some form of involvement of the central nervous system; spontaneous cure is said to take place in about a third of the remainder. It was said, in the days of arsenotherapy, that if treatment is begun, but not completed, the

death rate from neurosyphilis and cardiovascular syphilis may be higher than when the disease is untreated:[193] whether this view still holds today is uncertain.

In congenital syphilis, both tabes dorsalis and general paresis may occur. The histological features differ little from those in the adult forms of the disease. In juvenile paresis, however, the cerebellum tends to be involved to a greater extent than is usual in adults (Fig. 34.45).

It is now generally accepted that there are no special neurotropic strains of *Treponema pallidum*. Instances of conjugal and congenital neurosyphilis are sometimes regarded as evidence for the existence of such strains; however, the number of cases of neurosyphilis that can be traced to a single source of infection fails to give statistically significant support for this belief. Certainly, visitors who contract syphilis in the Orient, where tabes dorsalis and general paresis are not so commonly found in the local population, are as liable to suffer

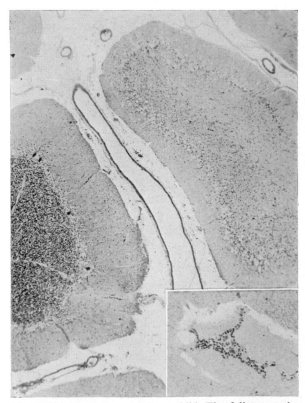

Fig. 34.45. General paresis in a child. The folium on the right of the larger picture shows extensive cerebellar cortical atrophy, with loss of Purkyně and granule cells, attributed to arteritis (which is illustrated in the inset): the folium on the left, although better preserved, shows partial loss of Purkyně cells. *Celloidin section. Nissl's stain.* × 30.

involvement of the central nervous system as those who contract the disease in occidental countries.

Another misconception is that patients with neurosyphilis rarely give a history of a rash in the secondary stage of the infection: this may be because of the time interval between the secondary stage and the advent of neurosyphilis, which may be many years, and because impairment of memory is so often symptomatic of the disease.

It is possible that a constitutional factor may determine involvement of the central nervous system: thus, several instances are on record of siblings with neurosyphilis whose initial infections were acquired from different sources. A constitutional factor might, moreover, explain the occurrence of congenital neurosyphilis. Possibly there is a racial predisposition to certain forms of syphilis: in oriental peoples and in the indigenous population of tropical countries, where syphilitic periosteitis, acute syphilitic meningitis and extraneural gummas are comparatively common, it is exceptional to see the forms of, for example, neurosyphilis that are seen in the indigenous population of Europe and among white people in general. In fact, the disease in the Orient today seems to conform more to the pattern in sixteenth century Europe than to that now typical in occidental countries. Observations in the southern states of the United States of America are sometimes said to indicate that neurosyphilis is commoner in the white population, but no relevant studies appear to have been made since those of Turner in 1930.[194] His conclusions are not wholly acceptable, because of the differences between his two groups in social status and in the standards of medical care available. There are no reliable figures to substantiate a former contention that the rarity of late neurosyphilis in the indigenous population of tropical countries is due to enhancement of specific immune-body production by the stimulating effect of sunshine on their skin.

The immune mechanisms in syphilis are in some way modified by pregnancy. It is an old observation that women who become pregnant shortly after acquiring syphilis are unlikely to develop neurosyphilis, whereas nulliparous women are as liable to neurosyphilis as are men. The ability to establish or maintain a degree of immunity to the treponemes is undoubtedly lowered by poor health, and also, it would seem, by trauma. The role of trauma in precipitating, or perhaps even in inducing, neurosyphilis in an infected person can be a matter of medicolegal importance. It has been suggested that the treponeme may become localized and multiply in any traumatized tissue, including the brain: other authorities maintain that the organism must already be established in the central nervous system before trauma can precipitate the onset of neurosyphilis. The possible aetiological role of trauma is comparable to that of alcohol, for symptoms of neurosyphilis may first appear—it is said—after a drunken debauch. In all such cases, it must be remembered that the injury or the drunkenness may be the result of neurosyphilis, not its precipitating cause; alternatively, either may be merely the circumstance that first draws attention to the presence of the disease.

WEST INDIAN AND SIMILAR NEUROPATHIES

A form of myelopathy histologically indistinguishable from Erb's spastic paraplegia (see opposite), but of uncertain causation, has been recognized in the Caribbean region: this brief account is included here for convenience. While an association with treponematosis (particularly yaws) has been suggested on clinical grounds, and in about half the cases is supported by the serological evidence, the disease cannot always be distinguished from a form of sensory neuropathy that occurs in the same population, often accompanied by blindness and deafness, with little serological evidence to suggest a treponemal infection and with a better prognosis for life.[195, 196] The aetiology and pathogenesis of this condition—if indeed it is a single entity—are obscure: studies to date do not suggest that dietary deficiency plays a part. A resemblance to neurolathyrism has suggested the possible importance of ingested toxins in its causation.

An identical paraplegic syndrome occurs in India.[197] In a similar condition in parts of Africa, a sensory neuropathy is commoner than paraplegia.[198, 199] The current view is that, despite the similarities, it is not justifiable to assume that the West Indian, Indian and African diseases are variants of the same process.[200, 201] It has been found in Nigeria that a cassava diet is correlated with the incidence of the ataxic syndrome: as cassava contains cyanide it is possible that the neuropathy may be related to chronic cyanide intoxication.[200, 201]

Histologically, there is demyelination of the corticospinal tracts and often of the posterior funiculi. In some instances there are mild inflammatory changes throughout the spinal cord, the small vessels being cuffed with lymphocytes. The appearance of binucleate neurons in the anterior grey columns of the spinal cord and of binucleate Purkyně cells has been described.

RICKETTSIAL ENCEPHALITIS

Typhus Fever

Typhus fever* is a louse-borne disease, caused by *Rickettsia prowazekii*. It is now rare in most parts of the world. It is a disease of wartime and famine,[202] particularly in temperate and cold climates; it occurs in epidemics among refugees and in armies devoid of proper hygiene. The case fatality rate is high, especially in older patients.

In fatal cases, the brain is almost always involved. The typical lesion is the *typhus nodule*, which consists of aggregates of glial cells, macrophages and lymphocytes in the adventitia of the cerebral arterioles; the endothelial cells of the affected vessels are swollen because of the presence of rickettsiae in their cytoplasm. Comparable juxta-vascular lesions are found in other organs, especially the heart and spleen, and also in the maculo-papular and petechial rash in the skin.

Rocky Mountains Spotted Fever[203] and Asiatic or Scrub Typhus (Tsutsugamushi Fever)†

Rocky Mountains spotted fever and Asiatic or scrub typhus are caused respectively by *Rickettsia rickettsii*, which is conveyed by the bite of ticks, and *Rickettsia tsutsugamushi* (*Rickettsia orientalis*), which is carried by mites; like all rickettsiae, these organisms are obligate intracellular parasites. Wild rodents are the natural reservoirs of both infections. The case fatality rate of both diseases ranges from 5 to 50 per cent; it has been appreciably higher in some outbreaks. The nervous system is commonly involved, and the histological appearances resemble those seen in classic louse-borne typhus fever. The lesions are widely scattered, but are most numerous in the brainstem, where scattered neutrophils may be present among the other cells in the nodules. In the earliest lesions, the minute intracellular organ-

* The word 'typhus', in many European languages other than English, if used without qualification means *typhus abdominalis*, which is typhoid fever. The rickettsial infection that in English we commonly refer to simply as typhus is more correctly named *typhus exanthematicus*. It is of some practical importance to English-speaking doctors to know that when patients whose native language is another European tongue give a past history of 'typhus' they are very likely to mean typhoid fever (Symmers, W. St C., *Curiosa*, chap. 20; London, 1974).

† See also page 633, Volume 2.

isms may sometimes be found within the endothelial cells of the blood vessels. In addition, there is a fairly widespread cuffing of blood vessels with lymphocytes and plasma cells. In Rocky Mountains spotted fever the inflammatory changes may be particularly marked, and there may be necrosis of the wall of the affected arterioles and venules.

ACTINOMYCETOUS AND FUNGAL INFECTIONS OF THE CENTRAL NERVOUS SYSTEM[204, 205]

Actinomycosis

Actinomycotic lesions of the brain and spinal cord are the result of blood-borne infection.[206, 207] In the brain they are usually subcortical. They form discrete, granuloma-like masses, riddled with multiple, intercommunicating foci of suppuration. Often the overlying leptomeninges are thickened; there may be a true leptomeningitis, which tends to remain localized. The primary focus is usually in the thorax or abdomen.

The cerebral 'actinomycoma', as—regrettably—it has been called, is composed of granulation tissue characterized by small pockets of pus and marked fibrosis, the honeycomb-like appearance so typical of this disease elsewhere tending to be reproduced in the cerebral lesions. Macrophages are numerous, and there may be occasional multinucleate giant cells. The characteristic 'sulphur granules', which are the yellowish colonies of the organism, *Actinomyces israelii*, can generally be found in the pus. The fine, branching mycelium is Gram-positive. The club-like endings that are often seen at the surface of the colonies are probably antigen-antibody complexes produced in the course of the reaction of the host tissues to the presence of the organism (Figs 34.46A and 34.46B).

Nocardiosis[208]

Nocardiosis is the infection caused by the actinomycete *Nocardia asteroides*, which differs from *Actinomyces israelii* in several ways, one being that it grows aerobically. It is Gram-positive (Fig. 34.46C) and often acid-fast (see Fig. 9.87 in Volume 2, page 617). The organism is usually abundantly present in bacillary form or as slender, short, branching filaments. The lesions are abscesses: these are often multiple, and larger than those of actinomycosis, and they lack the 'honeycomb' structure characteristic of the latter (Fig. 34.46D). Cerebral nocardiosis is usually a complication of nocardiosis of the lungs (see page 348, Volume 1).

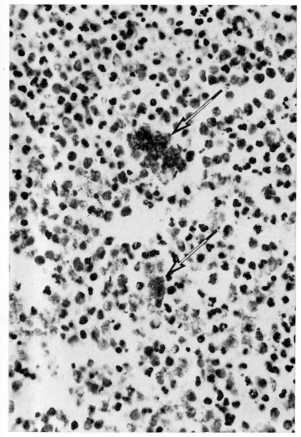

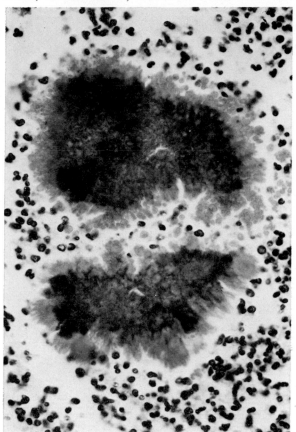

Fig. 34.46A.§ Two very small, early colonies of *Actinomyces israelii* (arrowed) in the contents of a rapidly developing abscess in the frontal lobe of a cerebral hemisphere. The organism was isolated in pure culture. The source of the infection was not discovered. The patient recovered after aspiration of the abscess and a prolonged course of anti-biotic treatment. The specimen photographed is a histological preparation of some coherent particles in the aspirated pus. Compare with Fig. 34.46B. *Haematoxylin–eosin.* × 400.

In many instances the infection is attributable to the adverse effects of drugs, corticosteroids in particular, on the body's ability to resist invasion by such organisms, which in these circumstances are classed among the causes of 'opportunistic' infections.*

Fig. 34.46B.§ Typical colony of *Actinomyces israelii* in one of several abscesses in the brain complicating actinomycotic infection of the lungs and pleural cavities. The darker (haematoxyphile) part of the colony consists of the tangle of filaments of the organism; the paler (eosinophile) peripheral zone—the zone of 'clubs'—consists mainly of a deposit of immunoglobulin on the fine filaments protruding from the deeper part of the colony. The apparent separation of the colony into two parts results from the 'folding' of this particular colony, the plane of the section passing through the interface between the folded parts. Comparison with the colonies in Fig. 34.46A, which is photographed at the same magnification, shows the great variation in size that may occur: the early, small colonies are readily overlooked, being liable to be mistaken for nondescript debris in the inflam-matory exudate. *Haematoxylin–eosin.* × 400.

Phycomycoses[209]†

The phycomyetoses are a group of infections— usually 'opportunistic'—caused by non-septate

* The expression 'opportunistic infection' is intended to indicate that the organisms responsible are, in the given circumstances, able to cause progressive infection only because resistance to their invasion has been undermined by other disease or by measures used in treating the latter.

† The phycomyetoses are still sometimes known by the name mucormycoses (Baker, R. D., in *Human Infection with*

Fungi, Actinomycetes and Algae, by R. D. Baker, chap. 21; New York, Heidelberg and Berlin, 1971), which strictly is appropriate only to the exceptionally rare infections that are caused by species of *Mucor*. More recently, the name zygo-mycoses has been proposed, consequent on a development in fungal taxonomy that treats the Zygomycetes—to which the fungi belong that hitherto have been named as causes of 'phycomyetosis'—as of full class rank (Reinhardt, D. J., Kaplan, W., Ajello, L., *Infection and Immunity*, 1970, **2**, 404).

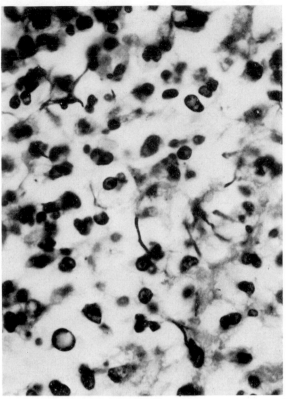

Fig. 34.46C.§ Fine, branching, Gram-positive filaments of *Nocardia asteroides* in purulent exudate at the periphery of a rapidly forming intracerebral abscess. The abscess was secondary to acute nocardial pneumonia complicating treatment of rheumatoid arthritis with large doses of corticosteroids. *Nocardia asteroides* is not always strongly or uniformly Gram-positive; its acid-fastness may be more helpful as a means to its demonstration (see Fig. 9.87, page 617 in Volume 2). *Gram stain.* × 1000.

myceliate fungi such as *Rhizopus* and *Absidia*. An important form of the disease is a subacute meningoencephalitis, which tends to be localized. In many cases the patients have had severe or badly controlled diabetes, or some other serious metabolic disturbance accompanied by acidosis, such as chronic renal failure. A syndrome of severe diabetes mellitus, orbital cellulitis and meningocerebral phycomycosis has been defined.[210] The intracranial infection is secondary to the orbital involvement, which itself is a result of spread of the fungus from the nasal sinuses. The organisms have a predilection for blood vessels, penetrating their walls, causing thrombosis, and colonizing the thrombus (Figs 34.46E and 34.46F).[209] The prognosis is very poor.

Cryptococcosis

The yeast, *Cryptococcus neoformans*,* which is believed to enter the body through the respiratory tract, has a predilection for the tissues of the central nervous system. Although modern antifungal drugs, such as amphotericin and flucytosine, have been curative in some cases, no wholly reliable means of treatment has been discovered. The infection has a worldwide distribution, and is not as uncommon as used to be thought. Cryptococcosis must always be remembered in the differential diagnosis of subacute meningitis and of expanding intracranial lesions.[211] Hodgkin's disease and other diseases of the lymphoreticular system, including sarcoidosis, predispose to cryptococcosis (see page 744, Volume 2). In many cases of meningocerebral involvement there is no evident cryptococcal infection elsewhere, but in others a lesion in the lungs or, occasionally, in some other part can be identified.

A curious feature of the cryptococcus is that it may not excite an inflammatory reaction: myriads of the organisms may be found in the greatly distended subarachnoid space, either on the surface of the brain or in the sulci, with scarcely any cellular reaction. Here and there, however, and especially round the penetrating arterioles, there may be accumulations of lymphocytes, and sometimes of macrophages and multinucleate giant cells, which may contain large numbers of engulfed organisms (Fig. 34.47). Foci of infection within the cerebrum often underlie the depths of a sulcus (Fig. 34.48); again, they are often devoid of any reaction round the organisms, or there is only a modest lymphocytic or giant cell response, with patchy fibrosis. Distension of the cerebellar sulci by the organisms is often a feature (Fig. 34.49). In the diffuser forms of meningocerebral infection, the meninges are thickened and opaque, particularly over the sulci; the infection is usually heaviest in the interpeduncular fossa and in the lateral sulci. The appearances can be mistaken for those of tuberculous meningitis or carcinomatous infiltration.

Because of the characteristic paucity of the cellular response to infection by *Cryptococcus neoformans* (Fig. 34.50), it is not surprising that the cell count in the cerebrospinal fluid is sometimes within normal limits; usually, there is a slight or

* Although *Cryptococcus neoformans* is the name now generally accepted, the older designation, *Torula histolytica*, is reflected in the formerly much used synonym for the disease, torulosis. Other names that are no longer current include Buschke–Busse disease and European blastomycosis.

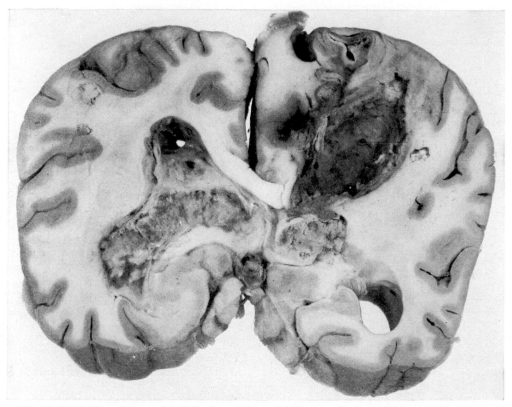

Fig. 34.46D.§ *Nocardia asteroides* infection of the brain. There is a large abscess in the white matter of the parietal lobe of the right cerebral hemisphere. In addition, there are multiple confluent abscesses in the choroid plexus in each lateral ventricle. The patient was a man, aged 55 years, with 9 weeks' history of progressive cerebral symptoms. A small pulmonary abscess was considered to be the portal of entry of the organism into the blood stream. Case reported by: Jacobs, S. I., Gibson, R. M., *J. Neurol. Neurosurg. Psychiat.*, 1963, **26**, 363; necropsy and histological studies by D. G. F. Harriman.

moderate increase in the number of lymphocytes. The organisms may be present in the fluid, yet, because they are not stained in the cell-counting chamber by the dyes used to colour the leucocytes, they may be overlooked, or mistaken for erythrocytes that have escaped destruction by the acetic acid diluent. The characteristic, thick, mucopolysaccharide capsule of the cryptococcus may not permit stains to penetrate readily into the cell body, particularly when examined in film preparations. However, the cryptococcus can easily be demonstrated if the cerebrospinal fluid is mixed with India ink or nigrosin. The mucoid capsule then stands out as a clear, light zone against the background of the dark fluid; the refractile, round or oval cell body of the fungus is visible within the capsule and ranges in diameter from 3 to 20 μm, with an average of 7 μm in many strains. The organisms are difficult or impossible to identify in dry, stained films.

In histological preparations the capsule of the cryptococcus usually renders the organism obvious (Fig. 34.47), and, because of its mucopolysaccharide nature, the capsular material—particularly where it is condensed at the surface of the cell body—stains well in Nissl (Fig. 34.50, insets), toluidine blue, periodic-acid/Schiff and mucicarmine preparations. In sections, as in the fresh state, the organisms vary much in size.

Chromomycosis (Cladosporiosis)

The chromomycoses (dematiomycoses) are caused by certain naturally pigmented fungi. In most cases the lesions take the form of warty granulomas of the skin (see Chapter 39, Volume 6), the infection following a penetrating wound by a thorn or the like. The organism most commonly concerned in cases of cutaneous infection is *Phialophora pedrosoi*, and this disease is seen most frequently in tropical and sub-tropical regions. In

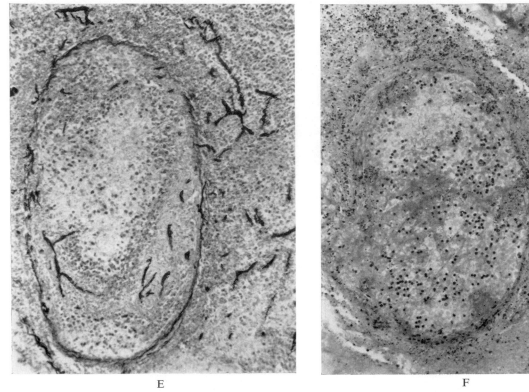

E   F

Figs 34.46E and 34.46F.§ Phycomycosis. Adjacent sections showing the same artery, occluded by thrombosis, with necrotic exudate in the surrounding subarachnoid space. × 135.

E. The hyphae of a phycomycete are clearly revealed in the Grocott–Gomori hexamine (methenamine) silver preparation.

F. The hyphae cannot be seen in the haematoxylin–eosin preparation.

exceptional cases the brain has become infected, presumably as a result of haematogenous spread of the organism from the skin. It is of more than passing interest that these pigmented organisms do not ordinarily produce mycelium when they infect the skin, where they appear in a yeast-like form: the intracerebral environment appears to favour germination of the chlamydospores, with mycelium formation.

A particular and very rare form of chromomycosis presents as a brain abscess caused by *Cladosporium trichoides*.[212, 212a]* The distinctive brown chlamy-

* After some years of vacillation, opinion among mycologists seems now to favour the view that *Cladosporium trichoides* is not a synonym of *Cladosporium bantianum* and that the latter is probably a distinct and unrelated species (Nomenclature of Fungi Pathogenic to Man and Animals, *Memor. med. Res. Coun.* (*Lond.*), No. 23, 4th edn, 1977; Emmons, C. W., Binford, C. H., Utz, J. P., Kwon-Chung, K. J., *Medical Mycology*, 3rd edn, page 471—Philadelphia, 1977). In this chapter, therefore, the name *Cladosporium trichoides* is adopted when referring to the organism that causes chromomycosis (cladosporiosis) of the central nervous system.

dospores and hyphae in the necrotizing granulomatous lesions enable the diagnosis to be made (Fig. 34.51). Cerebral chromomycosis has been a complication of cerebral infarction in a proportion of the cases on record.[212]

Histoplasmosis[213]

Histoplasmosis caused by *Histoplasma capsulatum* is ordinarily a benign, self-healing pulmonary infection (see page 355, Volume 1); exceptionally, it spreads to other organs. Involvement of the central nervous system is unusual. Cerebral involvement was found in 6 out of a series of 23 cases of the rare, fatal, disseminate form of histoplasmosis.[214]

The organisms are readily seen in sections stained with haematoxylin and eosin (Fig. 39.186, Chapter 39 in Volume 6). They measure about 5 by 3 μm and are generally ovoid, and they have a distinct, double-contoured capsule. The capsule is most readily seen when the organisms are few in number, and therefore not tightly packed. The

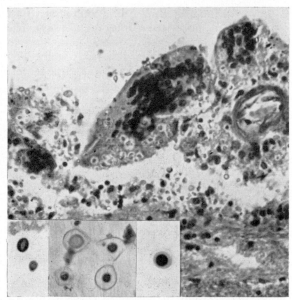

Fig. 34.47. Cryptococcosis. Multinucleate giant cells in the pia-arachnoid contain numerous organisms. Free-lying cryptococci are also present. Inset are further illustrations of the variety of appearances of the fungal cells. *Haematoxylin–eosin.* × 240 (insets × 400).

histoplasma, when infecting tissues, is a yeast-like, obligate intracellular parasite; the fungus also exists free in nature in a myceliate form with highly infective spores. Infection usually results from inhalation of contaminated dust, for instance that of gardens, outhouses or caves. The dried droppings of pigeons, starlings and bats are a good growth medium for the fungus and are a common source of the infection in those parts of the world where the disease is endemic. Histoplasmosis is an occupational hazard of archaeologists and spelaeologists in such areas.

Histoplasmosis is so prevalent in some parts of the United States of America that a large majority of the adult population give a positive skin reaction to histoplasmin. The disease is also endemic in various other parts of the world. It is rare in people who have never been to regions where the infection is endemic: when the infection occurs among such people it is the result of exposure either to laboratory cultures in the infective myceliate phase (saprophytic phase) or to imported materials contaminated by this form of the organism.

In the brain and spinal cord, as elsewhere in the body, the disease shows as discrete tubercle-like granulomas with occasional giant cells and sometimes central areas of necrosis. The organisms are usually to be found in clusters inside macrophages.

Meningitis may spread from a granuloma situated near the surface of the brain or spinal cord.

Coccidioidomycosis (San Joaquin Valley
near the surface of the brain or spinal cord.

Pulmonary infection by *Coccidioides immitis* is common in certain southern and south-western parts of the United States of America. The disease also occurs in parts of Central and South America. The organism is inhaled from the dry, dusty, spore-laden atmosphere that prevails in some seasons of the year. Primary pulmonary coccidioidomycosis is comparable in some ways to the primary lesion of tuberculosis, for the infection is ordinarily mild, and in some cases may cause no symptoms (see page 358, Volume 1). Most of those who have lived for some years in the San Joaquin Valley give a positive skin reaction to an extract of the organism (cocci-

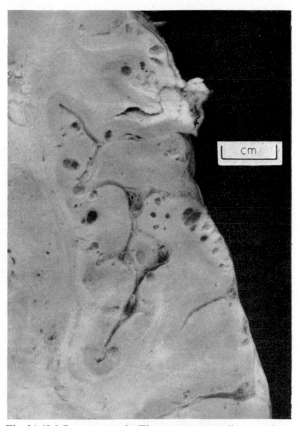

Fig. 34.48.§ Cryptococcosis. The numerous small excavations in the cerebral cortex are due to the presence of *Cryptococcus neoformans*. In the fresh state their contents appeared as clear or slightly milky, mucinous material ('slime cysts'): this material is formed of the capsules of the myriads of cryptococci that fill the excavations.

3

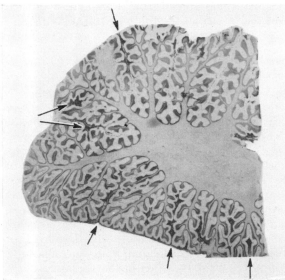

Fig. 34.49. Cryptococcosis. The cryptococci have spread into and distended the sulci (arrows). Because the fungi have retained the cresyl violet the expanded sulci with their contents have stained more heavily than the cells of the cerebellar cortex. *Celloidin section. Nissl's stain.* × 2.

dioidin). In a minority of cases, but least rarely in black patients, the infection spreads widely in the lungs. It may also be disseminated by the blood stream, with the appearance of lesions in any part of the body, including the meninges and brain. The organism, which measures up to 80 μm or more in diameter, is readily visible in sections stained by haematoxylin and eosin (Fig. 34.52). Its largest form produces numerous endospores: when the mature, spore-containing form ruptures, the endospores are liberated into the tissues and bring about a local extension of the infection.

The lesions are necrotizing, tuberculoid granulomas, and the organisms may be found in the necrotic centre of the focus or in surrounding giant cells. There is, in fact, a considerable histological resemblance to tuberculosis, but confusion between the two diseases is readily dispelled by finding the endosporulating spherules or the free-lying yeast forms.

'North American' Blastomycosis

The primary lesion of 'North American' blastomycosis is usually in the lungs (see page 359, Volume 1); infection spreads to other sites in the blood.[216] The metastatic foci are most commonly in the skin, and the disease rarely involves the nervous system. Its cause is *Blastomyces dermatitidis*. The disease is found only in parts of the Americas and of Africa (see also page 2415).

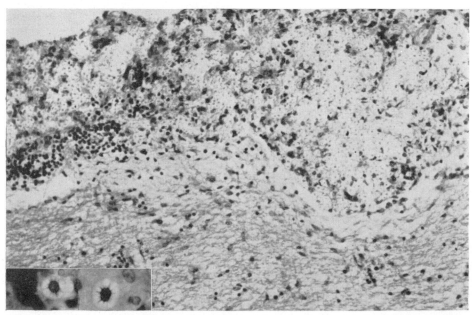

Fig. 34.50. Cryptococcosis. The leptomeninges contain innumerable cryptococci; there is little cellular reaction. The organism stains well with Nissl's stain (see insets), sometimes appearing to have spines: this appearance is due to irregular shrinkage of the capsular material during histological processing. Large picture: *haematoxylin–eosin*; × 180. Insets: *Nissl's stain*; × 450.

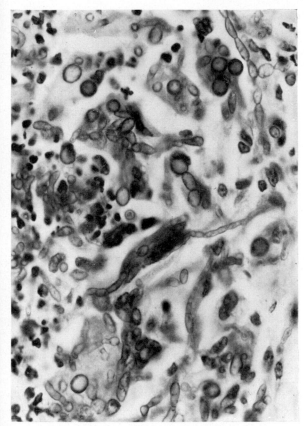

Fig. 34.51.§ Cerebral chromomycosis. Spherical cells and segmented hyphae of a brown fungus, microscopically identical with *Cladosporium trichoides*, in granulomatous tissue at the periphery of a cerebral abscess. The fungal elements are present both in giant cells and free in the tissue. Neutrophils are also seen. Case 1 in: Symmers, W. St C., *Rev. lyon. Méd.*, 1963, **12**, 979. *Mayer's haemalum* [omission of staining with eosin facilitates recognition of the brown fungus]. × 580.

The organism is not likely to be overlooked in the tissues: it is at least as large as an erythrocyte and may reach a diameter of 20 μm (Fig. 39.188, Chapter 39 in Volume 6). Many of the fungal cells are found to have been ingested by macrophages. They excite a tuberculoid granulomatous reaction, to which neutrophils characteristically contribute as well as epithelioid macrophages and multinucleate giant cells ('suppurating pseudotubercles'). Caseation sometimes occurs.

Other Fungal Infections

South American blastomycosis (caused by *Paracoccidioides immitis*), aspergillosis, candidosis and sporotrichosis are among other mycoses that have occasionally involved the central nervous system, usually in the course of dissemination by the blood stream.

ARACHNOIDITIS

The term arachnoiditis is used to denote an inflammation of the leptomeninges of undetermined type. The condition usually takes the form of a chronic granulomatous reaction in the leptomeninges, a variety of cells participating in the response: sometimes fibrosis is its major characteristic. It may be localized to the region of the optic chiasma or of the apertures of the fourth ventricle, or to the spinal theca, or it may be generalized throughout the subarachnoid space. Atypical forms of tuberculosis and syphilis have to be considered in the differential diagnosis of arachnoiditis, and it must be remembered that a negative Wassermann reaction in the blood and cerebrospinal fluid does not necessarily exclude syphilis.

Dense, fibrous arachnoiditis over the lower part of the spinal cord may follow trauma or the administration of a spinal anaesthetic or of other drugs or contrast media or it may develop for no apparent reason. A comparable condition can be

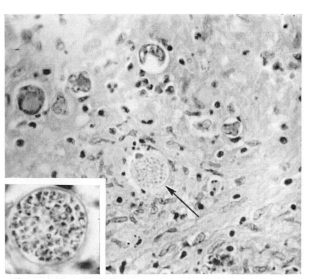

Fig. 34.52. Coccidioidomycosis. Several spherules of *Coccidioides immitis* are seen in this field from a granulomatous focus in the brain. They are surrounded by reacting Hortega cells. The arrow points to an endosporulating spherule; another is inset. *Haematoxylin–eosin.* × 100 (inset × 225).

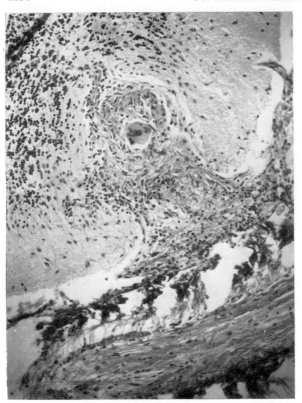

caused experimentally by the introduction of irritant substances into the theca.[217]

SARCOIDOSIS

Sarcoidosis is one of the causes of chronic arachnoiditis (Fig. 34.53). In occasional instances evidence of the disease elsewhere in the body may be hard to find. Meningeal sarcoidosis may have a clinical course of five years or more. The late stages are often characterized by hypothalamic symptoms that result from the predilection of the sarcoid granuloma for the structures round the third ventricle and in its floor (see page 1878, Volume 4). The lesions in the brain resemble those in other organs (see pages 747 and 753, Volume 2).

Fig. 34.53.§ Meningeal sarcoidosis. A small lesion has extended from the thickened pia-arachnoid through the molecular layer of the cerebellum toward the granular layer. A multinucleate giant cell is surrounded by epithelioid cells. *Haematoxylin–eosin.* × 130.

PROTOZOAL AND METAZOAL DISEASES OF THE CENTRAL NERVOUS SYSTEM

PROTOZOAL INFECTIONS

Amoebiasis[218, 218a]

Infection of the brain by *Entamoeba histolytica* is a rare complication of amoebic dysentery, and occurs late in the disease; indeed, cerebral amoebiasis may become manifest for the first time only after the intestinal lesions have apparently been cured. The cerebral lesion takes the form of an abscess-like necrotic focus. It is usually secondary to an amoebic 'abscess' of the liver (see page 1233, Volume 3), which may be symptomless and thus give no clue to the real nature of the brain lesion.

The neurosurgeon should always consider the possibility of this diagnosis if there is any past history of amoebic dysentery, or if, on reaching the abscess, he finds that the pus is 'creamy' and has a reddish tinge. The amoebae should be looked for in fresh wet films taken from the lining of the abscess.

Primary Amoebic Meningoencephalitis.[219–221]—This term has been applied to infection of the brain by species of free-living amoebae of the genera *Naegleria*[222] and *Hartmannella*. About 60 proven cases have been recognized since the disease was first described in 1965.[223] In most cases there has been a history of swimming or playing in brackish or stagnant water. The disease, which is probably worldwide in distribution, has an incubation period of no more than a few days. It is practically always rapidly fatal. The brain is swollen and congested and the appearances may resemble those of acute suppurative meningitis macroscopically. The olfactory bulbs and adjacent cerebral tissue are particularly severely affected, extensive necrosis and haemorrhage being a conspicuous feature in these parts. This reflects the pathway of infection, for the organisms enter the body through the nose, ascending the filaments of the olfactory nerves to invade the brain from the olfactory bulbs.

The organisms are most numerous in the circumvascular space (Fig. 34.54), where they have occasionally been mistaken for macrophages or cancer cells. Often there is little or no cellular

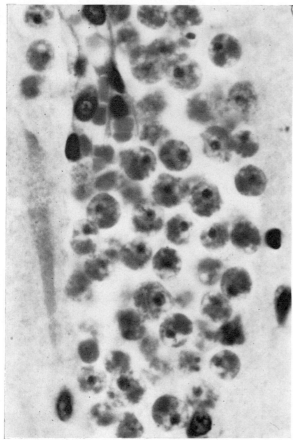

Fig. 34.54.§ Primary amoebic meningoencephalitis (infection by *Naegleria* species). The amoebae are massed in the circumvascular space and have invaded the adjoining substance of the cerebral cortex. The characteristic appearance of the nucleus, with relatively large nucleolus, fine nuclear membrane and surrounding halo of vacuolate cytoplasm, is seen in several of the parasites. There is an occasional leucocyte in the field but otherwise no evident reaction. From an unpublished case in the south-east of England (1975). *Haematoxylin–eosin.* × 1100.

reaction to their presence, particularly where they have invaded the cerebral tissue itself. Lymphocytes are sometimes present among the amoebae in the circumvascular space but they are greatly outnumbered by the organisms. Polymorphonuclear leucocytes are seldom conspicuous.

The rapidity of invasion and the extent of destruction make the prognosis very poor. Although the organisms may be destroyed by treatment with amphotericin, recovery from the infection may leave the patient severely and permanently crippled, mentally and physically.

Toxoplasmosis[224-226]

In 1937, Wolf and Cowen isolated *Toxoplasma gondii** from a fatal case of encephalitis in a child: this observation was the beginning of the present widespread interest in this infection.[227, 227a] In fact, however, the parasite had previously been found in man by Janků (see Chapter 40, Volume 6).[227b]

Toxoplasmosis is worldwide in distribution. It is most commonly recognized in the newborn, but primary infection may be seen in adults in the form of a continuous fever associated with pulmonary lesions or, oftener, with lymphadenitis (see page 654, Volume 2). In infants, the presenting symptom is usually hydrocephalus, caused by circumaqueductal gliosis, which obstructs the circulation of the cerebrospinal fluid. The region of the basal ganglia is another frequent site of involvement. If a toxoplasmic lesion reaches the surface of the brain, local leptomeningitis may result.

A notable diagnostic feature is the liability of toxoplasmic lesions to calcify. Foci have been seen radiologically as early as the third day of life, a finding indicating that the disease is congenital. A striking degree of choroidoretinitis is typical of toxoplasmosis and helpful in its diagnosis. Patients who have had congenital toxoplasmosis have been known to survive to early adult life.[228]

The toxoplasmas are usually about 2 μm in width and 4 to 6 μm in length. In histological preparations they often appear rounded or ovoid; they may form rosette-like clusters. In films, the free organisms are crescent-shaped, with pointed tips (their generic name indicates their resemblance to an archer's bow).

In infected brain tissue, toxoplasmas are often found in the form of cysts (Fig. 34.55A, insets), which develop within the cytoplasm of macrophages that have been colonized by the organisms. These intracellular parasitic cysts are usually found in foci of necrosis; they may be little larger than an erythrocyte, or they may be 30 μm or more in diameter. The cysts show up well with Leishman's stain, which colours the cytoplasm of the organisms blue and their chromatin red. They are also conspicuous in periodic-acid/Schiff preparations. Each organism is surrounded by a narrow, ill-defined halo. The trophozoites may also be found, but with difficulty, lying free in the inflamed tissues. They may be recovered by intraperitoneal and intracerebral inoculation of blood or cerebrospinal fluid

* The gondi is a North African rodent, from which the toxoplasma was originally isolated by Nicolle and Manceaux, in 1908 (Nicolle, C. J. H., Manceaux, L. H., *C.R. Acad. Sci.* [*Paris*], 1908, **147**, 763).

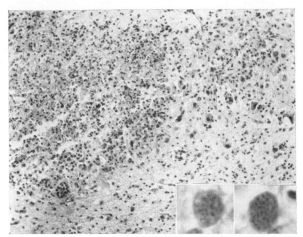

Fig. 34.55A.§ Toxoplasmosis. Necrotic lesion in the brain in which scanty toxoplasmas were found (two of the characteristic cystic forms of *Toxoplasma gondii* are shown in the insets). Adjacent neurons show marked chromatolysis. *Haematoxylin–eosin.* × 70 (insets × 400).

into young mice. The cerebrospinal fluid is often yellow; its glucose content may be reduced.

The individual lesions in the brain range from small foci of necrosis to a more chronic type of reaction in which proliferation of astrocytes is conspicuous. The more extensive necrotic lesions (Fig. 34.55) are apt to undergo cavitation, with widespread destruction of the brain substance. The brain may be much shrivelled, and somewhat spongy to the feel, and the greater part of the cranial cavity may, in fact, be filled with yellow fluid. Flecks of calcium are found round the lesions. When the central nervous system is heavily involved, lesions are usually numerous in other organs, including the heart (see page 46, Volume 1).

The mothers of infants with toxoplasmosis show no signs of active disease, although their serological reactions are always positive. In suspected cases, the mother's serum should be tested for specific antibodies; if the result is positive, the infant's blood should then be similarly examined. However, many adults give a positive reaction, and it has been stated that there is serological evidence of a past infection in from a quarter to half of the population of the United Kingdom.[229] Comparable figures have been reported from many parts of the world. No instance of infection of more than one infant in a family has been reported.

Malaria[230]

Cerebral malaria is a well-recognized and serious manifestation of infection with *Plasmodium falci-*

parum, the organism that causes malignant tertian malaria. The lesions in the brain are essentially ischaemic, and are due to the capillaries being blocked by masses of parasite-containing erythrocytes and by pigment derived from the breakdown of these cells. The brain is swollen, and the cortex of the cerebrum and cerebellum is much congested.

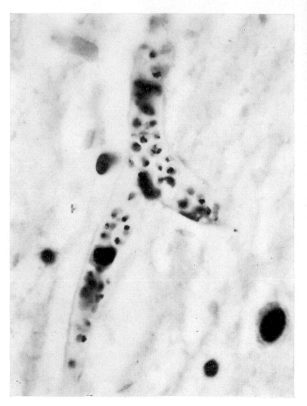

Fig. 34.55B.§ Cerebral malaria. The lumen of this capillary blood vessel in a tertiary lamina of the white matter of the cerebellum is filled with parasitized red cells (*Plasmodium falciparum* infection). Their content of pigment accentuates the appearance of the parasites. The patient was a business man whose flight from southern Africa to Europe made an unscheduled overnight stop in a malarial region. Although warned of the danger of not taking a prophylactic course of an antimalarial drug, he refused the treatment offered. When the symptoms of his illness began he suspected the correct diagnosis and went to a general hospital. He was referred, without investigation or treatment, to a fever hospital, where he had a convulsion while waiting to be seen by a doctor. The latter sent him on a 20 km drive by ambulance back to the general hospital for treatment as a case of cerebral malaria. The patient died half an hour after admission while doctors were still considering how he should be treated. An almost identical sequence preceded the death of another patient with cerebral malaria in the same country during the same year. *The patient with cerebral malaria will die unless adequate treatment is given without delay*, and without waiting for the result of laboratory investigations. *Haematoxylin–eosin.* × 950.

Petechial haemorrhages may be seen, and sometimes are very numerous, especially at the junction of the grey and white matter. As the parasites always remain inside the vessels they do not excite much local cellular response (Fig. 34.55B). The result of the obstruction of the many small vessels that are involved is widespread tissue destruction. The necrosis leads to proliferation and aggregation of Hortega cells—the so-called *Dürck nodules*.[230a] The Purkyně cells may be reduced in number and the surviving cells may show homogeneous or ischaemic change:[231] some of these changes could be due to hyperpyrexia.

Trypanosomiasis[232]

African Trypanosomiasis

The nervous system is regularly affected in trypanosomiasis. *Trypanosoma gambiense* is responsible for the central African variety of the disease that goes by the name of sleeping sickness (see footnote on page 2165). The severer East African form often kills the patient before neurological changes are noticeable: its cause is *Trypanosoma rhodesiense*.

In several respects there is a histological resemblance between the lesions of trypanosomiasis and those of general paresis, for the picture in both is that of a chronic meningoencephalitis. However, trypanosomiasis commonly involves the brainstem and spinal cord as well as the cerebrum. Trypanosomal myocarditis and general hyperplasia of lymphoid tissue are frequent features of the disease, especially in early cases. There is a diffuse thickening of the leptomeninges, numerous lymphocytes and plasma cells being found both in the pia-arachnoid and round the blood vessels of the cortex and white matter. Typical, though by no means pathognomonic, of this disease, are the large morular bodies, or 'mulberry bodies',* which have a diameter between twice and three times that of an erythrocyte: they are thought to be derived from plasma cells. They are most characteristic of infection by *Trypanosoma gambiense*. They are present in the leptomeninges and in the perivascular spaces. There may be degenerative changes in neurons, and Hortega rod cells (which should not be mistaken for trypanosomes) may be plentiful (see page 2096). Iron pigment is also found in the tissues.

* These bodies are also known as Mott bodies, after Sir Frederick Mott, who described them first (*Proc. roy. Soc. B*, 1905, **76**, 235). Mott was a founder of the Maudsley Hospital and pathologist to the London County Council Asylums Laboratory, which later became the Central Pathological Laboratory, attached to the Maudsley Hospital.

Trypanosomes may be found in the cerebrospinal fluid, which usually shows a moderate rise in its lymphocyte count. They have seldom been seen in histological preparations.

American Trypanosomiasis

American trypanosomiasis (Chagas's disease)[233,234] is caused by *Trypanosoma cruzi*. An acute form occurs in infants and is commonly complicated by encephalitis. A chronic form affects older children and adults and is comparatively seldom complicated by encephalitis. The disease involves the myocardium and the cardiac ganglia and conducting system and, in some cases, the myenteric plexus, resulting respectively in cardiac dysfunction (see page 46, Volume 1) and dilatation of the oesophagus, stomach or colon (see pages 1004 and 1103, Volume 3).[235, 236]

In the central nervous system the characteristic feature is a nodular proliferation of Hortega cells and, to a less extent, of astrocytes, accompanied by some accumulation of neutrophils. There may be small foci of necrosis and associated neuronophagia. The parasites, when demonstrable, are said to be in the cytoplasm of astrocytes; they are less often found in Hortega cells or capillary endothelial cells. The disease occurs throughout most of tropical South America, less frequently in Central America and rarely in North America. The vectors are large bugs that belong to the family Reduviidae; they infest the walls of clay-built houses and convey the infection to man from the animal reservoirs, which include rats, dogs, bats and armadillos.

METAZOAL INFESTATIONS

Cestode Infestation

Cysticercosis[237]

The central nervous system is liable to be involved when *Cysticercus cellulosae*, the larval form of *Taenia solium*, the pork tapeworm, is disseminated through the blood stream. The commonest source of this infestation is 'measly' (cyst-infested) pork, eaten raw or undercooked. When the ingested cysts reach the intestine of the new host, the larval worms are freed, and eventually one or more may develop into a mature tapeworm. Once this state is reached, fertile ova are produced by the parasite, and these are passed in the patient's faeces. If the patient ingests the ova as a result of faecal soiling of his fingers, 'somatic' (visceral) infestation may follow. The ova may also be transferred from person to person as a result of faecal contamination of food, either by an infested patient or through the intermediary of insects.

The capsule of the ovum is dissolved by the alimentary secretions and the contained embryo (onchosphere) escapes: after penetrating the mucosa of the intestinal tract, it enters the blood stream. The diameter of the larva is about 20 μm, and therefore the pulmonary capillaries tend to impede its passage to the systemic circulation; however, some larvae succeed in traversing the vasculature of the lungs and are arrested in the systemic circulation, notably in skeletal muscles and at the junction of the cerebral cortex and white matter.

Taenia solium is worldwide in distribution. Infestation in man is especially prevalent in Eastern Europe, South America and India. A history of infestation with mature tapeworms is obtained in about a quarter of the cases of somatic involvement. Ordinarily, it is *Taenia solium*, and not the much commoner beef tapeworm, *Taenia saginata*, that may become disseminated in larval form throughout the body in man. Thus, man is the definitive host of both these parasites, an occasional intermediate host of *Taenia solium*, and only exceptionally an intermediate host of *Taenia saginata* (see page 677, Volume 2).

Cerebral cysticercosis may be an incidental post-mortem observation. Sometimes it is found to be the cause of status epilepticus: this does not usually develop until some years, or even a decade or two, after the migration of the parasites (Fig. 34.56). The cysticerci are enclosed in a fibrous capsule, which may be partly calcified. They range from 3 to 10 mm in diameter and in most instances are multiple, from 20 to 50 being scattered, more or less evenly, throughout the cerebral hemispheres. Sometimes only a single cysticercus can be found in the brain. The parasite may lodge at some important site, such as the vicinity of the fourth ventricle: in such cases, symptoms—for instance, those caused by obstruction to the flow of cerebrospinal fluid— may develop while the larva is still viable and enclosed in its simple cyst. Rarely, the cysts may be clustered together on the basal surface of the brain, where a localized meningitis may result.

The early stages of encystment of the larvae are accompanied by an accumulation of lymphocytes and macrophages, often with the formation of multinucleate giant cells; sometimes eosinophils are a conspicuous feature of the cellular reaction. The cyst becomes walled off by fibrous tissue within

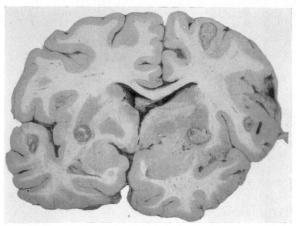

Fig. 34.56. Cysticercosis. The first symptom was a solitary epileptic attack while the patient, who was a soldier, was stationed in an area where infestation with *Taenia solium* is endemic. He remained free of attacks for eight years: they then recommenced and continued until his death, 20 years after the probable time of his initial infestation. There were about 40 calcified lesions in the brain and many more in the muscles, especially of the thighs. [The irregular alignment of the sagittal plane between the hemispheres is an artefact produced during preparation of the specimen.]

about 12 weeks of the arrival of the larva in the brain. The parasite is believed to remain viable for much longer: it has, for instance, been found alive after six years. In most cases of the disease symptoms do not appear until the larva dies, when a further inflammatory reaction develops, resulting in the formation of a larger fibrous scar round the dead parasite.

In the later stages of the disease, the dead parasite may not be recognizable; often, however, its typical hooklets may be identified in the small nodule that is all that remains of the lesion.

Cerebral cysticercosis occasionally presents as a complex racemose cyst within the ventricles or basal cisterns, leading to fluctuating hydrocephalus.[238, 239] Such cysts, which sometimes are multiple, have a smooth, semiopaque wall and consist of intercommunicating vesicles; they are readily confused with the racemose form of coenurosis (see below). Typical intracerebral cysticerci may be present within the substance of the brain in cases of intraventricular and intracisternal cysticercosis.

Cysticerci have been found in the subcutaneous tissue or in skeletal muscle in over half the cases with cerebral infestation. The upper limbs are affected oftener than the lower, and the nodules can usually be seen readily in radiographs, even before they become calcified.

Echinococcosis (*Hydatid Disease*)

Hydatid cysts of the brain are usually single, and may reach a diameter of several centimetres. They contain the onchospheres of *Taenia echinococcus* (*Echinococcus granulosus*), the dog and wolf tapeworm. The disease is worldwide in distribution, and is to be found especially in agricultural and sheep-raising communities, where dogs are very numerous. The fouling of watercress beds by infested dogs is a well-recognized, but now rare, source of infestation of man. Swallowed ova reach the small intestine: the liberated embryos pass through the mucosa to reach the portal blood stream, in which they are carried to the liver. In a small proportion of cases they reach the systemic circulation, and they may then pass through the lungs, eventually settling in the brain and other organs. A hydatid cyst in the meninges usually occurs as a unilocular lesion at the base of the brain, or it may take the form of a cluster of cysts of various generations. Rarely, the cyst forms within the spinal theca and may compress the spinal cord. The cyst wall is composed of two layers: the inner germinal layer, from which the brood-capsules and endogenous cysts develop, and the outer, chitinous layer, or ectocyst. There may be a well-marked cellular inflammatory reaction in the surrounding tissue, and in the brain this may be accompanied by proliferation of astrocytes. Sometimes, a distinct collagenous capsule eventually forms outside the chitinous ectocyst. The cyst fluid may contain free hooklets derived from the circumoral rings of the embryo worm. Man, pigs and sheep are the intermediate hosts of this parasite.

Coenurosis (Coenuriasis)

A second variety of dog tapeworm, *Multiceps multiceps*, has a similarly worldwide distribution,

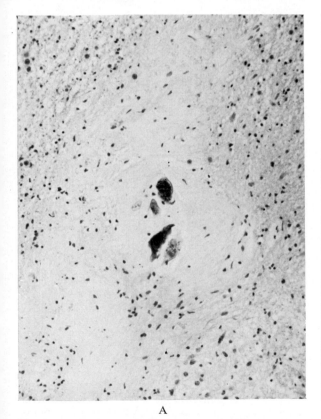
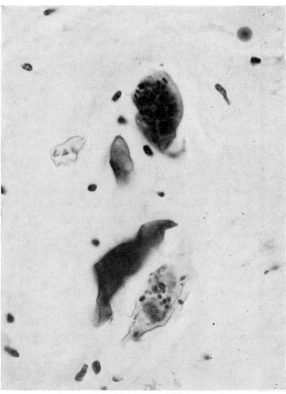

A   B

Fig. 34.57.§ Schistosomiasis of the spinal cord. Cluster of the distorted ova of *Schistosoma haematobium* in glial scar in vicinity of a posterior grey column of the lumbar region of the spinal cord. The patient had long suffered from a condition mimicking tabes dorsalis, without history or serological evidence of syphilis. He eventually developed paraplegia and died of acute bacterial infection of the urinary tract. Although he had last visited a country where schistosomiasis is endemic 25 years before his death, living adult schistosomes were found in the vertebral venous plexuses at necropsy. *Haematoxylin–eosin*. A: ×130; B: ×400.

3*

and, like the echinococcus, can infest man and other animals. The larval stage of the parasite is sometimes known as *Coenurus cerebralis*; this larva may develop in the brain of the intermediate host (usually sheep, but occasionally man, the latter especially in South Africa).[240, 241] It forms a semi-transparent bladder with as many as 400 scolices attached to its inner surface. The cyst is ordinarily solitary but racemose formations sometimes develop in the basal cisterns and are difficult to distinguish from racemose cysticercosis (see above).

Trematode Infestation

Schistosomiasis

The ova of the blood flukes may be carried in the blood stream to the meninges, brain and spinal cord (Fig. 34.57), where they excite a granulomatous reaction. The cells of the granuloma include lymphocytes, plasma cells and multinucleate giant cells; eosinophils may at first be plentiful. In the earlier stages of infestation, necrosis may occur in the tissue round the ova; later, fibrosis and calcification develop. *Schistosoma japonicum* has been found in the central nervous system oftener than *Schistosoma mansoni* and *Schistosoma haematobium*. Although the lesions have frequently been distributed widely through the brain, as is consistent with blood-borne dissemination of the ova from a distant source in the body, they are sometimes very localized: it has been suggested that in such cases the female fluke may lay her eggs while lying in a cerebral vein or venous sinus.[242]

Symptoms due to the presence of ova in the spinal cord or spinal nerve roots are a well-known, but infrequent, accompaniment of infestation by *Schistosoma mansoni*.[242a] They occur also, but more rarely, in cases of infestation by *Schistosoma haematobium* (Fig. 34.57). Although the granulomatous reaction to the presence of the ova within the substance of the cord is indisputably related to the development of symptoms in these cases, it is also possible that the severity of the reaction is accentuated by a local hypersensitivity response to the infestation.[242b]

Nematode Infestation

Round worms rarely give rise to lesions in the brain. In fatal cases of trichiniasis, *Trichinella spiralis* may sometimes be seen blocking a capillary or a terminal branch of an arteriole. The parasite excites an acute inflammatory reaction, usually with many eosinophils in the exudate, and there is often necrosis of the surrounding brain tissue.

Neurological symptoms have occurred in patients with *Toxocara* infestation and so cerebral lesions may be expected (Fig. 34.58).[243] The parasite has a predilection for the retina (see Chapter 40, Volume 6). [244]

Filariasis is accompanied only exceptionally rarely by involvement of the central nervous system. Both *Loa loa*[245, 245a] and *Wuchereria bancrofti*[245b] have occasionally caused encephalitis or encephalomyelitis, sometimes with meningitis. The histological changes have been widespread in such cases, as indicated by the presence of lymphocytes in the subarachnoid space, lymphocytic cuffing of blood vessels, and a general increase in the number of Hortega cells throughout the brain. Granulomatous lesions, with giant-cell formation, are present round the blood vessels.

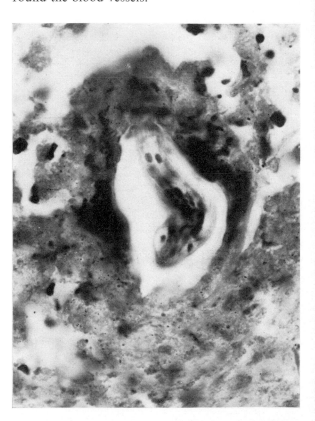

Fig. 34.58.§ Larva of *Toxocara* species in a necrotic focus in the brain of a boy, aged four years, the only child of parents who had brought him up in constant close association with large numbers of ill-cared-for dogs and cats. The child died of an obscure encephalitis-like illness accompanied by blindness. Larvae, identified as those of toxocara, were found in the retina of each eye and in multiple minute foci of necrosis in the brain. *Haematoxylin–eosin.* × 750.

VIRAL INFECTIONS OF THE CENTRAL NERVOUS SYSTEM[246]

Introduction

An important group of diseases of the central nervous system is caused by neurotropic viruses. Some of these viruses, such as that of rabies, affect nervous tissues only; others, particularly poliovirus, may damage a wider range of tissues, although the most serious lesions are in the central nervous system. A few viruses, notably those of measles and mumps, may involve the central nervous system as an infrequent complication of the illness that they ordinarily cause. There is much variety in the modes by which infection with neurotropic viruses is acquired.

A typical disease caused by a neurotropic virus, such as poliomyelitis, has a short incubation period, an explosive onset, and a predictable course, leading either to death or to recovery associated with formation of antibodies, disappearance of the virus and development of immunity. Diseases that follow this general pattern may be grouped arbitrarily as *conventional viral diseases* (this page): within the group there will be variations in the period of incubation, the severity of lesions and the degree of immunity.

It has long been recognized that varicella infection may differ considerably from this general pattern, may not be a solitary event, and may herald by many years the very different clinical syndrome of herpes zoster, due to persistence of the virus as a latent infection. More recently it has become evident that certain other viruses, such as those of herpes simplex and measles, that are also well known for acute effects, occasionally have comparably protracted and complex histories and, after a variable period, may also be associated with neurological damage. Such disorders will be considered as *latent viral diseases* (*persistent viral diseases*) (page 2156), with the reservation that current usage of the terms 'latent' and 'persistent' is not consistent: these designations may refer to the infection or to the disease or, since the states that the terms describe are not mutually exclusive, to both; further, they may imply that the virus is present but repressed, and also that it may or may not be identified or recovered. The problem of nomenclature has recently been discussed fully:[247] we shall take persistent to mean that infection is continuing, or permanent, and latent to mean that infection is present but not developed or manifest.

Neutrotropic viruses are among the causes of *opportunistic infections*: this aspect of viral infection may conveniently be considered in a separate subsection (page 2160).

The concept of *slow viral diseases*, stemming mainly from veterinary research, has become increasingly important over the past 20 years and has proved to have special relevance to human neuropathology. The concept can be reasonably well defined and, while there are important problems relating to the nature and action of the infective agents, consideration of the field as a whole and of the possible future implications is desirable (page 2161.)

There is also a miscellaneous group of *diseases presumptively or possibly caused by viruses*. Although these are in the main rare, they have important theoretical and practical implications. For convenience they are grouped in their own subsection (page 2165). Similarly, the neurological manifestations of *infection by chlamydiae* are considered at the end of this section (page 2169), although these organisms are no longer classified as viruses.

CONVENTIONAL VIRAL DISEASES

Poliomyelitis

(Anterior Poliomyelitis;* Infantile Paralysis; Heine–Medin Disease)[248]

There is pictorial evidence in Egyptian papyri that poliomyelitis existed in the days of the Pharaohs. The recognition of the disease as a nosological entity was due to the work of Heine, in Germany, in the 1830s;[248a] the foundation of much of our knowledge of its epidemiology was laid by Medin, in Sweden, some 50 years later.[248b]

Under natural conditions, poliomyelitis appears to be confined to man, although the possible existence of animal reservoirs cannot be excluded, especially in view of an immunological kinship between the poliomyelitis group of viruses and some viruses of mice, swine and birds. Poliomyelitis can be transmitted to animals, and Landsteiner and his colleagues, in 1909, laid the basis for our knowledge of its viral nature by their success in transferring the infection to primates by intraneural inoculation of Berkefeld filtrates of post-mortem material from human cases.[249, 250] In 1936, Sabin

---

* The designation 'anterior poliomyelitis' indicates that it is the anterior columns of the grey matter of the spinal cord that characteristically are affected in this disease. The simpler term 'poliomyelitis' is now more usual.

and Olitsky isolated the virus for the first time by cultivating it *in vitro* in nervous tissue obtained from human embryos.[251]

The Virus

Poliomyelitis virus is one of the smallest known, having a diameter of between 22 and 27 nm.[252, 253] It is an enterovirus of the picornavirus family, which also includes the echoviruses, Coxsackie viruses and rhinoviruses. It is symmetrical and probably icosahedral, and it has an inner core of which nearly two-thirds are composed of ribonucleic acid. This core is enclosed in a protein envelope that can be removed by proteolytic enzymes. After its removal, the core is still capable of replication: it is believed that the virus loses the protein envelope before it enters the cytoplasm of the host's cells.

A feature common to all viruses is their strict parasitism, for they depend for their reproduction on environmental factors to be obtained only within the living host cell; at other times, they survive in a state of suspended activity. Pathologically, one of the most important properties of the poliomyelitis virus is that the cells for which it has a special affinity are the motor neurons of the spinal cord and medulla and of the precentral gyri.

Many strains of poliomyelitis virus, of differing virulence, have been recovered from human sources: they have been given the name *Poliovirus hominis*, and all known strains can be classified into one or another of three types, the differences between which probably depend on the composition of their protein envelope. Type 1 ('Lansing') is common and is the most dangerous epidemic form. Type 2 ('Brunhilde') is perhaps commoner than type 1 and is less virulent; it has some antigenic resemblance to the virus of Theiler's mouse encephalitis, but there is no evidence that the mouse is a vector or reservoir of human poliomyelitis. Type 3 ('Leon') strains of poliomyelitis virus are not frequently found: they cause a severe form of the disease.

Epidemiology

In Britain, poliomyelitis is still mainly a summer and autumn disease that chiefly affects young children, but in recent years a larger proportion of cases has occurred among adults: this is an important change, because the case fatality rate rises markedly with age. The incidence of the disease differs from year to year, possibly because of variations in the summer temperature. The decline in incidence in the past few years is probably due to the widespread use of prophylactic vaccination: waning accept-ance of this means of protection by the population may reverse the effect (see Table 34.2). In general, the disease in England is commoner in southern counties; an unexplained feature of its epidemiology is its widely varying incidence in different, and often quite small, contiguous areas.[254]

Table 34.2. *Poliomyelitis in England and Wales, 1953 to 1975**

| Year | Notifications (acute cases) | | | Total deaths† |
	Paralytic	Non-paralytic	Total	
1953	2976	1571	4547	338 (320)
1954	1319	641	1960	134 (112)
1955	3712	2619	6331	270 (141)
1956	1717	1483	3200	137 (114)
Mass vaccination began in 1957				
1957	3177	1667	4844	255 (226)
1958	1419	575	1994	154 (129)
1959	739	289	1028	87 (66)
1960	257	121	378	46 (23)
1961	707	169	876	78 (59)
1962	212	59	271	43 (18)
1963	39	12	51	37 (3)
1964	29	8	37	28 (4)
1965	55	36	91	18 (3)
1966	19	4	23	21 (1)
1967	16	3	19	15 (1)
1968	19	5	24	15 (0)
1969	9	1	10	10 (0)
1970	6	0	6	19 (0)
1971	6	1	7	20 (3)
1972	3	2	5	15 (0)
1973	4	1	5	17 (0)
1974	5	1	6	23 (0)
1975	2	1	3	17 (0)
1976	10	3	13	‡25 ‡(2)

* *Report of the Ministry of Health for the Year 1961*, part 2, page 47; London, 1962. *The Registrar General's Statistical Review for England and Wales for the Year 1972*, part 1; London, 1974. *Statistics of Infectious Diseases: Notifications of Infectious Diseases in England and Wales, 1976* (Series MB2, No. 3); London, 1978.
† The number of deaths in the acute phase of the illness is given within brackets. All other deaths were due to the late effects of the disease.
‡ Provisional figures.

The incubation period of poliomyelitis is variable; it is usually 7 to 10 days, but extremes of four days to three weeks have been recorded.[255] The virus enters the body by way of the alimentary tract, either in droplets expelled from the mouth of carriers or in water, milk or food that has been contaminated directly, either by such droplets or, more usually, by infected faecal matter. Spread of the virus from faeces may also occur through the intermediary of coprophagic flies and, perhaps, of cockroaches. Once vectors have become infected with poliomyelitis virus, they may continue to carry it for the rest of their lives.[256] In view of the existence of a viraemia at one stage of the disease, it would seem that blood-sucking insects might occasionally transmit the infection, but this has not been proved. The sources of the infection and the modes of dispersal of the virus may well account for the characteristic rise in the incidence of the disease in the warmer months of the year.

Paralytic poliomyelitis is relatively rare in the indigenous population in the tropics, although in some areas its incidence has been high. It is commoner in North America, in the northern countries of Europe and in Australia than in most other parts of the world. The greater susceptibility of children in these areas has been attributed to two factors—neglect of breast feeding and the high standards of general hygiene and nutrition: both factors tend to postpone infection to a later and more vulnerable age.[257] In relatively less prosperous countries, babies appear not only to receive a more effective passive immunity from their mothers, but also to acquire, early in life, clinically inapparent, actively immunizing infections from their environment. Serological studies have shown that in some tropical countries in which poliomyelitis is ostensibly infrequent, almost all children over five years appear to have acquired an active immunity to the infection. In countries with a higher incidence of clinically apparent disease, immunity develops much more slowly in the population, and may never become complete, even among adults.[258, 259]

Periodical enhancement of the virulence of the virus is probably an important factor in determining the occurrence and extent of particular epidemics. Type 1 virus is responsible for most outbreaks, but some are due to the other types. The cross-immunity between the three types is considerable, so that infection by one, whether clinically recognized or not, may protect against the others. In fact, it would seem that paralytic attacks may be rendered milder by previous subclinical infection with one of the other types.[260]

The virus usually ceases to be recoverable from a patient's faeces about eight weeks after the onset of the disease, though in an important minority the period may be much longer.[261] The clinical condition of a patient gives no indication of his potential danger as a carrier, and an old belief that a patient may be regarded as no longer infective once he has recovered sufficiently to leave his bed is dangerously misleading. Of equal importance epidemiologically is the question of the stage in the incubation period at which a patient becomes infective. Clinical experience during epidemics has suggested that a person incubating poliomyelitis may spread the virus during a period of several days before the onset of paralysis. It seems likely that during most of the incubation period, virus multiplication is taking place within the infected epithelium of the intestinal tract, and that it is from these cells that virus escapes into the faeces. The virus can be recovered from the patient's faeces with some constancy, but it is in only a minority of cases that it can be isolated from the nasopharyngeal secretions.

In sewage, poliomyelitis virus only survives for a few days, but it may persist in water in the dark for several months. It is destroyed at $60°C$, and by ultraviolet light and oxidizing agents. It withstands drying and exposure to X-rays, ether and most common disinfectants. It survives well in a 50 per cent solution of glycerol in water.

Experimentally, poliomyelitis can be transmitted to primates by almost any route of inoculation, the most certain means being to inject an emulsion of infected spinal cord into the animal's brain. This technique was formerly much used: it seldom failed to convey the disease, the incubation period generally being from 7 to 14 days. Isolation and maintenance of the virus are now more conveniently and more cheaply accomplished by inoculating suitable infected material into tissue cultures of monkey kidney or of HéLa cells. This culture method, introduced in 1947, has proved of inestimable value in throwing light on the epidemiology and pathogenesis of poliomyelitis.[262]

Immunity

Infants seem to acquire a short-lived immunity from their mothers, although, as with other forms of congenitally transmitted passive immunity, this slowly falls to a negligible level after a few months. One attack of paralytic poliomyelitis almost always confers protection for life, but second attacks have been recorded: a second attack may well be due to a different type of the virus. After an attack, the virus-neutralizing antibody rises as a rule to a low maximum some two to four weeks after the onset of the illness, and gradually falls thereafter to very low or unmeasurable values. But even though the serum titres in such people may be very low, it seems likely that the specific sensitization of their antibody-forming tissues may suffice to promote a prompt and effective response to any further infection with the same type, even if incurred years afterwards.

Of the various measures devised for prophylaxis against poliomyelitis, the formol-killed virus has been most widely used. In the form in which it was originally developed by Salk in the United States of America, this vaccine contains the Mahoney strain of type 1, the MEF strain* of type 2, and the Sauket strain of type 3. The formolized vaccine used in Britain differs from the Salk vaccine in that the Mahoney strain is replaced by the less virulent Brunenders strain.†

Oral administration of live but attenuated strains of the three types of virus has proved to be an effective alternative to injections of the killed virus.[263, 264] Once within the bowel, the viruses multiply and evoke the formation locally of specific immunoglobulin class A (IgA) antibodies at protective titres. The employment of living virus given by mouth has an important advantage over the use of killed virus given parenterally, for it raises the resistance of the intestinal epithelium to any chance reinfection with a potentially pathogenic strain. Many infants protected in this way continue to excrete the strains of living virus for several weeks after ingestion of the immunizing material, but it is said that there is no danger to contacts, for the strains in the faeces retain their attenuated character.

After a prophylactic inoculation with a single dose of formolized vaccine, the titre of virus-neutralizing antibodies rises only slightly, and then declines slowly during the ensuing months. After a second dose, however, the titre rises to a peak of about 1 in 100 by the end of several weeks; it remains elevated for a few months, and never returns completely to the prevaccination level. The effect of a third, or booster, dose is to raise the antibody titre promptly to between 1 in 500 and 1 in 1000. The antibodies may then persist for months, and sometimes for years, at high titre.

Although active prophylaxis with formolized vaccines is not always successful in preventing paralysis in poliomyelitis, the frequency of this manifestation is greatly reduced by immunization.[265] In a study in the United States of America, it was found that the proportion of children who remained susceptible to poliomyelitis was reduced

* The 'MEF 1' strain was isolated by van Rooyen in 1943 from a man in the Middle East Forces: its name was derived from the initials of this military group.
† The Brunenders strain is so called because it is a modification developed by Enders from the Brunhilde strain; it is equally antigenic, but less virulent.

to 50 per cent by a single dose of Salk vaccine, to 8 per cent by three doses and to 5 per cent by four doses.[266] The efficacy of prophylactic inoculation was shown in the Mauritius outbreak of 1959: the incidence of poliomyelitis in children under the age of seven years who had been vaccinated was 2·3 per 100 000, in contrast to 279·1 per 100 000 in those of the same age who had not been protected in this way.[267]

Pathogenesis

It is believed that the lymphoid tissue in the wall of the intestine is the first part to be significantly involved by the invading virus, and that the infection then spreads in the lymph to the mesenteric lymph nodes, and, probably, in the portal blood stream to the liver. A stage of general viraemia is believed to occur only in those cases in which paralysis later develops. That this is the pathway of infection is supported by the observation that in fatal cases there is often swelling of the Peyer's patches in the ileum, and that this is associated with the occurrence of hyperplastic, reactive changes in the mesenteric lymph nodes and focal necrosis in the liver. There is never any evidence of injury to the intestinal epithelium.

It used to be thought that the virus of poliomyelitis gained access to the central nervous system along the olfactory nerves from the nasal cavity. This view has now been given up, for the virus has not been isolated from olfactory bulbs, although it is readily recovered from the affected parts of the brain itself.

How the virus reaches the affected neurons is not known. Before the occurrence of preparalytic viraemia was recognized, it had been postulated that the virus travels centripetally up major nerve trunks; however, the frequency in the early stages of the disease of pain in the regions that are subsequently affected by paralysis[268] suggests that the virus may enter the nervous system through dorsal root ganglia, where the barrier between blood and nervous system is known to be relatively ineffective (see page 2305).[269, 270]

There is evidence that physical fatigue influences the distribution of paralysis, which often particularly affects those parts that have recently been unduly active.[271] Trauma to a mucosal surface, such as occurs in tonsillectomy, apparently increases the chances that the disease may develop; in particular, the incidence of the bulbar form of poliomyelitis, which has a high mortality, is significantly raised among those who have tonsillectomy during an epidemic. Prophylactic inoculation against diphtheria and pertussis, especially if an alum-precipitated material is used, is also recognized to predispose to paralysis in the limb into which the injection is given—the so-called 'provocative poliomyelitis'.[272]

Clinical Features

Poliomyelitis is commonly ushered in by headache, vomiting, pain (particularly in the region in which paralysis later develops) and malaise.[273] It is noteworthy that in any epidemic the number of people who become infected, and who, in consequence, become temporary carriers of the virus, is very large in proportion to the number of patients with paralysis. Serious involvement of the central nervous system is relatively infrequent, and the non-paralytic form of poliomyelitis—the main symptoms of which are those of catarrhal inflammation of the upper parts of the respiratory and alimentary tracts—is the commonest manifestation of the infection during epidemics: the real nature of the non-paralytic illness often goes unrecognized.

In a large proportion of cases of paralytic poliomyelitis the fever is diphasic: the first phase is associated with general symptoms, and the second, which follows some days later, accompanies overt involvement of the central nervous system.

Structural Changes

In its paralytic form, poliomyelitis is an acute encephalomyelitis in which the nerve cells of the spinal cord, and especially those of the anterior grey columns, are mainly involved. In many fatal cases there are scattered lesions in the brainstem, dentate nuclei, roof nuclei of the cerebellum, thalami and motor cortex; symptoms rarely result from lesions in structures above the brainstem. The distribution of the affected neurons, even within the regions most heavily involved, is erratic. All the lesions appear to be of the same age, and this indicates that the cells involved are attacked virtually simultaneously.

The anatomical distribution of the lesions is curiously haphazard: strictly symmetrical involvement of the spinal cord is unusual. There is heavy involvement of the cervical and lumbar enlargements, but this is probably a reflection of the large number of neurons in the anterior grey columns in these segments of the cord. The most seriously affected segments are the second and third lumbar; in contrast, the third and fourth sacral segments are almost always spared. Neuronal damage in the fourth to sixth cervical segments, from which the phrenic nerves rise, and in the thoracic segments, which innervate the intercostal musculature, results in paralysis of the respiratory muscles, and is a commoner cause of distress in breathing than involvement of the respiratory centre in the medulla.[274] Although there seems to be no relation between the territories supplied by different blood vessels and the distribution of the lesions, it has been suggested that hyperaemia may facilitate the action of the virus. The effects of the virus seem to be influenced by the size of the neurons involved: the larger cells are particularly liable to injury, possibly because their greater content of ribonucleic acid allows the virus to multiply more actively. In cases in which neuronal damage had been only moderately severe, it was found that large nerve cells had disappeared while small ones had survived.[275] Neurons that ordinarily are specially susceptible to the virus can be rendered relatively resistant if their content of Nissl substance, which is rich in ribonucleic acid, is reduced by severing the axons.[276]

The distribution of atrophy in limb muscles in patients who have recovered from acute poliomyelitis can often be related to the number of segments from which their innervation is derived.[277] Thus, the tibialis anterior, the tibialis posterior and the long muscles of the toes, which are often paralysed, are supplied by neurons that are grouped in the spinal cord in short compact columns. In contrast, the flexors and adductors of the hip, although frequently affected, are seldom paralysed completely, and this may be attributed to the fact that they are innervated by neurons that are spread over a longer extent of the cord. It has been pointed out that the probability of recovery of any particular muscle can often be determined by consideration of the degree of involvement of the associated muscles:[277] thus, the peronei are less likely to recover if the long extensors of the toes are also affected than if they alone are paralysed.

Alterations in affected nerve cells (Figs 34.59 to 34.61) can be recognized histologically at least a day before the onset of paralysis clinically, and it is believed that the virus has been multiplying in their cytoplasm for a considerably longer period.[278] In experimental infections in primates, the first sign of the disease is found in the nerve cells and takes the form of severe chromatolysis, only the scantiest rim of Nissl substance remaining. Very soon after this—probably within a few hours—a marked inflammatory reaction develops round the blood vessels, and

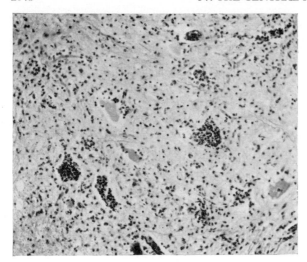

Fig. 34.59. Poliomyelitis: a few days after the onset of paralysis. The neurons in the anterior grey columns of the cervical enlargement of the spinal cord are undergoing dissolution and phagocytosis. Three of the nerve cells, exhibiting altered contour, loss of nucleus and Nissl substance, and homogenization of the cytoplasm, have attracted less phagocytic activity than the others. Part of the field is enlarged in Fig. 34.60A. *Haematoxylin–eosin.* × 130.

this is characterized by the accumulation of neutrophils, Hortega cells and lymphocytes in the circumvascular space and to some extent also in the general subarachnoid space. The neutrophils and Hortega cells soon move into the adjacent tissues and migrate toward the damaged nerve cells. On the second and third days after the onset of the paralysis the killed cells are almost completely obscured by the phagocytic cells that crowd about them (*neuronophagia*—Fig. 34.59).

It is certain that a large number of neurons is attacked by the virus (Fig. 34.62), and that by no

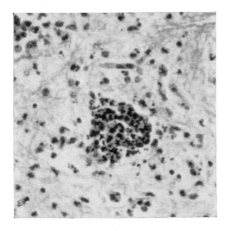

A

Fig. 34.60A. *Caption in adjoining column.*

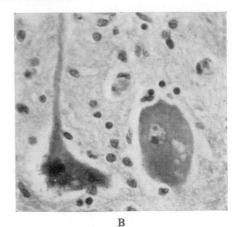

B

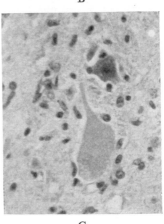

C

Fig. 34.60. *Motor nerve cells undergoing degeneration in poliomyelitis.* (A) Neuronophagia: the neuronal remnants are surrounded by neutrophils and Hortega cells. (B) Two severely altered neurons: the nucleus of the cell to the left is apparently in the process of being extruded and Nissl substance has disappeared; the neuron on the right shows altered outline, absence of Nissl substance, vacuolation of the cytoplasm, irregularity and thinning of the nuclear membrane, swelling of the nucleolus with alteration of its contour, and a small intranuclear inclusion body. (C) Two degenerate neurons surrounded by Hortega cells: the lower one has no nucleus and has lost all trace of structure. *Haematoxylin–eosin.* A: × 300; B: × 350; C: × 300.

means all of them succumb. The evidence for this view comes from studies in which infected animals have been killed at various intervals after the onset of symptoms; such investigations show clear evidence of recovery in some of the damaged nerve cells.[279, 280] Electron microscopy has shown that the synthesis and assembly of virus takes place in cytoplasm; there is also evidence that particles may be formed within the nucleus—eosinophile intranuclear inclusions are seen in some of the cells.[281] Occasionally, the cytoplasm of dead neurons is seen to be swollen, homogeneous and eosinophile,

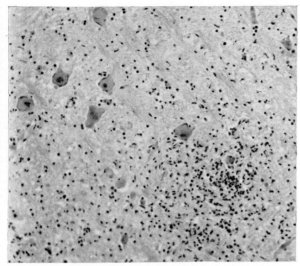

Fig. 34.61. Poliomyelitis. Small area of necrosis with adjacent neurons showing marked central chromatolysis. Death took place on the third day after the onset of bulbar signs. *Haematoxylin–eosin.* × 130.

and it may be vacuolate; although it is clear from the loss of the nucleus that such cells are dead, they fail to attract phagocytes, presumably because their autolytic products are not chemotactic (Fig. 34.59). The rapid loss of Nissl substance that is characteristic of infected cells may be a reflection of their inability to maintain their content of this material in competition with the demands of the virus for ribonucleic acid.

It used to be believed that local inflammatory oedema in the spinal cord was a significant factor in the pathogenesis of the paralysis. This view is no longer accepted, although there may indeed be a diffuse inflammatory exudate in the affected segments, with small haemorrhages in the anterior grey columns and in the white matter of the spinal cord.

When patients who have recovered from poliomyelitis die years later, from other causes, the anterior grey columns of the affected segments appear shrunken and gliotic, and contain many 'corpora amylacea' and, often, cyst-like spaces. Some surviving neurons of the anterior grey columns can usually be recognized in the affected areas (Fig. 34.63). Lymphocytic infiltration round the blood vessels and small focal accumulations of Hortega cells have been found as long as three years after the acute illness.[282]

Complications

Hypoxia and an accompanying retention of

carbon dioxide are important complications of poliomyelitis in those cases in which there is interference with breathing: they may appreciably contribute to the damage sustained by the tissues of the central nervous system, particularly the brainstem and the reticular formation.[283] These lesions in turn give rise to dysphagia, tachycardia and serious respiratory dysrhythmias.

In addition to the characteristic neurological manifestations, myocarditis may be a feature (see page 45, Volume 1). In the epidemic in Coventry, in 1957, cardiac lesions were found at necropsy in each of the five fatal cases and were regarded as a contributory cause of death.[284]

Functional Changes

Remarkably few studies have been made in which structural changes in neurons injured in the course of experimental infection with poliovirus have been correlated with functional impairment. It seems now to be evident that some damaged neurons in the spinal cord may continue to function, for it has been found in infected monkeys that impulses may still be discharged down the axon of such cells, as, for example, when the appropriate monosynaptic stretch reflex is excited by stimulation of the relevant afferent nerve fibres.[285] Later, if the injury to the neurons of the anterior grey columns becomes severer, this reflex gradually fails: the degree of its

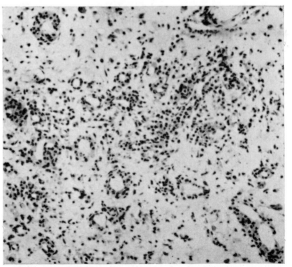

Fig. 34.62. Anterior grey column of spinal cord showing widespread loss of neurons and proliferation of blood vessels. Death occurred from pulmonary embolism six weeks after the onset of paralysis. *Nissl's stain.* × 150.

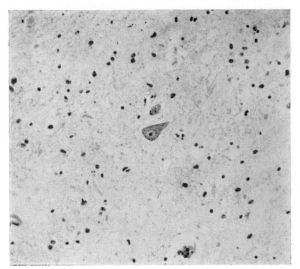

Fig. 34.63. Poliomyelitis. The patient had survived the attack for 45 years, and in this field in one of the anterior grey columns of the spinal cord a solitary healthy neuron is to be seen. The area consisted of spongy glial tissue with numerous 'corpora amylacea' situated peripherally. *Haematoxylin–eosin.* × 150.

failure is commensurate with the increasing inability of the cells to react to impulses that reach them by way of the corticospinal tracts from electrically stimulated areas in the contralateral motor cortex. When the acute phase of the disease is past, and the monkey shows signs of recovery, the motor units become capable of a slow, irregular (and easily fatigued) motor discharge. This is typical of the first few weeks of convalescence, and from then onwards the discharges become more regular, and further functioning motor units appear in other areas. The improvement continues for several months, after which there is no further restoration of the function of motor units.[286]

Apart from the improvement due to neuronal recovery, the partly paralysed muscles grow stronger by hypertrophy of those muscle fibres that have retained their innervation. It is also possible that some muscle fibres that have lost their original central connexions, because of the death of their motor neurons, may be reinnervated by axonal sprouts that develop at nodes of Ranvier in the course of healthy nerve fibres within the muscle itself (see page 2307).[287]

The Cerebrospinal Fluid in Poliomyelitis

It is usually, and properly, considered that *lumbar puncture should not be performed in a possible case of poliomyelitis unless the diagnosis is in doubt.* The procedure undoubtedly increases the liability to paralysis.

The pathological changes in the cerebrospinal axis in acute poliomyelitis are reflected in the cerebrospinal fluid. The pressure of the fluid is usually raised, and in patients with respiratory paralysis it may exceed 500 mm of water. On standing, a fine, fibrinous clot may separate, but this is not as characteristic as in cases of tuberculous meningitis (see page 2118). The number of cells in the fluid is raised to between $100 \times 10^6/l$ and $200 \times 10^6/l$ (between $100/\mu l$ and $200/\mu l$) during the early stages: most are lymphocytes. The count reaches its maximum in the preparalytic stage, and then falls rapidly, returning to within normal limits after four or five weeks. A count of $2 \cdot 5 \times 10^9/l$ (25 000/μl) is among the highest on record. In some cases the proportion of neutrophils may reach 15 per cent: this has no bearing on prognosis. Exceptionally, in mild cases, the cell count may be less than $5/\mu l$, but this is so unusual that alternative diagnostic possibilities should be considered. It should be realized, however, that the count may have returned to normal by the second day of paralysis, even when it was appreciably raised during the preparalytic stage. The leucocyte count in the blood is often normal, or it may be slightly raised; usually there is a relative lymphocytopenia, but in some cases there is slight lymphocytosis.

The protein content of the cerebrospinal fluid reaches its maximum (as much as $3 \cdot 0$ g/l) on about the tenth to the fourteenth day after the onset of clinical evidence of the disease, and thereafter falls slowly; the average value after eight weeks is about $1 \cdot 0$ g/l. The gammaglobulin fraction does not appear to rise, as shown by the Lange colloidal gold curve (see footnote on page 2121): electrophoretic studies in convalescent cases have not been reported. The chloride and glucose concentrations are usually within the normal range, as in the early stages of tuberculous meningitis.

The virus of poliomyelitis has been recovered from the cerebrospinal fluid only during the paralytic stage of the disease, when many neurons are undergoing dissolution.

Other Enteroviruses that Cause Paralysis and Encephalitis

An important group of enteroviruses has been named after the town of Coxsackie, in New York State, where Dalldorf, in 1947, isolated such a virus in the course of investigating an outbreak of a disease that had been regarded clinically as poliomyelitis.[288] The so-called *Coxsackie viruses* are the cause of various clinical syndromes. Coxsackie virus group B (type 7) and, very occasionally, other enteroviruses have caused illness indistinguishable from poliomyelitis. The best known, and commonest, of the diseases for which Coxsackie viruses are responsible is the painful, but ordinarily benign, condition that is known variously as epidemic myalgia, epidemic pleurodynia, 'devil's grip' and Bornholm disease (after the Danish island in the Baltic Sea where it was first described). Sudden outbreaks of this disease, with many cases, have been reported in military units.[289]

Coxsackie viruses may cause an acute (and often fatal) encephalitis and myocarditis in infants[290] (see page 45, Volume 1). They also cause meningo-encephalitis and meningomyelitis in babies, and non-suppurative meningitis.[291] The Coxsackie viruses have been divided into two groups. Group B viruses are the commoner, accounting for almost all cases of Bornholm disease and for most cases of respiratory tract infection, myocarditis, pericarditis and meningitis. Group A Coxsackie viruses most characteristically cause febrile illnesses with a vesicular eruption in the throat ('herpangina') or in the mouth and throat and on the palms and soles (a type of 'foot and mouth disease' in man that is, however, unrelated to the comparably named disease of animals). Several types of viruses from both Coxsackie groups have been associated with paralysis.[292] Coxsackie B5 infection may simulate encephalitis due to herpesvirus.[293]

The *echoviruses* (ECHO viruses) acquired their name from initial letters of the designation 'Enteric Cytopathic Human Orphan' viruses, used because they could not be classified with any of the previously recognized groups of viruses (they were called 'orphans' because the original isolates were not clearly associated with disease). Usually they cause nothing more than a mild, febrile illness, such as summer diarrhoea in children, or benign non-suppurative meningitis: some of them, however, particularly echovirus 9, have been found in cases of encephalitis (see page 2152).[294] The group has not generally been regarded as a cause of paralysis: however, paralysis was attributed to echovirus Frater in one case during an epidemic of 69 cases of aseptic meningitis in Scotland in 1959:[295] since then further examples have been attributable to echovirus 7 and other echoviruses.[295a]

Rabies[296]*

Rabies (hydrophobia, or lyssa) is a disease of world-wide distribution. It occurs in a great variety of

* The disease known as pseudorabies (Aujesky's disease) is referred to on page 2155.

mammals, both carnivorous and herbivorous. Rabies in man is almost always fatal. The infection usually results from the bite of a rabid dog or wolf, but in certain parts of the world other species of animals may be important—the jackal and the mongoose in India, the skunk and the squirrel in North America, the meerkat and the mongoose in South Africa, the vampire bat in Trinidad,[297] and the Arctic fox. Recently, pigs, goats, sheep and poultry have been implicated as carriers.[298] The diagnosis of rabies is apt to be overlooked, for the incubation period may be as much as a year; usually, however, the interval between the bite and the onset of symptoms is from one to two months, and it can be as little as 10 days. In general, it may be said that rabies comes on more rapidly after bites on the head than after bites on parts farther from the brain. Once the symptoms appear, the disease runs a rapid course.

Rabies had been almost eradicated from most of western Europe until, in recent years, it began to spread again, mainly across the continent from the east.[296] Reservoirs of potentially dangerous infection are now known to have persisted among the wild fauna in many regions of Europe.[298, 298a] The disease has not yet been eradicated from the American continents, and it is far from uncommon in eastern Europe, Asia, and Africa—indeed, wherever forests are so vast that it is impossible to control the reservoirs of infection among wild animals. It has been reported in Greenland.

In the British Isles the disease was eliminated by stringent quarantine regulations governing the importation of animals liable to convey the infection. It is becoming progressively more difficult to enforce these regulations, particularly because of increasingly easy access by privately owned small boats and other forms of unscheduled travel from the European mainland.

The last serious outbreak in Britain followed the smuggling of an infected dog at the end of the first world war: there were 318 known cases of the disease in dogs and eradication by strict enforcement of a muzzling order took 4 years. There were no cases of the disease in man during this epizootic in Britain. A similar outbreak among household pets in Amsterdam in 1962 led to the death of 5 people.[298]

Recent evidence indicates that the bite of an infected animal is not the only means of transmission of rabies, although it is the commonest and most important. Carnivorous animals may acquire infection from eating animals that have died of the disease. It seems that it may be conveyed from cave-dwelling insectivorous bats by droplet infection,[299] although ordinarily these animals pass the virus by biting. Fortunately, bat rabies is of reduced virulence, and human infection is a rare sequel of a bite by a rabid bat.

Structural Changes

Rabies is essentially an acute encephalomyelitis (Fig. 34.64). Collections of glial cells and Hortega cells in the grey and white matter, known as Babès's nodes,[300] are a characteristic—but not pathognomonic—finding; they are usually accompanied by an extensive lymphocytic infiltration. Sometimes the inflammatory picture is less marked.

There are two features in particular that distinguish rabies from other forms of encephalitis. First, the lesions tend to be most concentrated in the parts of the cerebrospinal axis that are in direct neural continuity with the site of the bite: this is because the virus travels up the regional nerve trunks, and, consequently, if the patient is bitten on a foot or leg the inflammation is severest in the lumbar enlargement and in the corresponding dorsal root ganglia.[301] It is not certain how the virus spreads along nerves, the possibilities being by way of Schwann cells, axons or endoneurium.[302] Second, large, acidophile, intracytoplasmic inclusion bodies (Negri bodies[302a, 302b]) are to be found, especially in the pyramidal cells of the hippocampi (Fig. 34.65). Negri bodies may be present in the cells of the cerebral cortex and in the Purkyně cells of the

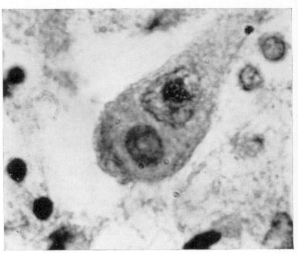

Fig. 34.65.§ Rabies. Large intracytoplasmic Negri inclusion body in a pyramidal cell of the hippocampus. *Haematoxylin–eosin.* × 550.

cerebellar cortex, but in the latter their presence may be masked by the adjacent granular cells, which, indeed, they not infrequently match in size. In general, Negri bodies are more plentiful in cases with a long clinical course; curiously, they are often present in parts of the brain that show little overt inflammation. They may be numerous or they may be scarce—in fact, they have not been found in some cases in which the circumstantial and clinical history has left no doubt of the accuracy of the diagnosis.

When rabies is suspected the diagnosis is confirmed most quickly, both in animals and in man, by the demonstration, at necropsy, of Negri bodies in smears from Ammon's horn or from the cerebellum: Mann's eosin/methylene-blue and Lendrum's phloxin-tartrazine methods are commonly used for this purpose. Fluorescent microscopy has also been recommended.[303] If these bodies cannot be found, animal inoculation studies are essential: for these purposes, fresh post-mortem material should be injected into mice. The hazards inseparable from the handling of such dangerous material must always be considered, and the strictest precautions must be taken to ensure the safety of the investigators.

Electron microscopy shows that Negri bodies consist of an inner core of rod-shaped, branching virus, embedded in an amorphous matrix;[304] the matrix may represent a deposit of viral antigens. Inclusions can be demonstrated with the electron microscope that are too small to be recognizable under the light microscope.

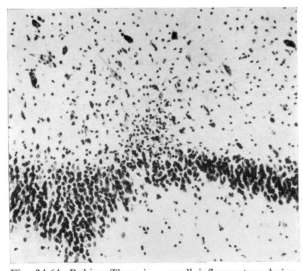

Fig. 34.64. Rabies. There is a small inflammatory lesion involving the granular layer of the dentate gyrus of the hippocampus. *Celloidin section. Nissl's stain.* × 100.

Immunization

In 1885, Pasteur introduced a method of prophylaxis against rabies that is analogous to Jenner's use of an attenuated vaccine to protect against smallpox. Pasteur used a strain of rabies virus—the *virus fixe*—of which the virulence had been greatly reduced by drying the spinal cord of rabbits that had died of experimentally induced rabies.[304a] The cords were dried in air over potassium hydroxide for a period ranging from one to 14 days: material from cords that had been dried for more than 7 days did not cause the disease in other rabbits; material from those dried for less than 7 days caused fatal rabies. The human patients were inoculated daily with a suspension of dried cord, starting with material that had been dried for 14 days and completing the course within two weeks with inoculation of material that had been dried for only one day. This Pasteurian prophylaxis was extensively used for many years, and the number of people who were inoculated ran into several millions; the original method has now been almost wholly discarded, however, owing to the risk of the so-called 'paralytic accident', a form of allergic encephalomyelitis that may follow the injection of emulsions of nervous tissue (see page 2258).[305, 306] Instead, increasing use is being made of attenuated rabies virus that has been cultivated on the chorioallantoic membrane of developing chick or duck embryo: such vaccines are devoid of the danger of inducing neural allergy. A further great advance in prophylaxis against rabies has been the introduction of hyperimmune antiserum, which, in a dehydrated form, retains its potency for years and can be stored at suitable distribution centres in countries in which the disease is rife.

The World Health Organization Expert Committee made authoritative recommendations regarding prophylactic immunization of those at risk and advised the use of nerve-tissue-free vaccine.[307] Combined vaccine and serum administration was advised for those known to have been exposed to the infection.

Virus B Encephalomyelitis

(Encephalomyelitis Caused by *Herpesvirus simiae*)

This very grave disease follows a bite by a monkey that harbours the virus.[308] It has an incubation period of 10 to 20 days, and takes the form of a progressive, ascending myelitis that culminates in encephalitis. Recovery has been reported in two cases;[309, 310] one of the patients later showed mental deterioration.[310] In the experimental disease in monkeys, large intranuclear inclusion bodies have been found in many nerve cells. Similar changes have been found in the naturally occurring disease in monkeys.[311] Virus B* (or *Herpesvirus simiae*), which is pathogenic for a number of mammalian species, has been much studied:[312, 313] it is a near relative of the herpes simplex virus, but of exceptionally high virulence. It also bears some resemblance to the virus of Aujesky's disease (pseudorabies), which is pathogenic in a wide range of domestic animals but not seriously so in man (see page 2155).

Virus B encephalomyelitis is an important occupational hazard for all who handle monkeys—several fatal cases have occurred among those engaged in testing poliomyelitis vaccines on these animals. Inclusion bodies have rarely been found in infected human tissues.[314]

Lymphocytic Choriomeningitis

(Benign Lymphocytic Meningitis)

This disease has been recognized as a nosological entity for many years.[315, 316] It owes its name to the fact that the infection is characterized by an intense lymphocytic infiltration of the choroid plexus, ependyma and meninges in mice and monkeys. It—and similar but less well defined viral infections—probably accounted for the majority of cases of supposed recovery from tuberculous meningitis in the days before the introduction of streptomycin. The causative agent was isolated in 1934 by Armstrong and Lillie,[317] and is now commonly known as the LCM virus. It is often present in the urine of the house mouse, which is probably the reservoir of infection. Instead of meningitis, LCM virus sometimes causes an influenza-like illness that, on occasion, has proved fatal. In cases with meningeal involvement, the virus can be recovered from the cerebrospinal fluid, and often from the pharynx and the blood. The diagnosis can usually be confirmed by the demonstration of a rising titre of specific neutralizing antibodies.

Clinically, most cases are of the 'aseptic meningitis' type (see next page): they are of moderate severity and recovery is usual, although adhesive

---

* The virus was designated 'virus B' because the surname of the first patient who was recognized to have the disease began with the letter B. This 'virus B encephalomyelitis' is distinct from Japanese encephalitis, which sometimes has been referred to as 'type B encephalitis'. See also page 2155.

arachnoiditis and secondary hydrocephalus are occasional sequelae. Useful necropsy studies have been few: they have confirmed the arachnoiditis in chronic cases; in acute cases they have shown necrosis and haemorrhage in the white matter, with some degree of leucocytic infiltration.

Mumps and Other Viral Infections That Cause Non-Suppurative ('Aseptic') Meningitis

Viruses other than the virus conventionally described as 'LCM virus' (see above) may give rise to benign lymphocytic meningitis. In Britain the commonest of these is mumps virus. There is lymphocytosis in the cerebrospinal fluid in over 30 per cent of cases of mumps. Mumps meningitis may occur in the absence of clinical evidence of parotitis. The meningoencephalitis that may be caused by the viruses of mumps and measles may present as a lymphocytic meningitis. Similarly, lymphocytic meningitis is known to have been caused by the viruses of poliomyelitis (particularly the Lansing strain of type 2), by all six types of Coxsackie B virus and by several types (particularly types 7 and 9) of Coxsackie A virus, by most members of the echovirus group, and by the virus of herpes simplex, Theiler mouse virus, and the virus of louping ill (which is closely related to the virus of Central European encephalitis).

Serotypes 4, 6, 9 and 30 of echoviruses have occasionally caused epidemics. Paralysis has been rare in these outbreaks, and death is exceptional. Necropsies have shown encephalitis to be present, as in cases of infection by LCM virus (see above).

The importance of early diagnosis between viral and bacterial meningitis is mentioned on page 2105.

The Arthropod-Borne Forms of Encephalitis
(Arbovirus Encephalitis)

St Louis Encephalitis

In 1933 and 1937 there were epidemics of encephalitis in St Louis and elsewhere in the state of Missouri, with a case fatality rate of about 20 per cent. The virus of this disease was isolated in 1935:[318] it is transmissible to monkeys, horses and mice, and is believed to be mosquito-borne, although the chicken mite has also been under suspicion as a vector. The disease differs from encephalitis lethargica (page 2165) in that there is more definite evidence of meningeal involvement, both clinically and histologically. The midbrain

lesions are more destructive than in encephalitis lethargica, but there is no liability to residual paralysis or Parkinsonism. As in encephalitis lethargica, there is a tendency for the basal ganglia and white matter to be affected also. No inclusion bodies have been observed in any type of cell in the brain; in a few cases, curiously enough, intranuclear inclusion bodies have been present in the renal epithelium.

Serological studies have shown the presence of antibodies to this virus not only in people who have had the disease, but also in a proportion of the inhabitants of Missouri who have no history of encephalitis, and, indeed, in a similar proportion of North Americans generally.[319] These antibodies have also been found in horses. Similar, if not identical, serological findings have been noted in eastern equine encephalitis, both in horses and in man (see below). Antibodies for St Louis encephalitis are present in a proportion of the indigenous population of East and West Africa, and cross-immunity has been demonstrated between the St Louis virus and the virus of West Nile fever. There also appears to be an immunological relation between the St Louis virus and that of Australian encephalitis (see opposite). Sporadic cases of St Louis encephalitis continue to be recognized in the midwestern parts of the United States of America. The disease has been reported in Trinidad, and it is believed that some cases may have passed unrecognized in Jamaica.[320]

Equine Encephalitis

Eastern Equine Encephalitis.—In the summer of 1938 a small outbreak of encephalitis occurred in Massachusetts. Most of the patients were children and the case fatality rate was high. Pathologically, this disease resembles that caused by the St Louis virus, but the degree of destruction of the brain is greater, and the accumulation of neutrophils amounts in places to abscess formation. Marked infiltration of the leptomeninges by neutrophils, with widespread degeneration of the neurons of the cerebral cortex, and sometimes of the Purkyně cells of the cerebellum, is typical of the disease. Its cause proved to be the eastern equine virus, which had originally been identified in 1930 as the cause of Kansas horse plague.[321]

The serological findings have been similar to, if not identical with, those of St Louis encephalitis, although the virus appears to be distinct. Sporadic cases of human encephalitis due to eastern equine virus continue to occur.

Western Equine Encephalitis.—There were sporadic cases of a different form of encephalitis in 1938, in Minnesota; in 1941, further cases were reported from this state and from North Dakota. The disease occurred mainly in farmers. In general, the case fatality rate was less than 10 per cent, but in a few subsequent outbreaks the rate has been appreciably higher. This variety of encephalitis has also been described in Canada. Its cause is a virus that was originally isolated from sick horses in 1931.[322] The lesions of western equine encephalitis are similar to those of the eastern form, but usually less severe.

The western equine virus has been isolated from man in various eastern areas of North America, and the eastern virus has been found in southern and central areas. It is clear that there is much geographical overlap between them.[323]

The Vectors and Reservoirs of Equine Encephalitis.—These equine infections, which appear to affect man only exceptionally, are mainly mosquito-borne; the chicken mite has also been incriminated in the spread of the western virus. Mammals other than horses may harbour the virus. In recent years the belief has gained ground that birds may be the main reservoir: a localized outbreak of eastern equine encephalitis involving horses and a few people in Jamaica in the autumn of 1962[324, 325] is believed to have resulted from migration of the palm warbler, coming to winter in the island.

There are many viruses that attack horses: one other—the Venezuelan equine virus, which antigenetically is close to the eastern equine virus[326]—has been isolated from a case of human encephalitis.

Californian Encephalitis

Californian encephalitis is, apparently, a distinct type of mosquito-borne virus encephalitis of man and other mammals. It has been recognized only in California.[327]

Japanese Encephalitis

Sporadic cases of encephalitis have been recorded in Japan since 1871, and in the past 100 years several epidemics have occurred, notably those of 1924, 1935 and 1948. Because the epidemic disease in Japan differed both clinically and pathologically from encephalitis lethargica—which also was believed to occur in that country—it became known for a time as 'type B encephalitis' to distinguish it

from the latter, which was designated 'type A encephalitis' (see page 2165). It has been known in the far eastern regions of the Soviet Union since 1938, when it occurred in epidemic form near Khasan,[328] where the Soviet Union borders on China and North Korea, not far from Vladivostok on the Sea of Japan. The Japanese disease has generally had a high case fatality rate. In outbreaks in Okinawa in 1945, and later in Korea, about 10 per cent of the United States servicemen who were affected died from the disease. The causative virus was isolated in 1939:[329] it is related to the viruses of St Louis encephalitis, West Nile fever and Australian encephalitis. Pigs and birds are believed to be the usual hosts,[330] and mosquitoes are the vectors.

Histologically, aggregates of Hortega cells are common in the cortex of both the cerebrum and the cerebellum. The disease superficially resembles acute poliomyelitis in that there is heavy involvement of the spinal cord. However, the changes in the cord are circumvascular in distribution rather than primarily related to neurons, and the involvement of the grey matter is more widespread, for the posterior grey columns and the nuclei dorsales (Clarke's columns) are affected in addition to the anterior grey columns. Involvement of the inferior olivary nuclei is a characteristic of the disease.[331]

Australian Encephalitis

Epidemics of encephalitis occurred in Australia in 1912, 1918, 1922 and 1926; their identity was never established, and the mystery of their nature is appropriately perpetuated in the name *Australian X disease*. It is probable that these epidemics were outbreaks of the disease that has become known as *Murray Valley fever* since an epidemic in that region in 1951. Murray Valley fever is caused by a virus closely related to that of Japanese encephalitis and less closely to those of St Louis encephalitis and West Nile fever.[332] The case fatality rate may exceed 40 per cent. There is widespread degeneration and death of neurons in the cerebral and cerebellar cortex and in the thalami.[333] The patients who survive are left seriously incapacitated.

Mosquitoes have been thought to carry the virus, and it has been noted that outbreaks of the disease have sometimes followed heavy flooding. Antibodies to the virus are carried by many Australians. Birds, horses and chickens also have these antibodies, and birds probably constitute a migrating reservoir of the virus. The disease has also been recognized in man in Papua New Guinea.

Louping Ill[334]

In the British Isles louping ill has been known for over a century as a disease of sheep of great economic importance. The name is derived from the curious staggering gait of the affected animal. The viral aetiology had been demonstrated by 1931.[335] The disease is transmissible to sheep, pigs and mice; inoculation of monkeys results in ataxia and tremors but no paralysis. The disease in sheep (and presumably in man) is transmitted by the bite of the vector, the tick *Ixodes ricinus*. Infections have occurred in sheep farmers, butchers, veterinary surgeons and laboratory workers, and are characterized by an influenza-like illness, followed by meningoencephalitis and occasionally paralysis (the disease can be mistaken for poliomyelitis): one fatal case has been recorded.

When invasion of the brain occurs in sheep and mice the resulting encephalomyelitis is accompanied by marked neuronal destruction, especially in the cerebellum and brainstem. There is less neuronal damage in pigs.

There is a close antigenic relationship between the virus of louping ill and the viruses of tick-borne encephalitis, especially the Central European type of the latter (see below).[336]

Central European Encephalitis (Russian Spring-Summer Encephalitis; Tick-Borne Encephalitis)

A form of encephalitis that was reported from Russia in 1935 was described as 'spring-summer encephalitis' because of the time of year when it is prevalent. It occurs also in Czechoslovakia, Poland, Hungary, Austria, Sweden and Finland, and it is now often known as Central European encephalitis. The so-called *Kyasanur Forest disease* in India is possibly a variant of the same infection. The disease may be conveyed by ticks, and rodents are the main reservoir. Some European cases have been ascribed to drinking the raw milk of tick-infested animals, usually goats that have themselves become infected by the virus. Several closely related strains of virus have been isolated from the tick-borne forms of encephalitis in Europe and Asia: they resemble that of *Omsk haemorrhagic fever* and also that of louping ill in sheep.[337]

The Powassan virus, isolated from a case of encephalitis in Western Ontario,[338] belongs to the same group of arboviruses but is antigenically distinct. The red squirrel appears to be a reservoir; a mite that infests it is the vector of this virus.[339]

Pathologically, Central European encephalitis somewhat resembles poliomyelitis, in that the neurons of the anterior grey columns of the spinal cord are heavily affected (Fig. 34.66), but, as in Japanese encephalitis (page 2153), those of the nuclei dorsales and of the posterior grey columns are also involved. The brainstem is also heavily affected, and changes are often noted in the thalami and in the cerebellum. In the cerebellum there is a considerable loss of Purkyně cells; glial nodules are found, particularly in the dentate nuclei. Neuronophagia is a marked feature. As in poliomyelitis, there is involvement of the Betz cells, but, in contrast to poliomyelitis, other parts of the cerebral cortex, including the occipital lobes, are also affected. Moreover, Central European encephalitis shows a greater degree of cellular infiltration of the spinal meninges.

Though the disease generally runs an acute course, it may sometimes last for as long as a year. Even in these cases, the lesions found at necropsy indicate that the inflammatory process remains intense and active throughout the course of the illness. Recovery is often accompanied by atrophy of the muscles of the neck and shoulder girdle. Interstitial myocarditis has been found in some cases.

Relationship of the Various Forms of Arthropod-Borne Viral Encephalitis (Arbovirus Encephalitis)

There are many viruses that can affect the nervous system, either directly or indirectly, and some of them appear to be related, possibly as variants of

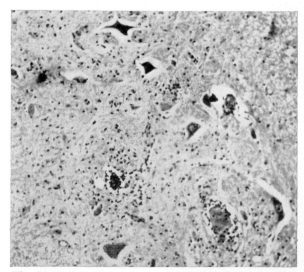

Fig. 34.66. Central European encephalitis. Involvement of neurons in the anterior grey columns of the spinal cord: one cell (below and left of centre) shows neuronophagia; others undergoing early degeneration are shrunken heavily. *Nissl's stain.* × 100.

one or more parent stocks. The viruses that are indigenous to the American continents produce a fairly constant pathological picture, with the horse rather than man as the proximate host and the mosquito as the main vector. Japanese encephalitis and Central European encephalitis have much in common pathologically, and it has been suggested that their respective viruses have a common origin, one variant having gone eastward and the other westward.[340] Certainly, there is some degree of cross-immunity between them. The Japanese infection, however, is spread by mosquitoes and the Central European infection by ticks. Indeed, epidemiologists tend to separate the forms of arthropod-borne virus encephalitis into two groups: tick-borne infection (Central European encephalitis, louping ill and several less well-defined conditions) and mosquito-borne infection (Japanese B, Australian and equine encephalitis, and a few other forms).

Nomenclature

The terminology of encephalitis is liable to cause confusion unless it is realized that the letters A and B have been applied to these diseases in different senses at different times. Originally, the terms encephalitis A and encephalitis B were used to denote encephalitis lethargica (page 2165) and Japanese encephalitis (page 2153) respectively. More recently, the arboviruses have been classified into groups A, B and C, and several others, distinguished by the properties of the viruses themselves and by their associated immunological reactions. More than 180 serotypes are now recognized.[341] Encephalitis due to viruses of the A group includes the three equine forms, while the viruses that cause the St Louis, Murray Valley, Japanese, Central European and kindred forms of encephalitis belong to the B group. It is confusing that the Coxsackie viruses have also been divided into groups termed A and B (page 2149). Furthermore, Cowdry distinguished A and B types of intranuclear inclusion bodies in viral diseases of the nervous system.[341a] Finally, to add to the confusion, a viral disease of monkeys that occasion-

* *Cowdry's type A inclusions* are eosinophile, spheroidal or ovoid, homogeneous or finely granular, well-defined bodies, usually single, and often surrounded by a clear halo. As they enlarge they displace the chromatin to the periphery of the nucleus. They are seen typically in infections by herpes simplex virus and by cytomegalovirus, and in subacute sclerosing panencephalitis (Figs 34.67 and 34.68, pages 2159 and 2160).
Cowdry's type B inclusions are eosinophile, small and spheroidal. They may be multiple in an affected nucleus. They do not displace the chromatin. They are seen typically in neurons infected by poliovirus (Fig. 34.60B, page 2146).

ally infects man, and that is characterized by the presence of Cowdry type A inclusion bodies, has been named virus B encephalomyelitis (page 2151).

Influenzal Encephalitis

Evidence of neurological involvement occasionally occurs during influenza: the role of the influenza virus in such cases is speculative. The clinical features are usually transient and the most consistent neuropathological changes in the rare cases in which death has been preceded by definite signs of meningoencephalitis have been congestion and oedema without histological evidence of inflammation.[342] Greenfield[343] described two cases of acute disseminated encephalomyelitis as a sequel to 'influenza'. Later, following the pandemic of Asian influenza in 1957–58, cases of 'perivenous' encephalitis, acute haemorrhagic encephalitis, and a Guillain–Barré type of encephalomyelitis were reported.[344–346] However, there is a widely recognized possibility that such cases of disease of the central nervous system in association with influenza, occurring during epidemics of the latter, when a large proportion of the population harbours the influenza virus, might be due to the coincidental presence of infection by a different causal agent; accidental contamination of brain tissue with influenza virus at necropsy is also difficult to exclude at such times. Another view, currently popular, is that influenza may trigger the onset of a so-called allergic or post-infective encephalomyelopathy.

Encephalomyocarditis

The viruses of the encephalomyocarditis (encephalo-cardiomyopathy, or ECM) group are generally regarded as immunologically indistinguishable strains of a single RNA virus.[347] All of them are highly infective for rodents, which are said to be the reservoir. Fatal disease is also caused in monkeys and pigs. In experimental infection of rodents and monkeys the virus causes inflammatory changes in the heart and brain, followed by necrosis. The cerebellar cortex is most intensely affected.

Strains of ECM virus have been implicated in cases of paralytic and non-paralytic meningo-encephalitis in man; human cardiac involvement has been reported. The histological changes in man have not been described.

Pseudorabies[348]

Natural infection by pseudorabies virus, a member of the herpesvirus family, occurs mainly in pigs, but also in cattle, dogs, sheep, cats and rats. The disease is also known as 'mad itch', infectious bulbar paralysis and Aujesky's disease (Aujesky[348a] first described it in 1902). Affected animals show evidence of severe pruritus at the point where the virus enters the skin, usually by way of an abrasion; this is followed by a rabies-like clinical picture, with bouts of frenzy, excessive salivation, paralysis, bulbar involvement and death. The histological lesions[349] vary: meningitis and encephalitis, with neuronal degeneration and necrosis, have been described in a range of combinations, depending on such factors as the species affected and whether the disease is naturally acquired or experimentally induced by subcutaneous or intracerebral inoculation. Neuronal vacuolation and intranuclear inclusions may be a pronounced feature. Human infection has occurred in laboratory workers and as a result of dog bites but the disease is not severe in man and fatalities have not been reported.

Marburg Disease[350]

In August, 1967, there was an outbreak in Marburg, in Germany, of a new disease that eventually affected 30 people, with seven deaths.[350, 351] The features included maculopapular and haemorrhagic skin rashes, lymphadenopathy, nasal and gastrointestinal haemorrhage, and signs of cerebral involvement.[351, 352] The neuropathological lesions[352, 353] were consistent with a viral encephalitis and included glial nodules, slight circumvascular infiltration with lymphocytes, and focal haemorrhages. The changes involved the whole brain, including the brainstem and sometimes the cranial nerves. The source of the disease proved to be wild-bred, recently imported, vervet monkeys (*Cercopithecus aethiops*) and those affected were either laboratory workers who had been in contact with the monkeys, or contacts of infected patients. The infective agent has since been isolated and is probably an RNA virus, somewhat similar to the rhabdoviruses of vesicular stomatitis and rabies,[351] but larger. The name *Rhabdovirus simiae* has been tentatively suggested:[352] this generic identification is debatable. The agent is still generally referred to as the Marburg virus (or Ebola virus, after the Ebola River, in Zaïre, where the natural infection of monkeys is prevalent).

This outbreak is of considerable significance, because it shows that unknown mortal diseases that are difficult to classify still exist, that all wild-caught animals should be adequately quarantined before use in the laboratory or as pets, and that the greatest care should be exercised in their handling.

A virus may persist in a permanently latent state; or it may persist over a short or long period in a latent state and at any time be activated by a particular event to cause acute illness; or it may persist in a continuously active state, causing uninterrupted chronic disease; or it may interact with the host in ways that indicate a deviation from these three clearcut situations. Some of the reasons for these different states are evident: others are far from clear. The course of infection by any virus depends on a number of independent variables, which include the type of virus, viral strain differences, the amount of virus entering the body, the route of infection, the species infected and the immunological state of the host.[355] The outcome depends on complicated interactions between these variables, and ranges from rapid death to absence of any apparent reaction by the host. The duration of infection differs from virus to virus and from host species to host species, and even from one case of infection to another caused by the same viral strain in the same species.

It is with the protracted time-spectrum that we are concerned in this section and in the section on slow viruses that follows. It is probable that latent neurotropic viruses remain latent in the nervous system and that cell-mediated immunity plays a major part in preventing their spread, whereas the presence of neutralizing (circulating) antibody does not inhibit such an occurrence. Diminution of the effectiveness of cell-mediated immunity can be important, therefore, in activating latent infection.[356]

Zoster[357]

Herpes zoster (zona; shingles) and herpes simplex (see opposite) are caused by different viruses. The virus of zoster can be seen under the electron microscope in fluid taken from skin vesicles and has been grown in cultures of human embryonic tissue. Meningoencephalitis is said to have been caused in the rhesus monkey by intracerebral inoculation of fluid from zoster vesicles.

It is now widely held that varicella (chickenpox) and herpes zoster are phases of the same infection.[358] *Herpesvirus varicellae* (varicella-zoster virus, or V-Z virus) is the cause of zoster, and zoster may be regarded as essentially a late (sometimes a very late) complication of chickenpox. Typically, the interval between an attack of chickenpox and the appearance of herpes zoster is 20 years or more. Virus from the skin lesions of the former probably ascends sensory nerves to a dorsal root ganglion (usually only one is affected), there to remain dormant. It is not known what determines the involvement of a particular ganglion: the nerves oftenest involved are those related to the skin areas where the rash of varicella is most prominent. Neutralizing antibody titres fall over the years following the attack of varicella, and it has been suggested that a level is reached at which there is no protection against the dormant intraganglionic virus. The virus is then able to reinvade the nerve root and trunk in some as yet obscure way. This explanation of the time relation between varicella and zoster is unsatisfactory in other respects: for instance, it is not usual for circulating antibody to prevent intracellular replication of virus.

When children and young adults are infected by this virus, the clinical consequence is much likelier to be varicella than zoster. Varicella is rarely complicated by any clinical manifestation of involvement of the nervous system. Older people who acquire infection by the virus are more liable to develop zoster (see also Chapter 39, Volume 6).

The typical segmental distribution of the rash of zoster reflects the distribution of the sensory nerves that have their neurons in the affected ganglion. Sensory ganglia of the cranial nerves, in particular the trigeminal ganglia, are occasionally involved.

The affected ganglion becomes enlarged, because of oedema and a heavy infiltration by lymphocytes and, sometimes, neutrophils. These changes doubtless account for the pain, which is often the earliest and most troublesome symptom. The inflammatory process spreads up the nerve root to the posterior column of grey matter in the spinal cord and down the sensory nerve to the skin. As in chickenpox, the epidermal vesicles are small and the fluid that they contain is identical with that in chickenpox vesicles. The characteristic icosahedral viral particles are readily identified under the electron microscope, enabling their differentiation from particles of variola and vaccinia virus. It is possible to demonstrate the virus in centrifugates of cerebrospinal fluid.

The inflammation may spread to the anterior grey column of the spinal cord. In one fatal case there were widespread lesions in the brainstem.[359]

In general, the older the patient, the likelier the development of troublesome neuralgia following the disappearance of the skin eruption. This postherpetic neuralgia eventually subsides; its long persistence has not been satisfactorily explained on anatomical or physiological grounds.

Encephalitis has been described in association with zoster:[360-362] the association does not mean that the encephalitis is necessarily due to the varicella-zoster virus itself.

Zoster Associated with Cancerous Involvement of Dorsal Nerve Roots.—The occurrence of zoster in association with cancerous infiltration of the corresponding spinal nerve roots or their ganglia is referred to in Chapter 39, in Volume 6. The role of the varicella-zoster virus in such cases is uncertain.

Herpes Simplex Encephalitis

A large proportion of the population is infected with herpes simplex virus (*Herpesvirus hominis*).[363] Infection results from contact with cutaneous or mucosal secretions of a patient with the disease (or of an asymptomatic carrier), or with contaminated fomites. Primary infection usually presents in early life as a gingivostomatitis, but may be subclinical or not recognized. Latent infection is then commonly initiated. Circulating antibody forms and protects against reinfection but not against recurrence of symptoms resulting from activation of the latent virus. Recurrent herpes usually manifests itself as 'cold sores' at the mucocutaneous junctions of lips and nose, and occasionally elsewhere.

There is evidence that the latent herpesvirus is located in the trigeminal ganglia of patients with recurrent herpes simplex of the facial region and not in the skin itself where the recurrent vesicles form.[364] Herpesvirus has been recovered from trigeminal ganglia after prolonged culture—10 to 45 days—*in vitro*. Some of these positive cultures were from the ganglia of people who had had no history of recurrent herpetic lesions: this is consistent with the view that permanent latency can occur, as had been suspected from the fact that 'normal' individuals may excrete herpesvirus in saliva. Little is known concerning the role of cell-mediated immunity in relation to latency.

For many years neurosurgeons have been aware that division of the sensory root of the trigeminal nerve may be followed by a crop of cutaneous vesicles in the territory of the divided root. This complication seems to be due to activation of latent herpesvirus by the operation and the subsequent migration of the virus along the sensory nerve fibres to the peripheral endings. Head injury, trauma to the face, ultraviolet light and systemic infection have also been accepted as activating factors. It is not known whether latent herpesvirus is present in the ganglia as intact infective virus, or as incomplete provirus with its genome RNA wholly or partly integrated with the chromosomal

DNA of the host cells, as occurs in tissue culture.

Infection of the central nervous system by herpesvirus presents in three forms—aseptic meningitis, acute encephalitis, and incidentally in the course of acute haematogenous viral dissemination.

Aseptic Herpesvirus Meningitis (see page 2152).—This is rare and not fatal. Its pathology is unknown.

Acute Encephalitis.[365]—This form of herpesvirus infection occurs mainly in adolescents and adults. It is probably a manifestation of activation of latent herpesvirus. It has become of considerable importance because of the possibility of the success of treatment, if instituted early, with iododeoxyuridine (IDU) and similar drugs, which are analogues of thymidine and interfere with DNA replication (herpesvirus is a DNA virus).[363] The clinical picture is usually that of an acute, catastrophic neurological illness, with a lesion of one temporal lobe, simulating neoplasm, haemorrhage or abscess. Pathological examination shows massive necrosis: this tends to be most marked in one (or both) temporal regions, is usually haemorrhagic, and involves both grey and white matter. Eosinophile intranuclear inclusions (type A—see page 2155) may be found in neurons and glial cells, but their demonstration can be difficult: nervertheless, it may be possible to suggest the diagnosis from examination of frozen sections or smears taken during operation. Rapid confirmation by the use of immunofluorescent techniques or electron microscopy is now possible,[363, 366] and is clearly necessary if there is to be rapid institution of drug therapy, as noted above. Herpesvirus particles have been seen with the electron microscope even after fixation of the brain tissue in formalin.[367]

In the absence of treatment the disease is fatal. It is not surprising that severe, permanent neurological disability is a sequel in some patients who survive as a result of treatment.

The relation of acute herpesvirus encephalitis to cases with similar clinical and pathological findings but without proof that the virus is responsible is discussed below (see 'acute necrotizing encephalitis'—page 2166).

Acute Disseminated Infection.[367a]—This form of infection by herpesvirus occurs in the newborn and is almost invariably fatal, causing focal necrotic lesions in many organs, including the lungs, liver and adrenals. The brain and spinal cord are less often and less severely involved but may show focal necrosis, inflammation and intranuclear inclusions.

Rubella[368, 369]

It is widely recognized that maternal rubella during pregnancy may have a direct teratogenic effect on the developing tissues of the embryo or fetus, malformation of the central nervous system being among the consequences. Intrauterine and perinatal infection with rubella may also occur and results in fetal and neonatal acute encephalomyelitis: the damage to the brain and spinal cord that is caused by this destructive infection may be distinguishable only with difficulty from the developmental abnormalities that are the result of interference with the normal embryological processes by rubella at an earlier stage. The wide range of malformations that have been recorded includes microcephaly, anencephaly, meningomyelocele, encephalomyelocele and agenesis of the corpus callosum. Other conditions attributed to rubella include retarded cerebral development leading to mental disorder, delayed myelination, abnormalities of gyral configuration, micropolygyria, subependymal cysts and juxtaventricular calcification. Cataract, congenital glaucoma and hearing defects have also been described.

The florid meningoencephalitis that occurs in the neonatal period[370] is probably due to activation of a latent infection acquired *in utero*. The brain in fatal cases has shown meningitis, angitis and multifocal parenchymal necrosis. Psychomotor retardation and severer mental changes occur in some children who survive congenital rubella encephalitis.

Cytomegalovirus Infection[371]

Infection with cytomegalovirus is common and takes several forms. It occasionally induces severe cerebral malformations in the fetus and it is also a cause of encephalomyelitis in the newborn: in these cases the infection is acquired transplacentally or during parturition. Fatal cases of perinatal infection show necrosis, circumvascular inflammation, astrocytic proliferation and intranuclear inclusions in neurons and in glial and endothelial cells. Juxtaventricular calcification and gliosis occur and can be difficult to distinguish from the corresponding effects of congenital toxoplasmosis (see page 2135) and of rubella (see above). Longer survival may be associated with microgyria, porencephaly, epilepsy and mental retardation.

Cytomegalovirus infection is commonly latent, at all ages. The virus is of relatively low pathogenicity.[372] Its dangers lie in the possibility of activation by immunosuppressive therapy or systemic disease, and in its transference by blood transfusion or organ transplantation: generalized infection, with brain damage, may then occur.

Subacute Sclerosing Panencephalitis

In 1933 and 1934 Dawson[373, 374] described a subacute form of progressive encephalitis in children in which type A intranuclear inclusions were found in the nuclei of neurons and occasional neuroglial cells. Many similar cases have since been described. In 1945, van Bogaert[375] described three cases of *subacute sclerosing leucoencephalitis* with similar clinical histories and with subacute inflammatory changes in the cerebral white matter, accompanied by marked gliosis and slight demyelination. Subsequently, examples were described with features both of Dawson's and of van Bogaert's cases: it is now generally accepted that there is a spectrum of changes that range from predominantly cortical involvement with many inclusions, through intermediate forms to predominantly subcortical involvement with marked gliosis and very few inclusions.[376] Most neuropathologists agree that all these cases may be grouped together under the term *subacute sclerosing panencephalitis* ('SSPE').

The neurological features of subacute sclerosing panencephalitis include involuntary myoclonic jerks, progressive dementia, pyramidal and extrapyramidal signs, a paretic Lange curve on examination of the cerebrospinal fluid (see footnote on page 2121), and a characteristic electro-encephalogram, with regular periodic complexes. Most cases occur between the ages of 4 and 20 years: death usually follows within two years of the onset, but spontaneous recovery[377] and clinical arrest[378] have been described.

Pathology

In addition to the intranuclear inclusion bodies (Figs 34.67 and 34.68), intracytoplasmic inclusion bodies may be seen in the neurons. In some cases, especially those of long duration, degenerative changes have been noted in the neurofibrils of the cortical neurons:[379, 380] these resemble changes typically found in Alzheimer's disease (see page 2275) and in the cells of the substantia nigra in cases of Parkinsonism following encephalitis lethargica (see page 2166).

Sections of the cortex may have a spongy appearance, as a result of the loss of neurons. They may also show a marked increase in the amount of the glial fibres, consequent on the proliferation of the astrocytes.

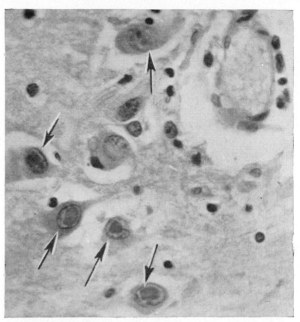

Fig. 34.67. Subacute sclerosing panencephalitis. Nerve cells containing inclusion bodies are arrowed: the inclusion bodies do not fill the nucleus completely. The nucleus of the cell at the top of the picture contains three inclusion bodies. *Haematoxylin–eosin.* × 420.

Demyelination and marked gliosis of the white matter, which are often features of subacute sclerosing panencephalitis, may result from infection and destruction of interfascicular oligodendrocytes. Oedema is believed to be another factor in the loss of myelin, and it is possible that hypoxic damage may be superimposed as a consequence of inflammation of blood vessels and narrowing of their lumen. The degree of gliosis is greater than might ordinarily be attributed to the myelin loss and is best demonstrated by comparing consecutive celloidin sections, one stained for myelin and the other for astroglial fibres (for instance, with Holzer's stain).

Pette-Döring Panencephalitis.[381]—The condition that goes by this name is a form of subacute encephalitis characterized by involvement of both the grey matter and the white matter of the brain, and with a predilection for the basal ganglia.[381, 382] The characteristic of this condition is the presence of 'micronodules' of glial cells and circumvascular cuffing, particularly in the dentate and inferior olivary nuclei and the spinal cord. Except for the fact that intranuclear inclusion bodies are not in evidence, this disease has much resemblance to

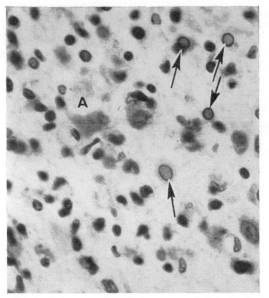

Fig. 34.68. Subacute sclerosing panencephalitis. Inclusion bodies are to be seen in the oligodendrocytes (arrows). A swollen astrocyte with eccentrically placed nucleus and copious cytoplasm is also seen (A). *Haematoxylin–eosin.* × 420.

subacute sclerosing panencephalitis: it is almost certainly a variant of the latter.

Aetiology.—Over the years evidence has accumulated that subacute sclerosing panencephalitis is a latent* infection of the brain by measles virus.[383–385] Measles virus has not been isolated from faeces or cerebrospinal fluid but measles antibody is demonstrable—often in very high titre—in the latter and in blood: in one case there was a sixteen-fold increase in the titre during the eight months of illness.[383] Controlled fluorescent-antibody tests commonly show neuronal staining. Paramyxovirus-like particles and nucleocapsids have been shown by electron microscopy of biopsy specimens of brain: a developmental sequence leading from nucleoliform to multitubular inclusions in the nucleus, and thence to cytoplasmic inclusions, has been suggested.[384] Various virus-like isolates have been made from cultures of brain cells in cases of subacute sclerosing panencephalitis;[385, 386] such cultures can transmit encephalitis to ferrets. These

* The term 'temperate' is sometimes used instead of latent in relation to subacute sclerosing panencephalitis and several other viral diseases. While usage is not consistent, 'temperate' generally implies that the viral material exists as incomplete provirus, integrated with host genome, with the implication that this state indicates a particular sort of latency.

isolates, unlike conventional strains of measles virus, remain bound to cells and are difficult to detect; their component units have different growth characteristics.

The immunological responses of patients with subacute sclerosing panencephalitis are perplexing. Although all patients have high antibody titres in serum and cerebrospinal fluid, their cell-mediated immune reactions are variable—they may show accelerated responses to measles antigen or varying degrees of hyposensitivity or even anergy to a range of test antigens. This suggests that the immunological mechanisms of affected patients are important in the pathogenesis of subacute sclerosing panencephalitis: a genetically determined variation in the host response to the virus may be more important than the strain of virus. Another facet that has been considered is interaction of two viruses present as a result of simultaneous infection (there is evidence that this may occur).[387, 388]

Another approach has been to use epidemiological methods.[389] The families of affected patients do not show evidence of inherited defects in antibody responses. There is a preponderance of cases in the south-east of the United States of America, males outnumbering females by three to one, with a history of measles before the age of two years in over half the cases, and an average age at onset of about seven years. No support was found for a suggestion that subacute sclerosing panencephalitis is acquired from animals.[390]

Crucial issues accrue from all these findings. We need to know how frequently measles infection is followed by viral persistence, how the virus reaches the brain, the in-vivo importance of incomplete forms of the virus and, most pressing, whether persistence follows the use of attenuated live-virus vaccine. In fact, six cases are known to have occurred within three weeks to three years of immunization.[391] Although recent discoveries have undoubtedly clarified certain aspects of the disease, some of its enigmas have been intensified.

'OPPORTUNISTIC' VIRAL INFECTIONS

The nervous system is peculiarly vulnerable to certain 'opportunistic' infections, particularly nocardiosis (see page 2126) and phycomycoses (see page 2127) and some infections that are caused by viruses. Diseases that reduce resistance to such infections include diabetes mellitus, leukaemia, lymphomas and conditions characterized by deficiency of immunoglobulins. A side effect of recent advances in the treatment of diseases that formerly were regularly fatal is that the patients may face a serious danger of developing 'opportunistic' infections. Those particularly at risk include patients under immunosuppressant treatment, patients receiving cytotoxic drugs or radiotherapy for various forms of cancer, and patients requiring continuous dialysis.[392] Further, new techniques and procedures have facilitated the transfer of infective agents from person to person: these potentially dangerous advances include organ transplantation, the use of complex equipment that may be difficult to sterilize effectively (for instance, apparatus for dialysis), and the use of large volumes of blood from a number of donors (especially during open heart surgery with extracorporeal circulation). Viruses of the herpesvirus group, the agent of serum hepatitis (type B hepatitis virus) and cytomegalovirus may be particularly important under such conditions.

Surgical developments could also make possible infection with previously unrecognized diseases, comparable to Marburg disease (see page 2156). The transplantation of organs of other primates into man could have serious consequences of this nature.

'Opportunistic' Infections by Conventional Viruses

It is recognized that patients with natural or therapeutically induced immunological depression have an increased susceptibility to conventional viral infections, including meningoencephalitis. Such patients should be protected from viral infection by all reasonable measures.

'Opportunistic' Reactivation of Latent Viruses

Latent viral infection may be reactivated during therapeutic immunosuppression: zoster and disseminated herpes simplex infection have occurred in such circumstances and been complicated by fatal encephalitis. Cytomegalovirus encephalitis has also occurred in patients after cardiac and renal transplantation; this may be due to transference of infection rather than reactivation of the virus.[393]

Progressive Multifocal Leucoencephalopathy as an 'Opportunistic' Disease[394, 395]

Progressive multifocal leucoencephalopathy is a rare demyelinating disease that occasionally occurs as the terminal event in the course of leukaemia and of such diseases of the lymphoreticular system as Hodgkin's disease and sarcoidosis. The lesions are scattered areas of demyelination that vary in size and tend to become confluent; the axons seem usually to be relatively unaffected. The astrocytes show bizarre cytoplasmic hypertrophy with duplication and enlargement of the nucleus, polyploidy and abnormal mitosis. Acidophile intranuclear inclusions are present, mainly in degenerate oligodendrocytes. The blood vessels are cuffed by variable numbers of lymphocytes, plasma cells and lipophages.

Electron microscopy in such cases[396–399] has shown that neuroglial cells within the foci of demyelination contain organized particles resembling papova or polyoma virions (Fig. 34.69). In animals these viruses are oncogenic under certain circumstances, inducing various carcinomas and sarcomas; little is known of their effects on the brain. A papova-virus-like agent, probably of a new type, has been cultivated from the brain in a case of multifocal leucoencephalopathy complicating Hodgkin's disease.[400] The virions were similar in size to those of members of the polyoma and simian vacuolating virus (SV40) subgroup of papoviruses.

It is not yet established that the virions are the mature phase of an infective agent that causes the demyelination and astrocytic transformation, or that they have been able to invade the brain as a result of immunological depression associated with disease of the lymphoreticular system and its treatment. They may be harmless 'passengers', or they may be a link in a multifactorial chain that induces demyelination.

SLOW VIRAL DISEASES[401, 402]

Visna and Maedi

The concept of slow viral infections was put forward in 1954 by Sigurdsson,[403] while working on unusual diseases of the nervous system and lungs of sheep in Iceland. These diseases are known by their respective Icelandic names, visna and maedi. He observed that they have a long period of incubation, perhaps corresponding to most of the animal's lifetime. Once signs appear, the condition follows a fairly regular, downhill course, with serious disability and eventual death. Natural infections are limited to a single host species and the anatomical lesions are localized to a single organ or tissue.

Since 1954, much has been learned about these diseases: the overall pattern still justifies their consideration as a distinct nosological group.

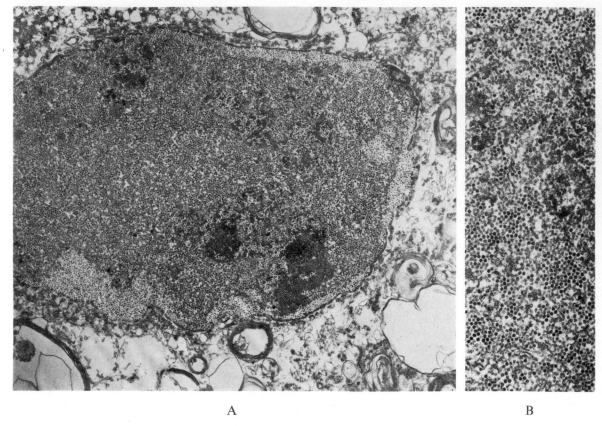

A   B

Fig. 34.69.§ Electron micrographs of the nucleus of a glial cell in a case of progressive multifocal leucoencephalopathy (post-mortem specimen). The nucleus contains numerous papovavirus particles. At the higher magnification (Fig. 34.69B) the virus particles are seen to be present in both spheroidal and filamentous forms. A: ×17 500. B: ×35 000.

There is a degree of variability of host immune responses and also, it seems, in the basic properties of the causative agents within the group as a whole. It has been suggested that a new type of self-replicating particle may be responsible for some slow infections; accordingly, terms such as 'causative virus' are sometimes modified to less closely defined alternatives such as 'causative agent'.

Visna and *maedi* have incubation periods up to four years. *Visna* results in weakness and paralysis, due to a granulomatous meningoencephalomyelitis that has a predominantly juxtaventricular distribution.[404] *Maedi* is a chronic progressive interstitial pneumonia characterized by severe breathlessness.[405] The infective agents contain ribonucleic acid and lipid, can be grown in tissue culture, are closely related antigenically, and are probably respectively neurotropic and pneumonotropic races of the same 'virus'. Affected animals show variable, often high, titres of neutralizing and complement-fixing antibodies: these are functionally inefficient

in protecting against and eliminating the virus. Visna virions contain RNA-dependent DNA-polymerase, which may be important in establishing the persistent state.

Rida is a third disease of sheep in Iceland. It resembles scrapie (see below) and is probably identical with it.[401]

Scrapie and Related Veterinary Diseases[401, 406]

Scrapie is a chronic neurological disease of sheep that derives its name from the fact that affected animals scrape themselves against suitably placed objects, denuding the skin of its fleece. They also show ataxia, wasting, weakness and altered behaviour. The main histological lesions are vacuolation of neurons, spongiform degeneration of the cerebral ground substance and proliferation of astrocytes. There is a particular tendency for the pons and cerebellum to be involved. The changes may be patchy in early cases; in advanced cases they are widespread.

Following attempts in 1935 to prepare a vaccine against louping ill from formolized brain tissue of sheep infected with that disease, it was found that sheep inoculated with this material developed scrapie after two and a half years' incubation.[407] It was assumed consequently that some of the sheep from which the inocula had been prepared were incubating scrapie. Further experiments confirmed that inoculation of material from sheep with scrapie induced scrapie in healthy sheep; they also showed that scrapie could be transmitted thus to goats, mice, hamsters and rats. The spongiform degeneration that characterizes the naturally occurring disease tends to be more pronounced in experimental scrapie.

The scrapie agent is filterable and probably less than 10 nm in diameter. It does not induce any form of inflammatory cellular infiltration in infected tissues and it is not antigenic. It has even stranger properties. Although widely distributed in most body tissues, it causes structural changes only in the central nervous system. It resists treatment with heat, ultraviolet light, acids, alkalies, X-irradiation, formalin, ribonuclease and deoxyribonuclease in concentrations that kill other known biologically active particles that are dependent on nucleic acid for replication. This suggests that the scrapie agent does not depend on the integrity of nucleic acid for replication:[408] the suggestion has been made that it may be a self-replicating polysaccharide.[401] It is closely associated with cell membranes and has not been separated from them by any means yet tried.

A *transmissible encephalopathy of mink* closely resembles scrapie in its clinicopathological features and in the immunobiological properties of the infective agent.[409]

Kuru[401, 410]

Kuru is a subacute disease that occurs among the Fore tribe and neighbouring peoples in the eastern central highlands of Papua New Guinea. Women aged from 16 to 40 are mainly affected; the disease occurs also in a small proportion of children of both sexes. Initial symptoms include tremor and difficulty in walking (the name of the disease is derived from the Fore word for 'shakes'). There is loss of insight and of emotional control, followed eventually by dementia and relentless deterioration to death, which usually occurs within four years. The pathological changes consist of vacuolation and loss of neurons, spongiform degeneration,

proliferation of astrocytes, gliosis, and phagocytic activity of Hortega cells.[411, 412] The lesions are widespread and especially severe in the cerebral cortex, basal ganglia and cerebellum. Argyrophile, periodic-acid/Schiff-positive, amyloid-containing, plaque-like structures are frequently seen and in some respects resemble the plaques of Alzheimer's and related diseases (see pages 2274 and 2275). A striking feature is the absence of significant inflammatory changes. Electron microscopy has not disclosed specific viral particles.[412]

Hadlow, in 1959, recognized the functional and pathological similarities between kuru and scrapie and made the prescient suggestion that it might be possible to transmit kuru to laboratory primates.[413] This hypothesis was confirmed in 1966 when the disease was serially passaged in chimpanzees and later in rhesus and various species of new-world monkeys.[412] The infective agent is present in many viscera (including the liver, kidneys, spleen and lymph nodes), although these organs are free from detectable pathological lesions. The disease can be transmitted by a single injection into the brain or elsewhere. Extensive searches for an antibody response to the agent have been unsuccessful.[414] As with scrapie, there are differences in the distribution and intensity of the histological changes in the brain in the natural and experimental forms of the disease.

Aetiology.—It has been suggested that cannibalism was responsible for the epidemic spread of kuru.[415] The disease apparently became manifest from 4 to 20 years after eating poorly-cooked brain and other tissues containing the infective agent. The very low incidence of kuru in Fore men, who tended not to indulge in this ritual, suggests that transmission other than by cannibalism was rare. The disease is gradually disappearing with the disappearance of cannibalism.[412] The way in which kuru is determined and expressed in the sexes at different ages, and in experimental animals, may be influenced also by genetic factors.[412]

Creutzfeldt–Jakob Disease[416]

It is now widely accepted that the term Creutzfeldt–Jakob disease[416a, 416b] is applicable to a number of variants that in the past have been considered separately under such names as subacute spongiform encephalopathy,[417, 418] Heidenhain's syndrome,[418a] subacute vascular encephalopathy and corticostriatospinal degeneration. The pathological changes, although basically similar, vary in distribution and severity, so accounting for the range of the clinicopathological differences that have been described. It is to be expected that as research progresses, and new data are revealed, some of the conditions that have been thought to be distinct entities will be shown to have common key-features, indicating that they are related variants and thus justifying their reclassification in a single category.

Clinical differences, especially in relation to early symptoms and signs, depend largely upon the part of the brain affected. Early visual disturbances may be related to involvement of the occipital region; early ataxia to involvement of the cerebellum; and early involuntary movements and spasticity to involvement of the basal ganglia and pyramidal tracts. The following parts may be involved, to a variable degree: cerebral and cerebellar cortex; hippocampi; putamina; pallidum; spinal cord; and caudate, amygdaloid, thalamic, subthalamic, dentate and brainstem nuclei.

On histological examination there are three cardinal features: first, spongiform degeneration (almost always present and often severe); second, neuronal loss and degeneration (cytoplasmic swelling or shrinkage, vacuolation of cytoplasm, nuclear shrinkage, satellitosis, neuronophagia); and third, astrocytic proliferation, with a variable degree of gliosis (Figs 34.70 and 34.71). The extent and combinations of these three features vary from

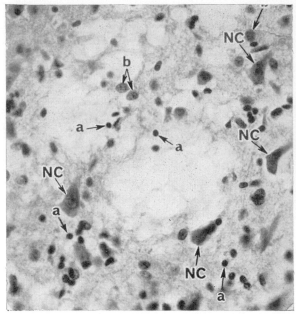

Fig. 34.71. Subacute spongiform atrophy showing nerve cells (NC) and coalescent vacuoles in the ground substance. The two nerve cells in the right lower quadrant are pathological. Nuclei of oligodendrocytes (a) and astrocytes (b) can also be seen. *Celloidin section. Nissl's stain.* × 280.

case to case: they are not always easily found. The disproportion between the neuronal and astrocytic changes in different cases fails to indicate which elements are primarily affected. The spongiform degeneration may be difficult to demonstrate, even in advanced disease, in which the pseudocystic spaces seem to collapse.[419] There has been controversy whether this spongiosity is due to swelling of the processes of neurons, of astrocytes or of both: although the question remains unsettled, recent studies with the electron microscope have suggested that the microcysts develop mainly in neuronal processes, from the combined effects of the 'clearing' of neuronal cytoplasm and of the formation of vacuoles in presynaptic and postsynaptic terminals.[412]

The similarities between Creutzfeldt–Jakob disease and kuru prompted experiments that led to the successful passage of the former in chimpanzees and in four species of new-world monkeys, the incubation period ranging from about 9 to about 30 months.[420] The infective agent resembles the kuru agent in its characteristics, including its lack of antigenicity. Two instances of accidental person-to-person transmission of Creutzfeldt–Jakob disease have been reported in which the infection must have been conveyed by electrodes implanted in the brain

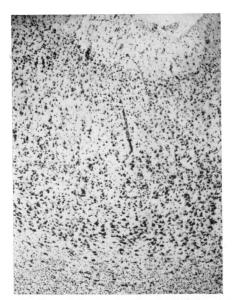

Fig. 34.70. Creutzfeldt–Jakob disease. Inferior temporal gyrus showing a considerable loss of cells in lamina III. *Celloidin section. Nissl's stain.* × 80.

in the course of a stereotactic electroencephalo-graphic exploration.[420a] The same electrodes had been used in the investigation of a patient with Creutzfeldt–Jakob disease 8 weeks and almost 11 weeks respectively before their implantation into the two accidentally infected patients. The electrodes were heat-sensitive and therefore were sterilized in formaldehyde vapour after cleaning with benzine and disinfection with 70 per cent ethanol. In another case the disease was transmitted by corneal transplantation.[420b]

It has been suggested that Alpers' disease (page 2273) may be similar in nature to Creutzfeldt–Jakob disease.[421, 422]

Slow Viruses as Possible Causes of Other Diseases of the Central Nervous System

In view of the fact that slow viruses neither induce infiltration of infected tissues by inflammatory cells, even in the presence of advanced degenerative changes, nor initiate a detectable host immuno-logical response, it is reasonable to suppose that other neurological diseases previously regarded as primary degenerations may also be associated with similar self-replicating infective agents. Among such diseases are the multiple sclerosis group (see page 2252), Parkinson's disease, Alzheimer's disease, Pick's disease and motor neuron disease. Transmission experiments to test these suggestions have not yet been successful.[423] As genetic factors may well influence the expression of slow virus diseases,[412] hereditary degenerative disorders such as Huntington's chorea and Friedreich's ataxia should also be investigated along such lines. It has been suggested that even ageing may be due to a slow virus.[401]

Certain transmissible agents that have been identified in 'slow' infections, such as visna and maedi, resemble conventional viruses in many respects, although the diseases that they induce are typical of slow infections as tentatively defined by Sigurdsson.[403] Other slow-infective agents, such as those of scrapie, mink encephalopathy, kuru and Creutzfeldt–Jakob disease, are quite unlike conventional viruses, particularly in their extraordinary powers of resistance and in their lack of nucleic acid, and it is a semantic point whether they are termed viruses or not: nucleic-acid-free, self-replicating macromolecules have been postulated by various authors,[412] and may include both proteins and polysaccharides. It is likely that the agents are not recognized as 'foreign' by the host and that for this reason an immune response does not occur:

overt disease develops when this tolerance breaks down.[424]

DISEASES PRESUMPTIVELY OR POSSIBLY CAUSED BY VIRUSES

Encephalitis Lethargica

The pandemic of encephalitis ('encephalitis A'; von Economo's disease) began in Europe in 1917.[425] Its onset preceded that of the great influenza pandemic, but in 1918 the two coexisted. The encephalitis reached England from the European mainland in 1917, and cases continued to be seen throughout the following decade.[426, 427] The disease occurred mainly in winter and early spring. In 1924, the peak year of the epidemic, over 5000 cases were reported in England and Wales, and the case fatality rate was about 35 per cent.

To this day, cases with an early clinical course similar to that of encephalitis lethargica are occasionally seen in Britain and elsewhere in Europe: these rare cases end in complete or almost complete recovery, and their identity with the epidemic disease is generally regarded as questionable. The same is true of the various poorly documented epidemics antedating the epidemic of 1917–24 that retrospectively have been regarded as outbreaks of encephalitis lethargica.[428]

Clinical Features

The most striking clinical feature of the disease was a persistent sleepy state, from which the patient could usually be roused, although with difficulty. It was aptly named encephalitis lethargica, and came to be widely known as 'sleepy sickness'.* In addition to the typical lethargy, an occasional but characteristic feature was the occurrence in some cases of a sustained spasm of one or more ocular muscles; this spasm was often accompanied by rotation of the head and trunk (oculogyric crisis). A peculiar feature of encephalitis lethargica was its tendency to be followed by a Parkinsonian state: this usually appeared within weeks or months of the acute illness, but in some cases not until after many years had passed. Postencephalitic Parkinsonism has been said to differ from Parkinson's disease (paralysis agitans) in four notable respects: (1) the

---

* 'Sleepy sickness' (encephalitis lethargica) and 'sleeping sickness' (trypanosomiasis, see page 2137) are, of course, completely unrelated, and neither is a cause of the peculiar condition narcolepsy, which also—confusingly—has been referred to as 'sleepy sickness' and 'sleeping sickness'.

characteristic predominance of rigidity over tremor; (2) the greater asymmetry of the involvement on the two sides of the body; (3) the greater tendency to excessive salivation; and (4) the frequent association with other neurological signs, and sometimes with psychiatric disturbances, indicative of widespread damage to the brain. However, although encephalitis lethargica affected mainly young adults, the differential diagnosis between postencephalitic Parkinsonism and Parkinson's disease was often difficult, particularly because the acute attack of encephalitis was commonly mild and its true nature not suspected until the sequelae developed, sometimes at an age more nearly approaching that at which Parkinson's disease occurs most frequently. The diagnostic differentiation of the two states has taken on a new significance in the light of recent epidemiological evidence that Parkinson's disease may be a result of an unsuspected infection by the causative agent of encephalitis lethargica followed by a long latent period (see page 2269).[429]

It seems that 'amyotrophy' (atrophy of muscles), affecting one or more limbs, also developed in some cases, years after the original illness.

Structural Changes

Pathological examination confirmed that the brainstem bore the brunt of the infection, as the symptoms suggested. The most prominent feature was destruction of the pigmented nerve cells, and this was associated with cuffing of the blood vessels by lymphocytes and, sometimes, plasma cells. In addition, there were often inflammatory foci in the circumaqueductal grey matter and in the basal ganglia, and sometimes in the cerebral cortex, the cerebral white matter and the spinal cord. In some cases, the destruction of the neurons was not accompanied by cellular infiltration.

The most characteristic histological change in the brain in cases of postencephalitic Parkinsonism is the result of damage to the neurons of the substantia nigra and substantia ferruginea. Macroscopically, this damage is reflected in the loss of the normal pigmentation of the midbrain (see page 2088). Microscopically, it is clear that many of the neurons of these parts have disappeared; some of those that remain show a peculiar degenerative change that involves the neurofibrils, which are thickened and matted together in tresses or whorls (neurofibrillary tangles).[430, 431] The pigment sometimes disappears completely from these cells, leaving a pale-staining globoid body in which the

swollen neurofibrils can be recognized in sections stained by haematoxylin and eosin. The loss of neurons is often asymmetrical. When Davenport's technique is employed the thickened fibrils may stand out vividly (Fig. 34.72). Cuffing of blood vessels with lymphocytes may be found many years after the commencement of the disease. In cases with amyotrophy a varying proportion of neurons of the anterior columns of the spinal cord is lost: the late onset of this sign has raised the possibility of delayed degeneration of neurons that had been damaged during the original attack, or even that there may be a persistent infection.

The Cerebrospinal Fluid

The number of cells in the cerebrospinal fluid was increased in most cases of encephalitis lethargica. The cells were usually lymphocytes, but neutrophils were present in those cases in which the injury to the tissue was more destructive. There was a slight or moderate increase in the concentration of protein in the fluid, and in most cases there was a first zone or mid-zone type of colloidal gold reaction (see footnote on page 2121).

Aetiology

Although McIntosh,[432] in 1920, demonstrated the occurrence of encephalitis in a monkey that had been inoculated with a filtrate of fresh human postmortem material, a viral origin for encephalitis lethargica has been generally regarded as unproved. The prevalence of the disease rose to epidemic proportions toward the end of a period of war and privation, but no particular predisposing factors could be incriminated. It is possible that the cases did not all have the same cause. In view of what is now known of the clinical and pathological features of herpes simplex encephalitis (see page 2157) it is unlikely that cases were due to postinfluenzal activation of herpes simplex virus, as Levaditi believed.[433] Another suggestion attributes the disease to some virus that is now extinct, or that no longer exists in the form in which it then occurred.

Acute Necrotizing Encephalitis

The term acute necrotizing encephalitis is applied to cases of encephalitis that are characterized by a particularly destructive reaction in the brain: the terminology is essentially morphological, for such cases do not appear to be caused by one specific type of virus (see note following *Polioclastic*

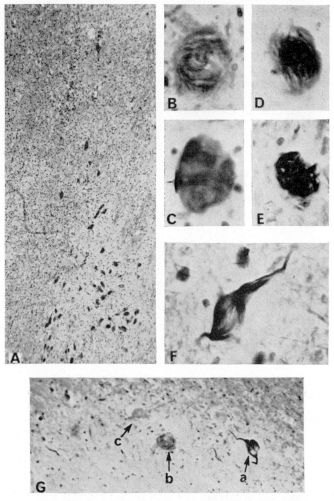

Fig. 34.72. A. Substantia nigra in a patient dying 35 years after epidemic encephalitis (von Economo's disease). Parkinsonism developed 10 years before death. In the lower part of the picture pigmented cells are present in fair numbers but above this many of them have disappeared. There is some free-lying pigment, presumably remaining from the destroyed cells. Glial cells are present in excess; there is also a little lymphocytic cuffing of blood vessels. *Celloidin section. Haematoxylin–eosin.* × 55.

B–F. Individual cells in locus coeruleus (substantia ferruginea) and substantia nigra from cases of post-encephalitic Parkinsonism, all showing neurofibrillary degeneration ('Alzheimer cell change'). B and C: *Celloidin sections; haematoxylin–eosin.* D, E and F: *Celloidin sections; Davenport's method.* × 400.

G. Cells in substantia nigra showing neurofibrillary degeneration with varying degrees of argyrophilia, cell 'c' being very pale. Such cells lose their pigment and often take on a globular shape ('b'). They can be identified in haematoxylin–eosin preparations (unlike the cells of the cerebral cortex showing neurofibrillary degeneration in Alzheimer's disease—see page 2275). *Celloidin section; Davenport's method.* × 150.

Encephalitis, below).[434, 435] The condition has been reported from many parts of the world, and occurs at any age. Some cases may well be instances of herpes simplex encephalitis in which inclusion bodies cannot be found (see page 2158). The temporal lobes and the insulae are particularly liable to be affected, and the involved areas are markedly reddened (Fig. 34.73).

The histological picture is one of acute disintegration of the affected parts of the cortex (Fig. 34.74), with extravasation of red cells into the necrotic areas in consequence of disruption of the walls of capillaries. The cerebral cortex is mainly involved, but there may also be widespread damage in the white matter. In sum, this is a form of encephalitis characterized by massive involvement of one or more lobes of the brain, although, as in all forms of encephalitis, lesions may also occur in the brainstem.

Polioclastic Encephalitis

The name polioclastic encephalitis was given by Greenfield to an acute disease in which the cerebral cortex is mainly affected, the brainstem and

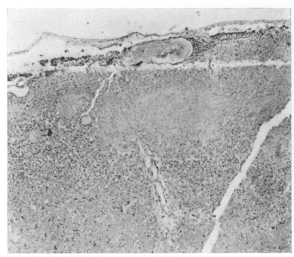

Fig. 34.74. Necrotizing encephalitis. A wedge-shaped area of necrosis involving the cortex lies deep to the pial surface. There is a widespread infiltration of the pia-arachnoid by cells, most of which are lymphocytes. *Haematoxylin–eosin.* × 30.

white matter being relatively spared.[436] Inclusion bodies are not found. A subacute form of this disease also occurs.

Note.—It should be emphasized that acute necrotizing encephalitis and polioclastic encephalitis are not nosological entities. Thus, if inclusion bodies are found in a case regarded morphologically as one of acute necrotizing encephalitis or of polioclastic encephalitis, the condition might be suspected, on histological grounds, to be respectively herpes simplex encephalitis or subacute sclerosing panencephalitis. The increasing use of electron microscopy and immunofluorescent techniques will help to clarify this problem.

Behçet's Disease

An interesting form of encephalomyelopathy has been described as a late complication of Behçet's disease[437] of the oral mucosa, genitalia and uveal tract (see Chapter 39, Volume 6). The encephalomyelopathy is characterized by multiple foci of softening, usually confined to the white matter. These foci seem to originate round small arteries and veins, although thrombosis has not been observed.[437a] Cuffing of blood vessels by inflammatory cells may be a conspicuous feature, and there may be extensive inflammatory changes in relation to the necrotic areas (Fig. 34.75). The nosological position of this condition is uncertain: although it appears to have

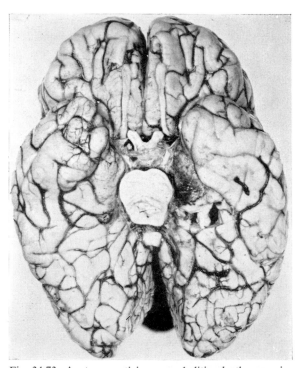

Fig. 34.73. Acute necrotizing encephalitis, death occurring on the seventh day. Note the marked inflammation of the uncus, particularly on the left. A piece of brain was removed for viral studies, which proved to be negative.

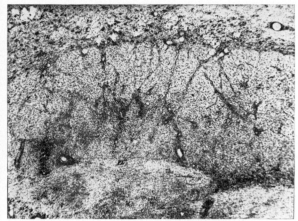

Fig. 34.75. Behçet's disease. Extensive inflammatory lesions in the pons. There is a diffuse infiltration by lymphocytes and macrophages, particularly round the blood vessels. Necrotic areas are bordered by accumulations of fat-laden Hortega cells. *Celloidin section. Nissl's stain.* × 30.

affinities both with the immune disorders of connective tissue and with the post-infection encephalo-myelopathies, the inflammatory features in the brain may be so marked that they strongly suggest a viral infection.

Myalgic Meningoencephalomyelitis

An extensive epidemic of a benign myalgic encephalomyelitis occurred among the staff of the Royal Free Hospital, London, in 1955, and was for some time known as 'Royal Free disease'.[438, 439] There seems to be little doubt that this was a viral infection, although no virus was isolated. Nothing is known of the pathological changes in the tissues.

The condition is now believed to be related to *Akureyri disease*, a clinically similar epidemic illness, called after the town in northern Iceland where over a thousand cases occurred in 1948.[440]

Infectious Mononucleosis

A strong link between the Epstein–Barr virus and infectious mononucleosis has been supported by virological, serological and epidemiological data.[451] It is probable that those cases of infectious mononucleosis in which the Paul–Bunnell test is positive are associated with infection by the Epstein–Barr virus; in cases in which the Paul–Bunnell test is negative the disease may be a manifestation of infection by other agents, among which cytomegalovirus and *Toxoplasma gondii* have been suggested (see page 648, Volume 2).[452]

Neurological complications occur in from 1 to 5 per cent of cases of infectious mononucleosis: they include meningitis, encephalitis and myelitis, and cerebellar, optic and peripheral neural symptoms and signs. The Guillain–Barré syndrome has also been recognized as a complication. The mortality rate rises from almost nil to about 15 per cent when the nervous system is involved.

In fatal cases the changes in the central nervous system are not usually impressive. They include congestion and oedema, patchy non-specific neuronal degeneration, minimal meningeal and circumvascular infiltration with inflammatory cells, and occasional circumvascular haemorrhages.[453, 454] The cases in which the Guillain–Barré syndrome has developed show lesions identical with those found in cases of this syndrome occurring without associated infectious mononucleosis (see page 2331).

Cat-Scratch Disease

Cat-scratch disease is usually a self-limiting disorder that follows a scratch or bite of a cat. It is characterized by pyrexia and malaise, and necrotizing lymphadenitis (see page 638, Volume 2). The aetiology is not known, although basiphile bodies resembling chlamydiae (see below)[455] and, more recently, particles resembling herpesvirus[456] have been found in lymph nodes. Neurological complications have sometimes occurred, usually about six weeks after the appearance of lymphadenitis: they have been described as encephalitis, meningitis, radiculitis and myelitis, but neuropathological assessments are not available.[457]

CHLAMYDIAL INFECTIONS

Psittacosis and Other Types of Ornithosis[458]

The causal agent of psittacosis was first isolated in 1930 by Bedson and his colleagues.[459] It has the characteristic property of producing basiphile cytoplasmic inclusions and elementary bodies. Its taxonomical position is intermediate between viruses and rickettsiae; it belongs to the same group as the organisms that cause lymphogranuloma inguinale (see page 634, Volume 2) and trachoma (see Chapter 40, Volume 6). In British practice it was for a time referred to by the name *Bedsonia*, but this is not in accordance with the conventions of microbiological nomenclature and generally it is now included in the genus *Chlamydia*.

Strictly, the name *psittacosis* relates to infection

contracted from psittacine birds (parrots and parakeets, including budgerigars) and *ornithosis* to infection from birds generally (pigeons, ducks and turkeys, and some gulls and other sea-birds). However, the two names are often used loosely as synonyms. The infection is characterized by bronchitis and bronchopneumonia (see page 325, Volume 1); it has a notable mortality. Neurological complications include meningitis and encephalitis.

The meningitis of chlamydial infection is often accompanied by a gelatinous exudate. Macrophages in the exudate may contain basiphile bodies.[460, 461] The picture may be similar to that of viral menin-gitis (see pages 2151 and 2152); the great majority of the cells in the cerebrospinal fluid may be lymphocytes. Circumvascular haemorrhage and some degree of circumvascular demyelination may occur in the brain; florid encephalitis is not a feature.

Lymphogranuloma Inguinale

Infection by the chlamydia of lymphogranuloma inguinale occasionally becomes generalized and is then liable to be complicated by meningoencepha-litis, which may be fatal. Neuropathological information is scanty but points to the occurrence of meningitis and focal cortical necrosis.[462]

VASCULAR DISEASES OF THE CENTRAL NERVOUS SYSTEM

The Blood Supply to the Brain

Blood reaches the brain through four large arterial trunks—the two internal carotid arteries and the two vertebral arteries. It has been estimated from the relative diameters of the vessels that about two-thirds of the total blood flow to the brain pass through the carotids and the rest through the vertebral arteries.[463] The caroticovertebral arterial supply is functionally a single system, and this is reflected in the pathology of the vascular diseases of the brain.[464] In health, the arterial circle of Willis, particularly the communicating arteries, ensures a well-distributed flow of blood to the various parts of the brain: the free anastomosis between the carotid and vertebral systems, which the circle provides, compensates for any restriction of the flow through the feeder channels that may accompany movements of the head and neck. To some extent, too, the arterial circle is the means of maintaining an adequate circulation through the brain when one, or even more, of its feeder arteries is obstructed as a result of disease. However, complete obstruction of an internal carotid or vertebral artery may seriously restrict the blood supply to the brain; this is particularly liable to be the case if the flow through the other vessels is deficient, as a result of local or general disease affecting the circulation, or if there is congenital hypoplasia or absence of any of the communicating arteries.

If there is much atherosclerosis of the vertebral arteries, the resulting oligaemia affects mainly the brainstem and cerebellum and the occipital lobes of the cerebrum.[465] These parts receive their blood supply from the vertebral arteries themselves, or from the basilar artery, which is formed by their junction, or from the terminal branches of the basilar artery (the posterior cerebral arteries). Atherosclerosis of the carotid arteries predisposes to oligaemic changes in the territories of the middle and anterior cerebral arteries; these oligaemic lesions tend to be multiple.

The superficial branches of the cerebral arteries spread over the surface of the brain in the sub-arachnoid space.[466] The divisions of these branches ramify in the pia before entering the brain as the cortical arteries. These cortical branches carry with them a pial investment; the space between this sheath and the wall of the vessel—the Virchow–Robin space—is continuous with the subarachnoid space: it contains cerebrospinal fluid and may be regarded as having much the same function as the lymphatic vasculature of other tissues. The cortical arteries supply the cerebral cortex and the white matter immediately under the cortex. The deep branches of the cerebral arteries arise in clusters from the circle of Willis and its branches, and particularly from the middle cerebral arteries; they penetrate the base of the brain as the central arteries, and supply the whole of the cerebrum with the exception of the cortex and the narrow sub-cortical zone of white matter.

Although anastomotic channels link the anterior, middle and posterior cerebral arteries and are readily demonstrable in injected specimens, they are inadequate to meet the circulatory demands of any part of the brain deprived of its blood supply by obstruction of any of these three vessels:[467] consequently, ischaemia necessarily results when one of them is occluded. The marked liability to ischaemic necrosis reflects the very high oxygen requirement of brain tissue; the great vulnerability of the brain to hypoxia allows little opportunity for an alternative blood supply to become effective in time to preserve any part of the organ should its normal arterial supply be cut off suddenly. It is unusual, even in young patients, for collateral circulation to open up sufficiently to compensate for sudden obstruction of a cortical or central artery.

The grey matter is considerably more vascular than the white matter, and is more susceptible to damage by hypoxia. Anastomoses between the cortical arteries and the central arteries are few,[468] and this deficiency contributes to the gravity of cerebral arterial occlusion.

When examining the brain for signs of vascular disease, the pathologist has to take into account the possibility that the cerebral circulation may have been adversely affected by disease elsewhere in the body. Small ischaemic softenings in the cerebral white matter may not be due to lesions of the cerebral vasculature itself, but to a sudden lowering of the systemic blood pressure, such as may be caused by myocardial infarction, by the injudicious use of hypotensive drugs or even by a general deterioration of the circulation during the last days of life. It cannot be too strongly stressed that the post-mortem study of any case of vascular disease of the brain is incomplete unless the carotid and vertebral arterial systems have been fully dissected. The commonest sites of occlusion of the internal carotid arteries are at their origin from the carotid sinuses and in the 'siphon' (the part passing through the cavernous sinus); these sites, and especially the latter, are not always adequately examined at necropsy—this being true of the quite easily accessible carotid trunks it is scarcely surprising that the vertebral arteries are rarely investigated.[469]

The Structure of the Blood Vessels of the Brain

The walls of the arteries of the brain are thinner than those of arteries of comparable calibre in other parts of the body. The normal basilar artery, for instance, is so translucent, and at necropsy often so collapsed, that it might be taken for a vein. The middle cerebral arteries, by contrast, are more tubular, and their wall is rather thicker. The arteries of the brain differ from those elsewhere in having only a single elastic lamina, which lies immediately outside the intima, and also in having only a very tenuous adventitia. Occasionally, too, their media is deficient, particularly at the points where the larger vessels give off their branches and where the

constituent vessels of the arterial circle of Willis unite: it is at these sites that the so-called congenital aneurysms are liable to form (see page 2179).[470]

The veins of the brain are in general similar in structure to veins elsewhere. The only peculiarity of the intracranial venous system is in the structure of the dural venous sinuses: their endothelial lining abuts directly on the tough fibrous tissue of the enclosing dural folds. The dural wall of certain sinuses is penetrated by small projections of the arachnoid: these are the arachnoid villi, through which the cerebrospinal fluid returns to the blood stream (see page 2198).

The Blood Supply to the Spinal Cord[471–473]

Three arterial trunks run the entire length of the spinal cord—the anterior spinal artery, formed inside the skull by the union of the anterior spinal branches of the right and left vertebral arteries, and the paired posterior spinal arteries, each of which is a branch of the corresponding posterior inferior cerebellar artery or of the vertebral artery itself. These three vessels are joined at intervals by from 7 to 10 branches of intercostal and lumbar arteries:[474] these feeder channels play an important part in maintaining the blood supply to the cord.

The arterial supply of the spinal cord in fact is a modification of the embryonic segmental supply: developmentally, the apparently continuous longitudinal vessels are no more than anastomotic channels between the segmental arteries. The blood flow is downward in the anterior spinal artery in the cervical region. Below this level the posterior branches of the spinal arteries, derived from the intercostal and lumbar arteries, accompany the nerve roots as the anterior and posterior radicular arteries: the extent to which these arteries supply the cord and the length and complexity of their course are very variable.

The spinal arteries are not always capable of providing an adequate anastomotic channel should one of the feeders be occluded: such an occurrence is, therefore, liable to be followed by segmental ischaemia of the cord and consequent paralysis.

Cerebral Vascular Lesions

Cerebral Atherosclerosis and Thrombosis

Obstruction of the lumen of a cerebral artery is usually due to the gradual enlargement of an atherosclerotic plaque—the immediate cause of complete occlusion is either intramural bleeding at the base of the plaque or, much oftener, thrombosis on its surface. Atherosclerosis tends to develop earlier in life in some arteries than in others: the internal carotid and vertebral arteries are likely to be affected first, followed by the basilar and middle cerebral arteries, and then by the posterior inferior cerebellar arteries (Fig. 34.76).[475] The other cerebral and cerebellar arteries are less liable to be affected (Fig. 34.77). Atherosclerotic changes appear first near the openings of branches or at the bifurcation of the vessels.

Thrombosis is particularly liable to develop in an atherosclerotic artery if there is a fall in blood pressure. This may occur in elderly people because of a sudden impairment of myocardial function, such as may result from coronary thrombosis; it may complicate general anaesthesia, and it may occur naturally when relaxing after a busy day, or during sleep. Patients whose blood clots unusually readily, for instance because of polycythaemia vera or because of some defect in the normal fibrinolytic activity of the plasma, are proner than others to develop cerebral arterial thrombosis. It seems likely, however, that in every case a defect in the endothelial covering of an atherosclerotic plaque initiates the formation of the thrombus.

Certain arteries, particularly the branches of the middle cerebral arteries, are liable to thrombosis, and the impediment to blood flow that results, although affecting perhaps only a small part of the

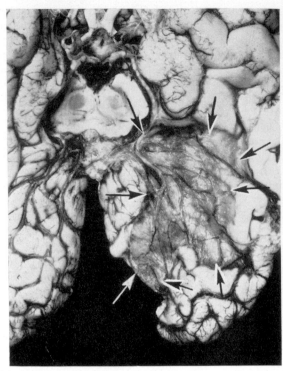

Fig. 34.77. Cerebral atherosclerosis, with an old area of infarction (outlined by arrows), due to thrombosis of the occipital branch of the left posterior cerebral artery. The anterior and left posterior communicating arteries are markedly atheromatous.

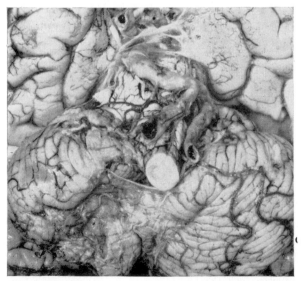

Fig. 34.76. Cerebral atherosclerosis. There is marked atheroma of the basilar artery, with an old ischaemic lesion in the territory of the right posterior inferior cerebellar artery.

brain, may cause serious incapacity. Indeed, the anatomical distribution of arteries in the brain is remarkably constant, and the functional disturbances that result from occlusion of their individual branches may be so well defined that the neurologist can say with confidence which vessel is concerned. Among the most important of these vessels is one of the striate branches (the so-called lenticulostriate branch) of the middle cerebral artery of each side: this vessel supplies the part of the internal capsule that is traversed by the axons of the motor cells in the precentral gyrus on their way to the anterior grey columns of the spinal cord. Occlusion of the striate portion of this artery suffices to destroy both the axons and the myelin sheaths in the affected part of the internal capsule, with consequent hemiplegia on the opposite side of the body (Fig. 34.78). The face, arm, trunk and leg may all be involved in this motor disorder; sensation is preserved because the afferent fibres are situated farther back in the internal capsule. The hemiplegia caused by thrombosis develops over a period of minutes, whereas that due to embolism is

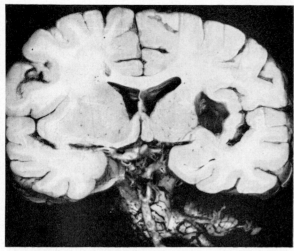

Fig. 34.78. Pseudocyst in the region of the external capsule, the result of thrombosis of one of the left striate arteries several years previously, giving rise to right-sided hemiplegia. There is also a small area of softening at the lateral extremity of the corpus callosum in the right hemisphere (on the left in the photograph). There is moderately severe atheroma of the basilar artery and of the arterial circle of Willis.

instantaneous. Once an infarct has developed, recovery of function in the infarcted tissue is not to be expected: the clinical improvement that is often observed during convalescence after a stroke is probably due to restoration of function in axons that had been temporarily paralysed by the swelling of the tissues in the vicinity of the infarct.

The hemiplegia that may occur in patients with tertiary syphilis in the third to fifth decade of life has a rather better prognosis than that complicating atherosclerosis: this is probably because the patients with syphilitic vascular disease are, on average, younger. Moreover, in syphilis the circulatory obstruction is, in part, the result of endarteritis and of oedema of the adventitia, both of which respond—the latter very quickly—to antisyphilitic treatment.

Cerebral atherosclerosis is often associated with atherosclerosis in other parts of the body, including the arteries of the limbs. Correlation between the occurrence of coronary atheroma and that of cerebral atheroma is usually close, although the severity of the disease tends to be greater in the former.[476] Occasionally, however, a person with marked involvement of the aorta and of the coronary arteries may have little or no disease of the cerebral arteries; the reverse may also be found. There is usually a close correlation between cerebral and retinal atherosclerosis. In a classic study of a group of patients with marked retinal athero-

sclerosis it was found that nearly half developed a cerebral vascular lesion within seven years of the discovery of the changes in the vessels in the eye.[477] Similarly, among patients admitted to hospital because of cerebral thrombosis or haemorrhage it was shown that 43 per cent had severe retinal atherosclerosis, 27 per cent had moderate or mild atherosclerosis, and the remaining 30 per cent had no apparent changes in their retinal vessels.[477]

Atheroma of the extracranial arteries is of paramount significance in the pathogenesis of cerebral infarction. Occlusion or a serious degree of stenosis was found in one or more of the major arteries in the neck in 58 of 100 cases with a clinical diagnosis of cerebral ischaemia.[478] In 18 the carotid arteries were affected alone and in 7 the vertebral arteries alone: in 33 both sets were affected. Infarcts were present in 35 of the 100 cases: these 35 cases between them presented a total of 74 separate cerebral infarcts. In all but 3 of the 35 there was significant stenosis (defined as a 50 per cent or greater reduction of the lumen) or occlusion of the extracranial arteries: in contrast, significant changes were found in the intracranial arteries in only 19 of the 35 cases (and the total of infarcts in these 19 was only 22). Significant disease of the intracranial arteries was lacking in no fewer than 16 (46 per cent) of the 35 cases with cerebral infarction. The most frequently diseased part of the internal carotid arteries was the sinus. In the vertebral arteries the atheroma was somewhat more widespread than in the carotids but generally involved the proximal 2 cm most constantly and severely. In 19 cases there was thrombotic occlusion of one or more extracranial arteries: cerebral infarction was present in all but four of these, and in two of the four it seemed probable that death had occurred before there had been time for gross changes to develop.

Distortion and obstruction of vertebral arteries can be produced or aggravated by osteoarthritis of the cervical spine.[479]

General factors that contribute to the occurrence of cerebral ischaemia include anaemia and loss of blood, hypoxia, hypotension and traumatic shock. Indeed, cerebral infarction rarely has a single cause: it is usually the outcome of a combination of the effects of systemic disease with circulatory inadequacy that affects the cerebral blood flow as a whole and that results from stenosis or total occlusion of extracranial or intracranial arteries, or of both, infarction being commoner in association with disease of the extracranial vessels.

The significance of incomplete stenosis in relation

to reduction in blood flow has been questioned as a result of experimental observation on the haemo-dynamic effects of increasing compression of the carotid artery.[480] It is possible that stenotic segments in the carotid and vertebral arteries in their cervical course may be likelier to predispose to thrombosis and embolus formation than simply to reduce blood flow by reason of the local narrowing of the lumen.

Occlusion of carotid or vertebral arteries may be found in patients who have shown neither clinical evidence of cerebral ischaemia nor necropsy evidence of infarction. Congenital and apparently symptomless anomalies of an internal carotid artery may be incidental findings at necropsy, even in old age. In such cases the development of ade-quate anastomotic channels is the determining factor: these are derived from three sources—the arterial circle, the meningeal anastomoses between the major arteries on the surface of the brain, and anastomoses between the internal and external carotid arteries. Collaterals develop much more effectively if the occlusion is gradual rather than sudden. The functional capacity of the arterial circle may be impaired by disease or by variations or anomalies[481] dating from early in development; congenital variations occur in at least 40 per cent of people. It is probable that occlusion of carotid or vertebral arteries is likeliest to cause infarction when the associated thrombosis leads to embolism, or when thrombus is propagated into the anterior and middle cerebral arteries or the basilar arteries, or when the other cervical arteries or the arterial circle are severely diseased or are affected by a significant developmental anomaly such as aplasia of an important segment.

Cerebral Embolism

Embolic occlusion of a cerebral artery is usually the result of thrombosis elsewhere. Five diseases are important in this connexion (see Chapters 1 and 3A): (1) infective endocarditis; (2) mitral stenosis complicated by thrombosis in the left atrium; (3) myocardial infarction, with thrombus formation on the endocardium covering the infarcted part; (4) thrombus formation on ulcerated atheromatous lesions in the aorta, or in the carotid sinus or the siphon (the petrous part of the internal carotid), in the vertebral or basilar arteries, or at points of branching of the arterial circle;[482] and (5) 'myxoma' of the left atrium.[483] The great majority of such emboli exert their effect solely through mechanical obstruction at the site where they lodge; sometimes,

as in cases of acute bacterial endocarditis, the embolus may contain pyogenic organisms and the resulting infarct may quickly become transformed into an abscess. Exceptionally, a thrombotic embolus reaching the heart from the systemic veins may pass through a patent foramen ovale to enter the systemic arterial circulation ('paradoxical em-bolism'). Cerebral emboli may originate in throm-botic lesions in the ascending portion of the aorta or in its arch, or in the carotid or vertebral arteries. Among the less common forms of emboli that may obstruct the cerebral blood vessels are aggregates of cancer cells, larvae of metazoal parasites, fat droplets, cholesterol crystals, gas bubbles, cotton fragments from swabs used to clean vascular catheters and, in cases of amniotic embolism (Fig. 34.79), clumps of epidermal squames and meco-nium.

The site of lodgement of an embolus will depend almost wholly on its size. Fragments of thrombus from the chambers of the heart are usually com-paratively large and are, therefore, likely to be held up in a main cerebral artery, particularly the middle cerebral artery or one of its larger branches. Smaller branches are specially liable to be involved when comparatively small fragments are detached from the vegetations in cases of infective endo-carditis of the mitral or aortic valve; in contrast, a larger embolus may block the main trunk of the artery itself, causing immediate hemiplegia and hemianaesthesia, and possibly hemianopia and vestibular disturbances—dysphasia will also result if the occluded artery is on the side of the dominant hemisphere (the left hemisphere in right-handed people). Sometimes, after an initial manifestation of embolism, there is a sudden improvement in the patient's condition, with disappearance of some of the symptoms, although leaving, perhaps, hemi-plegia and dysphasia. This amelioration may be explained by shrinkage of the embolus and perhaps also by relaxation of local arterial spasm: these changes allow the embolus to be driven farther into the vascular tree, thus re-establishing some circula-tion through a part of the brain that was, initially, ischaemic. Functional recovery in an area that has had its circulation restored in this way is only possible if the occlusion has been partial, and if the interval of time between the initial obstruction and the onward movement of the embolus has been so short that oxygen lack has not permanently damaged the neurons (see page 2097).

The smaller emboli tend to be arrested near to the junction of the grey and white matter of the cerebral hemispheres ('boundary zone lesions'), where the

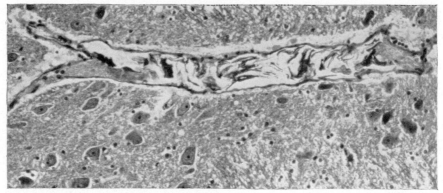

Fig. 34.79.§ Amniotic fluid embolism. A small vessel in the region of the nuclei pontis is plugged with desquamated fetal epithelium. Death occurred suddenly during the second stage of labour. *Haematoxylin–eosin.* × 150.

small cortical arteries, having passed through the grey matter, break up into their branches. This anatomical feature also accounts for the particular frequency with which pyaemic abscesses and secondary deposits of carcinoma are found in this boundary zone, which, for the same reason, is the most frequent site for the development of cysticerci (see page 2137).

A tendency for emboli to fragment and move farther distally in the vascular tree has an influence on the occurrence and course of oligaemia and on the extent of infarction. Fragmentation of emboli has been observed ophthalmoscopically in the retinal circulation during cerebral ischaemic episodes. Such emboli in the brain or retinae may be associated with transient clinical abnormalities that may clear completely, or clear and subsequently recur, sometimes in the same clinical form. Other transient attacks may not be associated with alteration in vascular patency but result from failure of the local homoeostasis. For instance, if artery walls are rigid as a result of disease, active compensatory changes may not be possible in the event of systemic hypotension or of a fall in cardiac output, or when the viscosity of the blood is increased or there is severe anaemia: the result may be a devastating haemodynamic crisis.

Infarcts of the Brain

A study published in 1964 showed that in the course of the five preceding years cerebral infarction had become commoner than cerebral haemorrhage as the cause of a 'stroke'.[484] In the 1930s haemorrhage was three times more frequent than infarction. The frequency of cerebral infarction rose abruptly in the period 1947–55, in notable contrast to the reduction in the number of cases of infarction in all the age groups at risk during most of the war years (1940–45). The war-time fall may have been due to suppression of atherosclerosis-induced thrombosis by the introduction (or removal) of some rapidly acting factor during those years: dietary changes are an obvious possibility, and stress and physical activity are among other possible factors. An increased awareness of the conditions that predispose to hypertension—for example, renal disease—and better treatment of hypertension have probably helped to reduce the incidence of cerebral haemorrhage over the past 30 years.

Cerebral infarction may be due to embolism, thrombosis and, perhaps, arterial spasm.

The occurrence of cerebral arterial thrombosis and infarction in otherwise healthy young women who have been taking oral contraceptive drugs has been reported with increasing frequency in recent years.[485–487] Although it has been disputed that these hormonal preparations are directly responsible for inducing such arterial occlusion,[488] controlled retrospective studies have indicated that women who take them face a sixfold increase in the risk of cerebral thrombosis.[487] Occlusion of the vertebral and basilar arteries has been particularly frequent under these conditions. Thirty-five per cent of thrombotic strokes in women aged from 15 to 44 have been attributed to oral contraceptives.[489] The evidence is still incomplete and it is important that material from fatal cases should be made available for neuropathological study whenever this is possible.

A fresh cerebral infarct appears at necropsy as a swollen, reddish area, spherical or ovoid in shape and softer than the surrounding brain: the comparative softness of the infarcted tissue becomes more apparent after the brain has been fixed in formalin. In the course of a few weeks the infarct shrinks, its margin becomes sharper, its central parts soften further and liquefy, and a yellow, gelatinous material occupies the resulting cavity. Eventually the infarcted tissue is replaced by a cyst-like space containing clear, yellow fluid.

Recent cortical infarcts are usually characterized by the presence of numerous minute foci of congestion on the surface of the affected convolutions and throughout their substance. Microscopically, there is engorgement of the arterioles and venules, and neutrophils and erythrocytes fill the circumvascular space; the nerve cells show varying degrees of ischaemic change. When, with time, the infarcted part of the cortex becomes completely softened, a thin layer of living tissue may remain immediately beneath the pia mater, separated from the subcortical white matter by a shrunken zone of necrotic tissue. The nerve cells disappear in the infarcted part (Fig. 34.80), and there is an accumu-

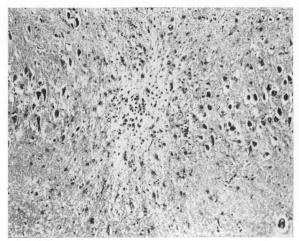

Fig. 34.81. Cerebral ischaemia due to atherosclerosis. There is a minute infarct involving the pyramidal cell layer of the hippocampus following occlusion of a small vessel. Nerve cells have been destroyed. Many of the Hortega cells that have migrated into the infarct contain haemosiderin, indicating that there has been a small leakage of blood. *Haematoxylin–eosin.* × 100.

lation of Hortega cells laden with fat or haemosiderin (Fig. 34.81).

Infarcts in the white matter may be multiple, giving rise to confluent foci of myelin loss that macroscopically resemble patches of diffuse sclerosis.

'Venous Infarcts'.[490]—Ischaemic changes in the cortex are sometimes the result of thrombosis of cerebral veins. The venous thrombosis may occur without other evidence of vascular disease, for instance in cases of polycythaemia vera or other conditions in which spontaneous coagulation of the blood is liable to occur. In other cases, cerebral venous thrombosis results from retrograde extension of thrombosis in the major dural sinuses (Fig. 34.82).

There are many causes of thrombosis of the dural sinuses and cerebral veins.[490] The condition may be secondary to otitis media, mastoiditis, meningitis, infection of the scalp or face, and bacteriaemia. It may complicate pregnancy or the puerperium, marantic states, head injuries and neurosurgical procedures. Oral contraceptive drugs have also been implicated.[491, 492]

Binswanger's Disease (Fig. 34.83).—Binswanger described a rare form of vascular encephalopathy associated with arterial hypertension and characterized by areas of ischaemic softening that may be confined to the white matter of the occipital and

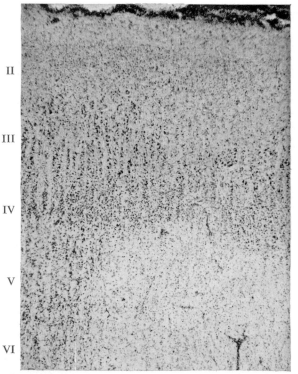

II

III

IV

V

VI

Fig. 34.80. Focal cortical infarction. There is a localized area of nerve cell loss in lamina V of the frontal cortex: only glial nuclei and blood vessels survive. This patient died of widespread cerebral ischaemia seven days after a subarachnoid haemorrhage. The Roman numerals indicate the cortical laminae. *Celloidin section. Nissl's stain.* × 30.

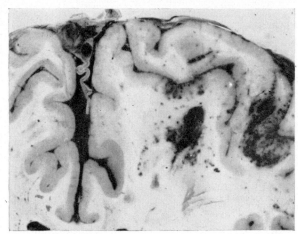

Fig. 34.82. Thrombosis of the superior sagittal sinus. This developed in a young woman one week after parturition. She died six days later. The haemorrhagic infarction in adjacent gyri involves both grey and white matter.

temporal lobes.[493] This condition is due in all probability to continued impoverishment of the white matter resulting from both a severe degree of atheroma of its nutrient blood vessels and a sudden, sustained episode of systemic hypotension. Other associations of causal factors, such as porphyria with atheroma, have been described.[494]

Infarcts of the Spinal Cord[471, 472]

Infarction of the thoracic or lumbar segments of the spinal cord may result when intercostal arteries are occluded by a dissecting aneurysm of the aorta. The whole cross-section of the cord may be involved, but the central grey matter is especially vulnerable. More localized infarction may follow occlusion of the anterior spinal artery, and this is especially likely to affect the upper part of the cord: in these cases, the posterior funiculi are spared. Thrombosis of the superficial veins[495] results in infarction of the white matter of the cord, often with sparing of the central grey matter: this condition has to be distinguished from involvement of the cord by an acute demyelinating disease.

Infarction in the distribution of the anterior or posterior spinal arteries can occur without occlusion of these arteries when the circulation in the larger radicular arteries that supply them is deficient, as may result from aortic disease involving the ostia of the intercostal or lumbar arteries or from embolism or surgical interference. Infarction may be precipitated by prolonged hypotension when the arterial supply is inadequate. When arterial in-

sufficiency is less severe focal microcavitation may result from local ischaemia.

Cerebral Arterial Haemorrhage

Massive haemorrhage into the substance of the brain is principally a disease of late middle age; it is usually associated with systemic arterial hypertension. The wall of a healthy artery does not give way under the force exerted on it by the blood inside, however high this pressure may be: rupture occurs only if there is some weakness in the arterial wall, the result either of a congenital defect or of an acquired disease—atherosclerosis is much the most important of these predisposing causes. It should be remembered that bleeding may also take place into a pre-existing lesion of the brain, such as a primary or secondary neoplasm, or an abscess or other focal infective lesion, the presence of which may be masked by the resulting clot; it is important, therefore, to search any clot for traces of a predisposing

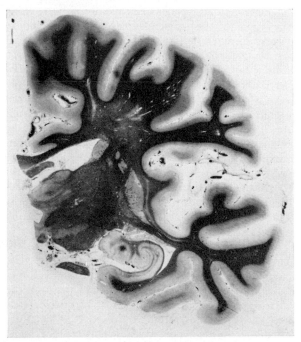

Fig. 34.83. Cerebral atherosclerosis. The patient, a woman of 52, was hypertensive. She had been admitted to hospital four years before death on account of depression, slurred speech and hemiplegia. She had a Parkinsonian facies. Streaky areas of demyelination in the centrum semiovale represent old haemorrhages. There is also more widespread demyelination. This combination of atrophy of white matter with extensive myelin loss and severe arterial degeneration, especially of the vessels in the white matter, is sometimes known as Binswanger's disease. *Celloidin section. Heiden-hain's stain.*

lesion, and material that has been evacuated surgically from a cerebral haematoma must always be carefully examined in the laboratory. More rarely, bleeding originates in a vascular hamartoma (see page 2181).

The commonest sites of haemorrhage in the brain: are (1) the lentiform nucleus (the so-called capsular haemorrhage, which usually comes from Charcot's 'artery of cerebral haemorrhage'—the 'lenticulostriate branch' of the middle cerebral artery); (2) the pons; and (3) the white matter of the cerebellum. Once bleeding begins it tends to track through the brain substance along the paths of least resistance; thus, a haemorrhage in the internal capsule extends down toward the brainstem, separating the fibres of the white matter. Alternatively, the haemorrhage may break into one of the lateral ventricles or the subarachnoid space.

Secondary brainstem haemorrhage should be distinguished from primary haemorrhage into the pons. Midbrain or pontine haemorrhages may be continuous with a primary massive intracerebral haematoma that has tracked caudally, usually along the line of the corticospinal tracts. Secondary brainstem haemorrhage can also result from circulatory disturbances induced by the presence of a primary intracerebral haematoma. Two sequelae of the latter are likely to throw an added stress on the vessels of the midbrain and pons: first, as a consequence of the rapid rise in supratentorial pressure that follows the initial haemorrhage there may be ischaemia of the vasomotor nuclei in the brainstem, resulting in further reflex elevation of the systemic blood pressure; second, deformation of the brainstem, resulting from its caudal displacement or from tentorial herniation, may impair the venous outflow or overstretch small perforating arteries.

It is unusual for a patient who has had a massive cerebral haemorrhage to survive for long. The haematoma grows progressively, although sometimes slowly, and eventually ruptures through the cortex or, more commonly, into a ventricle. This may happen within minutes of the onset of bleeding, or it may be delayed, occasionally even for some days. Haemorrhage within the substance of the brain is one of the causes of the presence of blood in the cerebrospinal fluid.

Signs of former small haemorrhages are sometimes found in the white matter in cases of cerebral atherosclerosis. Generally, these are subcortical and extend along the lines of the fibres. Macroscopically, they appear as red streaks or as yellow haematoidin-containing foci ('taches jaunes'). Histo-logically, there is clear evidence of earlier bleeding, for haemosiderin-laden phagocytes are present in large numbers, especially in the Virchow–Robin space. Another not infrequent finding is a glial scar along the transcortical part of the course of a penetrating artery that earlier has been occluded by a thrombus: collections of macrophages containing haemosiderin surround such vessels. The sites of these scars are often indicated by dimpling on the surface of the convolutions; if numerous, the surface of the cortex acquires a worm-eaten appearance ('état vermoulu').[496] This appearance is generally a result of hypertension, and the meningeal arterioles then show some degree of thickening.

Several theories have been offered to explain the mechanism of massive cerebral haemorrhage; in fact, the pathogenesis may well differ with age. It has been suggested that some haemorrhages follow thrombosis of an atherosclerotic artery, for the infarct that results from the thrombosis would be likely to deprive the adjacent unoccluded arteries and arterioles of external mechanical support, and thus weaken their resistance to the potentially disruptive force of the blood pressure. Such a sequence must be unusual, however, for a massive cerebral haemorrhage is rarely preceded, even briefly, by hemiparesis or other signs of vascular occlusion. The typical history in a case of cerebral haemorrhage is that an ingravescent coma has developed and been succeeded within a few hours by hemiplegia: this sequence is consistent with leakage of blood from a vessel and the gradual development of a haematoma.

Charcot and Bouchard,[496a] in 1868, were the first to claim that massive cerebral haemorrhage is the result of rupture of saccular aneurysms of miliary size; their observation has been confirmed repeatedly.[497–499] Others,[500] however, have concluded that the lesions described by Charcot and Bouchard were mainly 'false' aneurysms and that Green[497] in 1930 was the first to recognize the occurrence of true microaneurysms on the vessels concerned in such haemorrhages. Such lesions are likely to be destroyed by the haemorrhage and they are very difficult to demonstrate in ordinary histological preparations: they are best shown in their unruptured state by radiography after injecting the cerebral vessels with radio-opaque material.

It has been shown at necropsy that about 50 per cent of hypertensive patients have such microaneurysms compared with about 5 per cent of those who are normotensive.[501–503] The development of aneurysms is also related to age: 70 per cent of hypertensive patients aged from 60 to 65 have aneurysms in contrast to only 5 per cent of those under 50. Aneurysms were found in only 5 per cent of normotensive patients and then only among those over 65. No quantitative (histometric) differences have been demonstrated between the arteries of hypertensive patients with aneurysms and those of hypertensive patients without aneurysms, other than the presence of the aneurysms themselves.[504] Thickening of the media in hypertensive arteries is not related to age: however, the aneurysms are believed to result from the localized degeneration of the media, with loss of muscle and elastica, that occurs in older hypertensive patients (those aged over 50 years).

Cerebral arterial degeneration secondary to hypertension has been described by many authors.[505-507] The changes range from focal medial fibrosis to fibrinoid degeneration and necrosis: the latter changes are characteristic of the malignant phase of hypertension and most frequently affect the vessels in the pons, thus accounting for the relatively high incidence of primary pontine haemorrhage in cases of malignant hypertension.

Monoamine oxidase inhibitors have been blamed for some instances of cerebral and subarachnoid haemorrhage.[508] The bleeding in such cases is believed to result from a hypertensive crisis: this may be precipitated by sympathomimetic drugs, such as ephedrine, amphetamine and phenylpropanolamine, by imipramine, and by tyramine-rich foods, such as cheese, bean pods and yeast extracts, and some wines (particularly, it is said, Chianti). Tranylcypromine and other non-hydrazine monoamine oxidase inhibitors are likelier than the hydrazine derivates, such as phenelzine, to lead to this complication.[509]

Aneurysms of the Cerebral Arteries

Saccular aneurysms of cerebral arteries may arise in two ways: first, as a consequence of a defect in the arterial wall, often in association with atherosclerosis; and, second, following the lodgement of an infected embolus, such as may come from the heart valves in cases of infective endocarditis (the so-called 'mycotic aneurysm').

Fusiform aneurysms of the cerebral vasculature also occur, involving especially the basilar and internal carotid arteries.

'Berry' Aneurysms

The so-called 'berry aneurysms' are often regarded as congenital in origin, as was first suggested by Eppinger in 1887.[510] Turnbull described an instance in a child under the age of two years.[510a] They develop almost invariably at the bifurcation of arteries, and it is at such sites that the elastic lamina and the muscular coat may be defective or even absent. However, aneurysms are rare in comparison with the great frequency of such structural defects,[511] and it is necessary to look for some additional factor that may determine the development of the aneurysms at these sites of weakness. Similar defects have been recognized in extracranial arteries in man and in animals, but the development of aneurysms as a consequence of this anomaly is exceptionally rare outside the cerebral vasculature. It has been suggested that the determining factor is an acquired focal degeneration of the elastic elements in the congenitally defective vessel wall.[511] The importance of atheroma has been stressed and it has been noted that the incidence of the condition remains much the same from the fifth to the eighth decade.[470] In contrast, it has been considered that the majority of these aneurysms are due to an inherent congenital weakness and that atherosclerosis plays only a small role.[512]

There is a case for considering that most berry aneurysms may be acquired.[513, 514] The small congenital defects that are found in the media of cerebral arteries in the fetus differ from the larger defects in the arteries of adults that are believed to be the origin of the aneurysms. Small defects, which are numerous and apparently become more so with increasing age, occur throughout the arterial circle of Willis and are most frequent at the outer angles of the bifurcation of the vessels. In contrast, large defects are infrequent, particularly in the posterior part of the arterial circle, and they are situated mainly in the angle between the branches at the sites of bifurcation: it is here that berry aneurysms characteristically occur.

The age at which aneurysms are found favours an acquired origin: the mean age is 50, and only 20 per cent of the patients are under 40 and very few under 20.

It is possible that the relative importance of three factors—developmental weakness, atherosclerosis and hypertension—varies at different ages.[515] Subarachnoid haemorrhage from a berry aneurysm may occur in adolescents and young adults in the absence of local atherosclerosis. The possible importance of transient arterial hypertension is indicated by the frequency with which rupture of an aneurysm takes place during physical exertion or at a time of emotion, especially in young adults.[516]

Cerebral aneurysms may be multiple. Very rarely they are associated with aneurysms of the mesenteric or splenic arteries, or with other congenital anomalies, such as coarctation of the aorta or polycystic disease of the kidneys. Sometimes they are incidental necropsy findings. They occur most frequently on a middle cerebral artery, either at its origin from the internal carotid artery or where it branches, but they may be found in any situation on the arterial circle (Fig. 34.84) and on

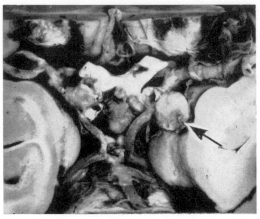

Fig. 34.84. Aneurysm (arrow) situated between the left internal carotid and posterior communicating arteries, pressing on and deforming the uncus. There are patches of atheroma in all the vessels of the arterial circle of Willis.

the larger vessels that join or leave the circle. The anterior cerebral arteries and the anterior communicating artery are more frequently involved than the posterior cerebral and posterior communicating arteries.

Intracranial aneurysms are the source of most subarachnoid haemorrhages. At operation, or at necropsy, the leaking aneurysm may be about a millimetre across, or, especially if there have been recurrent episodes of bleeding and thrombosis, its diameter may reach 2 cm or more. If the aneurysm is pedunculate the surgeon may be able to ligate its neck: oftener, however, it is sessile. At necropsy the aneurysm is not always apparent, because the blood in the subarachnoid space tends to hide it. As the search for the site of haemorrhage will be made still more difficult once the blood has been hardened by fixation of the brain in formalin, it is best to open the arachnoid membrane before fixation and wash the blood very gently from the subarachnoid space.

The aneurysm from which the bleeding has occurred may be collapsed, soft and flabby, or it may have a firm wall and be partly filled by laminated thrombus. Sometimes the tear in its wall may be obvious, and there may even be clot protruding through it. The haemorrhage may track into the substance of the brain itself. Histological study of the wall of the aneurysm near the point of rupture usually shows only a thin, collagenous membrane, devoid of muscle or elastic tissue.

Thrombosis may spread from the sac of an aneurysm into the artery from which it developed: cerebral infarction will then result.

The mortality of a first episode of subarachnoid haemorrhage is from 25 to 50 per cent: death usually occurs on about the ninth day.[517, 518] Many of those patients who survive the initial haemorrhage have a recurrence, usually within two weeks, and the second episode has a greater mortality than the first. The prognosis worsens with increasing age.[519]

The main consequences of rupture of berry aneurysms, apart from subarachnoid bleeding, are intracerebral haematoma and infarction of the brain.[520, 521] An *intracerebral haematoma* results either from direct rupture of an adherent aneurysm into the brain or from secondary extension of bleeding from the site of a subarachnoid clot; rupture into the brain occurs more frequently in cases of recurrent subarachnoid haemorrhage and the prognosis is thus particularly poor, fatal coma often resulting. The occurrence of *cerebral infarction* following rupture of a cerebral aneurysm was overlooked until comparatively recently:[520, 522–525] the lesions are patchy and easily escape recognition in the unfixed brain; they are most numerous in the territory of the aneurysm-bearing artery but may occur elsewhere, even in the opposite hemisphere. The cause of the infarcts is not established: factors such as secondary vasospasm, arterial compression by subarachnoid haematomas and the effects of anaesthetic drugs or arteriography have been considered—indeed, multiple and varying factors may well be involved. The infarcts have a notably adverse effect on prognosis; they are also an important cause of residual disabilities, which are observed in as many as 70 per cent of the patients who survive. It has been suggested that vasoconstrictor substances, such as serotonin, are released from subarachnoid clots and induce spasm,[526] and that antivasospastic drugs may therefore be of use in some cases: experimental studies have not substantiated this.[527]

Mycotic Aneurysms

When an embolus contains bacteria of low virulence, such as *Streptococcus viridans* in vegetations detached from the heart valves in subacute infective endocarditis, it is exceptionally rare for an infective lesion to develop at the site of impaction. However, if the organisms succeed in colonizing the thrombus that forms in the lumen of the occluded artery proximal to the embolus itself, the resulting focus of infection may lead to weakening of a small segment of the arterial wall and the local development of a saccular aneurysm (the so-called mycotic aneurysm—see pages 37 and 147, Volume 1). Mycotic aneurysms may also form as the result of impaction of infected emboli that originate in thrombosed pulmonary venules in cases of empyema or pulmonary suppuration.

Rupture of a mycotic aneurysm of a cerebral artery results in haemorrhage, which generally proves fatal. At necropsy, it may be difficult to find the sac.

This diagnosis must be considered in any case of intracranial haemorrhage, particularly when there is evidence of bacterial infection of the heart, lungs or pleurae.

Fusiform Aneurysms

The internal carotid and basilar arteries are specially liable to atherosclerosis, and in severe cases this may lead to much tortuosity and dilatation, amounting sometimes to the formation of a fusiform aneurysm (Fig. 3.15, page 129, Volume 1). This type of dilatation predisposes to thrombosis.

Dissecting Aneurysms[528–530]

Dissecting aneurysms of cerebral arteries result from haemorrhage between the media and the intima, with extension of the bleeding along the plane of cleavage. The dissection is usually accompanied by thrombotic occlusion of the arterial lumen. Infarction of the tissue supplied by the affected vessel follows in most cases. The middle cerebral artery is most frequently involved. Young adults and children account for a considerable proportion of the patients. In some cases hypertension, atherosclerosis, syphilis or trauma have been cited as causal agents: in others no such factors are identified and in general the cause of the condition remains unknown. The plane of cleavage is different from that in aortic dissecting aneurysms, in which the dissection is within the media.

Dissecting aneurysm of a cerebral artery is readily overlooked. The frequency of secondary thrombosis in the lumen accounts for the large proportion of cases in which the outer limit of the cleavage plane is mistaken for the periphery of the true lumen. Careful histological study of thrombosed cerebral arteries, with awareness of the need to make this distinction, is required: this is particularly so in the case of young patients dying with cerebral infarction.

Vascular Malformations

There is a group of benign tumour-like lesions that are the result of faults in the embryonic development of the vasculature of the meninges and brain. These hamartomas* are sometimes of no apparent importance. In other instances they undergo thrombosis and occasionally they are the source of intracranial bleeding.

Meningocerebral Vascular Hamartomas. — The angiomatoid hamartomas of the brain are composed of closely packed blood vessels so intricately intertwined that they have been likened to a tangle of worms. Capillary and cavernous haemangiomas of the type commonly seen in the skin and the liver are rarely found in the brain. The vessels forming the meningocerebral hamartomas usually have thin walls, composed of fibrous tissue and lined by normal-looking endothelium. Glial tissue intervenes between them, and corpora amylacea and foci of calcification are often present among the glial fibres. Occasionally, the vessels have thick walls, which may then contain smooth muscle; elastic fibres are usually sparse.

These congeries of vessels are generally buried within the substance of the cerebral cortex; they maintain an attachment to the pia deep in a sulcus in their immediate vicinity. They occur most frequently in the territory of the middle cerebral artery (Fig. 34.85). Over the years they tend to enlarge, but this seems to be the outcome more of slow, passive distension of the vascular channels than of proliferative growth. Slowing of the blood flow and thrombosis commonly follow. Thrombosis is succeeded by organization, and, in the course of the latter, fibrosis may extend for a short distance into the surrounding brain substance: this small collagenous and glial scar may provoke epileptic attacks. Foci of calcification may be found in the brain adjoining the affected parts.

* The name hamartoma was coined by Albrecht to denote any benign tumour-like mass that is formed of a mixture of differentiated tissues of the types that are normally constituents of the part in which the lesion is present (Albrecht, P., *Verh. dtsch. path. Ges.*, 1904, **7**, 153).

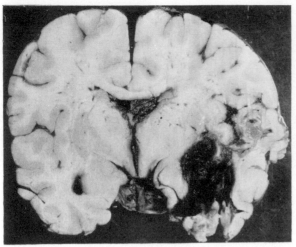

Fig. 34.85. Intracerebral angioma. Fatal bleeding resulted from rupture of the angioma (which can be seen above and lateral to the haemorrhage, situated in the distribution of the left middle cerebral artery). These malformations are often deep-seated, but always attached to the leptomeninges. The brain is swollen, the surface being flattened and the ventricular cavities (which contain blood) diminished and distorted. There is herniation of the left cingulate gyrus toward the other side below the level of the falx.

These angiomatoid malformations are often amenable to surgical removal, but the surgeon must be prepared to find that the extent of cortical involvement is considerably greater than the clinical manifestations suggest.

Sturge–Kalischer–Weber Syndrome.[531, 531a] — The association of a vascular hamartoma—usually a 'port wine naevus'—in the skin of the face or scalp with a developmental vascular anomaly of the leptomeninges on the same side was first recognized by Sturge,[531b] in 1879, and by Kalischer,[531c] in 1897. General recognition of the syndrome dates from the account by Parkes Weber in 1929.[532] The intracranial lesion usually takes the form of a superficial capillary or venous malformation, confined to the leptomeninges and most frequently situated over the posterior half of the cerebrum, particularly over the vertex. The condition may be associated with abnormal tortuosity of the retinal vessels or with the presence of retinal angiomas (see von Hippel–Lindau disease, Chapter 40, Volume 6).

Cobb's Syndrome.—Cobb's syndrome[533] is a condition comparable to the Sturge–Kalischer–Weber syndrome, but involving the spinal cord. The meningeal vascular malformation is in the pia-arachnoid over part of the cord, and the accompanying cutaneous naevus is in the territory innervated by one or more of the corresponding spinal nerve roots.

Telangiectases.—Small collections of dilated capillaries or venules are occasionally found in the substance of the brain. They occur particularly in the white matter, including the corpus callosum, but may be found anywhere in the brain. A notable site is the pons, a fact that may be relevant to the pathogenesis of some cases of pontine haemorrhage.

Arteritis

Giant Cell Arteritis ('Temporal Arteritis')[534]

In a proportion of cases of giant cell arteritis (see page 140*) there is involvement of the vertebral arteries, or of intracranial arteries, particularly the posterior cerebral arteries: this may result in infarction of part of the brain. Blindness is a common complication of this disease:[535] it may result from arteritis of the retinal arteries or from ischaemic changes in the optic pathways in the brain. The association of 'polymyalgia rheumatica' ('polymyalgia arteritica') with giant cell arteritis is mentioned on page 2371.

Polyarteritis

Involvement of the cerebral arteries is said to occur in nearly a quarter of all cases of polyarteritis[536] (see page 142*), but it is not always conspicuous. In fact, the relative infrequency of lesions in the central nervous system contrasts with the often heavy involvement of the nutrient arteries of the major nerve trunks of the limbs (see page 2310).

Thromboangitis Obliterans

The cerebral vasculature is affected in exceptional cases of thromboangitis obliterans (Buerger's disease —see page 138*). The changes in the vessels at the surface of the brain are unlikely to be overlooked: the affected vessels appear prominent and are remarkably firm to the touch. A distinctive type of cortical atrophy may develop in the brain in these cases, involving specially the boundary zones between the areas supplied by the main cerebral arteries.[537]

Purpuric Conditions Affecting the Brain

Thrombotic Thrombocytopenic Purpura

The bizarre, fluctuating neurological signs that complete the pathognomonic clinical tetrad of thrombotic thrombocytopenic purpura are the

* In Volume 1.

manifestations of transitory episodes of focal ischaemia caused by the typical thrombotic micro-angiopathy; their tendency to be evanescent is explained by the partial restoration of the circulation that accompanies retraction of the obstructive platelet thrombi. The other components of the tetrad are the acute febrile course of the illness, haemolytic anaemia and thrombocytopenic purpura (see page 493, Volume 2).[538] The characteristic vascular lesions (Figs 8.40A and 8.40B, page 494) are almost confined to the grey matter.[539]

'Brain Purpura'

'Brain purpura' is a non-specific descriptive term, applicable to any condition of the brain that is characterized by the occurrence of multiple petechial haemorrhages. The petechiae may be numerous or few. They are usually confined to the white matter, a feature that has been attributed to the supposedly greater fragility of the capillaries in this tissue.

There are many causes of petechial haemorrhages in the brain. *Cerebral malaria* (page 2136), *acute haemorrhagic leucoencephalitis* (page 2252) and *thrombotic thrombocytopenic purpura* (above) are notable examples. There are usually quite widespread petechiae in the brain in fatal cases of *hypertensive encephalopathy*: experimental evidence[540, 541] supports the view that these are the result of a combination of factors—vascular spasm, increased capillary permeability, focal oedema, fits and hypoxia. *Fat embolism* is another cause (see page 2194): the presence of fat emboli can be confirmed at necropsy by examining frozen sections stained with one of the Sudan dyes. Petechiae are often present in the brain after a severe *injury to the head*, but in such cases they tend to be localized, occurring particularly in the posterior part of the corpus callosum (see page 2187); they are usually associated with contusions to the surface of the brain. Petechial haemorrhages in the brain due to a head injury may, of course, be accompanied by others due to fat embolism complicating fractures of bones elsewhere.

Brain purpura may be due to *viral infection*, and efforts to isolate a virus should always be made in any case in which there is no obvious cause for the petechiae.

Petechial haemorrhages may result from *poisoning*, for example by carbon monoxide or by phosphorus. They may also occur in eclampsia and uraemia.

Allergic sensitivity to drugs is another infrequent but important cause. Of drugs in current use, penicillin is probably the one best known to have such an effect. Formerly, this type of drug-induced encephalopathy was most frequently a complication of treatment with certain organic arsenicals, particularly neoarsphenamine, which was widely used in the treatment of syphilis and some other diseases in the days before the introduction of the antibiotics. As in haemorrhagic leucoencephalitis, the underlying lesion is necrosis of the walls of small blood vessels, particularly venules (see page 2252).

Brain purpura may also be a manifestation of a general state of *hypoxia*, but petechiae are less frequent in the brain in such cases than in the epicardium and pleurae. Petechiae also occur in cases of the primary and secondary forms of *thrombocytopenic purpura*, and in certain other disorders of the blood, notably *leukaemia*. Very rarely, *anticoagulant therapy* may be complicated by brain purpura, which, in exceptional cases, becomes confluent and leads to death. It may be noted here that, in general, patients under treatment with anticoagulants are no more liable to suffer haemorrhage into the brain or its coverings than other people: however, when bleeding occurs from other causes, including vascular disease and trauma, it is likely to be more extensive and progressive.

Widespread petechiae may appear in the brain in some cases of *convulsions*: they may be found, for instance, when death has occurred during electroconvulsive therapy,[542, 543] or after the administration of convulsant drugs. They are unusual, however, when convulsions have been a manifestation of hypoglycaemia or of status epilepticus in idiopathic epilepsy.

EFFECTS OF TRAUMA ON THE CENTRAL NERVOUS SYSTEM[544–548]

The brain and spinal cord are encased in bone, cradled by the dural membrane and tentorium, and cushioned by the cerebrospinal fluid: they thus have a threefold natural protection from all but

the severest injuries.* If violence is sufficiently severe to fracture the skull or vertebral column and

* A fourth line of protection, in the form of a crash helmet, is a legal requirement for the motor cyclist in the

tear the dura mater, laceration of the brain or cord may result from the penetration of a foreign body or fragment of bone, with the likelihood of haemorrhage and infection. Even if the dura is untorn, and even when the skull is unfractured, there may be serious bleeding, and this may be mainly superficial to the dura or mainly deep to it: haemorrhage in the latter situation (*subdural haemorrhage*) is the more usual, and results from a tear at a point where a cerebral vein opens into one of the dural sinuses. An *extradural haemorrhage* is due to tearing of one of the meningeal arteries, usually the middle meningeal artery, where it lies in its bony canal. Injury to the middle meningeal artery is commonly associated with a fracture; for instance, it is sometimes the result of a blow on the side of the head, such as may happen to boys on the games field: inattention to the possibility of this complication has cost the lives of many children.

Whether or not the skull is cracked, there is at the instant of its impact with an unyielding object a very great rise in intracranial pressure, and a spread of pressure waves throughout the brain, which, although of momentary duration, may cause widespread damage to delicate blood vessels, and consequent injury to the glial cells and neurons dependent upon them. Experiments on dogs have shown that the increase of pressure inside the skull as a result of an impact may be from 1 to 7 kg per square centimetre.[549] This stress accounts for the fact that damage to the brain is often greater in a closed head injury than had been expected: failure to demonstrate a fracture of the skull does not exclude the possibility that an injury has caused serious intracranial damage.

Concussion

There have been many explanations offered for the instantaneous and profound loss of consciousness that occurs in so many cases of severe head injury. Some authors have postulated that concussion is a manifestation of ischaemia caused by paralysis of the cerebral vasculature, which may be directly due to the physical shock or the result of a reflex inhibition of vasomotor tone. The latter possibility seems unlikely in view of the paucity of vaso-

constrictor nerves to the cerebral blood vessels. Injection studies made on brains freshly removed after death in cases of concussion have demonstrated foci in which the capillaries have failed to fill with the perfused fluid; it has been supposed that these foci, which are distributed irregularly throughout the grey matter, represent sites of ischaemia caused in some unexplained way by the injury, but this suggestion is controversial.

The frequent finding of red cells and plasma in the circumvascular space, especially in the white matter, suggests that rupture of capillaries may be a widespread occurrence at the time of injury (Figs 34.86 and 34.87). It seems unlikely, however, that cerebral vascular disturbances can account for the instantaneous loss of consciousness; it has, therefore, been suggested that unconsciousness is the result of actual physical jolting of the neurons themselves.[550] Consciousness is lost immediately if a fast moving pendulum is allowed to strike and push forward the head of an animal; when the head is fixed, and therefore fails to move, consciousness is not lost.[551] Under these conditions concussion is attributable to the effect of the abrupt acceleration of the head (*acceleration concussion*).

Electroencephalographic studies on animals subjected to head injury under experimental conditions show that from the instant of impact all electrical activity ceases, and that it does not return until consciousness is recovered. Disturbance of the normal polarity of the neurons has been suggested as the physical basis of concussion, for often no abnormality can be detected in the brain either

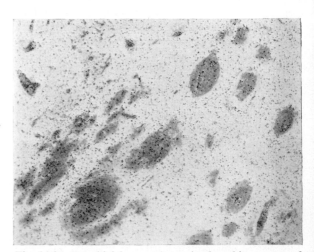

Fig. 34.86. Petechial haemorrhages in the white matter of the frontal lobe of a boy who died six hours after being run over. Blood has already found its way into the circumvascular spaces. *Haematoxylin–eosin.* × 40.

United Kingdom, and affords some protection against the risk of serious head injury, as Sir Hugh Cairns hoped (Cairns, H., *Brit. med. J.*, 1941, **2**, 465). Comparable protective measures should be devised for all people who are engaged in work rendering them liable to head injury. Protective helmets are increasingly used by building workers and others who may be endangered by falling material.

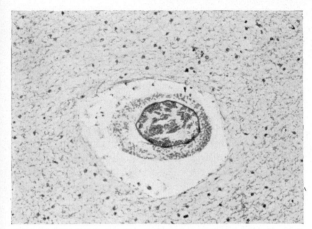

Fig. 34.87. Blood vessel in white matter of a girl who died 24 hours after a street accident. Blood has found its way into the circumvascular space, probably because of a rupture proximal to this point. The vessel wall is thinned and stretched and the blood contained within the lumen is sludged. There is oedema of the white matter and swelling of the oligodendrocytes. *Haematoxylin–eosin.* × 100.

macroscopically or microscopically. The concussion may last only for a short time, as, for instance, in the knock-out sustained while boxing.

Concussion is said also to result when neurons of the upper part of the brainstem are affected by the pressure gradients that develop in the region of the craniospinal junction almost instantaneously after the impact.[552] Death may be immediate if the neurons of the cardiac and respiratory centres are paralysed by the transmitted pressure wave. Concussion is often accompanied by vasomotor changes, such as constriction of the peripheral vessels, and this has been attributed to hypothalamic influences of a supposedly protective kind.[549] This immediate *medullary shock* has, of course, to be distinguished from the generalized delayed shock reaction that may complicate any severe trauma.

It has been shown in various animals that the neurons of the reticular formation and of other brainstem nuclei lose their Nissl substance within 14 hours of a severe injury to the brain.[553] This may indicate that the Nissl substance has been utilized in repairing the axon. The observation is of interest, for there is histological evidence in man that, in some cases, the axons may indeed bear the brunt of the disturbance and become functionless in large numbers.[554, 555] Studies of the brains of patients who, from the moment of injury to the head, had presented a sustained picture of complete mutism with quadriplegia showed that there may be marked loss of myelin in the white matter, especi-

ally in the posterior part of the frontal lobes and in the parietal lobes; in the less severely affected areas this is not easy to recognize with ordinary myelin stains, but it becomes obvious if the Marchi technique is used.[554] There is usually also a loss of nerve cells in the thalami in these cases, due to damage to the thalamocortical fibres in the initial stages of the injury. In view of the bulk of the average axon relative to that of its associated perikaryon, it probably would bear the brunt of the damage. The fine, delicate dendrites may also be vulnerable.

Clusters of microglial cells and axonal 'retraction bulbs' and 'retraction balls' are found in the brainstem and cerebral hemispheres of patients who have sustained concussion, recovered consciousness and then died of other causes.[556] Retraction balls are beads of eosinophile and argyrophile axoplasm that escape soon after an axon is severed (see page 2187): before the ball separates, the proximal end of the severed axon may be seen to be bulbous. It has been suggested that concussion may also be associated with reversible lesions, perhaps resulting from stretching rather than tearing and disintegration of nerve fibres, or from interruption of synapses or displacement of cell organelles.[557] While the brainstem is regarded as the essential site involved in concussion, the retrograde and other types of amnesia and the confusion that are often such notable clinical signs suggest more widespread dysfunction and cerebral disturbance.

Contusion and Laceration of the Brain

A *contusion* of the brain consists of a cluster of more or less confluent petechiae associated with a variable degree of necrosis (necrosis may accompany even very minor bleeding). A *laceration* is a severer lesion, characterized by tearing of the cortical surface and overlying pia-arachnoid: it is likely to be accompanied by subarachnoid or subdural haemorrhage. In civilian practice, damage to the brain is usually caused by the impact of the moving skull against a stationary object, as, for instance, in a fall downstairs or from a ladder, or in being thrown to the ground from a bicycle. Most head injuries sustained in motor-car accidents are also of this nature. A typical feature of these *deceleration injuries* is the presence of the so-called *contrecoup lesion*, which is a contusion of the aspect of the brain diametrically opposite to the point of impact (Fig. 34.88). The contusion of the brain just deep to the point of impact is known as the *coup lesion*: it is usually considerably smaller than the contre-

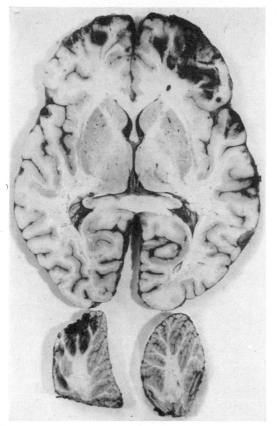

Fig. 34.88. Contrecoup contusions, most marked in the left frontal lobe (right of photograph), resulting from impact on the right side of the occiput on falling from a ladder. Note that on both sides the temporal lobes are involved in addition to the frontal lobes. The 'coup lesion' is in the right lobe of the cerebellum. *Note*: The photograph shows the undersurface of the slices of the brain.

coup contusion. When the fall or blow is on the back of the head, the contrecoup contusions are at the tips of both frontal and temporal lobes, and on their undersurface. Similarly, if the point of impact is over the right occipital lobe, the contrecoup contusions will be severest in the left frontal and temporal lobes, perhaps with small lesions on the right side. If the fall or blow is on to the left temporal region, the contrecoup will be under the right temporal bone. If, however, it is the forehead that is struck, contrecoup lesions are not likely to be found, but only the direct contusions involving predominantly the frontal lobes (see below).

Several theories have been advanced to explain the pathogenesis of coup and contrecoup contusions. In fact, when the body is falling backward, the brain keeps pace with the skull until the moment when the occiput hits a fixed object and progress of

the skull is immediately checked: the brain, because of its momentum, continues its onward movement, striking against the inside of the skull and thereby sustaining a local, direct contusion. The more serious lesions are at the opposite end of the brain and result from the continued movement over the uneven, stationary surface of the anterior and middle fossae, with consequent tearing of many of the fine blood vessels in the pia-arachnoid. When the point of impact is over the forehead, a contrecoup lesion does not usually develop, for the undersurface of the occipital lobe slides over the smooth surface of the resilient tentorium cerebelli. The sliding movement of the brain due to its momentum within the abruptly decelerated skull has been observed experimentally through lucite windows inserted in the cranium.[558]

Apart from the gliding movement of the brain, there are other important forces at work at the time of impact of the skull with an unyielding object. One is the transmission of force through the skull and brain, and this, too, can play a part in the causation of the coup and contrecoup contusions. It is possible that the shock waves are propagated through the substance of the brain in the same direction as the applying force; alternatively, they may spread in all directions round the skull from the point struck, and meet again at a diagonally opposite point.

There remain two further explanations of the coup-contrecoup phenomenon. The first is that, under certain circumstances, the skull, when struck, is momentarily deformed, behaving as would a hoop, with the result that the opposite surface of the brain is exposed to the forceful impact of the adjacent aspect of the cranium, which is abruptly drawn in to compensate for the compression deformation of the skull as a whole. This theory is complicated by the fact that the cranial 'hoop' is not uniformly resilient. The second possibility is that the axis of the brain within its dural sling may, again under certain circumstances, be violently twisted at the moment of an impact. It is generally held that this second explanation is of considerable importance, for a shearing type of stress could account for the frequency with which subdural haematomas occur, the cerebral veins being torn as they cross from the subarachnoid space to enter the dural sinuses.[559, 560] In a record of the movement of the brain, filmed through lucite inserts, there was no rotatory movement when the fixed head was struck but when the head was free to be thrust forward by the striking object, the brain was seen to undergo a sudden movement of partial rotation on its vertical axis.[558] This shearing injury may be important even in seemingly trivial impact injuries. In other experiments lesions have been produced by rotational acceleration and deceleration of the head, without impact:[561, 562] this situation occurs in certain types of head injury in man—for instance, in the so-called 'whiplash' injury, in which momentum (or inertia) and the mobility of the cervical spine allow the head to be abruptly accelerated in relation to the trunk when movement of the latter is suddenly stopped, as occurs in certain types of high-speed traffic accident.

Severe blows on the vertex may be transmitted through the brain to the brainstem as it passes through the tentorial opening, resulting in contusion of the cerebellar tonsils where they are pressed against the base of the skull near the foramen magnum: in such cases, there may also be contusions in the dorsal part of the medulla.[563] Contusions are also commonly found in the upper part of the pons (Fig. 34.89). The disorganization of the brainstem,[564] and specifically of the reticular formation, that results from the bleeding and associated oedema, has been blamed for the profound disturbance of consciousness that occurs in so many cases of head injury: this is in accord with current views on the pathogenesis of concussional coma (see page 2184). In fatal cases, petechial haemorrhages may be found in the white matter, and particularly in the posterior half of the corpus callosum. Gross swelling of the cytoplasm of the oligodendrocytes is an almost constant histological finding, even in the absence of petechiae.

Both the contusions and the petechial haemorrhages are caused by rupture of the walls of small blood vessels, with extravasation of blood into the circumvascular space. If the patient survives, the blood pigments are gradually removed by Hortega cells; when death occurs, even many years later, as a result of some other cause, haemosiderin will sometimes be found in the circumvascular space. A small contusion can probably heal completely. Larger lesions may be followed by atrophy of the cortex, with yellowish discoloration of the overlying pia-arachnoid. Histologically, there may be a dense gliotic scar at the surface of the brain, with collections of haemosiderin-laden macrophages (Fig. 34.90); deep to the scar there is a zone of astrocytosis in the remnant of the cortex. Collagen, originating from the fibroblasts in the adventitia of torn blood vessels,[565] may contribute to the formation of a cortical scar, but usually to a small extent only (Fig. 34.91). A collagenous scar may also result from a cortical laceration: such a scar may become attached to the dura, particularly when this membrane is torn or there is a subdural haematoma. A meningocortical scar is likely to become an epileptogenic focus (*traumatic epilepsy*).

Damage to nerve fibres may be very widespread even when there is little macroscopical evidence of haemorrhage or other abnormality.[557] Retraction balls[566, 567] mark sites of axonal severance (see page 2185) and remain visible for many months. Their number and local concentration depend on mechanical factors such as the direction of shear strains relative to alignment of fibres. Retraction balls are not always to be found at sites of injury; in particular they may be absent in the vicinity of contusions or haemorrhages. The distal ends of severed axons undergo Wallerian degeneration (see page 2187):[568, 569] after several weeks stainable lipids are present, although they may be difficult to demonstrate, particularly in relation to short fibres or tracts.

It will be apparent, therefore, that in injuries in which the moving head has struck a stationary or almost stationary object (the so-called deceleration injury), there are two important considerations for the surgeon, irrespective of whether or not there

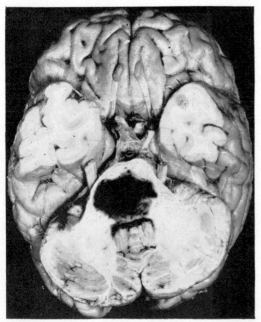

Fig. 34.89.§ Pontine haemorrhage which has reached the surface and spread into the subarachnoid space and also into the fourth ventricle, following a blow on the vertex, not at the time regarded as serious. Death occurred after 18 hours. There were also petechial haemorrhages in the splenium of the corpus callosum.

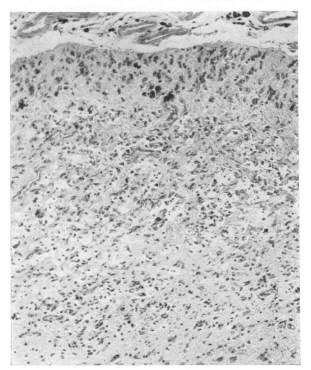

Fig. 34.90. Frontal cortex in a case of traumatic dementia. Death occurred many years after the accident. The cortex is largely destroyed and the outer part consists mainly of glial tissue in which most of the cells are macrophages containing blood pigment. Phagocytosed pigment and thickened blood vessels are seen in the fibrotic meninges. Deep to the spongy remains of the cortex there is marked proliferation of the astroglia. *Haematoxylin–eosin.* × 100.

has been a fracture of the skull. The first is to determine the precise point of the impact on the skull, and if possible the direction of the force. The second is to assess the potential efficacy of the 'brain cradle' in relation to the particular injury. A study of these factors will indicate the likely sites of the coup injuries, and the possibility of contrecoup contusions, and of dural or extradural bleeding. In this connexion, it should be emphasized that the falx cerebri and the tentorium cerebelli are remarkably taut membranes, and serve to protect the adjacent parts of the brain from injury.

Subdural and Extradural Haematomas

Subdural Haematoma

Subdural haematomas are a common complication of head injury. In a series of 151 fatal cases of head injury, a subdural haematoma was present in 34.[570] In 30 of these 34 cases, the collection of blood was over the front half of the brain, and could have been

exposed and removed if a frontoparietal trephine opening had been made 5 cm from the midline on each side. It is important for those who deal with cases of head injury to appreciate both the frequency of this sheering lesion and the fact that the haematoma is so often in a situation where it is readily accessible to surgical treatment, with a good chance of cure (Fig. 34.92).

Extradural Haematoma

Extradural haematomas are considerably less frequent than subdural haematomas. Their prognosis is less favourable, even when the source of the bleeding (usually the middle meningeal artery) can be found and dealt with surgically, for they are likelier to be associated with severe contusions or laceration of the brain.

Effects, Causes and Course

An expanding subdural or extradural collection of blood presses on the brain. In young adults, the symptoms of compression appear soon; in old people, whose brains have shrunken with ageing, the subarachnoid space is larger, and the haematoma can continue to expand for a longer period before causing symptoms. Subdural haematomas may enlarge rapidly, and are then liable to be complicated by transmission of raised pressure to the structures in the posterior fossa, resulting in haemorrhage into the brainstem and the development of a cerebellar pressure cone. In other cases,

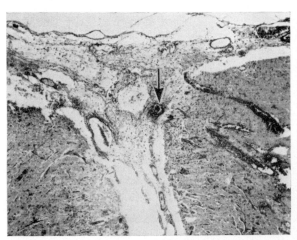

Fig. 34.91. Early meningocortical adhesions: proliferating capillaries have spread from the leptomeninges into the cortex. Death took place 23 days after fracture of the skull. There is thrombus in one of the vessels (arrow). *Haematoxylin–eosin.* × 40.

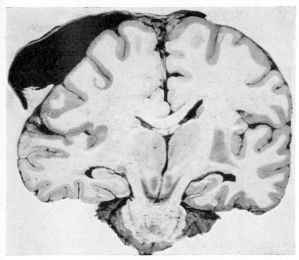

Fig. 34.92. Right-sided frontoparietal subdural haematoma displacing the midline structures to the left (right of the picture), distorting and narrowing the ventricles and causing herniation of the cingulate gyrus below the falx to the left. There was a much smaller subdural haematoma on the opposite side. The patient was a man of 64 who had complained of a sudden headache 10 weeks earlier. There was no history of trauma.

a subdural haematoma grows slowly, sometimes over a period of days, or even weeks, so that the patient, if he is conscious, and his doctor are apt to overlook the significance of the injury that caused the haemorrhage. Subdural haematomas may result from injuries other than those that involve the head directly; for instance, they may complicate a heavy fall or a severe jolting of the whole body. It is of great practical importance in diagnosis to appreciate that patients whose memory is impaired, either because of the lesion or in the ordinary course of ageing, may be unable to remember the injury.

The dura mater is a tough, almost avascular, mainly collagenous membrane: it contains few fibroblasts and so is not well fitted for ordinary reparative processes. When oozing of blood takes place from the point where a vein opens into a sinus, the haematoma forms between the dura mater and the underlying, intact arachnoid. The commonest site is beside the superior sagittal sinus. Repair is probably initiated by adventitial cells round the injured vessel, and in the course of about 10 days an investing layer of fibroblasts spreads over the inner aspect of the clot. These cells only rarely become attached to the underlying, highly vascular arachnoid, but they grow into the superficial portion of the clot, which thus begins to

undergo organization. By the end of three or four weeks, organization has progressed considerably, and the deep aspect of the clot is bounded by a fibroblastic capsule that is clearly demarcated from the underlying arachnoid. A similar layer of fibroblasts spreads over the outer aspect of the clot, and separates it from the inner surface of the dura. In fact, if it is examined at this stage, the partially organized haematoma can be stripped from the dura mater.

In the clot itself, vascularization, fibrosis and liquefaction take place side by side, but as long as there are fragile young blood vessels within the organizing area there is a risk of further oozing of blood. Thus, a subdural haematoma is always liable to grow larger, and until it has been removed it remains a threat to the patient's life. It is a matter of judgement when it should be removed, and in view of the constant hazard of further bleeding these patients should be under constant observation until the lesion has been dealt with.

Intradural Haematoma

Some haematomas are neither subdural nor extradural but within the dura, splitting it into two layers. These intradural haematomas are particularly likely to be found in old people, in patients with dementia, and in chronic alcoholics.

Subdural Hygroma

Considerable clinical interest has been attracted by a condition that may closely simulate a subdural haematoma:[571] following a head injury, a localized subdural collection of yellowish fluid with a high protein content is found. It is important to recognize this lesion because the simple procedure of withdrawing the fluid may bring about a rapid improvement in the patient's condition, with a return to consciousness. Exposure to blast is now a well-recognized cause.[572] It has been suggested that the fluid collects as a result of a valve-like tear in the arachnoid, which allows cerebrospinal fluid to pass only outward into the subdural space. The presence of a subdural hygroma does not exclude the possibility that a subdural haematoma is also present: the two conditions have been known to coexist.

Effects of Trauma on the Brainstem[573]

The occurrence of brainstem lesions after head injury in man has been reviewed by Tomlinson,[573] who discussed the possibility that stem lesions are the basis of temporary unconsciousness in concussion and can be equated with the lesions that accompany experimental concussion in animals. Information concerning stem lesions due to relatively minor head injury is fragmentary, depending on opportunities to study such cases when death has occurred from other causes.

Two types of haemorrhage, primary and secondary, are recognized to occur in the brainstem as a result of injury. Primary haemorrhages may be obvious to the naked eye or only of microscopical extent. They are present in practically every case in which death has occurred within a few hours of injury, although their detection depends on the thoroughness of the examination. There is a tendency for the upper part of the brainstem to be particularly involved, especially the grey matter round the ventricle and aqueduct and the periphery of the midbrain and pons. Such haemorrhages are not usually extensive in patients who die quickly. Small infarcts may be found in the same parts in the case of those patients who survive longer, which suggests that they result from similar but less severe stresses.

Secondary haemorrhages are associated with tentorial herniation and caudal or lateral displacement of the brainstem: they occur particularly in the central tegmental structures in the midbrain and pons. The lesions are usually visible macroscopically and may measure a centimetre or more across. Small secondary haemorrhages in patients who survive longer are usually associated with infarcts of variable extent. The haemorrhages and necrosis may extend into the hypothalamus or the thalami in severe cases. Secondary lesions are probably due to distortion and tearing of arteries rather than obstruction of veins.

When patients have lived for days or weeks after such injuries retraction balls (see page 2185) are usually found at necropsy in the upper part of the pons and in the midbrain. In those who have survived for months or longer, in coma or with incapacitating dementia, there is evidence of Wallerian degeneration of descending or interconnecting fibre tracts, with secondary atrophy of the related neurons. There is a good correlation between the lateral and peripheral evidence of damage caused by the primary haemorrhages and the areas where most retraction balls and tract degeneration are found.

Fractures of the Skull and Their Complications

A fracture of the skull may be directly responsible for various types of injury to the brain: these include laceration, haemorrhage, infection, introduction of air, escape of cerebrospinal fluid, rupture of cranial nerves, and the establishment of an arteriovenous anastomosis. The commonest is haemorrhage, which may take many forms.

Fractures of the skull are not always demonstrable by radiological examination during life. Some, and especially those of the base, are not immediately apparent even at necropsy: the dura, therefore, should always be carefully stripped off and the bone tapped, so that any difference in note on the two sides may be detected and investigated. The temporal bone should be examined with especial thoroughness. The squamous part of the temporal bone is particularly vulnerable: even in adults it may be of little more than eggshell thickness. Sometimes there is a history of an injury that sounds quite trivial—for instance, a child knocked over while at play, or a boy struck on the head by a ball—yet the fracture resulting from such an injury, unless promptly recognized, may prove rapidly fatal. The parietal bone, too, is often surprisingly thin and therefore liable to fracture.

Haemorrhage Complicating Fracture

A fracture of the skull may amount to no more than a crack, without alteration in alignment, yet deep to it there may be potentially serious bleeding because of tearing of a branch of a meningeal artery or vein lying in one of the vascular grooves crossed by the fracture line. Such possible sites of haemorrhage may be recognized if the lines of fracture, as shown by X-rays, cross the vascular grooves. If there is a comminuted fracture, a fragment of bone may be pressed firmly against the dura and thus prevent free bleeding from a torn vessel: haemorrhage may occur when the fragment is lifted by the surgeon.

When the dura is torn, blood will almost certainly collect in the subdural space, forming a subdural haematoma (see page 2188). Serious as this complication is, the position must be regarded as even more dangerous when the arachnoid is also ruptured, for then there will also be bleeding into the subarachnoid space. If the pia is injured, its repair is liable to result in the formation of a meningo-cortical cicatrix: this may eventually lead to the occurrence of epileptiform seizures.

Infection Complicating Fracture

Any compound fracture of the skull may be followed by the entry of micro-organisms into the cranial cavity; because of the greater likelihood of rapid dissemination, this complication is particularly serious when there has been a tear in the arachnoid. The organisms may enter with a foreign body, or on fragments of scalp or hair, or in the air that has been admitted. When a fracture involves the frontal, ethmoid or sphenoid bones, organisms in the nasal air sinuses may find their way into the subarachnoid space. A fracture of the skull, or tearing of the meninges, therefore, whether clinically apparent or not, is attended by a special risk of infection, which continues until such time as the fracture has healed: this may be a matter of many weeks.

If micro-organisms have entered through the arachnoid, they may spread rapidly throughout the subarachnoid space, causing meningitis. They may penetrate the pial membrane, especially if it, too, has been damaged: this may result in the development of a cerebral abscess.

When a foreign body penetrates through the skull, dura and pia-arachnoid into the brain, contaminating micro-organisms may give rise to liquefactive necrosis of the cerebral tissue, which soon protrudes through the opening (*traumatic encephalocele*). The swelling is particularly marked when gas-forming bacteria are among the invaders. In the early days of cranial surgery, this protrusion of a spongy mass of softened brain was known as 'fungus cerebri'. Sometimes, *Clostridium tetani* is carried into the brain and gives rise to the rapidly progressive form of tetanus known as *cerebral tetanus*.

Aerocele

When a fracture involves an air sinus, or the vault of the skull, and is accompanied by tearing of the dura mater and pia-arachnoid, air may find its way into the brain (*aerocele*). These aeroceles are apt to rupture into a ventricle. Their danger lies in the possibility that the air may contain bacteria, which, although not ordinarily pathogenic, may give rise to infection when introduced into the peculiar environment provided by the brain and meninges (see pages 2108 to 2110).

Leakage of Cerebrospinal Fluid

A common complication of a fracture of the skull is the escape of cerebrospinal fluid, either down the nose (*cerebrospinal rhinorrhoea*), when the fracture has involved the ethmoidal, frontal, or sphenoidal air sinuses, or through the external auditory meatus (*cerebrospinal otorrhoea*), when the temporal bone has been fractured. Cerebrospinal rhinorrhoea is commoner than cerebrospinal otorrhoea, but the latter is the more serious, perhaps because there is so often an associated fracture of the base of the skull. Both conditions are liable to be complicated by meningitis.

Arteriovenous Aneurysm Complicating Fracture

Tearing of the internal carotid artery within the cavernous sinus may give rise to an *arteriovenous aneurysm*. Rapidly fatal bleeding takes place if there is avulsion of any of the larger vessels within the cranial cavity.

Injury to the Cranial Nerves and to the Pituitary Circulation

The violence of an injury may be sufficient to rupture cranial nerves or damage the infundibulum, with consequent pituitary infarction (page 1879, Volume 4). The olfactory nerves are particularly liable to be damaged, probably because of their long course and slender structure and of the frequency of contusion of the undersurface of the frontal lobes. Permanent loss of smell (anosmia) is not unusual after a head injury. The facial nerve may be injured in its canal (the Fallopian canal) in the petrous part of the temporal bone and oculomotor paralyses result from tearing of the third, fourth or sixth cranial nerves. Deafness and blindness, from injury to the vestibulocochlear and optic nerves, are occasional sequels. At necropsy, lesions of the nerves are not always recognized, partly because they may be obscured by a haematoma, and partly because the fibres may be torn without disruption of the nerve sheath. Facial palsy sometimes develops some hours after an injury to the petrous portion of the temporal bone: this delayed form of paralysis, from which recovery may in time take place, is usually the result of pressure by a blood clot.

Reaction of Brain Tissue to Traumatic Haemorrhage

When interpreting the histological appearances in some cases of injury to the brain, the pathologist may be puzzled by what seems to be a disparity between the degree of tissue reaction and the time that has elapsed between the injury and death. Thus, in the brain of a patient who has survived for, say, eight days, a haemorrhage may be present round which there is practically no cellular response. It is important to realize that not all the abnormalities found at necropsy date from the time of the accident: there are, in fact, many secondary changes—among them thrombosis, infarction and haemorrhage—and one or more of these late events may have led to the patient's death. Sometimes the secondary manifestations develop a long time after the original injury.[574] Nonetheless, there is so often a surprising lack of reaction round traumatic haemorrhages in the brain that it seems possible that some effect of the injury may depress the activity of the Hortega cells, astrocytes and vascular endothelium in the vicinity of the lesion.

Direct Injuries to the Brain

As well as the so-called deceleration injuries (see page 2185), so common in civil life, the head may be injured by a moving object when it is itself more or less at rest. Thus, the skull may be penetrated by a bullet or fragment of metal, or it may be fractured by an object striking it. The nature of the resulting injury will depend on the size, shape, consistency and velocity of the object.

In the case of a bullet it will depend, too, on the distance between the muzzle of the gun and the scalp. A bullet may traverse the brain and ricochet back into it from the inside of the skull on the opposite side. In general, greater damage is inflicted on the inner table of the skull than on the outer table, and although the entry wound in the latter is generally sharply outlined and of about the same diameter as the bullet, the former may be splintered and fragments of bone driven into the brain. Occasionally a bullet will destroy a large part of one or both frontal lobes and yet the patient survive. If fired at close range, a bullet causes more disruption to the brain than when fired at long range. The bullet itself is believed to be sterile, because of the high temperature to which it has been raised by friction in the gun barrel and in its passage through the air, but its track within the brain may be infected by fragments of headwear, hair and skin that it carries in.

When the head is hit by a relatively slow-moving heavy object, the injuries are nearly always localized to the region of impact; contrecoup injuries are unusual in these cases.

Crushing Injuries to the Brain

The brain may be injured by crushing between two unyielding surfaces. While crushing injuries are occasionally sustained in accidents, by far the commonest form of crushing of the brain is that which takes place while the fetal head is passing through the birth canal.

There are many types of birth injury of the brain, some of which have been discussed under the heading of perinatal hypoxia (see page 2102). The infant's head may be seriously damaged during birth, especially in breech presentations, and there may then be extensive and fatal bleeding from injured veins, particularly those near the free edge of the tentorium, which is very liable to be torn. Minor degrees of injury, giving rise to no immediate symptoms, also occur. It is known that fresh blood may be found in the cerebrospinal fluid of some apparently normal newborn babies if the fluid is examined immediately after birth, or the fluid may be yellow if examined a few days later, when the red cells have broken down. Birth trauma is a hazard of forceps delivery, and especially of the application of 'high forceps'. Apart from damage due to bleeding within the cranial cavity, an infant delivered by forceps may be subjected to a variety of other neurological risks, including damage to the brachial plexus. The late consequences of damage to an infant's brain are potentially serious;[575] cerebral birth injuries are believed to be frequent causes of defective postnatal development of the brain through interference with the cerebral circulation.

Repetitive Injuries to the Brain

There is a special type of cerebral damage that is due to repetitive trauma. Such injuries are an occupational hazard of boxers, amateur as well as professional, and the evidence indicates that repeated knockouts (concussion), or repeated pummelling of the head without loss of consciousness, may render boxers liable to a progressive and disabling encephalopathy. There is unequivocal evidence that some boxers develop a clinical disorder that mainly has a neuropathological basis.[576] The severity of this condition varies greatly, ranging from a slight clumsiness of speech or movement, with or without loss of memory, to an ataxic-dysarthric dementia with Parkinsonism.

Four main pathological changes have been recognized in these boxers' brains.[576] They are:
1. *Abnormalities of the septum pellucidum*. The laminae of the septum pellucidum are fenestrate in most cases and the average width of the septal cavity is three times greater than in the brain of men who have not boxed. The fornix tends to be detached from the undersurface of the corpus callosum. The pathogenesis of these changes is obscure. Atrophy

of brain tissue and ventricular enlargement are associated features.

2. *Cerebellar scarring.* Glial scarring occurs most commonly in the cerebellar tonsils. There is a related increase in the distance between Purkyně cells, especially in the ventral parts of the cerebellum. No significant scarring is found in the cerebral hemispheres.

3. *Degeneration of the substantia nigra.* There was absence of macroscopical pigmentation in 4 of 15 cases showing clinical Parkinsonism; the amount of pigment was reduced in 7 of the other 11. Neurofibrillary tangles (see page 2275) are common in the substantia nigra in such cases; in contrast, Lewy bodies—which are numerous in this region in cases of paralysis agitans (see page 2267)—have not been found in boxers' brains.

4. *Regional occurrence of neurofibrillary tangles.* Tangles are abundant in the temporal lobes of the cerebral hemispheres, especially their medial parts; the parietal and occipital lobes are relatively or wholly free from this type of neuronal change. Argyrophile plaques (see page 2274) are rare or absent.

Serious permanent damage to the labyrinths may also develop insidiously in these men. Such cases, in fact, provide further evidence of the direct effects of mechanical forces on nerve cells and their processes (see pages 2185 and 2187).

Post-Traumatic Oedema of the Brain

Authorities differ in the importance they attach to oedema of the brain in the period that follows a head injury. It has been suggested that in adults oedema is less important than in children, in whom the brain may swell considerably, even after a seemingly slight injury, impairing cerebral function accordingly. The swelling is apt to be progressive, and may no longer be localized to the vicinity of focal lesions. When such a brain is examined after fixation, the cerebral cortex will be found to be stretched over the greatly swollen white matter. The convolutions are flattened and the sulci largely obliterated. Histologically, plasma that has escaped through the vessel walls is seen to fill the circumvascular spaces in the white matter (Fig. 34.93). The astrocytes, even by the end of 24 or 48 hours, are swollen, with clearly visible cytoplasm and peripheral displacement of the nucleus, which usually is enlarged. The oligodendrocytes, too, are swollen, and their enlarged nuclei are surrounded by a halo-like clear area, so that they may be difficult to distinguish from normal astrocytes. In the medulla

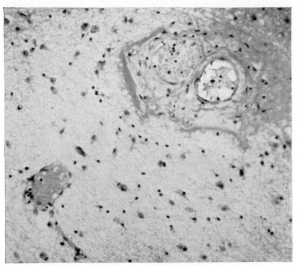

Fig. 34.93. Oedema of the white matter in the brain of a two-years-old boy who died 36 hours after a fall. Extravasation of plasma and swelling of astrocytes are seen. *Haematoxylin–eosin.* × 100.

and pons the neurons may appear as if compressed by interstitial accumulation of fluid. When the oedema resolves the white matter shows a variable degree of atrophy: it stains less intensely and less variably, and there is usually no significant degree of Sudanophile degeneration, although secondary gliosis may be pronounced.

It is uncertain how much of the increase in the volume of the brain is due to the accumulation of fluid within the glial cells and how much to fluid in the intercellular spaces. A breakdown of the blood–brain barrier, with consequent accumulation of extracellular fluid, has been demonstrated after injury to the brain by cold.[577] Recent work suggests that fluid may leak from vessels in destructive lesions and seep into the extracellular compartment of the adjacent white matter, where the vessels are normal. This seepage is aggravated by hypertension.[578] Swelling of the brain following trauma has been attributed to low oxygen tension in the blood. It may also complicate burns in children, usually developing from 24 to 48 hours after the accident.[579, 580]

Injuries Involving the Hypothalamus and Pituitary

The problem of injury to the hypothalamus and pituitary has recently been reviewed on the basis of a series of 15 cases involving the former and 158 involving the latter, correlating the clinical evidence of hypothalamic-pituitary defects with the lesions found.[581] The supraoptic nuclei were particularly vulnerable, being affected by haemorrhage, infarction or suppuration, in this order of frequency. The paraventricular nuclei were similarly but less frequently and less severely affected. Haemorrhages and infarcts were found in the infundibulum and lateral parts of the hypothalamus, although infrequent in the mamillary bodies.

Fresh haemorrhage was often found in the posterior lobe of the pituitary; this leads to atrophy and haemosiderosis at a later stage. Axonal damage was indicated by the finding of retraction balls and retained neurosecretory material. The anterior lobe of the pituitary was massively infarcted in some recent cases, consistent with severance of portal vessels in the infundibulum. In chronic cases atrophy of the pars distalis was an inconstant finding.

Clinical evidence of hypopituitarism was related to damage in the hypothalamic region (where the substances that control the release of the adenohypophysial trophic hormones are produced) and to the adenohypophysis (where the trophic hormones themselves are produced). Diabetes insipidus was related to damage to the supraoptic nuclei and the tracts connecting them to the hypothalamus, which are the source of antidiuretic hormone and its pathway respectively. Damage in the vicinity of the third ventricle affected temperature regulation.

Fat Embolism of the Brain[582, 583]

Fat droplets may enter the blood from the bone marrow, especially as a result of accidents that involve the long bones. It may also take place after blast injuries or severe damage to adipose tissue or to a fatty liver. Under these circumstances, venous channels are torn, and fat droplets extruded from the cells of the crushed tissue enter the vessels; when bones are damaged, clumps of haemopoietic cells may accompany the fat. It has been claimed that plasma 'lipomicrons' are the main source of the emboli, fusing in some way to form larger globules; this is debatable, and experiments on dogs with fractured femurs suggest that the emboli resemble marrow fat rather than plasma fat.[584] In surviving patients, the presence of fat droplets in the lungs may be shown by the demonstration of Sudanophile globules in the sputum. If much fat reaches the blood stream, some of it may find its way through the vascular bed of the lungs into the systemic circulation. It may thus reach the kidneys, and fat globules may then appear in the urine. Fat was found in the lungs in the great majority of a series of 100 cases of fat embolism, and in the organs supplied by the systemic circulation in a quarter of the series.[585]

When fat emboli are held up in the small, delicate vessels of the brain, the vascular stasis leads to damage to the endothelium of the occluded vessels, small focal haemorrhages resulting. Numerous vessels are affected, particularly in the white matter, and there is often very extensive and severe 'brain purpura' (Figs 34.94 and 34.95) (see page 2183). If the patient survives, the fat is removed by phagocytes and carried back to the blood stream. Cerebral symptoms due to fat embolism usually appear within a few hours of the accident but may be delayed for a day or two. Sudden death occurs if the emboli cut off the blood supply to vital centres in the medulla oblongata.

More recently it has been postulated that cerebral signs of fat embolism—such as delirium and coma —are due to general hypoxia and not to direct effects of emboli.[586] However, the haemorrhagic lesions in the brain are related histologically to vessels occluded by fat emboli and are unlike the lesions that are characteristic of general hypoxia

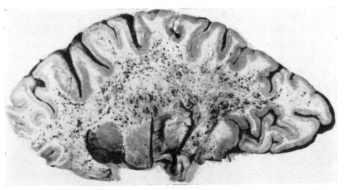

Fig. 34.94.§ Fat embolism. The petechial haemorrhages are confined to the white matter.

(see page 2097). General hypoxia, therefore, probably worsens the ischaemic effects of cerebral fat emboli but is not the main cause of the cerebral lesions. Administration of oxygen has been shown to improve the mental state of some patients.

Fat emboli may also be numerous in the posterior lobe of the pituitary gland: this may explain the development of diabetes insipidus in some patients who survive.[587] Such lesions may also influence renal tubular function by altering the secretion of vasopressin.

Episodic Deficiency of Cerebral Blood Flow Complicating Head Injury

Head injury may be complicated by episodic inadequacy of the cerebral blood flow.[588] This is probably a result of the very high intracranial pressure that develops in some cases. Secondary vasodilation and an accompanying increase in intracranial blood volume, with traumatic oedema, are factors that may be responsible for the increase in pressure. As a result, boundary zone lesions (see page 2174), characteristic of deficient cerebral arterial blood flow, can be identified if appropriate techniques are used, particularly examination of large histological sections.[589] These changes can occur in the absence of occlusive intracranial and extracranial arterial disease.

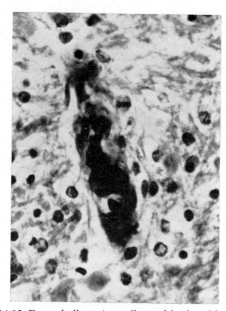

Fig. 34.95. Fat embolism. A small vessel in the white matter is plugged with fat. Symptoms developed 12 hours after a street accident; death occurred seven days later. *Frozen section. Sudan IV; haematoxylin.* × 300.

5

Injury to the Central Nervous System by Irradiation and Other Physical Agents

Ionizing Radiations.[590]—The brain and spinal cord may be seriously damaged in the course of deep X-ray therapy of lesions in their vicinity. The manifestations of the injury to the nervous tissue are usually a delayed sequel of the exposure.[591, 592] The essential changes are hyaline degeneration of the wall of blood vessels and necrosis of surrounding nervous tissue.

The practical applications of atomic energy, the development and stockpiling of atomic weapons and the hazards faced by astronauts have engendered much experimental work on the effects of various forms of ionizing radiation.

Electricity and Lightning.[593]—When death is due to electrocution, the only abnormality visible in the brain may be hyperaemia, possibly with petechial haemorrhages. If the discharge was directed through the brain, as in death due to lightning, there may be charring or widespread fissuring of its surface.

Laser Beams.—Haemorrhage and necrosis have been found in the brain and spinal cord of animals exposed to laser beams.[593]

Heat.—In heat stroke,[594] the brain is swollen and there may be petechial haemorrhages in the white matter and in the vicinity of the third ventricle. The neurons swell, and some, especially the Purkyně cells, may undergo lysis.

Encephalopathy Complicating Burns.[595, 596]—Convulsions, delirium and coma may complicate burns, especially in children. The onset of the encephalopathy may be delayed for days or weeks. If the patient survives the other effects of burning, recovery from the encephalopathy is usual, although there may be sequelae such as hemiplegia, dysphasia and blindness.

In fatal cases the brain is found to be swollen and congested and shows features of raised intracranial pressure; haemorrhagic and thrombotic lesions have been found (detailed histological studies have not been recorded). The pathogenesis of this condition has not been established and many factors may be involved—dehydration, hyperpyrexia, bacterial toxaemia and acute arterial hypertension (which is not uncommon in burned children) are possibilities that need consideration.

Ultrasound.[597]—Ultrasonic radiation, when directed through trephine openings on to a focal point within the white matter, has a very destructive effect on tissues of all types. A surrounding zone of oedema, together with activation of astrocytes, has been observed following the therapeutic use of ultrasound as an alternative to surgical lobotomy.[598]

Injuries to the Spinal Cord[599]

The spinal cord may be injured directly or indirectly, the latter being the more usual.

Direct injuries do not necessarily damage the dura, which throughout the length of the spinal column is tough and elastic; in cases of penetrating wounds, however, the dura is often lacerated. When the cord is injured directly, whether by a severe blow, by shot, or by a knife wound, one or more nerve roots may be interrupted.

Most injuries to the spinal cord are secondary to blows on other parts of the body: they are not necessarily accompanied by injury to the spinal column. When, in such cases, the dura is incised surgically at the level indicated by the symptoms, the only visible abnormality may be a localized swelling of the cord. When the trauma is more extensive, haemorrhagic softening of the grey matter of the cord may be found if a period of about 12 hours has elapsed since the injury; this softening usually extends for some distance beyond the level of the injury, both upward and downward.

Fracture-dislocation of the spinal column, with compression of the cord, is a common result of forcible flexion of the spine: in such cases it is generally found that the spinal column has snapped in the mid-thoracic region. A blow that causes sudden extension of the neck, such as a punch on the chin, or a dive into shallow water, or even one that causes sudden flexion of the neck, may break the second cervical vertebra: this injury may result in quadriplegia.

The mechanism of the central softening and haemorrhage, ranging from minute to very extensive lesions, that occur in the cord at the site of a vertebral injury, or sometimes in the absence of evident skeletal injury, cannot always be adequately explained. Distortion of a vertebral artery may be a factor in some cases of cervical dislocation. Local and individual variations in the blood supply to the cord may be important (see page 2171).

Prolapsed Intervertebral Disc[600, 601]

One of the commonest of neurological complaints results from herniation of the nucleus pulposus of an intervertebral disc through part of the anulus fibrosus—the so-called 'slipped disc' (see page 2507). The nucleus pulposus develops from the notochord, and forms the central portion of the disc. As a result of injury or of lifting heavy weights, part of the nucleus pulposus may be forced through a weak place in the anulus, and it may then compress a nerve root. The condition generally affects the lumbar part of the spine, although occasionally it occurs in the neck. Formerly, the significance of the injury was often overlooked: such patients were then believed to be suffering from sciatic neuritis ('sciatica'), and alleviation of the symptoms often followed rest in bed for some weeks or months. Today, recovery may be expedited, in the more serious cases, and prognosis improved, by surgical intervention to relieve the pressure.

When examined histologically, the prolapsed fragments of the disc are usually seen to be devitalized, only a few normal cells remaining. Sometimes, however, as a result of chronic irritation, the material shows evidence of vascularization, and there may be macrophages containing haemosiderin—a sequel of former bleeding. The pathologist who sees many surgical specimens from cases of prolapsed intervertebral disc learns the importance of being on the lookout for unexpected instances of granulomas, such as tuberculosis, and of tumours, such as metastatic carcinoma or myeloma, all of which may simulate prolapse of the nucleus pulposus, both clinically and at operation.

Osteophytosis of the Cervical Spine

The spinal cord is sometimes damaged by osteophytes growing from the posterior surface of the bodies of the vertebrae (see page 2504). The cervical segments are most vulnerable to such injury.[602] The damage may be strictly local; sometimes, however, the anterior spinal artery is affected, and spreading thrombosis within it may lead to infarction of the cord.[603]

DEVELOPMENTAL ANOMALIES[604-607]

Various malformations of the central nervous system may arise during its complicated development. Some of these are incompatible with prolonged post-natal life; others are associated with imbecility or idiocy, or with neurological disorders of a less severe kind that become manifest some time after birth. Occasionally, an individual may go through life with a minor malformation—a partial defect of the corpus callosum, for instance —without any apparent handicap.

These malformations may be the result of various adverse influences which, in the severer forms, usually act on the embryo early in the course of development, when the rudiments of the organs are appearing. Comparable disturbances can be induced experimentally in animals, and it has been found possible to reproduce some of the malformations found in man by exposing the animal embryo to such damaging agents as hypoxia, nutritional deficiencies and excesses, antimetabolites, hormonal derangements and ionizing radiations.[608-611]

Viral Infections as Causes of Malformation.—Infection of the mother, during the first trimester of pregnancy, with the virus of rubella or with some other viruses, including cytomegalovirus, can lead to serious malformation of the fetus.[612, 613] Viruses can pass the placental barrier in the early stages of pregnancy: those of mumps, rubella and poliomyelitis, and cytomegalovirus, have been isolated from the placenta and the embryo or fetus when the mother has become infected during pregnancy. The earlier in pregnancy the mother is infected, the greater the likelihood of major malformations of the embryo. Not all viral infections of the mother lead to interference with the normal development of the embryo, and evidence is still far from complete as to the extent and frequency of the hazard of many of these conditions. For instance, there is good evidence that influenza virus may cross the placental barrier but none that it causes any harm to the developing embryo or fetus.

Drugs as Causes of Malformation.—Thalidomide (alpha-phthalimidoglutarimide), a non-barbiturate hypnotic and sedative, was synthetized in 1953. It became generally available in the Federal Republic of Germany in 1957 and in the United Kingdom in 1958. By 1961 it was recognized to be responsible for a range of malformations, the most obvious of which were failure of proper development of the limbs.[614, 614a] In December, 1961, the drug was withdrawn from sale in Britain. As late as 1973 the birth in England of a baby with rudimentary arms and legs (phocomelia) was attributed to the administration of thalidomide to the mother while resident, early in her pregnancy, in another country where the drug was prescribed for its

effects in suppressing lepra reactions from which she suffered during treatment of leprosy.[615] Other therapeutic agents with known teratogenic effects include mustine (nitrogen mustard), aminopterin, azathioprine, actinomycin D and other antineoplastic agents.

Genetically Determined Malformation.—Some of the malformations discussed below have a genetical aetiology. The role of chromosomal anomalies in the pathology of development is becoming increasingly recognized: of the neurological disorders of this type, Down's syndrome is still the best authenticated (see page 2204).

Agenesis and Related Defects

The term *agenesis* is applicable when any defined structure has failed to develop. The severest form of agenesis in the central nervous system is *anencephaly*, in which most of the brain is absent and the spinal cord and pituitary are also often much malformed (see also pages 1877 and 1933, Volume 4); this anomaly, which is usually associated with grave defects in the bones of the cranial vault, is now generally regarded as the outcome of an early defect in the closure of the neural tube. More limited varieties of agenesis, though seldom compatible with survival for more than a few hours, are those associated with *cyclopia* (see Chapter 40, Volume 6); in this condition, the single eye may be accompanied by *arrhinencephaly*, and the frontal lobes may be represented only by a single large vesicle. Less grave forms of agenesis include fusion of the two frontal lobes, with absence of the anterior part of the falx cerebri and failure of development of the anterior part of the corpus callosum.

Somewhat later in the course of embryogenesis, disturbances of development may result from the failure of some of the neuroblasts to reach their destined places in the cerebral cortex at the end of their migration from the vicinity of the primitive cerebral vesicles, where they are formed. This failure of development of the neuroblast mantle is known as *dystectogenesis*. In a pronounced form it gives rise to *lissencephaly*, a condition in which the whole or part of a cerebral hemisphere, when stripped of meninges, presents a smooth outer surface instead of a convolutional pattern (Figs 34.96 and 34.97). This condition, in which the brain is usually small (*micrencephaly*), is also known as *agyria*. When such a brain is sliced for macroscopical examination, its grey matter appears unusually conspicuous, and prolongations from it

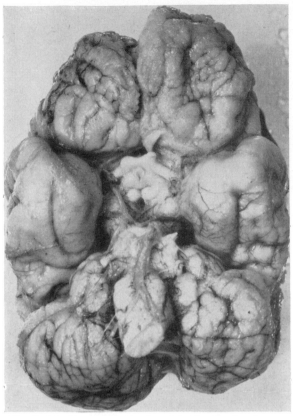

Fig. 34.96. Abnormally developed brain showing in some places numerous malformed convolutions (micropolygyria) and elsewhere—for instance, on the under-surface of the temporal lobes—absence of convolutional pattern ('agyria'). Death occurred at the age of four months.

often extend into the underlying white matter. Sometimes a distinct layer, intermediate both in colour and nerve cell content, is visible between the grey matter and the white matter. A commoner form of dystectogenesis is the condition known as *microgyria*, in which the convolutions are small and often unusually numerous (*micropolygyria*), with loss of the normal gyral pattern in the affected areas (Fig. 34.96). Micropolygyria is especially common in the parietal area; it is to be distinguished from atrophy of the cortex due to ischaemia. *Heterotopia* of grey matter, in the form of collections of neuroblasts or neurons in the white matter, is sometimes found, particularly toward the occipital poles; the foci may, rarely, be large enough to be seen by the unaided eye.

Porencephaly, or *schizencephaly*, is a condition in which one or more horns of a lateral ventricle are distended; the overlying grey matter and white matter are rudimentary or even absent. The

ventricular cavity may, in fact, be separated from the subarachnoid space by no more than its ependymal lining and the pia mater. True porencephaly is believed to be due to an error of development, and may be associated with microgyria. It must be distinguished from the dilatation of a ventricle that may follow trauma, infarction or infection (the so-called encephaloclastic or secondary porencephaly).[616]

Hydrocephalus[617–619]

The cerebrospinal fluid is secreted mainly by the choroid plexuses, particularly in the lateral ventricles, although some is added by percolation along the Virchow–Robin space. A contribution to the fluid may be made by the neural parenchyma, the ependyma and the vessels in the subarachnoid space.[620] From observations when the fluid has been allowed to drain freely externally, it is believed that a volume of about 500 ml may be secreted daily; this is about three times the total volume present in the ventricles and the cranial and spinal subarachnoid space under normal conditions. The fluid passes through the third ventricle and the aqueduct into the fourth ventricle, whence it escapes into the basal cisterns through the median and lateral apertures. From the basal cisterns it passes by way of the opening in the tentorium cerebelli to percolate slowly through the subarachnoid space over the surface of the cerebral hemispheres; it also passes down into the spinal subarachnoid space. It eventually returns to the blood, mainly through the arachnoid villi, which

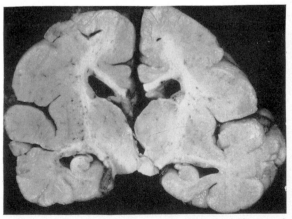

Fig. 34.97. Lissencephaly. The surface of the brain is smooth and the sulci are few in number and mostly shallow ('agyria'). The cortex is unusually deep and in places shades almost imperceptibly into the white matter. There has been a failure of migration of neurons to the cortex.

are essentially diverticula of the subarachnoid space that cross the subdural space to penetrate the dura mater and protrude into the venous sinuses;[620a] the specialized mesothelial cells that cover the villi fuse with the endothelium of the sinus. The largest villi are the arachnoid granulations (Pacchionian corpuscles[620b]). Some fluid may be absorbed from the subarachnoid space along cranial and spinal nerves and directly into blood vessels.

Obstruction to the flow of cerebrospinal fluid may be at one or more of three sites. First, the aqueduct or the apertures in the roof of the fourth ventricle may be obstructed: this is referred to as *non-communicating hydrocephalus*—dye injected into a lateral ventricle does not find its way into the spinal fluid. In this form, fluid accumulates under pressure within the ventricles (*internal hydrocephalus*). Second, the blockage may occur at the level of the subarachnoid cisterns or of the tentorial incisure: this is a *communicating hydrocephalus*—dye passes from the lateral ventricles and the subarachnoid space into the spinal fluid. Third, absorption into the venous sinuses may be impaired, so that fluid collects in the subarachnoid space over the vertex of the brain in the form known as *external hydrocephalus*: this too is a communicating form of hydrocephalus.

Hydrocephalus may result from obstruction of the cerebrospinal fluid pathway by fresh or organized inflammatory exudate or by a tumour. It may also be due to some congenital anomaly. Hydrocephalus due to a congenital malformation usually becomes manifest in the neonatal period; often, indeed, it is apparent at birth. In these cases, steps must be taken to exclude the presence of other congenital causes of obstruction, such as infection (toxoplasmosis or syphilis, or a prenatal bacterial meningitis), or occlusion of the aqueduct following bleeding. The commonest causes of congenital hydrocephalus are the Arnold–Chiari malformation (see below) and forking of the aqueduct (see page 2200). In occasional cases, hydrocephalus caused by congenital malformations does not become apparent clinically for many months, and even, exceptionally, for years.

The measurements in Table 34.3 of the circumference of the head of normal children at various ages are useful in the assessment of the degree of hydrocephalus in an affected child.

Arnold–Chiari Malformation[621]

In the Arnold–Chiari malformation, part of the medulla oblongata and part of the vermis of the

Table 34.3. *Mean Circumference (in Centimetres) of the Head of Normal Children at Various Ages*[*]

Age	Boys	Girls
0–1 month	36·0	35·0
2–3 months	39·0	38·4
5–6 months	41·9	41·1
6–9 months	43·5	44·0
9–12 months	45·5	44·7
12–24 months	47·2	47·6
2–3 years	48·9	48·3
5–6 years	50·6	49·5
9–10 years	51·4	51·2
13–14 years	53·6	52·0

* Myers, B., *Brit. J. Child. Dis.*, 1926, **23**, 87.

cerebellum, sometimes with the caudal end of the fourth ventricle lying between them, are to be found below the level of the foramen magnum, in the spinal canal (Fig. 34.98).[622] The foramen magnum is effectively plugged by these structures, so that the cerebrospinal fluid is unable to escape through the apertures in the roof of the fourth ventricle. As the ventricles and the aqueduct dilate under the pressure of the fluid, which continues to be secreted by the choroid plexuses, the membranous bones of the still immature skull separate, and the scalp becomes stretched and thinned, especially over the greatly expanded fontanelles. Concurrently, the pressure of the retained fluid in the dilated ventricles stretches the surrounding brain, causing extreme atrophy of its substance: as a result, hardly any of the white matter may remain, the cortex is reduced to a thin rim, and the basal ganglia are compressed almost beyond recognition.

At necropsy, the Arnold–Chiari malformation is

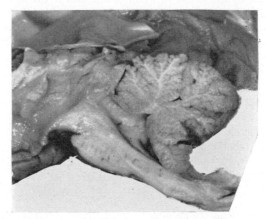

Fig. 34.98. Arnold–Chiari malformation. The pons is flattened; the medulla and cerebellar tonsils protruded below the level of the foramen magnum.

displayed to best advantage when the brain and spinal cord are exposed in continuity from behind. It can then be seen that the upper cervical nerve roots have to run upward to reach the intervertebral foramina instead of taking their usual downward course. A characteristic notch is visible on the anterior aspect of the cord at the point where the lower part of the medulla oblongata overrides it. The posterior fossa of the cranial cavity is small, and so is the tentorium cerebelli, which is attached close to the margin of the abnormally large foramen magnum. The tentorial incisure (the opening bounded by the free edge of the tentorium) is also enlarged.[623]

If the brain affected by this malformation is removed from the skull by the usual necropsy method, the cut through the neuraxis (which ordinarily is made through the upper part of the spinal cord, at the level of the foramen magnum) is likely to pass through the attenuated and displaced medulla oblongata instead.

A meningomyelocele, usually in the lumbar region, is a constant accompaniment of the Arnold–Chiari malformation.[624] Indeed, the finding of a spinal meningocele at birth strongly suggests that this malformation is also present: if hydrocephalus is not already apparent, its development may be expected. The finding of mere dimpling of the skin over the lumbar part of the spine, with its suggestion of spina bifida occulta, does not carry the same serious implication. The Arnold–Chiari malformation is liable to be accompanied by other developmental defects of the central nervous system and of the skull and spinal column; micropolygyria (see page 2198) was noted in all of a series of 20 cases, craniolacunia (defects in the bones of the vault of the skull) in 15 of them, and hydromyelia (see page 2204) in 8.[625] In addition, there may be abnormalities of other parts of the body: bilateral hydronephrosis, associated with hypertrophy of the wall of the urinary bladder, has been observed particularly often, and may be a result of a disturbance of bladder control secondary to malformation of the spinal cord (the so-called 'neurogenic bladder'—see page 1520, Volume 4).

The cause of the Arnold–Chiari malformation is obscure, but it has been suggested that the elongation of the brainstem may result from failure of the pontine flexure to form.[626]

The so-called Chiari type 2 malformation* is of

different nature and may be secondary to congenital hydrocephalus. In these cases, the prolapse of the brain substance through the foramen magnum involves the cerebellar tonsils and not the vermis, and the fourth ventricle is not drawn downward and included in the extruded cone. The condition is not associated with any variety of myelocele. It may not become manifest until the second decade or later.

Forking of the Aqueduct (Double Channel Aqueduct)[627]

Occasionally, the aqueduct is composed of two channels: the dorsal one has an irregular outline when seen histologically in cross section, while the ventral one is usually a mere slit. The two small channels together prove insufficient for the free passage of cerebrospinal fluid: internal hydrocephalus results.

Other Forms of Congenital Obstruction of the Aqueduct

Rarely, a minute septum lies across the caudal end of the aqueduct and causes hydrocephalus. The obstruction may be incomplete, and the ventricular dilatation may then be so slow in development that the onset of symptoms is delayed until early adult life.

Congenital stenosis of the aqueduct is a rare, and sometimes hereditary, malformation.[628] It has to be distinguished from obliteration of the aqueduct by surrounding gliosis, which may be developmental in origin, as in central neurofibromatosis, or a sequel of local inflammation. It seems surprising that during fetal life the aqueduct should sometimes fail to adapt its calibre progressively to the pressure of fluid within it. This fluid is formed, at first, by transudation through the ependymal cells; it starts to flow through the neural tube very early in development—probably by the fourth week of embryonic life, when the neural folds have just united to form the tube.[629] When investigating cases of supposed congenital stenosis, great care must be taken to ensure that sections are taken precisely at right angles to the line of the aqueduct. The appearances in sections cut in an oblique plane are often misleading. Moreover, the aqueduct

---

* It should be explained that the Arnold–Chiari malformation was first recorded by Chiari in 1891 (Chiari, H., *Dtsch. med. Wschr.*, 1891, **17**, 1172); he also described the type 2 anomaly and a third anomaly (the third example was

an occipital meningoencephalocele). His further report on 'types 1 and 2' followed in 1895 (Chiari, H., *Denkschr. Akad. Wiss. Wien*, 1895, **63**, 71). Meanwhile, in 1894, Arnold reported an instance of what Chiari called the 'type 1' malformation (Arnold, J., *Beitr. path. Anat.*, 1894, **16**, 1).

must be examined at closely spaced intervals, and the appearances must be carefully compared with those of normal brains that have been fixed and sectioned by the same method. It is important to appreciate that the normal aqueduct narrows at not less than two points in its centimetre-long course.[630]

Congenital Obstruction of the Apertures of the Fourth Ventricle (Dandy–Walker Syndrome[618, 631])

In this condition, the apertures of the fourth ventricle are obstructed and fluid is consequently retained in the ventricles. The obstruction may take the form of a septum across the median aperture; much oftener it is due to atresia (congenital failure of the apertures to develop).[618, 631, 632] In either case the effect is to obstruct the flow of the fluid from the fourth ventricle: if this occurs early in embryonic life the posterior part of the vermis fails to develop completely.[633]

Other Causes of Congenital Hydrocephalus

Occasionally, cases of hydrocephalus are seen in which no obstruction can be found either in the ventricular system or at its apertures: a failure of the subarachnoid space to form normally, or a failure of the mechanism by which cerebrospinal fluid is absorbed, has been postulated to explain such instances.

In the anomaly known as *platybasia*, the flow of cerebrospinal fluid may be seriously impeded by pressure on the apertures in the roof of the fourth ventricle as a result of a congenital upward displacement of the foramen magnum. The name describes the flattening of the clivus* that is associated with the bony malformation. In some of these cases there is a marked depression of the anterior surface of the pons, due to moulding over the odontoid process of the atlas vertebra, which is displaced upward through the foramen magnum: this is the so-called 'basilar impression' of the pons.[634] 'Occipitalization' of the atlas and the Klippel–Feil anomaly,[634a] in which several cervical vertebrae are fused or lacking, may also be present.

Hydrocephalus is an occasional accompaniment of *achondroplasia*.

In some cases of faulty development of the brain, the ventricles are dilated, especially in *lissencephaly* (see page 2197). The hydrocephalus is probably

---

* The clivus (of Blumenbach) is the slope, formed of the basal parts of the occipital and sphenoid bones, that extends upward from the anterior border of the foramen magnum to the dorsum sellae.

compensatory, and secondary to the deficiency of cerebral tissue.

Spina Bifida

The term spina bifida is applied to malformations involving the spinal cord and vertebral column that range from unimportant, minor abnormalities to gross lesions that are incompatible with survival. In all types, the primary defect is usually a failure of fusion of the neural plate and tube early in embryonic life; this is followed by malformation of the mesodermal bony structures of the region. It may be noted that spina bifida is often only one of a number of congenital defects involving various body systems in such cases.[635] Recent studies on chick and rat embryos and on human material provide convincing evidence that the condition may result from apparently spontaneous reopening early in embryonic life of a previously closed neural tube.[635a, 635b]

In its least serious form, *spina bifida occulta*, there is incomplete closure of one or more of the vertebral arches. The site of this bony defect is often marked by a small dimple or a hairy or pigmented mole in the overlying skin. When the bony defect is larger, the meninges may herniate from the spinal canal and thus create a *meningocele*, which can be recognized as a soft, fluctuant swelling under the skin, usually in the lumbar or sacral region. In this form, the spinal cord is not seriously affected, and lies more or less normally in the depths of the spinal canal. In a more serious and commoner variety, *meningomyelocele*, the spinal cord is involved, and portions of its posterior funiculi may be stretched out in the wall of the subcutaneous cystic swelling. The severest and rarest form is *rachischisis*, in which the spinal canal is open to the exterior, either for a short distance or over its whole length: the spinal cord is exposed, and is almost always grossly deformed, its central canal often being open posteriorly throughout its length; the rest of the cord is flattened against the meningeal lining of the anterior wall of the vertebral canal.

Malformations that are not immediately fatal may have two serious effects: first, neurological disability resulting from the regional disorganization of the spinal cord and its nerve roots; and second, predisposition to bacterial infection of the meninges, particularly when there is some defect of the overlying skin.

Epidemiology.—The epidemiology of congenital defects of the neural tube, especially spina bifida and anencephaly, has been widely studied. Such factors as race, social class, maternal age and parity, family history, geography and water-hardness have been thought to play a part. A more recent hypothesis is that there may be an association with the occurrence of potato blight (an infection of the potato plant caused by the fungus *Phytophthora infestans*).[636]

Tuberose Sclerosis

(Epiloia; Bournville's Disease[637])

Tuberose sclerosis is a heredofamilial disease characterized by malformations of various parts of the body. The malformations are usually hamartomas—tumour-like masses of irregularly arranged but well-differentiated tissues of the same types as those that make up the normal structure of the affected part. Abnormalities of the central nervous system are only one feature of the wide-spread distortion of organ development that is characteristic of tuberose sclerosis.

Genetical studies have shown that tuberose sclerosis occurs sporadically as the result of the appearance of a dominant mutant gene. The affected children are usually, but not always, imbecile.[638, 638a] Epilepsy may become manifest even before there is evidence of mental defect.

During childhood, a charcteristic focal fibrosis of the dermis of the face, misleadingly known as adenoma sebaceum, often develops (see Chapter 39, Volume 6). This is an inconstant feature.

Macroscopically, the brain may be normal in size or rather small. There may be a number of small, slightly umbilicate, firm white areas in some gyri; sometimes a whole gyrus may be broadened and white. These are the gliotic foci that are characteristic of the disease (Figs 34.99 and 34.100).[639] The lining of the lateral ventricles, especially the floor, is characteristically roughened: this appearance has been likened to the wax that has run down the side of a guttering candle (Fig. 34.100). Calcium salts tend to be deposited in these areas, which often become visible in radiographs: this feature has to be distinguished from the juxta-ventricular calcification that may follow intra-uterine infection by rubella virus. Occasionally, gliotic foci are present in the white matter also, particularly in the cerebral hemispheres, but some-times in the cerebellum and brainstem; they are often more easily felt than seen.

Histologically, the changes in the cerebral cortex indicate a disturbance in the development of its lamination at a very early stage of embryonic life.

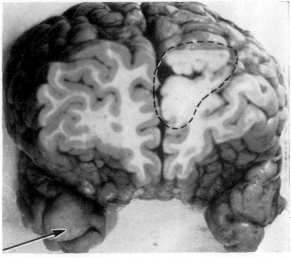

Fig. 34.99.§ Tuberose sclerosis. The arrow points to a nodular swelling on one of the gyri. The dotted line defines an area where most of the cortex is absent, its place being taken by dense gliotic scar tissue.

In the depressed scars, the normal differentiation between grey and white matter may be wholly lost, and the absence of neurons may be striking. The extensive gliosis is associated with proliferation of astrocytes. Scattered throughout the plaques of gliosis in the grey matter there are curious globoid cells (Fig. 34.101), which are sometimes very large and may have spike-like cytoplasmic protrusions: in some respects these cells resemble astrocytes, and in others they resemble neurons, and their peculiar hybrid appearance suggests that the anomaly dates back to the time of differentiation of the primitive medullary epithelium. The gliotic foci in the white matter do not always contain the globoid cells, but there are many astrocytes and these may be un-usually large. Flecks of calcium salts are often present in the gliotic tissue. An analogous glial mass may be found in the retina, where it forms the lesion sometimes known as a *phacoma* (see Chapter 40, Volume 6); its presence may prove of value in the clinical diagnosis of the disease. Rarely, a glioma arises in one of the gliotic areas, particularly in the floor of the lateral ventricles.

The most frequent anomalies elsewhere in the body in cases of tuberose sclerosis include renal tumours, which are often bilateral and of embryonic type.[639, 640] Multiple renal tubular adenomas are a commoner feature. Nodular myocardial hamar-tomas containing abundant glycogen may be present: these were formerly misinterpreted as rhabdomyo-mas (see pages 66 and 81, Volume 1). In the lungs

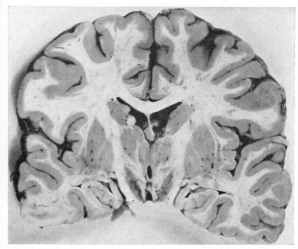

Fig. 34.100. Tuberose sclerosis. Note the nodular protrusions on the lateral walls of the ventricles, giving rise to a corrugated appearance ('candle guttering'). These subependymal areas of gliosis often calcify and they may then be identified radiologically. The cortex of the right inferior temporal gyrus (left side of the photograph) is deficient and its place is taken by dense gliosis. The patient, an imbecile, died at the age of 21 years.

there may be many small cysts and bronchial hamartomas. Osteoporosis occurs, especially in the small bones of the hands: it is uncertain whether this is a primary effect of the disease or secondary to malnutrition or physical inactivity.

The finding of any of these malformations during investigation of cases of imbecility is helpful as an indication of the likelihood of tuberose sclerosis. However, tuberose sclerosis may exist with no anomalies other than those in the brain.

Central Neurofibromatosis

The rare condition that is sometimes referred to as central neurofibromatosis, or Wishart's disease,[641] may occur in association with neurofibromatosis of the peripheral nerves (von Recklinghausen's* disease of nerves), or it may exist without the latter. It is usually associated with anomalies of development of the nervous system, and sometimes with multiple gliomas. It is characterized by tumours of the vestibulocochlear nerves, multiple meningiomas, and multiple tumours of spinal nerve roots. The disease tends to give rise to symptoms early in adult

* Von Recklinghausen described the disease of peripheral nerves in 1882 (Recklinghausen, F. von, *Ueber die multiplen Fibrome der Haut und ihre Beziehung zu den multiplen Neuromen*; Berlin, 1882). It had previously been illustrated by Tilesius in 1793 (see footnote on page 2338), by Walther in 1814 and by R. W. Smith, of Dublin, in 1849.

5*

life and it may be familial. The tumours, although usually referred to as neurofibromas, have features that relate them both to meningiomas and to neurolemmomas: however, there is, in general, a more widespread deposition of collagen than is usual in either of these types of neoplasm. In spite of this fibrous component, the tumours are often soft. Those on nerve roots, like the tumours of peripheral nerves in von Recklinghausen's disease, often have a fusiform outline (see page 2339).

Syringomyelia

Syringomyelia, which is characterized by a tube-like cavity in the spinal cord, is probably developmental in origin, for it is sometimes associated with neurofibromatosis and malformations of the skeleton. The clinical signs of the disease generally appear in adolescence or early adult life. Less often, the defect is in the medulla oblongata—*syringobulbia*.

The cavity, or 'syrinx', is generally largest in the cervical region of the spinal cord, which, in consequence, may appear fusiform (Fig. 34.102). It usually lies within the grey matter, often apart from

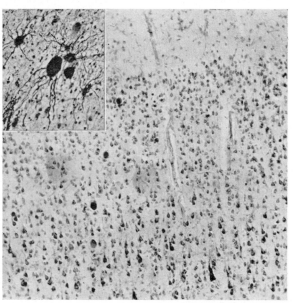

Fig. 34.101. Tuberose sclerosis. The field illustrated is from part of the cerebral cortex in which the abnormality is of moderate severity only: there is a reduction in the number of nerve cells in laminae III and IV. Occasional large globoid cells are present. *Haematoxylin–eosin.* × 100.

Inset: Globoid cells stained to show their processes. These cells are of bizarre character, with resemblances to both nerve cell and astrocyte. *Frozen section. Bielschowsky's stain.* × 180.

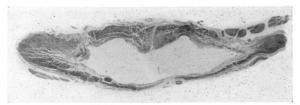

Fig. 34.102.§ Syringomyelia. Cervical region of the spinal cord. The patient was a middle-aged man who had been incapacitated for many years. The cord is much distorted, through artefact; this does not obscure the relative size and position of the syringomyelic cavity. ×4.

and behind the central canal, compressing both it and the nerve fibres that convey the sensations of pain and temperature as they cross in the anterior white commissure to enter the spinothalamic tracts. For this reason, the earliest signs of the disease are disturbances of these types of sensation: for instance, a cook repeatedly burns her hands, because the afferent element in the protective withdrawal reflex has been lost, or a young factory worker suffers repeated injuries to his fingers because the deficiency in pain sensibility deprives him of the stimulus to take greater care.

As the cavity enlarges, it may compress the anterior grey columns. When the lower cervical segments are so affected, the muscles of the forearm and the intrinsic muscles of the hand—notably those of the thenar eminence—become atrophic. Syringomyelia is the classic cause of the 'claw hand' deformity (*main en griffe*). In time, fibres in the long tracts may become involved, notably those of the corticospinal tracts, the spinocerebellar tracts and the posterior funiculi: the symptomatology of the disease therefore becomes more diverse, and signs of disability appear in the legs as well. Nystagmus, which is a fairly constant sign, results from the destruction of fibres that enter the medial longitudinal fasciculus from the vestibular nuclei.

The upper end of the cavity is usually at the level of the second cervical segment, but a slit-like extension sometimes continues upward into the medulla oblongata and may reach the pons. In such cases, there may be involvement of the hypoglossal and facial nerves, and even of the ophthalmic nerves (the ophthalmic divisions of the trigeminal nerves), the fibres of which descend to synapse with the lowermost cells of the spinal nucleus of the ipsilateral trigeminal nerve in the first cervical segment of the spinal cord. The maxillary and mandibular nerves terminate above this level and are unaffected.

The cavity generally contains clear, yellow-tinted fluid, of variable protein concentration.

Syringomyelic cavities have also been found in association with an ependymoma or haemangioma.[641a] The cavity in such cases is usually in the lumbosacral region, extending over a few or many segments and not necessarily in continuity with the tumour. It is not known whether syringomyelia precedes the development of the tumour or is a sequel of its presence.

Hydromyelia is the name given to the dilatation of the central canal of the spinal cord that is sometimes found in association with meningomyelocele and the Arnold–Chiari malformation (see page 2199), particularly in older patients.

A cavity within the spinal cord may also be the end-result of a haematoma. An intramedullary haemorrhage tends to track along the cord in the line of the columns of nerve fibres: when the blood forming the haematoma has broken down its place is taken by yellow fluid occupying a longitudinally disposed cavity.

Pathogenesis.—It has been suggested that most, if not all cases of syringomyelia are the result of longstanding hydromyelia, originating in embryonal life through overdistension of the neural tube.[642] The hydromyelia is caused by obstruction to the outflow of the cerebrospinal fluid from the fourth ventricle because of inadequate drainage through its roof, with the consequence that the cerebrospinal fluid pulse wave is transmitted into the central canal of the spinal cord. At a later stage a breach develops in the ependyma, allowing lateral dissection of the wall of the hydromyelic canal by the pulsating fluid. The cavity thus formed is later separated by gliosis from the central canal, which eventually becomes obliterated. The histological features of syringomyelia are thereby established. In those cases in which the median aperture of the fourth ventricle is patent syringomyelia may result from arachnoiditis involving the roof of the ventricle or from obstruction of the aperture by abnormally situated cerebellar tonsils. Surgery is of great value in many cases.[643]

Down's Syndrome (Mongolism)[644, 644a]

Down's syndrome is a manifestation of an error in chromosomal separation during the formation of the germ cells.

Cytogenetics[644b–644d]

In the normal human karyotype (46,XY), every somatic cell contains 22 paired chromosomes and two sex chromosomes, a total of 46. Each parent normally contributes a complete half set (23 chromosomes) to the offspring. In 'squash' preparations of dividing nuclei the individual chromosomes are seen to have a distinctive length and shape: for identification, they have been numbered, in decreasing order of length, from 1 to 22, leaving X and Y to denote the two sex chromosomes.

In the common form of Down's syndrome, which is most frequent among infants borne by mothers towards the end of reproductive life, and which is not familial, there are 47 chromosomes in each somatic cell—three of them of the type numbered 21 (47,XX,21+ or 47,XY,21+).[645, 646] This trisomy arises through the failure of the two chromosomes of pair 21 to separate during oogenesis, with the consequence that the ovum contains both chromosomes of pair 21 instead of only one, and contributes both of them to the zygote that follows fertilization by a normal sperm.

There is an infrequent form of Down's syndrome, occurring without relation to maternal age, and often familial. In this form, 'squash' preparations show that 46 chromosomes are present in dividing somatic cells, but analysis of their length and shape show that an extra chromosome 21 is attached to the end of one of the other chromosomes. Hence, although 46 chromosomes are counted, the genetic material of chromosome 21 is triplicated within each somatic cell instead of duplicated as in the normal state. This condition is known as *translocation Down's syndrome*. Chromosomal examination of the parents of these patients often shows that the somatic cells of one of them have only 45 chromosomes, and that this apparent deficiency is again due to the fusion of number 21 to one of the other chromosomes (usually to a chromosome of the 13-15 group): such a parent has little or no loss of chromosome material and is clinically normal. When gametes are formed there are four possible combinations. If the gamete receives a 21 and, say, a 15 the result will be a normal child. If it receives a 15 and no 21 the zygote will be non-viable. If it receives a composite 15²¹ chromosome and a chromosome 21 the child will have translocation Down's syndrome (46,XX, 15²¹ or 46,XY,15²¹). In the event of the gamete receiving a composite 15²¹ and no 21 the child, like the parent, will be a translocation carrier. If the mother is the composite 15²¹ translocation carrier the incidence of Down's syndrome in her children will be the expected one in three; but if it is the father the chances are that the children will be either normal or translocation carriers.[647] An example of Down's syndrome apparently with normal chromosome karyotype has been recorded.[648]

Neuropathology

There have been many reports of structural abnormalities in the brain of patients with this disease: these have sometimes been attributed to maldevelopment and sometimes to ischaemia. They include micrencephaly, the presence of undeveloped neurons, widespread absence of the neurons of the third cortical lamina, defective myelination, and fibrillary gliosis of the white matter. The only specific peculiarity, however, is the characteristic shape of the posterior part of the brain, which has had to adapt itself to the almost vertical disposition of the occipital bone that is a typical feature of the cranium in this condition. Smallness of the cerebellum and undue narrowing of the superior temporal gyrus are also characteristic, but these features may be seen in the absence of Down's syndrome.[649]

The association of argyrophile plaques and neurofibrillary tangles with Down's syndrome is of interest;[650] a series of 45 cases was reviewed in 1969.[651] The lesions are similar to those of Alzheimer's disease (page 2274) and it has been stated that Alzheimer's disease is present in every patient with Down's syndrome who is over 35 years old.[652] Severe mental deterioration is frequently observed in patients with Down's syndrome who survive until puberty: hormonal factors may be important in this development, and the changes that bring Alzheimer's disease into consideration may also be relevant, although the latter may be present without clinical evidence of dementia. Nothing is known about the relation, if any, between the development of plaques and tangles and the differences in karyotype that are represented by the occurrence of Down's syndrome in association with simple trisomy and with translocation. There is evidence that variations in physical characteristics and in development may be related to chromosomal differences.[653]

The Brain in Mental Deficiency[654]

Many forms of idiocy and imbecility have their origin in embryonic life and are recognizable at birth or soon afterwards. Some of them, like phenylketonuria (see page 2239) and the various cerebral lipidoses (see page 2235), may become apparent in infancy. However, the lipidoses sometimes remain clinically silent until childhood or even later.

Gross errors of development, such as microgyria and porencephaly, will be obvious when the brain is examined at necropsy, and so will the major anomalies of cortical lamination and the glial patches typical of tuberose sclerosis (see page 2202). For the rest, the neuropathologist who is called upon to investigate the brain of a mentally defective patient must rely upon histological material. He will gain much help from the stains that selectively demonstrate glial fibres and myelin in thick celloidin sections; Nissl stains will be needed for the study of the nerve cells. Haematoxylin–eosin preparations are of most value in the recognition of inflammatory states, tumours and other types of reaction that are not peculiar to the central nervous system.

TUMOURS OF THE CENTRAL NERVOUS SYSTEM

Many types of 'space-occupying lesion' are met with in the central nervous system. Some of these are granulomas, usually infective or parasitic: they have already been considered. Others are neoplasms, some of which originate in the central nervous system while the rest arise elsewhere and involve the brain or spinal cord, or the meninges, by direct extension or by metastasis. There is also a miscellaneous group of developmental lesions that present as solid or cystic masses and that may appropriately be considered in this section; they are infrequent in comparison with true neoplasms. We use the term tumour, therefore, to refer both to true neoplasms and to this miscellaneous group; in accordance with custom, we do not include infective, granulomatous and other such masses under this term.

It is intended to discuss here the tumours that involve the central nervous system with the exception of those that arise in the pituitary gland (see page 1880, Volume 4) and pineal body (see page 2070, Volume 4). There have been many classifications of the primary neoplasms of the brain. It is not proposed to review them here: full accounts have been given by Russell and Rubinstein[655] and by Zülch.[656] The following classification is employed:

Tumours Involving the Central Nervous System

(Excluding Tumours of Pituitary and Pineal Origin)

A. Primary tumours—

   1. neuroectodermal tumours—

      (a) gliomas:

         (i) glioblastoma multiforme
        (ii) astrocytic glioma
       (iii) oligodendrocytoma
       (iv) ependymoma
        (v) papilloma of choroid plexus
      (vi) mixed glioma

      (b) neuronal tumours:

         (i) ganglioneuroma and ganglioglioma
        (ii) neuroblastoma
       (iii) medulloblastoma

   2. mesodermal tumours—

      (a) meningeal tumours:

         (i) meningioma
        (ii) sarcoma
       (iii) melanoma

      (b) neurolemmal tumours

      (c) blood vessel tumours:

         (i) haemangioblastoma
        (ii) blood vessel hamartoma

      (d) tumours of reticuloendothelial cells

B. Secondary tumours

C. Miscellaneous tumours and cysts of developmental origin:

   1. craniopharyngioma
   2. colloid cyst
   3. 'cholesteatoma' and dermoid cyst
   4. chordoma.

PRIMARY TUMOURS

Neuroectodermal Tumours

The medullary epithelium differentiates to form both the neurons and the neuroglial cells, the latter eventually developing into astrocytes, oligodendrocytes and ependymal cells.

Gliomas

The gliomas are primary tumours of neuroglial cells, and in their cellular structure they may resemble any of the three main types of these cells. They are by nature invasive, and their complete surgical removal is often difficult or impossible. Their prognosis depends less on the type of tumour than on its site of origin, its capacity to attract attention by causing significant symptoms at an early stage in its growth, and its accessibility to the surgeon. For example, a slowly growing, well-differentiated tumour in the pons may have a graver prognosis than a more rapidly growing tumour in a frontal lobe, which is surgically accessible.

Glioblastoma Multiforme

By far the commonest of the gliomas is the glioblastoma multiforme, a rapidly growing tumour that is rarely amenable to surgical treatment. It is sometimes seen in childhood, but its incidence is greatest in the fourth and fifth decades. It is usually in the cerebrum, and symptoms are seldom present for more than a few months before the patient is obliged to seek medical attention.

Glioblastomas are found oftenest in the white matter of the frontal lobes, the septum pellucidum, the basal ganglia, the hypothalamus and the corpus callosum. The callosal glioblastomas may radiate out into the white matter of the centrum semiovale on both sides, giving rise to an appearance sometimes described as the 'butterfly tumour'. Occasionally, glioblastomas arise in the white matter of one hemisphere and spread through the corpus callosum to the opposite side. Sometimes, they are peripherally situated in the parietal or temporal lobe, and at first sight appear to be removable. However, it is always difficult to define where the glioma ends and uninvolved white matter begins. Macroscopically, these growths are mainly pale yellow, with salmon pink areas scattered through their substance. They are soft and often haemorrhagic (Fig. 34.103).

Histologically, a glioblastoma multiforme has several characteristic features: (1) cellular pleomorphism; (2) the presence of primitive glial cells; (3) the presence of multinucleate tumour giant cells; (4) endothelial proliferation in the blood vessels, with or without thickening of the connective tissue round them; (5) areas of necrosis; and (6) regimentation ('palisading') of the tumour cell nuclei round blood vessels and at the periphery of necrotic areas (Fig. 34.104). Many of the cells resemble spongioblasts, which are the somewhat spindle-shaped, earliest precursors of the astrocytes (Fig. 34.105). For the rest, the cellular component

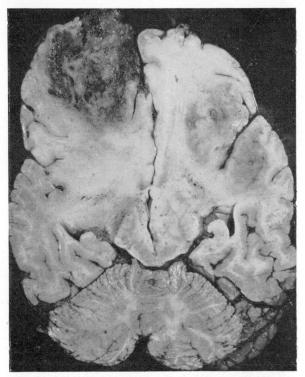

Fig. 34.103. A haemorrhagic glioblastoma multiforme is present in the left frontal cortex; on the opposite side there is a glioma (of similar microscopical structure) astride the lateral sulcus. Multiple gliomas are uncommon: when present, they are not always of the same histological type. Two apparently separate tumours may prove on careful examination to be continuous with each other.

of the tumour ranges from cells with an abundance of cytoplasm, an eccentric nucleus and some discernible similarity to the astrocyte (Fig. 34.106), to cells of such bizarre appearance as to make any comparison with normal glial cells impossible. Others may have cytoplasmic processes attached to blood vessels: these cells resemble astroblasts, which are cells at a stage of maturation intermediate between spongioblasts and astrocytes. Mitotic figures are common.

It has been suggested that all glioblastomas develop from astrocytomas; however, it cannot be denied that other types of glial cell could be their origin in some instances. There have been occasional reports of slowly growing tumours that at biopsy have been found to be astrocytomas or oligodendrocytomas, and that eventually—perhaps years later—became transformed into rapidly growing tumours with the histological characteristics of a glioblastoma multiforme. There is, however, no evidence that this sequence is the rule:

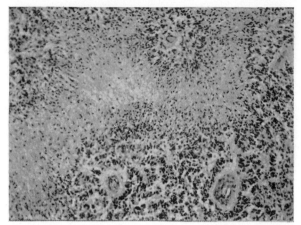

Fig. 34.104. Glioblastoma multiforme showing an area of necrosis with bordering 'palisades' of tumour cells. The tumour cells close to the thick-walled blood vessels probably survive because of their proximity to the blood supply. *Haematoxylin–eosin.* × 120.

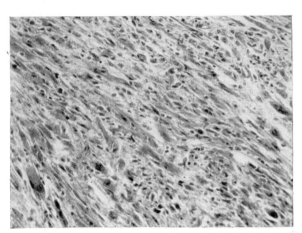

Fig. 34.105. Malignant glioma composed of spindle-shaped cells (spongioblasts). Note the giant multinucleate form toward the bottom left-hand corner. In other parts of the specimen the cells were more pleomorphic and all the features of a glioblastoma multiforme were present. *Haematoxylin–eosin.* × 120.

indeed, a survey of 129 cases of glioblastoma indicated that 78 (60 per cent) were glioblastomas *ab initio*.[657] These tumours, therefore, are assigned to a category of their own, for they are too un-differentiated to be considered among any of the types of tumour composed of cells resembling mature glial cells.

Proliferation of the endothelium of the blood vessels is a regular, and often striking, feature of glioblastomas (Fig. 34.107): it obstructs the blood flow and predisposes to thrombosis, and therefore to ischaemic necrosis of the parts of the tumour supplied by the affected vessels. Necrosis of the tumour tissue is often accompanied by haemorrhage. On rare occasions, malignant change seems to take place in the vessels, producing a mixed tumour with both glioblastomatous and angiosarcomatous elements.

Astrocytic Gliomas: (a) Astrocytoma

The second commonest tumour of the glioma group is the astrocytoma. Macroscopically, it generally appears as a solid, whitish, ill-defined tumour, difficult to distinguish from ordinary white matter, except that it usually feels softer and has a finely granular appearance. Sometimes the tumour is firmer; in other instances it contains many small, cyst-like spaces, which may be confluent (Fig. 34.108). When very slow growing it may show a little calcification (Fig. 34.109).

Various histological types of astrocytoma have been recognized: protoplasmic, fibrillary, pilocytic, gemistocytic and anaplastic (see below). However, these tumours often show much variation in structure from one part to another: mixed forms are common, and many are so ill-differentiated as

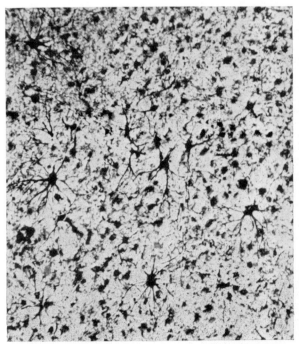

Fig. 34.106. Glioblastoma multiforme: the tumour cells are derived from the astrocyte series but have abnormally large cell bodies and show great variation in the number and shape of the processes. *Frozen section. Cajal's gold sublimate.* × 150.

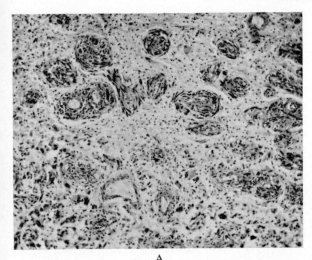

A

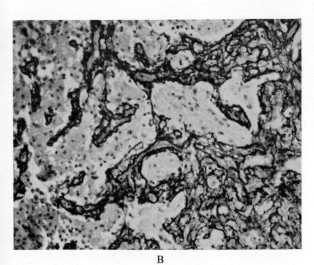

B

Fig. 34.107. Glioblastoma multiforme showing very marked endothelial proliferation in the blood vessels, many of which are occluded. Scattered pleomorphic cells of glial origin are to be seen, especially at the bottom of 'A'. A: *Haematoxylin–Van Gieson*; × 100. B: *Reticulin*; × 150.

to merge into the category of glioblastoma multiforme.

Protoplasmic Astrocytoma.—This type is composed of cells that have a close resemblance to the normal astrocyte. The nuclei are more conspicuous than those of normal cells; they stain more darkly, and vary much in size and shape. The cytoplasm is usually clearly discernible, but cytoplasmic processes are few and are separated from each other by minute spaces (Fig. 34.109) that, on becoming confluent, gradually develop into pseudocysts.

Fibrillary Astrocytoma.—This type contains an abundance of astroglial fibrils, although the cells themselves are sometimes quite small. The fibrillary astrocytomas are white; because of their fibrillary structure they are rather firm.

Pilocytic Astrocytoma.—This variant is characterized by elongation of its cells, and particularly of their nuclei (Fig. 34.110). The paucity of the cytoplasmic processes, which are both long and

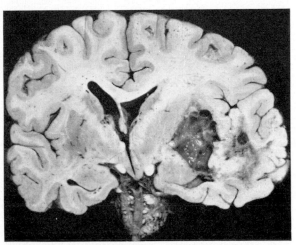

Fig. 34.108. A large and mainly pseudocystic astrocytoma in the left cerebral hemisphere. It has produced so much swelling that the ventricular cavities are displaced and the septum pellucidum is well across the midline. Above the corpus callosum the left cingulate gyrus has herniated across the midline below the free edge of the falx cerebri. The true extent of a tumour of this type, when examined histologically, is often far greater than naked-eye inspection would suggest.

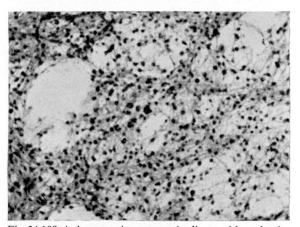

Fig. 34.109. A slow-growing astrocytic glioma with coalescing pseudocystic spaces. Note the fine glial processes and the variation in the size of the nuclei. This is a so-called protoplasmic astrocytoma. There is one small deposit of calcium (centre of picture). *Haematoxylin–eosin.* × 175.

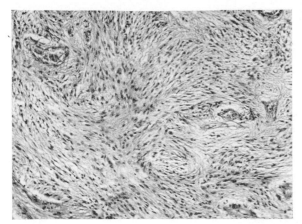

Fig. 34.110. Astrocytoma composed of small cells with fine hair-like processes (pilocytic type). It bears a superficial resemblance to a neurolemmoma. *Mallory's phosphotungstic acid haematoxylin.* × 100.

fine, and their arrangement often give the cells a bipolar appearance.

Structures known as 'cytoid bodies' or Rosenthal's fibres[658] are commonly present in pilocytic astrocytomas. They are tapering or beaded masses of homogeneous, opaque, eosinophile appearance, situated in the cytoplasm of the tumour astrocytes: they are particularly well seen in sections stained with phosphotungstic acid haematoxylin, which colours them dark purple. Electron microscopy shows them to occur in relation to a well-marked formation of glial filaments in the astrocytes:[658a] they are osmiophile and distinct from, although merged with, the glial filaments. They are considered to be degenerative in nature. Identical structures are seen in occasional gliomas of other types and in foci of longstanding reactive gliosis (for instance, adjoining syringomyelic cavities).

Gemistocytic Astrocytoma.—In this form, the cells are greatly swollen (Fig. 34.111). The nucleus is eccentric, varies much in size and shape, and contains a prominent nucleolus. The cytoplasmic processes are few in number. The tumour is usually very cellular and the cells are packed closely. It presents macroscopically as a soft, grey mass.

Anaplastic Astrocytoma.—The commonest variety of astrocytoma is the poorly differentiated and rapidly growing tumour described as anaplastic. It may show features of any of the four types already described, together with cellular pleomorphism, proliferation of blood vessels and necrosis. In rapidly growing astrocytomas, mitotic figures may be found. It is often difficult to distinguish histo-

logically between anaplastic astrocytoma and glioblastoma multiforme (Fig. 34.112); prognostically, the distinction is unimportant.

General Comments on the Astrocytomas.—Astrocytomas in particular sites may show distinctive pathological features. For instance, a slowly growing and usually 'cystic' variety of astrocytoma is found typically in the cerebellum in children and adolescents, and occasionally in young adults (Fig. 34.113). Sometimes, almost the whole of the cerebellar tumour undergoes pseudocystic degeneration, only a single nodule remaining in the wall of the cavity. These tumours are composed mainly of small cells, which resemble a type of astrocyte that is peculiar to the normal cerebellar cortex. They may also contain pilocytic and other forms of astrocyte.

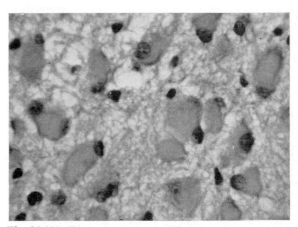

Fig. 34.111. Tumour composed of large swollen astrocytes ('gemistocytic' astrocytoma). *Haematoxylin–eosin.* × 360.

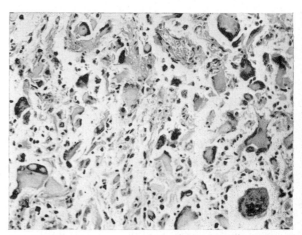

Fig. 34.112. Tumour composed of bizarre cells, many of them multinucleate: this is part of a glioblastoma multiforme. *Haematoxylin–eosin.* × 150.

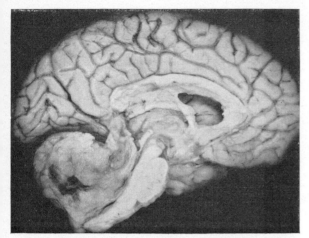

Fig. 34.113. Slow-growing pseudocystic astrocytoma occupying most of the midline of the cerebellum and obstructing the aqueduct, thereby giving rise to dilatation of the third and lateral ventricles. The patient was a girl, aged 17 years, who complained of severe headache and visual failure.

Another part in which astrocytomas are particularly likely to arise is the brainstem. The brainstem tumours may occur at any age, even as late as the eighth decade: they are especially common in young people. They have sometimes been grouped with the polar spongioblastomas (see next page), because the tumour cells of the brainstem astrocytomas are spindle-shaped: however, it seems very likely that this appearance of the cells results from their adaptation to the anatomical peculiarities of the pons, where some axons run longitudinally and others transversely. The tumour cells thus tend to be moulded lengthwise in the plane of the fibres between which they grow. This interpretation has been supported by the observation that in tissue cultures these spindle-shaped cells, while retaining their neoplastic features, revert to the ordinary shape of astrocytes.[659]

In children, the region of the third ventricle is another site in which astrocytomas are especially likely to develop.

The glioma of the optic nerve, the commonest tumour of this structure, is an astrocytoma. It arises oftenest in childhood (see Chapter 40, Volume 6). It tends to grow through the sheath of the nerve, and may sometimes closely simulate a meningioma. Several histological varieties have been described, the commonest being composed of closely packed, spindle-shaped cells with readily demonstrable intervening glial fibrils: these cells are usually regarded as astrocytic.

Astrocytomas are commonest, however, in the cerebrum. They may be found in any of the regions in which glioblastoma multiforme arises (see page 2207), but the parietal lobe and the frontal lobe are their most usual locations. The fibrillary astrocytoma is the commonest variety in the cerebrum. The tumour may be localized or it may spread diffusely through its surroundings: it is often impossible to distinguish a boundary between the neoplastic and normal tissues. When an astrocytoma invades the cortex, as sometimes happens, the nerve cells often persist, apparently unaffected, among the tumour cells. Endothelial proliferation is often seen in the blood vessels of astrocytomas.

The incidence of the slower growing types of astrocytoma is greatest in the third decade. The prognosis worsens as the age at the onset of symptoms rises.[660]

An occasional but important source of diagnostic confusion in biopsy practice is the tumour-like arrangement and cytological characteristics of astrocytes in the tissue bordering on some inflammatory lesions of the brain (Fig. 34.114).

Astrocytic Gliomas: (b) Astroblastoma

The term astroblastoma was included in the classification of gliomas set out by Bailey and Cushing,[661] and it has been retained by Russell and Rubinstein.[662] Kernohan and his colleagues,[660] however, placed the astroblastomas among the astrocytomas. The diagnostic feature of the astroblastoma is the rosette-like arrangement of the tumour cells round the blood vessels, each of the cells having a broad attachment to a vessel wall. Pure tumours of this type are rare: they usually occur in the cerebral hemispheres of young adults. Ordinarily, they grow slowly. Sometimes, parts of a glioblastoma multi-

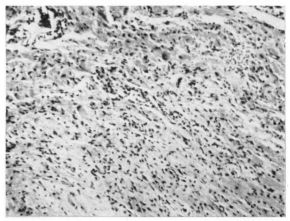

Fig. 34.114. Simulation of a tumour by reacting astrocytes (upper part of picture) at the margin of an inflammatory lesion in the brain. *Haematoxylin–eosin.* × 100.

forme or of an astrocytoma show this arrangement of the neoplastic astrocytes.

Astrocytic Gliomas: (c) Polar Spongioblastoma

This is a rare malignant tumour that arises in the region of the third or fourth ventricle in young people. It has a pronounced tendency to infiltrate along the ependyma and in the meninges. It is composed of cells with tapering ends that resemble bipolar spongioblasts; their nuclei are arranged in palisade fashion.[663]

Oligodendrocytoma

The oligodendrocytoma is a relatively uncommon tumour in spite of the fact that the oligodendrocyte greatly outnumbers the other cells of the brain. It arises as a rule in the cerebral white matter, especially that of the frontal lobes, and it generally becomes manifest in adult life. Sometimes, the tumour protrudes into the lateral ventricle. In children, it is often situated in a thalamus.[656] The patient's symptoms usually suggest that the growth has been developing slowly over a long period, often for years.

The cut surface of an oligodendrocytoma is generally pink or red, and its outline is rounded and fairly well defined (Fig. 34.115). It may be gelatinous in parts, or it may feel gritty because of numerous flecks of calcification in its substance. The presence of the calcium salts may facilitate localization of the tumour by X-ray examination. Although calcification is usually most marked in the outer margin of the tumour, the size of the growth sometimes proves to be appreciably larger than is shown radiographically.

Tumour oligodendrocytes may differ little from normal oligodendrocytes (Figs 34.116 and 34.117): the nucleus of each is surrounded by a halo of clear cytoplasm, and as the cells may lie grouped together the histological appearance has been likened to a honeycomb. The size and shape of the nuclei vary, usually more so in the central parts of the tumour than near its edge, where it may not be possible to distinguish the tumour cells from normal oligodendrocytes. Astrocytes are sometimes present in these tumours, singly or in small clusters; it is debatable whether they should be regarded as tumour astrocytes or as a manifestation of a reactive proliferation of glial cells in response to the presence of the tumour. A typical feature of the oligodendrocytoma is the arrangement of its plentiful blood vessels, which tend to branch at

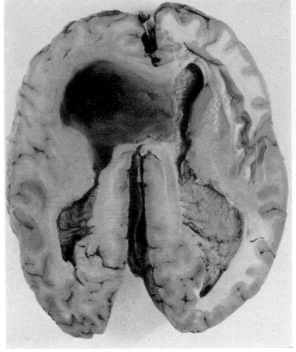

Fig. 34.115. Oligodendrocytoma. The tumour is sharply defined, deep-seated and well vascularized. Flecks of calcification were visible radiographically.

right angles. Endothelial cell proliferation, often so conspicuous in astrocytomas, is unusual unless the tumour is undergoing malignant change. Calcification occurs so commonly that it may be regarded as a feature typical of the oligodendrocytoma: it appears as fine lamellae of calcium salts within the walls of blood vessels, or as coarse clumps within the tumour tissue in their vicinity. In some tumours, fine deposits of calcium may be found outlining individual tumour cells or their nuclei.

Although most oligodendrocytomas grow slowly, occasional mitotic figures may be found. After attempts at surgical removal, the tumour may become less differentiated: mitotic figures are then more plentiful, the cells are less well formed, and growth proceeds rapidly. In fact, parts of such tumours may be difficult to distinguish from a glioblastoma.[664]

Ependymoma

Ependymomas develop from the lining of the ventricular system (Fig. 34.118) and, as might be expected, they commonly grow into the ventricles. However, not all tumours that appear to arise from

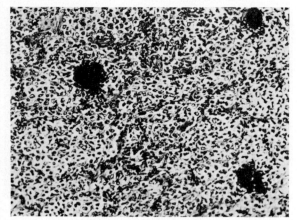

Fig. 34.116. Oligodendrocytoma showing irregular foci of calcification, and small, thin-walled, branching blood vessels dividing the tumour in a characteristic way. The cell nuclei may be pleomorphic as here, but characteristically they are round. Each nucleus is surrounded by a clear halo ('boxing' of nuclei—see Fig. 34.117). *Haematoxylin–eosin.* × 80.

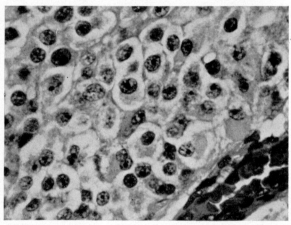

Fig. 34.117. Oligodendrocytoma showing typical 'boxing' of nuclei within clear cytoplasm. An occasional tumour cell is seen to have abundant opaque cytoplasm. *Haematoxylin–eosin.* × 400.

the ventricular walls are ependymomas: some are astrocytomas, developing from subependymal astrocytes. Glioblastomas and oligodendrocytomas, although arising at a greater distance from the ventricles, may also in time protrude into their cavity.

The ependymoma is a slowly growing tumour occurring mostly in young people. Its cells are typically epithelial in appearance and arrangement and may be grouped round small spaces that resemble glandular acini: sometimes they are regularly arranged in a rosette-like pattern round blood vessels (Fig. 34.119). When typical and slowly growing, ependymomas are easy to recog-

nize, but in their rarer, more anaplastic forms they may resemble the glioblastomas. In the majority of these tumours, and most constantly in the slowly-growing varieties, minute granules, called *blepharoplasts*, may be seen near the nucleus of some cells.[665] The blepharoplasts correspond to the basal bodies, which are seen under the electron microscope to be the point at which the ciliary shafts terminate. Light microscopy often fails to disclose them, particularly in biopsy specimens, even when sections are stained with Mallory's phosphotungstic acid haematoxylin, for which the blepharoplasts ordinarily have a strong affinity. This stain will

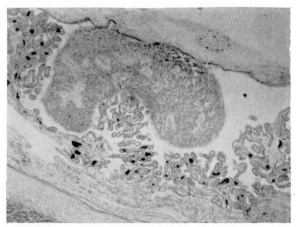

Fig. 34.118. Minute ependymoma discovered by chance in a lateral aperture of the fourth ventricle. *Celloidin section. Nissl's stain.* × 40.

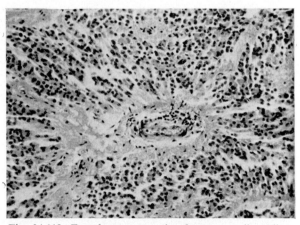

Fig. 34.119. Ependymoma: cords of tumour cells radiate round a blood vessel ('pseudorosette', or 'gliovascular system'). The tumour illustrated was in the thoracic part of the spinal cord. Its effect was comparable to transection of the cord. A syringomyelic cavity extended through several segments of the cord above and below the level of the tumour. *Haematoxylin–eosin.* × 135.

often also reveal glial fibres among the cells that form the circumvascular rosettes.

Ependymomas occur in any of the ventricles; they arise most frequently in the fourth ventricle. They are also the commonest variety of intramedullary tumour of the spinal cord, in which they occur oftenest in the lumbosacral and cervical regions. An ependymoma of the spinal cord is likely to be associated with syringomyelia (see page 2204).

Some ependymomas have a papillary form, and it is important to distinguish them from papillomas of the choroid plexus and from metastatic deposits of papillary adenocarcinoma. The name *myxopapillary ependymoma* is reserved for a form of this tumour that arises in the filum terminale (Fig. 34.120): mucoid degeneration of the fibrous stroma is a feature characteristic of ependymomas in this situation and seen only exceptionally when they arise elsewhere.

The term *subependymoma* has sometimes been given to an ependymoma in which there is a diffuse proliferation of subependymal fibrillary astrocytes among the ependymal tumour cells. Occasionally, such tumours are small and symptomless; they may be multiple, and they occur oftenest in the fourth ventricle.[666]

Papilloma of the Choroid Plexus

The simple papilloma arising from a choroid plexus is not uncommon. It is formed of epithelial cells that are arranged regularly, usually in a single layer, on the delicate connective tissue stroma of the papilliform processes. It occurs most frequently in young adults. Its commonest site is the fourth ventricle (Figs 34.121 and 34.122); it may cause

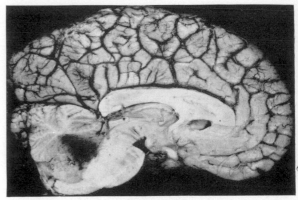

Fig. 34.121. Choroid plexus papilloma of fourth ventricle. It has spread up the aqueduct and caused dilatation of the third and lateral ventricles.

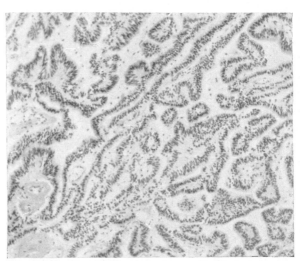

Fig. 34.122. Choroid plexus papilloma: histological appearance of tumour illustrated in Fig. 34.121. *Haematoxylin–eosin.* × 70.

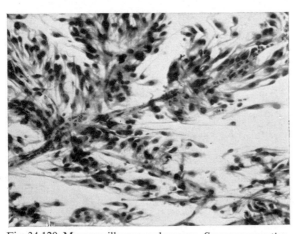

Fig. 34.120. Myxopapillary ependymoma. *Smear preparation. Mallory's phosphotungstic acid haematoxylin.* × 150.

intermittent obstructive hydrocephalus, and sometimes blindness due to herniation of the optic recess and consequent pressure on the optic chiasma or optic nerves. It may also arise in the lateral ventricles, notably in the trigone; it is a rarity in the third ventricle.[656]

The tumour sometimes occurs in early childhood, and it may be congenital. It secretes cerebrospinal fluid, and the resulting overproduction may give rise to hydrocephalus in infancy or even in late fetal life.

The cells of the choroid plexuses are specialized ependymal cells, and the tumours that arise from them might therefore appropriately be classified among the ependymomas. In an ependymoma, however, occasional glial processes are found, and these are absent from the choroid papillomas.

Papillomas of the choroid plexuses are difficult to remove. They tend to recur after attempted excision.

Other tumours and tumour-like lesions of the choroid plexuses include meningiomas (particularly in the lateral ventricles), haemangiomas, xanthomatous nodules and metastatic carcinoma. Metastatic carcinoma requires very careful consideration in the differential diagnosis of choroid papilloma.

Mixed Gliomas

In general, although there may be considerable variation in the intimate structure, and particularly in the cytology, of any example of a glioma, each tumour is composed essentially of cells that are typical of the form that it represents. However, mixed gliomas are by no means rare: the commonest combination is the presence of oligodendrocytomatous foci in an otherwise typical astrocytoma, which may belong to any of the mature or poorly differentiated types. A mixture of oligodendrocytoma and ependymoma is seen occasionally.

Prognostic Grading of Biopsy Specimens

Efforts that have been made to grade biopsy specimens of astrocytic and other gliomas for purposes of prognosis[667, 667a] have proved to be of limited value because of the variation in histological appearances that may be found in sections of different parts of a single tumour. However, it is of some help to the neurosurgeon to know to which of the four grades defined by Kernohan and his colleagues[667] the biopsy sample conforms: if it is to grade 1, he may hope for a relatively favourable prognosis; if it is to grade 4, he knows at once that the tumour is rapidly growing. The Kernohan grades indicate increasing degrees of malignancy as shown by histological appearances, ranging from well differentiated to anaplastic: however, the grading of individual cases, in biopsy material, is relevant only to the appearances in the sample examined and takes no account of variation in the degree of anaplasia that may exist elsewhere in the tumour.

Aetiology of Gliomas

Little is known of the pathogenesis of gliomas. The view that they originate from embryonic rests has little to support it. Likewise, no significant association has been observed between the development of gliomas and the presence of chronic inflammatory disease of the brain or of metabolic abnormalities.

There is no convincing evidence that trauma plays any part in the causation of gliomas. It is not uncommon, however, to obtain a history of a blow on the head, with symptoms dating from that time. In such cases the clinical course is often rapid—perhaps only a few weeks—and it is improbable that even the most malignant glioma could grow so quickly to the size found. It is generally believed that the head injury in such patients may have precipitated thrombosis in the vessels of a pre-existing glioma, or caused haemorrhage into its substance or rupture of thin septa of tumour tissue separating pseudocystic spaces, with consequent sudden appearance or aggravation of symptoms. It must be remembered, too, that the patient may have received his injury because of a neurological disability caused by the tumour: for instance, he may fail to avoid a blow because his field of vision is limited by homonymous hemianopia caused by an otherwise symptomless tumour involving an optic radiation, or he may be unable to save himself from a fall because his control of balance is disturbed.

Efforts to induce gliomas experimentally by introducing oncogenic substances into the brain have met with some success. In adult mice, several investigators have reported that the application of benzpyrene, dibenzanthracene and methylcholanthrene to the white matter and to the ependyma has been followed by the growth of astrocytomas, oligodendrocytomas and ependymomas.[668, 669] In adult rats, in contrast, only methylcholanthrene caused tumours to develop, none resulting from the application of dibenzanthracene or of benzpyrene.[670, 671] There are well-recognized differences in the susceptibility of different species to particular oncogenic chemicals, and this may account for these differing findings.

In recent years considerable attention has been centred on the ability of N-nitroso compounds (nitrosamines and nitrosamides) to induce tumours of the central and peripheral nervous system in animals.[672] The administration of a single dose of ethyl nitrosourea to pregnant rats induces a high yield of neural tumours in the offspring; newborn rodents are also highly susceptible to a single dose of this compound,[673] and the tumours that result have a particular tendency to arise from the subependymal plate, a site of active cell division in the normal neonatal brain. The possibility that nitroso compounds may be environmental contaminants can be viewed only with anxiety.

Neuronal Tumours

Ganglioneuroma and Ganglioglioma

A *ganglioneuroma* (neurocytoma) of the brain is a slowly growing tumour composed of neurons. The cells may be multinucleate, and although of bizarre appearance they may contain Nissl substance and even develop neurofibrils (Fig. 34.123). When neoplastic glial cells are also present, the tumours are called *gangliogliomas.*

Both these types of tumour are rare. They may occur in any part of the brain, but most frequently in the floor of the third ventricle, the hypothalamus, and the frontal and temporal lobes. They grow slowly, and are usually seen in the third decade of life. They are usually well circumscribed and firm, but they may be cystic. They are liable to be misinterpreted as an astrocytoma that has invaded an area containing neurons, or as a gemistocytic astrocytoma, the swollen cells of which have a superficial resemblance to nerve cells. They are occasionally found in the cerebellum, where they may present as a nodule in the cortex.[674]

Ganglioneuromas may also arise in the dorsal root ganglia, where they may grow so large that they compress the spinal cord and greatly expand the related intervertebral foramen. They form one variety of 'dumb-bell tumour': the other, the commoner, is a neurolemmoma (see page 2222).

Malignant change has been seen in ganglioneuromas, and in the nerve cells and the glial cells in gangliogliomas.[675] The pathologist must be on the look-out for nerve cells in any glioma, for their presence may have diagnostic importance. They are most readily distinguished from swollen astrocytes by their well-marked nucleolus and the presence of Nissl substance. It must be remembered that normal neurons may become incorporated in the substance of any variety of glioma as it invades the brain.

Neuroblastoma

Neuroblastomas (as distinct from medulloblastomas showing neuroblastic differentiation) rarely occur in the central nervous system. They usually appear during the first decade. They are well circumscribed but tend to spread by the cerebrospinal fluid pathways. The cells are uniform, polygonal or spheroidal, and have a clear nucleus with a prominent nucleolus. Various stages of differentiation toward mature neuron formation may be seen, although mature Nissl material is rarely found. The diagnosis can be difficult and debatable, depending on the demonstration of rosettes and the identification of neuroblasts with the help of silver impregnation techniques.

Medulloblastoma*

This distinctive tumour arises almost exclusively in the cerebellum. It is rarely seen after the age of 20 years, and it is commonest under the age of 10 years. It occurs oftener in boys than in girls. About three quarters of all medulloblastomas are midline tumours;[676] the rest arise in one of the cerebellar hemispheres or in the cerebellopontine angle. The tumour forms a soft, friable, greyish mass, with areas of necrosis. It grows quickly, and may cause symptoms suggestive of tuberculous meningitis or of the posterior basic type of meningococcal meningitis. It tends to protrude into the fourth ventricle, sometimes closing it, and it may spread widely within the subarachnoid space.

The medulloblastoma is a highly cellular growth and differs from almost all other primary tumours of the central nervous system in being markedly radiosensitive. The cells are small and have nuclei that are round or somewhat elongated, and usually hyperchromatic; the cytoplasm is scanty (Figs 34.124 and 34.125). Although they are arranged irregularly there is usually evidence of the tendency of the cells to form rosette-like groupings. Neurons of a primitive type are sometimes present: the

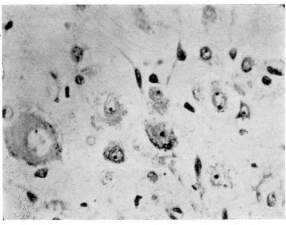

Fig. 34.123. Ganglioneuroma of frontal lobe. The tumour consists of nerve cells of various sizes and shapes, many of them containing Nissl substance. Some glial cells are also present. *Nissl's stain.* × 280.

* The name medulloblastoma, introduced in 1925 (Bailey, P., Cushing, H., *Arch. Neurol. Psychiat.* [*Chic.*], 1925, **14**, 192), is in general use. It is somewhat unsatisfactory in that there is no embryonic cell—or other normal cell—that is known as a medulloblast.

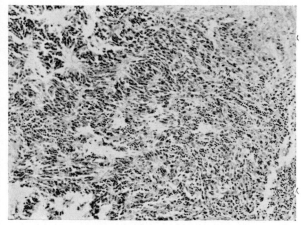

Fig. 34.124. Medulloblastoma invading cerebellum. The small round granule cells of the cerebellar cortex can be seen (bottom right quadrant) among the invading pleomorphic and primitive cells of the tumour. Note the tendency of the tumour cells to form rosettes. *Haematoxylin–eosin.* × 100.

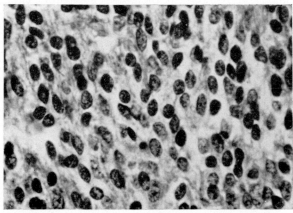

Fig. 34.125. Medulloblastoma. The nuclei are small, oval, undifferentiated and variable in their staining intensity; glial processes are scanty. *Mallory's phosphotungstic acid haematoxylin.* × 360.

embryonic medullary epithelium, of which the medulloblastoma is the neoplastic derivative, is the precursor of neurons as well as of glial cells. Delicate argyrophile fibrils can be seen in the tumour cells that form the rosettes; the fibrils occupy the same relative position in these cells as the fibrils in normal embryonic neuroblasts at an early stage of differentiation. Histologically, there is a close resemblance between the medulloblastoma and the adrenal neuroblastoma (see page 1963, Volume 4).

It has been suggested that the medulloblastomas originate from the cells that constitute Obersteiner's external granular layer in the cerebellum of the fetus and newborn infant and that migrate inward to join the definitive granule cell layer during the early months of life. A recent case report gives considerable support to this hypothesis: a medulloblastoma in a neonate merged with the external granular layer, the latter showing irregular proliferation.[677] Comparable tumours have been induced by the administration of ethyl nitrosourea.[677a]

General Observations on the Neuroectodermal Tumours

The ability of a glioma to spread by seeding is of considerable practical importance, and is determined by the situation of the growth rather than by its histological type. A glioma of any sort that has broken through the ependymal wall of one of the ventricles may shed cells into the cerebrospinal fluid: these may become implanted and grow in the wall of this or another ventricle or in the subarachnoid space, and particularly in the subarachnoid space of the spinal meninges. Ependymoma of the fourth ventricle and medulloblastoma are the tumours that are likeliest to be disseminated over the surface of the spinal cord by way of the cerebrospinal fluid. In fact, such seedlings are so common in cases of medulloblastoma that a prophylactic course of X-irradiation of the spinal canal is commonly given when the presence of this tumour has been established. A glioma that reaches the surface of the brain may spread by infiltration of the meninges: this is rarer and more localized than the comparable invasion of the meninges by metastatic carcinoma.

Rarely, a glioma is found in the nose, usually in the form of a polyp.[678] In almost all such cases a meningoencephalocele has presented through the floor of the ethmoidal sinus, and the tumour has arisen in this misplaced tissue. In the exceptional cases, the tumour arises from glial tissue that has been misplaced as part of a local malformation of the brain and skull (see page 224, Volume 1).

Gliomas do not naturally metastasize to parts of the body outside the central nervous system, although when a glioma develops in a teratoma—for instance, in an ovarian dermoid—it may metastasize through lymphatics to the regional lymph nodes (see Fig. 9.161, page 714 in Volume 2), and by the blood stream. After craniotomy, however, gliomas have been known to invade the adjacent soft tissues of the scalp and neck; medulloblastomas are particularly prone to spread in this way and may then metastasize, especially to lymph nodes and to bones.[679] Medulloblastomas may also metastasize to the lungs as a complication of a surgical ventri-culovenous shunt, performed to relieve internal hydrocephalus.[680]

Glioma cells may be found in the cerebrospinal fluid obtained by lumbar puncture: however, it is difficult or impossible to distinguish them from other types of tumour cell. The cell count of the cerebrospinal fluid is raised in some cases of glioma, especially those involving the optic chiasma and the corpus callosum: most of the cells are lympho-cytes, and their presence simply reflects a reaction to the presence of the tumour. Sometimes neutro-phils or macrophages may also be found in the fluid, and this suggests that the tumour is necrotic, and therefore almost certainly malignant. Malig-nancy is also suggested if the cerebrospinal fluid is yellowish and contains an increased amount of protein. Discoloration of the fluid contained in the cystic parts of a slowly growing astrocytoma, how-ever, has no prognostic significance.

Gliomas occasionally appear to be multiple. Sometimes these seemingly distinct gliomas prove to be, in fact, constituent parts of a large, single tumour that has spread from one lobe to another, perhaps then appearing in two separate places in one slice of brain. Even in cases in which no macroscopically visible link can be shown between two tumour masses, it is sometimes possible to show that they are connected by a slender intervening tract of neoplastic cells that is only recognizable microscopically. Bearing these possibilities in mind, however, genuine instances of double, and even multiple, gliomas do occur. In such cases the tumours usually have the same histological struc-ture, and most frequently they are glioblastomas. Occasionally, a glioblastoma may coexist with a slowly growing astrocytoma, or an ependymoma or an oligodendrocytoma with an astrocytoma or a glioblastoma.

Mesodermal Tumours

Meningeal Tumours

Meningioma

The commonest of all meningeal tumours are the meningiomas. Because of their attachment to the dura mater and of the histological appearance of their commonest variety (Figs 34.128 and 34.129) these tumours used to be described as dural endotheliomas. However, they are now known to develop from the specialized arachnoid cells of the villi that project into the lumen of the dural venous sinuses (Fig. 34.126; and see page 2198). The

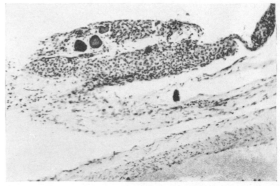

Fig. 34.126. Large arachnoid granulation (Pacchionian body) projecting into the lumen of the superior sagittal sinus of an elderly man. It is composed of specialized arachnoid cells and contains a few psammoma or 'brain-sand' bodies. This might be regarded as an early stage in the formation of a meningioma. *Haematoxylin–eosin.* ×95.

tumours may arise wherever arachnoid villi occur, and they are sometimes multiple. Their commonest site is in relation to the superior sagittal sinus (Fig. 34.127), but they may also arise in relation to the other main venous sinuses. The sites next in frequency to the superior sagittal region are the sphenoid ridges, the tuberculum sellae, the olfactory grooves and the posterior cranial fossa. A menin-gioma sometimes arises over the lateral cerebral sulcus, or in the vicinity of the foramen magnum or

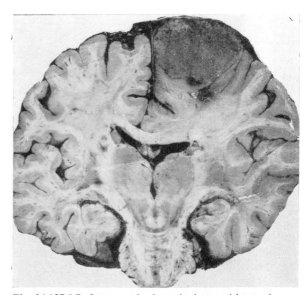

Fig. 34.127.§ Left parasagittal meningioma with attachment to dura mater and falx cerebri. The patient was a man, aged 72, admitted to hospital in status epilepticus. Several days previously he had been brought to the hospital after a fit but had refused investigation. The lateral ventricles are distorted and compressed. There is herniation of the cingulate gyrus.

in the cerebellopontine angle (Fig. 34.128). Occasionally, one develops near the optic foramen, growing outward from the sheaths of the optic nerve into the orbit (see Chapter 40, Volume 6). In the spinal canal, meningiomas may arise from the dura over the lateral aspect of the spinal cord, and from the arachnoid tissue in the dural reflections over the spinal nerve roots, especially in the thoracic region. Exceptionally, a meningioma may originate in the choroid plexus of a lateral ventricle.

Meningiomas most frequently first cause symptoms during the fifth or sixth decade. However, their presence may not be manifested until old age, and they are sometimes found *post mortem* in elderly people who have not been known to have symptoms attributable to the tumour. They are uncommon before the age of 40 years. Women tend to be affected oftener than men, and the clinical effects of these tumours tend to worsen during menstruation and pregnancy, possibly due to the changes in fluid balance that characterize these states.[681]

Meningiomas grow slowly. Their surface may be smooth or nodular. They tend to be somewhat flattened because of their position between skull and brain, which makes it easier for them to expand laterally, between these structures, than to grow uniformly in all directions. In those cases in which the tumour assumes a more spherical form, it creates a corresponding cup-like depression in the underlying brain. Rarely, the tumour grows in the form of a flat mass in the meninges (meningioma *en plaque*).

The substance of a meningioma is usually firm, although when it is examined after incision of the capsule it often proves to be friable. The microscopical picture of the majority of meningiomas is that of a benign neoplasm: yet in spite of these appearances, the tumour may grow into the overlying bone, the infiltration being accompanied by reactive hyperostosis of the outer surface of the skull. The tumour has been known to perforate the bone (see page 2221).

Several histological types of meningioma have been described; the microscopical appearances often vary in different parts of a single tumour. The two commonest varieties, together constituting about 65 per cent of meningiomas, are the syncytial type, in which poorly-defined polygonal cells are arranged in sheets (Fig. 34.129), and the transitional type, in which whorl formation is the main feature (Fig. 34.130); intermediate and combined forms are common. Those that arise in the posterior fossa tend to be fibrous, and contain reticulin and collagen (Figs 34.131 and 34.132). Others, notably those of the spinal meninges, are often abundantly stippled with fine, gritty particles: these particles are the so-called 'brain sand', or 'psammoma bodies', and each is the end result of calcification in an obliterated capillary blood vessel that forms the core of the whorled collections of tumour cells that are so distinctive a feature of many meningiomas (Fig. 34.130).

Intracranial meningiomas are usually well vascularized tumours, and this may enable their situation to be revealed precisely by arteriography. Some, in fact, are so vascular that they have been described as angioblastic (Fig. 34.133), and there may be serious bleeding from such growths if they are inadvertently incised or torn while being resected. Meningiomas, especially those of the angioblastic type, may contain groups of cells that, in paraffin wax sections, have a small eccentric nucleus and clear cytoplasm (Fig. 34.134): in frozen sections, these cells contain abundant Sudanophile fat. Ossification is sometimes found (Fig. 34.135).

A sharply outlined intranuclear vacuole is sometimes present in the tumour cells, and gives a characteristic crateriform appearance to the nucleus. Not infrequently, bizarre giant cells, with very large, hyperchromatic nuclei, are present, but,

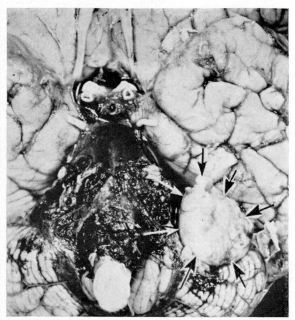

Fig. 34.128. Left cerebellopontine angle tumour (defined by arrows): it proved to be a meningioma. It was an incidental finding in a patient who died from a ruptured intracranial aneurysm. Note, incidentally, the marked thickening of the internal carotid arteries.

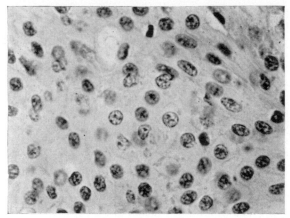

Fig. 34.129. Meningioma of 'syncytial type' showing fairly uniform, oval or round, vesicular nuclei, and ill-defined cell outline. The cells are arranged in a regular pattern and in places tend to run in strands. It was on account of this appearance that these tumours gained the name of dural endothelioma. *Haematoxylin–eosin.* × 360.

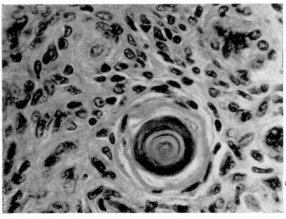

Fig. 34.130. Meningioma of transitional type showing typical whorl formation. These concentrically arranged structures become calcified in old and slow-growing tumours, especially those arising over the spinal cord: their gritty feel earned them the name 'psammoma'. *Haematoxylin–eosin.* × 360.

provided there is no other sign of pleomorphism or anaplasia, such cells have no serious significance (Fig. 34.136). Meningiomas occasionally contain collections of melanin-filled cells, a finding that reflects the occurrence of melanoblastic cells in the normal pia-arachnoid.

Rarely, meningiomas undergo malignant change. There is no variety that is particularly liable to become malignant. The histological features that may indicate malignancy include cellular pleomorphism, hyperchromasia of the nuclei, the presence of numerous mitotic figures, and areas of

necrosis. As mentioned above, the presence of large, bizarre cells is not in itself evidence of malignancy. A tumour that is histologically benign may sometimes recur after surgical resection, but this is generally due to incomplete removal of the original growth. A parasagittal meningioma, for example, may have spread along the interior of the superior sagittal sinus, and this intravascular extension may be the origin of local recurrent growths. Even histologically malignant meningiomas very seldom give rise to metastasis, apart from seeding within the subarachnoid space. The benign meningioma does not invade the brain, although it often compresses it; the malignant

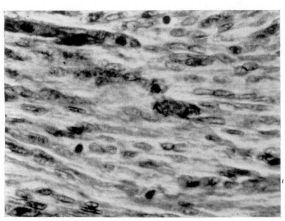

Fig. 34.131. Fibroblastic type of meningioma. Most of the nuclei conform to a regular pattern, but some are larger and more deeply-staining than others. Whorling is not evident. *Haematoxylin–eosin.* × 360.

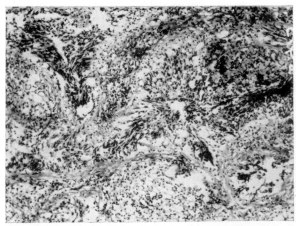

Fig. 34.132. Meningioma. A rare variety showing marked palisading of nuclei in places, the cells being long and thin as in the fibrous type of meningioma. In addition there are many water-clear cells with small nuclei. *Haematoxylin–eosin.* × 100

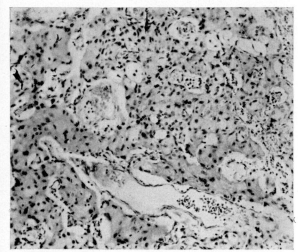

Fig. 34.133. Meningioma of the so-called angioblastic type, with many small vascular spaces separating the sheets of tumour cells, the cytoplasm of which is uniformly eosinophile. *Haematoxylin–eosin.* × 100.

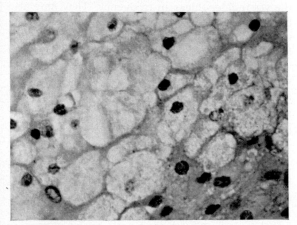

Fig. 34.134. Cells with vacuolate cytoplasm in part of an angioblastic meningioma. The vacuoles contained fat before it was removed during the processing of the tissue. Such 'xanthomatous' form of degeneration is common in this variety of meningioma. *Haematoxylin–eosin.* × 360.

meningioma, in contrast, is often invasive. Both types, benign and malignant, may spread into the diploic space of the adjacent bone, and may penetrate the base of the skull or protrude into the air sinuses.

Sarcomas

In addition to the malignant meningiomas, some rare types of meningeal sarcoma require mention. Fibrosarcomas may arise in the leptomeninges. More rarely, leptomeningeal sarcomas are pleomorphic, and contain many giant cells. Both these

types of tumour begin as a localized thickening of the leptomeninges and eventually compress and invade the cerebrum or the cerebellum.[682] They may respond to radiotherapy.

Melanosis and Melanoma

It is important to note that melanin-containing cells are normally present in small numbers in the pia-arachnoid, particularly over the anterior surface of the pons and on the spinal cord: they are commoner in dark-skinned people.

Meningeal Melanosis.—This is a rare condition in which there is widespread but patchy blackening of the leptomeninges as a result of hyperplasia of the pigmented cells. Occasionally, an apparently benign, tumour-like aggregate of melanin-laden cells is found, either in association with melanosis or as an isolated condition.

Meningeal Melanoma.—Malignant melanoma has been known to develop as a complication of melanosis or of the benign tumour-like pigmented lesion of the meninges referred to above. It should be noted, however, that primary meningeal melanomas are much rarer than metastatic involvement of the meninges by melanomas that originate elsewhere.

Neurolemmal Tumours (Schwann Cell Tumours)

Neurolemmomas* arise from the cells of the neurolemma, or nerve sheath. It is believed that the cell

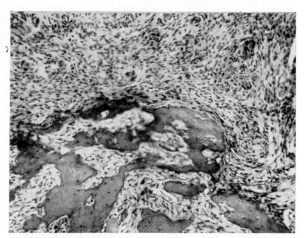

Fig. 34.135. Meningioma showing ossification. *Haematoxylin–eosin.* × 100.

* This name is variously spelt neurilemoma, neurilemmoma, neurolemoma and neurolemmoma. The last of

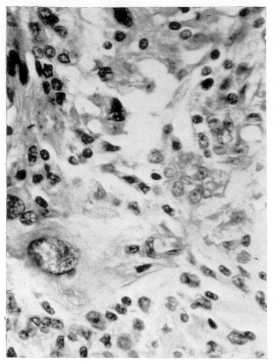

Fig. 34.136. Meningioma showing cellular pleomorphism. One cell is of gigantic proportions. This tumour was slow-growing. It was readily removed and there was no recurrence. *Haematoxylin–eosin.* × 360.

of origin is the Schwann cell, and the name Schwann-oma is sometimes given to the tumours. They are also known as neurinomas. They may arise in any part of the course of any nerve trunk, cranial or spinal (see also page 2334).

The commonest intracranial site of neurolem-momas is the vestibulocochlear nerve. The vesti-bulocochlear neurolemmoma is generally single, but bilateral tumours are not very rare. Usually, the tumour arises where the nerve enters the internal acoustic meatus, and if it grows into the meatus the latter becomes gradually enlarged in a funnel-shaped way: when this enlargement can be shown radiologically it is of much diagnostic importance. In most cases, however, the tumour grows inward and comes to fill and expand the cerebellopontine

angle* distorting the brainstem and the trigeminal and other cranial nerves, which become stretched over its surface. Because the tumour originates from the sheath of the nerve, and not within its substance, the characteristic symptom of tinnitus, with progressive nerve deafness, comes on only when the nerve itself becomes compressed. Indeed, these tumours may be encountered without any history of symptoms referable to involvement of the nerve from which they arise. Stretching of the trigeminal nerve over the tumour, however, often results in early loss of the corneal reflex; later, all the divisions of this nerve become affected. Com-pression of the facial and glossopharyngeal nerves is also liable to give rise to abnormal physical signs. Sometimes the presenting symptoms are the result of compression of the brainstem. On occasion, quite small tumours cause marked internal hydrocephalus.

Neurolemmomas are occasionally found on other cranial nerves, the trigeminal being next to the vestibulocochlear in frequency. They may also be found on spinal nerve roots at any level, some-times compressing the spinal cord and sometimes forming a 'dumb-bell tumour', so-called because it is constricted where it passes through the inter-vertebral foramen. Sometimes a neurolemmoma of a cranial nerve or of a spinal nerve root is found unexpectedly at necropsy, having caused no symptoms.

Neurolemmomas are generally solid and fibrous, although they may undergo central liquefactive necrosis. Histologically, they consist of interlacing bands of spindle-shaped cells; when a band is cut transversely, the cells forming it appear round. A feature typical of these tumours is the tendency for the nuclei of adjacent cells to be aligned in columns parallel to one another ('palisading' of the nuclei—Fig. 34.137): this arrangement is seldom absent, and it is of help in diagnosis. A similar alignment of nuclei, however, is often seen in leiomyomas, and this must be borne in mind when a particular tumour has developed at a site where it might have arisen either from a nerve sheath or from smooth muscle. The finding of intercellular reticulin fibres is sometimes said to help in the identification of neurolemmomas, but it should be noted that this is also a feature of the fibrous type of meningioma; further, it is of no aid

these forms is the one used in this book, although the spelling neurilemoma is the original form, introduced in the classic account of this tumour (Stout, A. P., *Amer. J. Cancer*, 1935, **24,** 751). There is a useful note on these spellings in: Beattie, J. M., Dickson, W. E. Carnegie, Drennan, A. M., *A Textbook of Pathology—General and Special—for the Use of Students and Practitioners*, 5th edn, edited by W. E. Carnegie Dickson, vol. 2, page 1310 (footnote); London, 1948.

* It should be emphasized that by no means all cerebello-pontine angle tumours are neurolemmomas. A meningioma may arise in this region (Fig. 34.128); a medulloblastoma, an ependymoma or any other tumour of the adjoining parts may protrude into it.

in distinguishing neurolemmomas from leiomyomas.

Intracranial neurolemmomas very rarely undergo sarcomatous transformation.

Blood Vessel Tumours

Haemangioblastoma

The cerebellum is the commonest site of the haemangioblastoma. The tumour is usually said to be a true neoplasm of blood vessel origin, arising from capillaries of the pia, but doubt about this view will remain until the similarities between the haemangioblastoma and the so-called angioblastic meningiomas (page 2219) have been explained.[656] It has been suggested that the angioblastic meningioma may also be of pial origin.

The cerebellar haemangioblastoma may appear as a solid mass or it may be cystic. The cystic type has to be distinguished from a cerebellar astrocytoma (see page 2210): however, the solid tumour nodule in the wall of a cystic angioma is bluish or purple, while the corresponding nodule in the astrocytomatous pseudocyst is white.

The haemangioblastoma is said to arise from misplaced vascular mesoderm, and thus to be developmental in origin. As it is a progressive lesion, although growing only slowly, it has been regarded by most authorities as a true neoplasm rather than as a hamartoma (see footnote on page 2181). Symptoms due to its growth usually appear first in early adult life. Polycythaemia is an occasional concomitant of this tumour.

A haemangioblastoma is always well circumscribed. Its solider parts are composed of small, endothelium-lined, blood-containing spaces. These channels are packed closely, but between them there is a considerable amount of reticulin, and there may also be interstitial collections of large mononuclear cells that contain Sudanophile fat.

Von-Hippel–Lindau Syndrome.—Lindau[683] noted an association of retinal angiomatosis (von Hippel's disease[684]—see Chapter 40, Volume 6) with cerebellar haemangioblastoma, and that other developmental amomalies, including cystic disease of the pancreas and of the kidneys, are to be found in such cases. Syringomyelia is sometimes present also. The von-Hippel–Lindau syndrome is rare (see Chapter 40, Volume 6), and most cerebellar haemangioblastomas are not accompanied by angiomatosis or other malformations.

Blood vessel neoplasms similar to those that occur in the cerebellum have been found more rarely elsewhere in the central nervous system, notably in the medulla oblongata and the spinal cord. They hardly ever occur above the level of the tentorium, but they have been described in the occipital lobe.

Blood Vessel Hamartomas.—These tumour-like lesions are discussed on page 2181.

Lymphomas (Including 'Hortega Cell Tumours')

The classification and identification of lymphomas involving the central nervous system are no less confused and confusing than when these tumours arise elsewhere (see page 777, Volume 2). Conventionally, the tumours arising in the central nervous system are considered to fall into two main groups—tumours of Hortega cells, and other lymphomas. They will be considered here in that order.

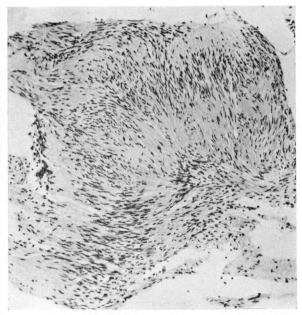

Fig. 34.137. Neurolemmoma (Schwann cell tumour). The cells tend to run in strands rather than form whorls as is so commonly seen in meningiomas, and the palisading or clustering of nuclei (shown here) is very characteristic. The tumour may grow from the sheath of any intracranial, intraspinal or peripheral nerve. *Haematoxylin–eosin.* × 80.

'Hortega Cell Tumours' (Tumours of the Reticuloendothelial Cells of the Central Nervous System)

The Hortega cell is the representative of the reticuloendothelial system in the brain and spinal cord.

It, or its forerunners, gives rise to tumours that have been recorded under various names, including *histiocytic lymphoma, reticulum cell sarcoma, perithelial sarcoma* and *microglioma*. When the tumours in the brain are multicentric the condition has been described as *microgliomatosis*.[685–687] As it is desirable to use the term glia only for the supportive elements of the central nervous system, which are of ectodermal origin (the astrocytes and oligodendrocytes, and their cytoplasmic processes—see pages 2078 and 2083), the names microglioma and microgliomatosis are unsatisfactory. Further, these terms fail to indicate the essential relationship between these forms of neoplasm of the central nervous system and their counterparts that arise in the lymphoreticular system elsewhere in the body. The name adopted in this chapter is 'Hortega cell tumour', but it should be noted that this is used as a convenient designation to cover lesions of all degrees of malignancy, and without particular regard to the relative proportions of differentiated Hortega cells and of 'primitive' or immature forms of these cells.

These tumours usually develop in middle-aged adults. As the history is generally short and the tumours may be multiple, the condition is commonly confused with secondary carcinoma. The tumours arise in any part of the brain, but most notably in the basal ganglia. In some patients similar tumours are present in the lymph nodes, spleen and other parts of the lymphoreticular system, and occasionally in the heart and kidneys. In these cases, it is clear that the involvement of the brain is one of the manifestations of a systemic disease of the lymphoreticular system, and not primarily a disease of the central nervous system.

Some authorities have sought to draw a fine distinction between a tumour that is formed of mature Hortega cells and one formed of supposedly less mature cells.

The histological appearances of these tumours may resemble those of the rare, true reticulum cell sarcomas (histiocytic lymphomas) that arise elsewhere in the body (see page 851, Volume 2). Survival of cells in the immediate vicinity of the blood vessels in the tumour when those farther from the vessels have undergone necrosis results in a distinctive histological picture (Fig. 34.138), to which the now obsolete name 'perithelial sarcoma' was given. The tumour spreads along the circumvascular spaces in the brain, and its presence leads to a characteristic response by the astrocytes, which swell and become globular.

Many of the cells in these tumours are demon-

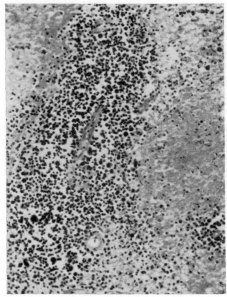

Fig. 34.138. Hortega cell tumour of the brain ('microglioma'). The tumour is composed of round cells, varying in size. The cells farthest from the blood vessels have died, and consequently there is a characteristic pattern of necrosis round viable tumour tissue centred on the vasculature of the growth. *Haematoxylin–eosin.* × 100.

strated by the silver impregnation methods that are used to display Hortega cells. This poses the question whether the cells that are so displayed are, in fact, tumour cells, or whether they are non-neoplastic histiocytes engaged in scavenging, just as they would (although usually in smaller numbers) in the neighbourhood of any necrotic tumour in the brain. Lymphocytes, plasma cells and other non-metallophile cells are also dispersed in varying numbers throughout the reticuloendothelial tumours. The amount of reticulin is likewise variable; it is usually greatest in the vicinity of blood vessels. The metallophile Hortega cells are recognizable in haematoxylin–eosin preparations by their characteristic elongated, twisted or lobed, dark-staining nuclei.

Other Lymphomas Arising in the Central Nervous System

Lymphomas other than 'Hortega cell tumours' (see above) arise in the brain and spinal cord only with exceptional rarity. Their cytogenesis in the nervous system is uncertain. They are seen with particular frequency among the tumours that develop as a complication of long-term therapeutic immunosuppression following organ transplantation:[687a] in such cases the microscopical appearances are often those of the immunoblastic sarcomas (see page 849, Volume 2); lymphocytic lymphomas, undifferentiated lymphomas and histiocytic lymphomas—that is, 'Hortega cell tumours' —also occur in the brain in these patients.

Involvement of the Central Nervous System by Lymphomas Arising Elsewhere

Any lymphoma, wherever it arises, may come to involve the central nervous system. The frequency of such involvement varies to some extent with the type of the lymphoma.

Hodgkin's Disease.—Hodgkin's disease seldom involves the central nervous system. When it does so, the lesions are most frequently spinal in situation, with local invasion of the meninges, particularly as a consequence of spread of the disease from a vertebral body. However, intracerebral and intracerebellar tumours may occur.[687b, 687c]

Lymphomas Other than Hodgkin's Disease.— *Lymphocytic lymphomas* (see page 821, Volume 2) are less unlikely than Hodgkin's disease to involve the meninges and the parenchyma of the central nervous system.[687d]

Follicular lymphoma (see page 835, Volume 2) is among the rarest lymphomas to be found in the parenchyma of the central nervous system. In contrast, *Burkitt's lymphoma* involves the brain with considerable frequency (see page 829, Volume 2, and Table 9.15, page 831).

Immunoblastic lymphomas (page 849, Volume 2) involve the central nervous system with much the same frequency as lymphocytic lymphomas. A considerable proportion of the tumours that in the past were called reticulum cell sarcomas might now be regarded as immunoblastic lymphomas.

METASTATIC TUMOURS IN THE CENTRAL NERVOUS SYSTEM

The brain is a common site for metastatic deposits of tumours, particularly in cases of carcinoma of bronchus, breast, kidney, colon and nasopharynx.[688] Melanoma (Fig. 34.139) of the skin or eye and choriocarcinoma of the uterus also have some predilection for the brain. Both in general hospitals and in neurological centres, carcinoma of the

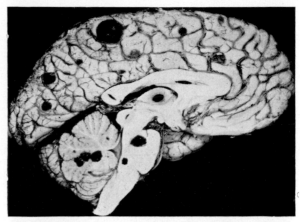

Fig. 34.139. Multiple metastatic deposits of melanoma: the site of the primary tumour was never convincingly determined. Some of the deposits contain less pigment than others.

bronchus is by far the commonest source of secondary deposits in the brain in men: the various histological types of bronchial carcinoma seem about equally liable to spread to the brain.[689] The neurological manifestations often present clinically at a time when the primary tumour in the bronchus is still silent. In contrast, manifestations of secondary deposits of mammary carcinoma are very seldom evident before the primary growth has been recognized and treated. For this reason, their significance is rarely in doubt, and these patients are seldom subjected to neurosurgical procedures.

Estimates of the frequency with which bronchial cancer metastasizes to the brain range from 20 to 40 per cent of the cases.[690] There are probably two reasons for this high incidence: first, the brain has an abundant blood supply, and second, tumour cells that enter the blood stream from a primary growth in the lungs do not have to pass through the pulmonary capillaries, which act as a filter for tumour cells carried in the systemic venous circulation from other parts of the body. About two thirds of all secondary tumours in the central nervous system are in the cerebrum and about one third in the cerebellum.[691] A rare distribution of metastatic tumours is illustrated in Fig. 34.140.

Metastasis to the brain may take place by a variety of routes when the primary tumour is in a part of the body other than the lungs. Secondary deposits in the lungs may be the source of the further metastasis to the brain; alternatively, tumour cells or tumour may traverse the pulmonary circulation. Another possible pathway is the

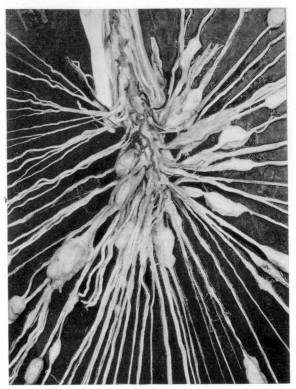

Fig. 34.140. Deposits of tumour in the cauda equina resulting from spread in the cerebrospinal fluid from a metastatic growth in the choroid plexus of the left lateral ventricle. The primary tumour was an anaplastic carcinoma of bronchus. The patient presented with a cauda equina syndrome of sudden onset.

vertebral venous plexus. A very rare route is through a patent foramen ovale into the left atrium.

Carcinoma of the thyroid may spread up the carotid sheath. A carcinoma of the air sinuses or middle ear, or a sarcoma arising in the skull itself, may invade the brain by direct spread through the dura.

The secondary deposits in the cerebrum are generally multiple. They develop from tumour cells that lodge as emboli in arterioles, particularly at the junction between the grey and white matter. They may be of different ages, and the smallest deposits may elude discovery by naked-eye examination. In view of this and of the likelihood that other organs —notably the adrenals in cases of carcinoma of the bronchus—are also involved there is little chance that a deposit in the brain that comes to the attention of the surgeon is the sole instance of spread from the primary tumour. However, it is well known that the rate of growth of metastatic

deposits of some types of tumour is unpredictable, and many years may separate the removal of the primary growth and the appearance of its secondaries. In such instances, it must be assumed that the tumour seedlings were already *in situ* when the primary was excised, and that their growth was for long inhibited by unknown factors, which eventually ceased to act. While melanoma is the classic example of a tumour that may present a long delay between removal of the primary growth and the development of clinical signs of metastasis, similar intervals may be observed in occasional examples of other types of cancer, particularly adenocarcinoma of the kidneys, although carcinoma of the breasts and even of the bronchi must also be mentioned.

A metastatic deposit may be removed from the brain before the primary tumour has been recognized, and it is sometimes possible then to proceed with the excision of the primary tumour itself. A remarkable case of successful surgical treatment of a secondary tumour in the brain illustrates this rare occurrence. A medical practitioner developed symptoms of a tumour in the frontal lobe of one cerebral hemisphere: the lobe was resected, and the tumour was found to be a keratinizing squamous carcinoma. Reappraisal of chest radiographs disclosed collapse of the lingula of the left lung: at the patient's insistence, the lung was removed, and the obstructing mass proved to be a primary keratinizing squamous carcinoma. The patient died from unrelated causes 18 years later, at the age of 72: he had maintained a busy general practice throughout this time; there was no further evidence of cancer after removal of the lung.[692] It is such rare exceptions that may encourage the surgeon to remove a secondary tumour that he has reason to hope may be solitary.

Secondary tumours in the brain are usually spherical, firm and greyish. They often appear well circumscribed, and the surgeon may be tempted to shell them out; it is impossible to eradicate the disease in this way since the growth infiltrates the nearby brain substance.

In some instances the deposits may liquefy. If composed of mucus-secreting cells, they may exude mucinous fluid when incised: this mucus is likely to enclose viable tumour cells and, if allowed to contaminate the operation site, may be the source of further growths.

Tumour emboli occasionally lodge in the blood vessels of the leptomeninges, and may then give rise to cancerous infiltration without the development of any discrete foci within the brain substance

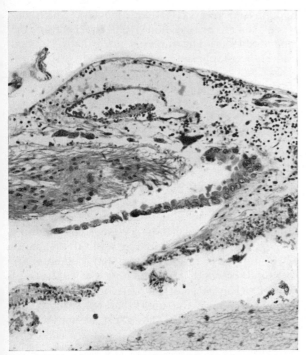

Fig. 34.141. Malignant epithelial cells in the leptomeninges spreading out in linear fashion. These cells had been identified during life in the cerebrospinal fluid of a patient who had presented with symptoms and signs of subacute meningitis. The primary tumour was in a bronchus. *Haematoxylin–eosin.* × 125.

are readily distinguished from arachnoid cells and macrophages by the size, and, often, the hyperchromasia of their nuclei, and also by their pleomorphism, and their tendency to occur in clusters. In some cases, the total cell count in the fluid may be little, if at all, raised, but a search of the deposit may reveal the presence of unmistakable cancer cells and so indicate the diagnosis. Clustering of cells in the cerebrospinal fluid is sometimes assumed to indicate malignancy, but this is a dangerous generalization, for macrophages may also be found in clumps. A helpful point in the diagnosis of carcinomatous invasion of the meninges is a reduction in the concentration of glucose in the cerebrospinal fluid.

Metastatic tumours in the skull or dura mater may press on or invade the brain. Mammary cancer is among the most frequent sources of such deposits.

The spinal cord is seldom involved by metastasis, although the spinal theca may be invaded in the course of direct extension of a bronchial carcinoma. Compression of the cord is not uncommonly caused by extradural masses, including secondary deposits of carcinoma (Fig. 34.143), Hodgkin's disease and other lymphomas, particularly follicular lymphoma. The cord may also be injured by the deformation and collapse of vertebral bodies containing secondary deposits or involved in such multicentric forms of neoplasia as myelomatosis.

(Figs 34.141 and 34.142). Oftener, however, the tumour cells reach the subarachnoid space as a result of direct spread from a subcortical deposit. The condition of carcinomatous infiltration of the meninges,[693] if widespread, is sometimes known as 'meningitis carcinomatosa': the term is usually regarded as a misnomer as the condition is neoplastic and not primarily inflammatory, although the tumour cells are commonly accompanied by a moderate accumulation of lymphocytes and, occasionally, plasma cells. Similarly, an occasional finding of widespread microscopical infiltration of the brain by carcinoma cells has been referred to as 'carcinomatous encephalitis';[694] in this condition there may be so heavy an admixture of lymphocytes and plasma cells that the tumour cells are difficult to see and may be overlooked. The presence of the inflammatory cells may indicate an immunocellular response.

In cerebral carcinomatosis, and notably in meningeal carcinomatosis, the cell count in the cerebrospinal fluid is often raised, and a proportion of the cells may be identified as tumour cells. They

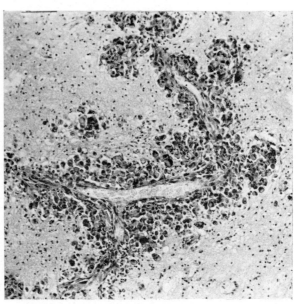

Fig. 34.142. Metastatic tumour cells in the circumvascular space are invading the substance of the brain. The patient had a carcinoma of the thyroid gland. *Haematoxylin–eosin.* × 125.

6

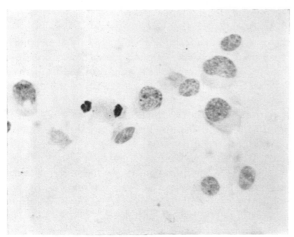

Fig. 34.143. Film preparation (smear) of extradural carcinoma in the thoracic spine of a woman in her sixties. The cells have a large nucleus and are of irregular and atypical appearance: one is undergoing mitosis. The primary tumour was in a breast. *Haematoxylin–eosin.* × 750.

MISCELLANEOUS NEOPLASMS AND CYSTS OF
DEVELOPMENTAL ORIGIN

Craniopharyngioma and 'Craniopharyngeal Cysts'

Craniopharyngiomas are so named because they are believed to originate in the craniopharyngeal canal; this is considered to be the vestige of the hypophysial recess (Rathke's pouch), which develops as an evagination from the roof of the stomatodaeum. The tumours are usually situated above the diaphragm of the sella turcica (suprasellar), but a few are within the fossa (intrasellar) or even within the sphenoid bone. Solid and cystic forms, papillary cystic forms, and mixed forms are recognized, and the tumours may be benign or malignant (see also page 1881, Volume 4).

'Craniopharyngeal Cyst'

The cystic lesions may be unilocular. The unilocular cyst is lined by epidermoid epithelium. It contains clear or cloudy, colourless or brown fluid containing cholesterol crystals, and there may be deposits of calcium in the wall. If the lining epithelium is keratinized the cyst contents are semisolid or solid, and resemble the contents of epidermoid cysts in other parts of the body. It is doubtful whether the unilocular cysts should be regarded as neoplasms. They are sometimes termed *craniopharyngeal duct cysts* and *suprasellar epidermoids.*

Craniopharyngioma

The solid craniopharyngiomas are true neoplasms (Fig. 34.144). They are composed of a meshwork of epithelial strands enclosing a fibrous stroma. The

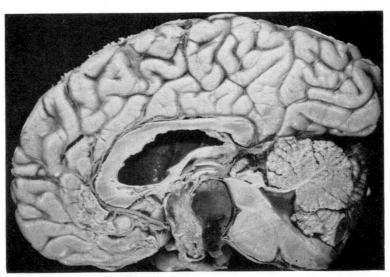

Fig. 34.144. Craniopharyngioma. The patient was a plump girl, 54 inches (137 centimetres) tall, who was 17 years of age when she first menstruated. At the same time she began to develop headaches, and this was followed soon afterwards by blurring of vision. She died a year later. The tumour has grown down to compress the optic chiasma from behind: the anterior part of the tumour is solid and the posterior part cystic. See also Fig. 29.5, page 1882 in Volume 4.

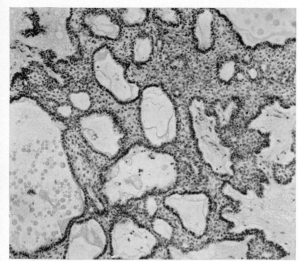

Fig. 34.145. Craniopharyngioma with a cribriform pattern of cystic spaces containing mucoid material and surrounded by masses of cells resembling immature squamous epithelium. See also Figs 29.6 and 29.7, page 1883 in Volume 4. *Haematoxylin–eosin.* ×70.

strands consist of a single outer layer of columnar cells on each side and an intervening mass of polygonal cells (Fig. 34.145). Keratinization is rarely found. The appearances resemble certain types of basisquamous carcinoma of the skin and may be reminiscent of ameloblastoma (adamantinoma) of the jaws; indeed, the name adamantinoma is sometimes given to them. Pseudocysts may result from liquefaction of the central parts of the epithelial masses. Coagulation necrosis and calcification may occur in the epithelial areas, and calcification or a foreign body type of granulomatous reaction may develop in the stroma.

Although these lesions originate in the midline, they often grow more toward one side than the other. They enlarge very slowly: most of the patients are in the second or third decade of life when symptoms first appear. The manifestations are those of pituitary dysfunction and may include obesity, somnolence and headache, dwarfism, and diabetes insipidus. There may be pressure on the optic chiasma. Exceptionally, craniopharyngiomas have been observed in middle-aged and even elderly people.

Colloid Cyst (Paraphysial Cyst)

The name colloid cyst is given both to a simple dilatation of the blind end of the paraphysis (an embryonic epithelial evagination of the roof of the anterior end of the third ventricle) and to the commoner condition of cystic distension of other embryonic outpouchings of the diencephalon.[695] Whatever its origin, the cyst is usually solitary. Because of its situation, it is liable to act as a ball valve over the interventricular foramina, so causing symptoms of intermittent hydrocephalus (Fig. 34.146). Its wall is lined by low columnar epithelium. The contents of the cyst are an opaque, firm, light grey, proteinaceous material.

'Cholesteatoma' and Dermoid Cyst

The so-called 'cholesteatoma' is really an epidermoid cyst: it occurs most frequently in the cerebellopontine angle (Fig. 34.147), or in relation to the pituitary gland or its vicinity. It arises from ectopic islands of stratified squamous epithelium. Symptoms usually appear in middle life. The cyst tends to send out prolongations widely into the brain substance. It contains a pearly mass of hyaline keratinous material mixed with cholesterol and other lipids. Similar cysts sometimes occur in the spinal canal, compressing the cord.

True *dermoid cysts*—that is, cysts lined by skin, with hair follicles, sebaceous glands and other cutaneous appendages—have occasionally been found in the posterior fossa of the skull. They

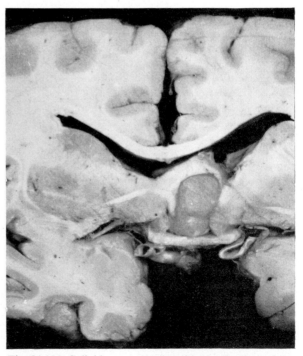

Fig. 34.146. Colloid cyst occupying the anterior part of the third ventricle.

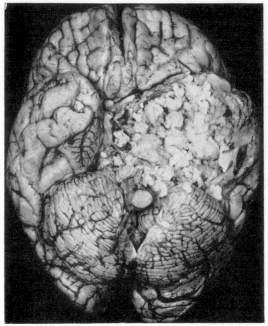

Fig. 34.147. Epidermoid cyst ('cholesteatoma'). Most of the temporal lobe and much of the occipital lobe have been excavated.

occur also, but less frequently, in the spinal canal, where they may be associated with spina bifida.

Chordoma

Although the chordoma is not a tumour of the nervous system, its clinical manifestations are mainly neurological and it is conveniently considered here (see also page 2475). It is a rare tumour, arising from a remnant of the notochord;[696] it usually does not give rise to symptoms until middle life. It occurs most commonly in the sacrococcygeal region; other sites are the dorsum sellae, the basilar part of the occipital bone and the body of the sphenoid bone. Sometimes small notochordal remnants, known as ecchordoses, are found at necropsy in these sites in normal adults.

It is noteworthy that chordomas do not ordinarily arise from notochordal remnants in the cervical, thoracic, or lumbar parts of the spinal column— for instance, the traces of notochordal tissue that are so common in the substance of the nucleus pulposus of the intervertebral discs of children. Schmorl's nodes[696a]—projections of the intervertebral discs into the adjacent vertebral body— sometimes contain material that appears to be derived from the notochord.

The sacrococcygeal chordoma is a lobulate tumour of gelatinous appearance, mainly soft, but with solid areas of cartilaginous consistency. It arises from the anterior surface of the lower part of the sacrum, and it may become adherent to structures in the pelvis, often involving the sacral nerve plexus and causing great pain.

An intracranial chordoma may occupy a wide area of the dorsum sellae, and for this reason it is commonly referred to as the spheno-occipital chordoma. It compresses and invades the anterior surface of the medulla oblongata and the emerging cranial nerves, giving rise to multiple palsies as well as to symptoms of raised intracranial pressure. Although slow-growing, it is locally invasive and difficult to eradicate. Very rarely it may metastasize.

Histology

Chordomas are readily recognizable histologically (Fig. 34.148). They are derived from what is essentially a primitive type of embryonic cartilage,[697] and they consist of a mucinous matrix in which the tumour cells lie haphazardly.[697a] The cells are usually large, their nucleus is vacuolate, and there are often mucin-filled spaces in the cytoplasm, the margins of which may be so indefinite that the appearances are those of a syncytium. Because of the bubble-like character of the vacuoles, the cells have been called *physaliphorous cells*: they were so named by Virchow, who studied them first in the condition that he described as ecchondrosis physaliphora, a chordoma-like nodule

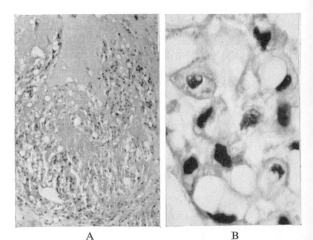

A   B

Fig. 34.148. Chordoma. A: Mass of mucinous material surrounded by clusters of tumour cells. B: The so-called physaliphorous (bubble-bearing) cells are characterized by the coarse vacuolation of their cytoplasm, and often by finer vacuolation of the nucleus. *Haematoxylin–eosin.* A: ×70; B: ×430.

—now often referred to as an ecchordosis—on the clivus of Blumenbach (see footnote on page 2201).[697b] Several histological varieties of chordoma exist, including papillary and glandular forms. It is usually possible, however, in any of these varieties to find fields that have the characteristic structure of mucinous matrix and physaliphorous cells. The fact that the matrix is neither stained by phospho-tungstic acid haematoxylin nor impregnated by silver methods for reticulin is helpful in distinguishing chordomas from chondromas.[698]

General Observations on Expanding Intracranial Lesions[699, 700]

Within the rigid confines of the cranial cavity, any expanding lesion is liable to bring about pathological changes, even in parts of the brain that it does not directly involve. An expansive lesion on one side of the brain—whether neoplasm, granuloma or haematoma—will displace the midline structures to the other side; it will tend to compress, and may even obliterate, the ipsilateral ventricle, while indirectly causing much distortion of the contralateral ventricle. The cingulate gyrus on the side of the mass is often pushed across below the free edge of the falx cerebri, and sometimes the prolapsed portion may be forced upward and thus bent sharply on itself (see Fig. 34.27, page 2111; Fig. 34.85, page 2182; Fig. 34.92, page 2189; Fig. 34.108, page 2209; and Fig. 34.127, page 2218).

Apart from the pressure that it exerts on nearby structures, a tumour may cause swelling of the adjacent white matter, and on occasion this may involve almost an entire hemisphere. Oedema is particularly liable to develop in cases of malignant glioma of the frontal lobe, even if the tumour is only small: should such a growth be situated near the frontal pole, the accompanying oedema may extend as far back as the level of the splenium of the corpus callosum. The oedema is thought to be due to venous stasis and increased permeability of the capillary endothelium. The fluid collects between the myelin sheaths, and also seemingly within the cytoplasm of the oligodendrocytes and astrocytes. The presence of the excess fluid, whether intracellular or extracellular, or both, appears to stimulate the astrocytes to lay down glial fibres in the affected parts. The separation of the myelin sheaths from one another, as a result of the oedema, makes preparations stained for myelin appear unusually pale. If so much fluid collects that the blood supply to the white matter is impaired, a local breakdown of myelin may follow.

A tumour of the cerebellum or in the fourth ventricle may cause expansion of the whole hind brain and force the cerebellar tonsils into the foramen magnum: this 'pressure cone' impedes passage of cerebrospinal fluid through the apertures of the fourth ventricle. Cerebrospinal fluid continues to be secreted by the choroid plexuses, and hydro-cephalus will therefore follow, with dilatation of the lateral and third ventricles and of the aqueduct. The development of hydrocephalus necessarily entails a progressive reduction in the amount of cerebral white matter: in infants, in whom swelling is not limited by a rigid skull, the cerebral cortex may become obviously thinned.

Blindness is sometimes a symptom of intracranial tumours: it may be due to several causes, one of which is distension of the optic recess of the third ventricle, with consequent pressure on the optic chiasma. Pressure on the optic chiasma is also responsible for blindness in cases of pituitary tumour, which thus is associated with bitemporal hemianopia. A tumour that encroaches on the optic radiation will give rise to a homonymous hemianopia affecting the visual fields of the opposite side. The commonest cause of blindness is papilloedema, which may be consequent upon venous stasis affecting the optic nerve, or due to an extension of the oedema of the white matter that so often accompanies the presence of a tumour (see above).

Any large supratentorial mass will also have the effect of pushing the upper part of the brain through the tentorial opening, so that the free edges of the tentorium press on the uncus, the hippocampus and the cerebral peduncle on one or both sides. The pressure marks are commonly bilateral, but are much more marked on the side of the tumour. The same is true of uncal herniation and of the rarer hippocampal herniation, which occurs when the tentorium cerebelli has an unusually wide opening. Indentation of the peduncle is usually unilateral: it is known as *Kernohan's notch*[701] and is the cause of the contralateral hemiparesis often found in association with expanding supratentorial lesions. The severity of the secondary disturbances in the displaced parts of the brain could depend, to some extent, on the size of the tentorial opening, which varies from individual to individual:[702] the smaller the opening, the more marked the distortion of the herniated parts. The displacement of the brain downward into the opening results in venous congestion of its infratentorial portion, and this may lead to the development of areas of infarction and, in some cases, to rapidly fatal haemorrhage into the brainstem. The secondary vascular effects are found most frequently in the reticular formation and in the tegmentum: pressure on the vessels crossing the subarachnoid space and entering the brainstem may be their cause.[703] The free edge of the tentorium may not only indent the peduncle but it may also compress the third cranial nerve and the posterior cerebral artery. Obstruction of the posterior cerebral artery results in ischaemia of the medial part of the occipital lobe, including the calcarine cortex. Other effects of the downward displacement of the brain include stretching of the fourth and sixth cranial nerves, and necrosis of parts of the pituitary[704] due to interference with its blood supply (see page 1879, Volume 4).

It sometimes happens that the midbrain is pressed upward by an infratentorial growth. The possibility of this so-called *reversed cone* should be borne in mind, because tapping the lateral ventricles—a life-saving procedure in cases with downward herniation—is likely to be followed by a rapid deterioration in the patient's condition. In cases of infratentorial tumours, therefore, the aim must be to reduce the pressure in the fourth ventricle.

It should be added that minor degrees of protrusion of the unci through the tentorial opening, or of the cerebellar tonsils through the foramen magnum, may take place after death. The possibility of this artefact must be considered when assessing the significance of displacement of these parts of the brain.

There may be serious consequences if a large quantity of cerebrospinal fluid is removed rather quickly by lumbar puncture in a case of raised intracranial pressure. The main danger is that the reduction of pressure in the spinal theca may lead to the cerebellar tonsils being forced into the foramen magnum, so obstructing the normal flow of the cerebrospinal fluid, or even causing sudden death from ischaemia of the vital centres in the brainstem. For this reason, it is inadvisable to remove cerebrospinal fluid for diagnostic purposes in patients with an intracranial tumour, unless a neurosurgical service is immediately available and the procedure is under neurosurgical supervision.

INBORN ERRORS OF METABOLISM

The concept of genetically determined metabolic diseases was put forward by A. E. Garrod in 1908;[705] his views have acquired great importance in relation to many aspects of medicine. Originally, only four diseases in this category were recognized: albinism, alkaptonuria, cystinuria and pentosuria. When the second edition of *Inborn Errors of Metabolism* was published, in 1923,[706] Garrod was able to include two more diseases, haematoporphyria congenita and congenital steatorrhoea. The neurological symptoms accompanying some cases of porphyria congenita had by then been recognized, but, save for amaurotic familial idiocy, the various forms of mental retardation associated with anomalies of metabolism still awaited discovery. Although Meckel, in 1816,[707] and Mansfeldt, in 1826,[708] had described albinism as a 'malformation by arrest', intending by this expression to indicate a congenitally determined defect of metabolism, it was Garrod who saw in this group of inherited diseases the manifestations of genetically conditioned failures of specific enzymes.

The conditions to be described here are the leucodystrophies, the neuronal lipidoses, and various enzymal disorders, many of which have come to light in recent years. The leucodystrophies and the neuronal lipidoses are often grouped together.

THE LEUCODYSTROPHIES[709]

The so-called leucodystrophies are chronic diseases that are characterized by extensive derangement of the white matter. Deficient myelination is the main feature: the axons show a variable degree of degeneration, which usually is greater than in the primary demyelinating diseases. Characteristically, the optic radiations are relatively seldom involved. Although they have sometimes been regarded as demyelinating diseases, these conditions are now widely believed to be the outcome of an inherited fault in myelination: the term leucodystrophy, introduced in 1928 by Bielschowsky and Henneberg,[709a] seems, therefore, to be appropriate.

The recognized forms of leucodystrophy fall into five main groups—Pelizaeus–Merzbacher disease, Krabbe's disease (globoid cell leucodystrophy), metachromatic leucodystrophy, Alexander's disease (fibrinoid leucodystrophy), and spongiform degeneration of the white matter. These will be considered here.

Pelizaeus–Merzbacher Disease[710]

Merzbacher,[710a] in 1908, described a form of diffuse sclerosis in a family that had previously been observed by Pelizaeus.[710b] The family history suggested that the disease was determined by a sex-linked recessive gene: most of the affected patients were males and the disease was apparently transmitted by healthy females. In a family studied more recently it appears that 27 males have been affected in seven generations.[711]

Pelizaeus–Merzbacher disease is very rare. Its earliest manifestations usually are seen toward the end of the first year of life. The deficiency of myelin is widespread, but it is noteworthy that islands of normally-staining myelin persist round some of the blood vessels: this may also be observed, although in less marked form, in some cases of diffuse sclerosis (Schilder's disease—see page 2259). In contrast to Schilder's disease, in which they are only rarely involved, the arcuate fibres (U-fibres), immediately deep to the cerebral cortex, are often affected in Pelizaeus–Merzbacher disease. Clinically, the frequency of symptoms referable to the brainstem differentiates this condition from Schilder's disease.[711]

Krabbe's Disease
(Globoid Cell Leucodystrophy)[712, 713]

This variety of leucodystrophy is characterized by the presence in the white matter, and elsewhere in the brain, of large cells that are distended with fine granular material (Fig. 34.149). These cells, 20 to 25 μm in diameter, and sometimes multinucleate, tend to be clustered near blood vessels. Because of their striking appearance, the condition has been termed *globoid cell leucodystrophy*.[713] It is commonly familial. The whole of the white matter may be affected, but the condition usually begins in the occipital lobes. Its manifestations are generally recognized during the first year of life, but they may be delayed until later in childhood.

The origin of the globoid cells has been disputed, but they are now generally believed to be Hortega cells.[714, 715] They are numerous in affected parts of the white matter, and their presence is associated with a marked local deficiency, or even absence, of myelin. The material inside the cells stains grey with Sudan black B, and gives a positive periodic-acid/Schiff reaction; it is believed to be a protein-bound glycolipid, histochemically similar to the cerebrosides of myelin.[716] A case of this disease has been recorded in which comparable intracellular

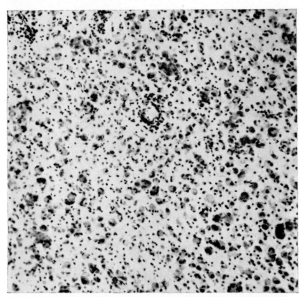

Fig. 34.149. Leucodystrophy, globoid cell type. The characteristic histological feature of this disease is the presence of 'globoid cells'—often, as here, arranged in clusters. There is no demonstrable myelin and no Sudanophile material. Blood vessels in the white matter are cuffed with lymphocytes. *Celloidin section. Nissl's stain.* × 100.

accumulations of the glycolipid were found in the lungs, spleen and lymph nodes.[717]

In some patients, melanosis of the skin, with atrophy of the adrenals, has been present (adreno-leucodystrophy).[718]

The neurochemistry of Krabbe's disease is not fully understood. There is a general loss of phospholipids and a smaller decrease in the amount of cerebrosides and sulphatides in the white matter of the brain. The fall in sulphatide content is proportionately greater than the fall in cerebrosides,[719] although it is not clear whether this is due simply to deficient sulphuric acid esterification of cerebroside galactose. A marked deficiency in the cerebroside sulphotransferase content of the white matter has been found in this disease.[720] More recently, the missing enzyme has been identified as galactocerebroside beta-galactosidase.[721]

There is no increase in the amount of cholesterol esters in the brain.

Globoid cells, or something very similar to them, have been produced by injecting cerebroside into the cerebral white matter and into the liver and spleen of normal rats.[721a]

Metachromatic Leucodystrophy

This disease is characterized by pallor of the myelin[722] and the presence in the white matter of many small bodies that are metachromatically stained purple by Nissl methods and give a positive periodic-acid/Schiff reaction. This metachromatic material contains a lipid fraction that is partly soluble in fat solvents and can thus be seen only in frozen sections. This lipid fraction is not Sudanophile. Such Sudanophile material as may be present is confined to the circumvascular space. Peripheral nerves are also affected (see page 2329).

Metachromatic material may also be found in the interstitial substance of the central nervous system in some cases of multiple sclerosis and of diffuse sclerosis: occasionally, indeed, it is a striking histological feature in these conditions. Metachromatic leucodystrophy is distinguished by the fact that there is no Sudanophile material associated with the well-marked and wide-spread metachromasia.

The disease appears to be a true inborn error of metabolism, with a familial transmission as a recessive trait. Although the total amount of glycolipids present is usually normal it is made up mainly of sulphatide instead of neutral cerebrosides, apparently through deficiency of sulphatase. True myelin lipids (neutral cerebrosides, phospholipids and cholesterol) are decreased in amount in the white matter while hexosamines are increased. The excess sulphatides do not stain metachromatically with Nissl methods in all cases, but they always give a characteristic golden brown metachromasia with cresyl violet in 1 per cent acetic acid (the von Hirsch–Peiffer reaction).[723]

Three main varieties of metachromatic leucodystrophy are recognized, differing in the age of onset. The condition can be diagnosed with the help of assay of the urinary content of arylsulphatases.[724]

Late Infantile Variety of Metachromatic Leucodystrophy.—This condition seems to have been first recognized independently by van Bogaert and Scholz[725] in 1932 and by Greenfield[726] in the following year. The gross appearance of the sliced brain may be normal, but microscopical studies, preferably on celloidin-embedded material, show widespread absence of myelin. Usually, only the optic radiations and a few other groups of fibres that normally become myelinated early in life are stained in the myelin preparations.[727, 728] It is, in fact, those parts of the brain that ordinarily undergo myelination comparatively late in development that tend to be affected. The fault in myelination is related to virtual absence of oligodendrocytes[729] and a variable degree of damage to axons. How-

ever, as Greenfield, who did so much to elucidate the nature of this disease,[729] was careful to point out, the white matter may mistakenly be thought to be 'rotten' because of the paucity of cells within it. The astrocytes may be hypertrophied, and there is well-marked gliosis.

The metachromatic substance is scattered throughout the affected white matter, and is particularly abundant round blood vessels, where it appears as globular bodies. Similar material is present in the cytoplasm of Hortega cells in the affected parts. The metachromasia may be difficult to demonstrate, especially in material that has been embedded in paraffin wax. Demyelination and the presence of metachromatic material may be detected in the peripheral nerves, and this may be a useful diagnostic procedure.[730] Rectal biopsy has also been successfully employed for this purpose, comparable changes being seen in the myenteric plexus. Occasionally, a metachromatic lipid is present in the renal tubules, the portal tracts and the wall of the gall bladder (see page 1323, Volume 3): this substance may not be identical with that in the brain. Metachromatic material has been found in the urine.[731]

Juvenile Variety of Metachromatic Leucodystrophy.—This form of the disease differs from the late infantile variety in three respects: the oligodendrocytes are less consistently absent in the unmyelinated areas, the arcuate fibres are less often affected, and metachromatic material may be found distending nerve cells, particularly those of the brainstem and dentate nuclei.[732]

Adult Variety of Metachromatic Leucodystrophy.—This rare form, which has sometimes been called Ferraro's leucodystrophy, is distinctive only in its later age of onset.[733]

Alexander's Disease (Fibrinoid Leucodystrophy)

This is an infantile form of leucodystrophy that is readily recognized histologically because of the presence of acidophile material deposited at the surface of the brain and round its blood vessels. It is occasionally familial. The brain is enlarged (megalencephaly). Alexander, who first described the condition,[734] believed that the acidophile material resulted from 'fibrinoid degeneration' of the astrocytes. It has been identified as related to neurokeratin. The suggestion has been made that the footplates of the astrocytes fail to deal effectively with the abnormal material, which reaches them from elsewhere in the brain and which they should transfer to the blood.[735]

The fibrinoid material is apparently similar in origin to the 'cytoid bodies' (Rosenthal fibres) that are a familiar feature of many pilocytic astrocytomas and in some other conditions in which there is marked formation of glial filaments in the cytoplasm of astrocytes (see page 2210).

Spongiform Degeneration of the White Matter

It is convenient to consider the so-called spongiform degeneration of the white matter among the leucodystrophies. It is a rare and sometimes familial disease found in infants; it is also known as Canavan's disease, although it had been recognized before Canavan described it in 1931.[736]

The main feature is a sponge-like atrophy of the white matter—a change that may extend into the deeper layers of the cortex. The astrocytes exhibit little reaction, except in the cortex, where their numbers may be increased and their nuclei notably big and pale. As in certain other leucodystrophies, the optic radiations are usually unaffected. The axons are little, if at all, involved. Affected infants generally die within six months to two years.

There are two other features of this disease. First, the cerebrospinal fluid is often under raised pressure. Second, the spongiform appearance of the white matter is associated with a similar change in the pallidum and in the fibre tracts in the ventral part of the pons and in the spinal cord.

There are various views about the pathogenesis of spongiform leucodystrophy. It has been attributed to: (1) neonatal hypoxia; (2) oedema due to abnormal permeability of the 'blood–brain barrier'; and (3) a congenital defect in the metabolism of the cerebral lipids. The last of these views is supported by the finding that the brain lipids of a child who died with this disease at the age of two years had the chemical constitution typical of those of a normal seven-months fetus. This suggests that there had been some defect in myelination.[737] However, the second theory is usually favoured:[738] its basis is the increased weight of the brain, the enlargement of the skull and the raised pressure of the cerebrospinal fluid.

Although, on clinical grounds, spongiform degeneration may be considered among the leucodystrophies, the constant finding of changes in the grey matter puts this disease in a position intermediate between the other leucodystrophies and the heterogeneous group of metabolic diseases that affect neurons. It is notable that similar changes

have been found in the brain in cases of 'maple sugar urine' disease (page 2240), phenylketonuria (page 2239) and homocystinuria (page 2240).

(page 2240), phenylketonuria (page 2239) and homocystinuria (page 2240).

THE NEURONAL LIPIDOSES AND OTHER
STORAGE DISEASES
(LYSOSOMAL ENZYME DEFICIENCIES)

These uncommon disorders are characterized by an abnormality of the metabolism of the neurons that, in many instances, leads to an accumulation of some metabolite in their cytoplasm. As a group, they are sometimes known as the neuronal storage diseases; the term poliodystrophy has also been used, by analogy with leucodystrophy, to indicate that it is the grey matter that is affected. Although the materials that collect in the cells are usually lipids, this is not always so, and the term lipidosis is inappropriate for the group as a whole. It is noteworthy that the neurons often share their abnormality with the reticuloendothelial cells of the lymphoreticular system in general (see pages 757 to 767, Volume 2).

These diseases are of much interest to the geneticist, for, like the leucodystrophies, they often exhibit a marked familial incidence, with a recessive form of inheritance. Each of them may be regarded as manifesting a defect in the functioning of a specific enzyme system, with a corresponding anomaly among the chemical constituents of the neurons.[739] In general, the enzymes concerned would normally be present within lysosomes:[739a] it has been suggested therefore that the diseases that result from their deficiency should be called lysosomal enzyme deficiencies[739b] or lysosomal diseases.[739c]

Amaurotic Familial Idiocy

Amaurotic familial idiocy is the name for a group of hereditary storage diseases in which the abnormality is confined to the tissues of the central nervous system and the eyes (see Chapter 40, Volume 6). In most cases the material concerned is a ganglioside. The three essential clinical features are indicated by the designation amaurotic familial idiocy.[740] It was recognized independently by Warren Tay, in 1881, and Bernard Sachs, in 1887. Tay observed the characteristic cherry-red spot in the macula of an idiot who had muscular hypotonia.[741] Sachs described the histological changes in the brain;[742] in later studies, which firmly established the familial nature of the disease, he concluded that it was the outcome of an arrest of development. The red macular spot, which is typical of the infantile form

6*

of the disease is, in fact, a relative accentuation of the normal red colour of the macula in contrast to the pallor of the surrounding retina, which is greyish-white because of the accumulation of lipid-containing macrophages (see Chapter 40, Volume 6).[743]

The brain may be small and much underweight, or its overall size may be normal apart from the diminution of the optic nerves and maybe of the cerebellum. Exceptionally, the brain may be abnormally large (a weight of 2300 grams has been recorded in a child aged 29 months[744]—see Table 34.1, page 2077): on cutting across the enlarged brain in the coronal plane, however, ventricular dilation is clearly evident.

Histologically, the nerve cells of the cortex are greatly swollen because of the accumulation of ganglioside within them: this lipid appears as a finely granular material, which is insoluble in alcohol and xylene, and stains poorly with Sudan dyes and osmium tetroxide. It gives a distinct, but not intense, positive periodic-acid/Schiff reaction. It displaces the nucleus and neurofibrils to the periphery of the cell, and all traces of Nissl substance are lost. The lipid occurs not only in the perikaryon but also in the dendrites: sometimes the amount accumulated in the latter matches that in the former. A remarkable appearance results when these distended cells are present in abundance in the cortex.

The number of Hortega cells is increased, and they contain Sudanophile material as well as the ganglioside. They tend to collect in clusters, particularly in the thalami. Such Hortega cell clusters are sometimes termed 'Russell bodies', a name that is misleading, for there is no relation between them and the familiar Russell bodies of plasma-cell origin that are a feature of many chronic inflammatory lesions in any part of the body (see Fig. 4.5, page 206, Volume 1).

There is a moderate proliferation of astrocytes in the affected tissues. Poverty of myelin may be noted throughout the brain and spinal cord. In the cerebellum the Purkyně cells are filled with ganglioside. So, too, are the ganglion cells of the retina. The meninges are usually thickened, and may contain macrophages in which small amounts of ganglioside are present.

The ganglioside, usually G_{M2}, that collects in the cells in amaurotic familial idiocy is a complex lipid composed of sphingosine, hexoses, chondrosamine and neuraminic acid.[745] It appears to differ only slightly from that present in normal brains.

It has been suggested that the missing enzyme in this disease may be one that normally splits off chondrosamine during the formation of cerebrosides.[746]

Varieties.—Several varieties of amaurotic familial idiocy have been distinguished—congenital,[747] infantile ('Tay–Sachs disease'),[741, 742] late infantile,[748] juvenile (Batten–Mayou disease[749, 749a]—also known as Vogt–Spielmeyer disease[749b, 749c]) and adult (Kufs' disease) (see Chapter 40, Volume 6).[750]

There are often minor chemical, and sometimes histological, differences between individual cases: sometimes these distinctions are specific to certain affected families. Batten–Mayou disease and Kufs' disease are peculiar in that the substances that accumulate are not gangliosides but a mixture of ceroid and lipofuscin.[750a, 750b]

The congenital variety has been recognized in only one family, and its features were distinctive in several ways.[747] Most patients with the infantile or late infantile variety of the disease are Jewish; the course of these forms is shorter, the neurons are greatly distended with the lipid, and the red macula is conspicuous. In contrast, few of the older patients are Jews; the course in these varieties is longer, neuronal changes are less marked and there is often atrophy of the cerebellum. In place of the red macula, the eye changes in these older patients take the form of a fine pigmentation that begins in the macula and spreads later to the whole retina: this is associated with degeneration of the outer layer of the retina and of the rods and cones (see Chapter 40, Volume 6).

Ultrastructural studies show swollen lysosomes that appear as membranous cytoplasmic bodies: these are probably peculiar to Tay–Sachs disease. They are found in neurons and glial cells and contain G_{M2}.

About half of the circulating neutrophils and some monocytes contain conspicuous cytoplasmic granules that are azurophile or, sometimes, basiphile. The lymphocytes often contain vacuoles: the contents of these vacuoles have no affinity for fat stains although electron microscopy seems to show that they contain lipid.[751]

In Tay–Sachs disease there is an almost complete absence of aldolase from the serum.[752] In other forms of amaurotic familial idiocy the amount of this enzyme in the serum is little if at all reduced.

Niemann–Pick Disease

In Niemann–Pick disease,[753, 753a] the reticulo-endothelial cells of the liver, spleen, lymph nodes and bone marrow gradually become distended with sphingomyelin (see page 761, Volume 2) The accumulation begins early, and splenomegaly and hepatomegaly usually become evident during the first year of life. The central nervous system tends to become affected late in the course of the disease, and death may take place before it is noticeably involved. Survival beyond early childhood is exceptional.[753b] The disease is commoner in Jews, but the proportion of Jewish patients is smaller than in amaurotic familial idiocy. The red macular spot is also less common than in that disease.

Sphingomyelin accumulates in the ganglion cells in the cerebrum and in the Purkyně cells in the cerebellum. It is soluble in alcohol and it does not give a positive periodic-acid/Schiff reaction. The latter reaction is positive in the affected cells when, as occurs in some cases, a glycolipid is also present.[754] There is some evidence that Niemann–Pick disease is related to Gaucher's disease and to amaurotic familial idiocy, for in one case sphingomyelin was found both in nerve cells and in the Kupffer cells of the liver, while the spleen contained a neutral glycolipid indistinguishable from that stored in Gaucher's disease.[755]

In the central nervous system it is the nerve cells that are primarily involved in Niemann–Pick disease, and not the Hortega cells, although these are the homologues of the reticuloendothelial cells elsewhere in the body. As in amaurotic familial idiocy, the Hortega cells may contain the lipid, but their involvement is subsidiary to the neuronal lipidosis.

It has been shown that the erythrocytes of patients with Niemann–Pick disease contain only very low levels of the enzyme that splits phosphoryl choline from sphingomyelin. This supports the view that the disease is a failure of sphingomyelin catabolism, with consequent accumulation of the phospholipid in the tissues.

Gaucher's Disease

The central nervous system is consistently involved in infantile Gaucher's disease, a condition determined by a recessive mode of inheritance (see page 759, Volume 2).[756] The material that collects is mainly a protein-bound glycolipid (cerebroside); it gives a positive periodic-acid/Schiff reaction. The affected nerve cells are vacuolate. In some cases there are widespread degenerative changes in neurons that do not contain the abnormal material; these changes are particularly marked in the dentate nuclei.

Hunter-Hurler Syndrome[757–759]

The conditions that are now included under the name Hunter–Hurler syndrome are those that formerly were referred to as 'gargoylism', an insensitive designation that should be abandoned. Other names for these conditions include Hurler–Pfaundler disease,[758, 759a] lipochondrodystrophy and chondro-osteodystrophy (Ellis–Sheldon disease [759b]). They are rare heredofamilial diseases, in which mucopolysaccharides are deposited in many neurons in the central nervous system (Fig. 34.150), in macrophages throughout the lymphoreticular sys-

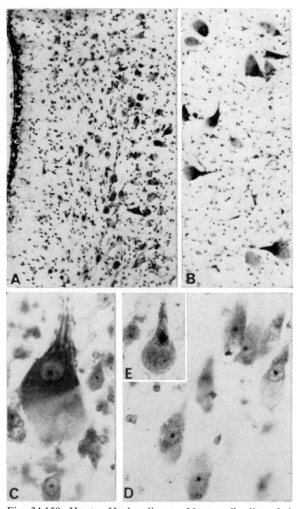

Fig. 34.150. Hunter–Hurler disease. Nerve cells distended with periodic-acid/Schiff-positive material that contains sphingolipid and mucopolysaccharide. *Periodic-acid/Schiff; haematoxylin.* A: Paraventricular nucleus; × 100. B: Nucleus of hypoglossal nerve; × 100. C: Betz cell; × 400. D: Pyramidal cells in hippocampus; × 400. E: Ganglion cell from lamina V of cerebral cortex; × 400.

tem, and in cartilage and bone. The involvement of the cells of cartilage and bone accounts for the characteristic skeletal deformities.[760]

When fibroblasts from the skin of patients with the disease are grown in tissue culture, metachromatic granules containing acid mucopolysaccharide accumulate in them. Such granules do not accumulate in normal fibroblasts in cultures. The granules are in lysosomes, which presumably lack the enzymes necessary for catabolism of the material concerned.

Metabolic disorders of connective tissues have lately been classified in four groups—mucopolysaccharidoses (see Chapter 40, Volume 6), Ehlers–Danlos syndrome (see Chapter 39, Volume 6), Marfan's syndrome (see page 82, Volume 1), and Ehlers–Danlos syndrome combined with Marfan's syndrome.[761] The mucopolysaccharidoses are subdivided into six types and two variants: of these, Type I corresponds to Hurler's disease and Type II to Hunter's disease.* Hurler's disease has an autosomal recessive form of inheritance. Hunter's disease, which is some five times rarer than Hurler's disease, has an X-linked recessive inheritance.[761]

The intracellular material that accumulates in Hurler's disease is probably a mixture, for it appears to contain sphingolipid as well as the mucopolysaccharide that is now named glycosaminoglycan. It has been suggested therefore that two series of enzymes are at fault in this disease.[762]

Two macroscopical abnormalities are sometimes found in the central nervous system—fibrosis of the meninges and enlargement of the circumvascular spaces in the central white matter of the cerebral hemispheres and in the white matter of the gyri.[763] The enlargement of these spaces is clearly visible in sections stained for myelin.

Hand–Schüller–Christian Disease

Except in very rare instances,[764] the central nervous system is not directly affected in this disease (see

* The other types of mucopolysaccharidosis in this classification (reference 761 on page 2289) are: Type III, Sanfilippo's syndrome (Sanfilippo, S. J., Podosin, R., Langer, L. A., Jr, Good, R. A., *J. Pediat.*, 1963, **63**, 837) [heparan sulphate mucopolysaccharidosis]; Type IV, Morquio–Ullrich syndrome (Morquio, L., *Arch. Méd. Enf.*, 1929, **32**, 129; Ullrich, O., *Ergebn. inn. Med. Kinderheilk.*, 1943, **63**, 929) [keratan sulphate mucopolysaccharidosis]; Type V, Scheie's syndrome (Scheie, H. G., Hambrick, G. W., Barness, L. A., *Amer. J. Ophthal.*, 1962, **53**, 753) [dermatan sulphate and heparan sulphate mucopolysaccharidosis]; and Type VI, Maroteaux–Lamy syndrome (Maroteaux, P., Lamy, M., *J. Pediat.*, 1965, **67**, 312) [dermatan sulphate mucopolysaccharidosis]. See also Chapter 40, in Volume 6.

page 763, Volume 2), but there may be tumour-like aggregates of cholesterol-laden histiocytes in the bones of the skull or in the dura, and these, if they press on the brain or cranial nerves, may cause neurological disturbances. This is prone to happen when the deposits are within the orbits or near the sella. In the early stages, the presence of the cholesterol may lead to the accumulation of eosinophils and giant cells, and the true nature of the disease may be overlooked. In its later stages, the cholesterol deposits may be obscured by an intense fibrosis.

Fabry–Anderson Disease ('Hereditary Dystopic Lipidosis')[765–767]

This metabolic abnormality is associated with attacks of burning pain and paraesthesiae in the extremities, diminished sweating, proteinuria, diabetes insipidus and macular or papular skin lesions ('angiokeratoma corporis diffusum', or Fabry's disease—see Chapter 39, Volume 6).

The neuronal involvement is largely restricted to cells of the autonomic nervous system but the abnormal material—probably a sphingolipid[767, 767a]—is also to be found in some cells of the amygdaloid, preoptic and paraventricular nuclei, the thalami, the subicula and the substantia nigra. This lipid may also be found in the cells of the intima and media of arterioles.

Glycogen Storage Diseases

Glycogen is rarely present in nerve cells in these conditions, except in a familial variant characterized by involvement of the myocardium and of voluntary muscle.[768] In this form, now often referred to as Pompe's disease (see page 44, Volume 1), the nerve cells of the spinal cord, especially those of the anterior grey columns, are involved (Fig. 34.151); those of the cortex have been affected only exceptionally. The deficiency appears to be of an alpha-glucosidase but the mechanism by which glycogen is stored is not known.[769]

OTHER METABOLIC DISTURBANCES

There are several diseases characterized by defects in metabolism that are not associated with progressive intracellular accumulation of metabolites. Like the lipidoses, some of these diseases have been attributed to lack of specific enzymes, and often the defect is shown by the presence of abnormal substances in the blood and, usually, in the urine.

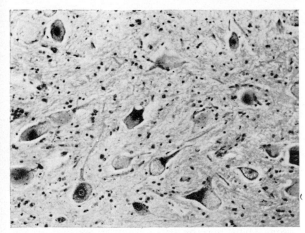

Fig. 34.151.§ Glycogen storage disease (Pompe's disease) involving neurons in one of the anterior grey columns of the spinal cord. The material distending the cytoplasm gave positive reactions for glycogen. *Haematoxylin–eosin.* × 100.

Phenylketonuria (Phenylpyruvic Oligophrenia) and Other Anomalies of Amino Acid Metabolism

In 1934, Fölling discovered that the urine of certain idiots and imbeciles contained relatively large quantities of phenylpyruvic acid.[770] The patients are fair-haired, and have a delicate, pale skin and blue eyes. It is now believed that this syndrome results from lack of the enzyme that effects the hydroxylation of phenylalanine to tyrosine.[771] In consequence, phenylalanine accumulates in the tissues, and, after deamination, is passed in the urine, mostly in the form of phenylpyruvic acid. There is a simple test for this substance—the appearance of a greenish colour after the addition of a few drops of ferric chloride to *fresh* urine. Unfortunately, since the urine may not contain phenylpyruvic acid for some weeks after birth, the anomaly cannot be recognized by examination during the first days of life. If the disorder is recognized early in infancy, and the amount of phenylalanine in the diet is severely restricted, the formation of phenylpyruvic acid is correspondingly reduced: in consequence, mental retardation may be lessened[772] and the pigment content of the hair and skin becomes more normal.

The defect is transmitted by a recessive gene. The affected baby is generally undersized, because the amount of tyrosine available is insufficient to meet normal growth requirements.

The structural changes in the brain in these cases are not well defined. Most observers have recorded some deficiency of myelination, but only in those parts of the brain that are not normally myelinated until after birth. The deficiency may be recognizable only in celloidin sections. Its significance is obscure.

Other Forms of Aminoaciduria

Three major abnormalities of the central nervous system have been recognized in association with diseases due to enzymatic defects in amino acid metabolism: impaired maturation resulting from interference with the development of the brain in the last trimester of intrauterine growth; defective myelination; and spongy degeneration of both the grey matter and the white matter, possibly the effect of impaired protein synthesis on glial cells. These abnormalities have been seen in varying degree and combination in some of the following conditions.

The 'Hartnup Syndrome'. [773]*—This rare familial disease is characterized by a pellagra-like photosensitive condition of the skin, attacks of cerebellar ataxia during exacerbations of the dermatitis, and a constant renal aminoaciduria.[774] The amino acid pattern in the urine is specific. There is a corresponding reduction in the plasma amino acids. The pellagra-like state is attributable to abnormalities of tryptophan metabolism: defective absorption and transport of tryptophan in the small intestine have been demonstrated;[775] this is only one of several similar deficiencies of amino acid transport. The cerebellar signs and transient psychotic disturbances that sometimes accompany them may be caused by some form of intoxication by metabolites, such as indole, tryptamine and tyramine, formed by bacterial action on the excessive amounts of amino acids in the contents of the colon.[776] Histopathological studies have not been reported. Consanguinity in two of the families in which the disease has been recognized[774, 777] suggests that a rare recessive gene is almost certainly responsible.

Oculo-Cerebro-Renal Dystrophy (Cerebro-Oculo-Renal Dystrophy; Lowe's Syndrome).[778, 779]— These names are given to a syndrome comprising glaucoma and other severe ocular abnormalities, mental retardation, and severe renal tubular defects

---

* This name gained currency because the nature of the disease did not indicate any simple alternative: another familial affliction has thus come to be generally known by the family's name. 'H disease', Hart's syndrome (after the physician who recognized the syndrome—reference 774 on page 2289) and 'pellagra/cerebellar-ataxia/renal-aminoaciduria syndrome' are among the synonyms.

accompanied by aminoaciduria. The neuropathological changes have included widespread lack of myelination, spongy transformation (status spongiosus) of both grey and white matter, loss of Purkyně cells, and proliferation of astrocytes, especially in the white matter.[780]

'Maple Syrup Urine' Disease.[781]—This is a familial cerebral degenerative disease caused by defective metabolism of branched-chain amino acids (valine, leucine and isoleucine). The block is at the stage of oxidative decarboxylation and as a result certain organic acids accumulate in the blood and are passed in the urine. These substances give the urine a distinctive smell, like that of maple syrup. Affected babies cease to thrive soon after normal birth, become lethargic, develop muscular rigidity and fits, and die within weeks or at most a few months. The disorder is inherited as an autosomal recessive character. There is widespread and severe spongy degeneration of the grey and white matter throughout the central nervous system, with gliosis and defective myelination.[782]

Miscellaneous Varieties of Aminoaciduria.[783, 784]— There are many other diseases characterized by disordered metabolism of amino acids, and mental retardation is an accompaniment of most of them. Some of the better known are arginosuccinic aciduria,[785] histidinuria[786] and homocystinuria:[787] all are rare, although homocystinuria, an autosomal recessive disease due to the absence of cystathionine-β-synthase,[788] is second only to phenylketonuria (page 2239) in frequency among the inherited errors of amino acid metabolism.

It should be remembered that congenital defects are often multiple, and that congenital biochemical disorders may be associated with structural malformations that are not pathogenetically related to them. It follows that neurological disturbances accompanying a biochemical anomaly do not necessarily have a biochemical basis.

Wilson's Disease (Hepatolenticular Degeneration)

In 1912, Kinnier Wilson[789] described a progressive neurological disorder of adolescents and young adults that is characterized by extrapyramidal rigidity, choreoathetosis, dysarthria and cirrhosis of the liver (see page 1278, Volume 3). A ring of greenish or brownish discoloration (the Kayser–Fleischer zone[789a, 789b]) is often present in the outer part of the cornea. Aminoaciduria is commonly found. The serum copper level is lowered. The disease is determined by a rare recessive gene for which these patients are homozygous.[790]

The changes in the brain include shrinkage and brown discoloration of the corpora striata and, often, cavitation of the putamina. Microscopical examination of the latter shows the so-called Alzheimer type II astrocytes.[791] These cells are larger than normal astrocytes, and have a large vesicular nucleus with a distinct nuclear membrane and one or more prominent nucleoli; in Nissl preparations, yellowish granules can often be seen in their ill-defined cytoplasm. The subthalamic nuclei may be atrophic and show a characteristic brownish discoloration. Copper-containing material may be deposited round the capillaries in the putamina. There may be much loss of neurons in the affected centres. Peculiar, very large, oval cells, with finely granular cytoplasm and a small nucleus, are found in the thalami, pallidum and substantia nigra; they are said to occur only in this disease, and are known as Opalski cells.[792] They may be histiocytes.[793]

The essential disorder in Wilson's disease is considered to be lack of caeruloplasmin (an alpha globulin) to bind the copper that is normally transported from the intestines in a loose, temporary chemical association with the plasma albumin.[794, 795] In Wilson's disease the amount of caeruloplasmin in the serum is low, and there may be none: consequently, when the copper is released from the albumin, it is partly excreted in the urine and partly deposited in the liver, in the corpora striata and putamina, and in the posterior limiting lamina of the cornea (Descemet's membrane) (see Chapter 40, Volume 6).

The aminoaciduria in Wilson's disease is believed to be due to an associated inability of the renal tubules to reabsorb amino acids that have been excreted in the glomerular filtrate. The concentration of amino acids in the blood is not raised.

Galactosaemic Oligophrenia

Mental deficiency may accompany this inborn error of metabolism The nature of the changes in the brain and the reason for the mental retardation are unknown.[796] Enlargement of the liver, jaundice and cataracts occur in some cases. The defect, which is believed to be in the conversion of galactose l-phosphate to glucose l-phosphate, is determined by a recessive gene. Galactose is found in the urine. Limitation of the intake of galactose is the basis of treatment: early recognition of the disease is imperative if there is to be a chance of preventing irreversible mental deficiency. Histologically, gliosis of the white matter with some pallor of myelin staining has been reported, together with an increase in the lipochrome content of neurons and a loss of Purkyně cells and, to a lesser extent, of granule cells in the cerebellum.[797]

Porphyric Myelopathy and Encephalopathy

Neurological disturbances are not part of the rare and florid variety of porphyria, congenital erythropoietic porphyria (haematoporphyria congenita, or Günther's disease[798]), which is conveyed by a recessive gene and is characterized by excessive production of photosensitizing porphyrinogens (see page 471, Volume 2).

Acute Intermittent Porphyria ('Swedish Porphyria')

Motor paresis with paraesthesiae and sensory loss in the extremities may occur in acute intermittent porphyria.[798a] This is a condition often precipitated by the administration of sulphonamides or barbiturates to susceptible people, usually in the third and fourth decade of life. Episodes of abdominal pain with vomiting, vertigo and tachycardia are the usual early symptoms; ataxia, a depressive state, confusion and even convulsions may develop. Episodes of hypertension may occur. The blood pyruvate level after taking glucose may be abnormally high. The urine may go dark on standing, due to the presence of porphobilinogen and its metabolic precursor, delta-aminolaevulic acid: usually this happens only during the attacks. Susceptibility to the condition is inherited as a dominant characteristic.[799]

Histologically, there may be a patchy loss of myelin in the peripheral nerves (see page 2319) and in preganglionic and sympathetic fibres, without loss of axons. In the brain, small areas of infarction and neuronal loss may be found: these have been attributed to hypoxia, possibly consequent on vascular spasm. In the spinal cord, the neurons of the anterior grey columns are much swollen; there is chromatolysis and vacuolation of their cytoplasm. Severe chromatolysis may also occur in the cells of the medulla oblongata. Porphyrins may be demonstrated in the adventitia of some of the blood vessels of the brain and spinal cord, and in a proportion of Hortega cells.

Other Forms of Porphyria

Neurological symptoms may occur in the hepatic-cutaneous varieties of porphyria, both in the acquired form, which may develop in alcoholics whose livers are already damaged—for instance, in Bantus (Bantu porphyria[799a])—and in the dominantly inherited form (the 'South African' familial porphyria—porphyria variegata), in which there is an excess of protoporphyrin and coproporphyrin in the faeces (see also page 2319).[800]

Hallervorden–Spatz Disease[801]

This is a rare, and sometimes familial, disease that is included among metabolic disorders with questionable justification. The patients are usually adolescents who present extrapyramidal symptoms, particularly muscular rigidity and choreoathetosis.

Macroscopically, the brain presents reddish-brown discoloration of the pallidum and substantia nigra. Histologically, these parts of the brain contain much iron pigment, most of it extracellular, but some in neurons, astrocytes and Hortega cells. The nerve cells of the cerebral cortex and the Purkyně cells are those likeliest to be involved, and after gradual atrophy the affected cells may eventually disappear. Globoid bodies, similar to those found in neuroaxonal dystrophy (see below), are present in large numbers in the pallidum and the substantia nigra.

The disease runs a slow course, and death is usually due to inhalational pneumonia resulting from the dysphagia that is associated with the extrapyramidal disturbance.

'Neuroaxonal Dystrophy' (Seitelberger's Disease)

Seitelberger described a rare form of idiocy in young girls that appears to be related to Hallervorden–Spatz disease.[802, 803] It is characterized by a symmetrical, brownish-pink discoloration of the pallidum: histological examination shows abundant Sudanophile fat in the neurons of these structures, with deposits of iron pigment round blood vessels and in some astrocytes. The most striking finding, however, is the occurrence in the grey matter, especially of the pulvinaria and of the dorsolateral part of the brainstem, of peculiar rounded masses ('globoid bodies'): these are believed to be focal swellings of the axons, and they may reach a diameter comparable to that of the body of the nerve cells. The posterior roots of the cervical part of the spinal cord are also affected. Atrophy of the vermis of the cerebellum and loss of myelin in the fasciculi graciles have also been described. Seitelberger regarded this 'neuroaxonal dystrophy' as an infantile form of Hallervorden–Spatz disease, for similar axonal swellings have been recorded in the latter.[804]

It has been suggested that there may be an association between Hallervorden–Spatz disease, Seitelberger's disease and Unverricht's myoclonic epilepsy (see below).[805] In addition, Seitelberger's disease is possibly related to Tay–Sachs disease, for the axonal swellings contain a lipoglyco-protein.[805]

Unverricht's Syndrome

Myoclonus is a manifestation common to many conditions in which the cerebellum has been damaged. One of these, known as Unverricht's syndrome (myoclonic epilepsy),[806] is inherited as a Mendelian recessive, and affects boys oftener than girls. It runs a clinical course of a decade or longer. The spasmodic movements affect mainly the proximal muscles of the limbs; in the course of time, ataxia, dementia and, sometimes, pyramidal tract lesions develop.

A characteristic, but inconstant, finding in the brain in Unverricht's disease, and peculiar to it, is the presence in the cytoplasm of many of the neurons, especially those in the dentate, olivary and red nuclei, the substantia nigra and the thalami, of large, rounded bodies that give the staining reactions of amyloid. These are the so-called Lafora bodies (Fig. 34.152).[806a, 806b] They may be

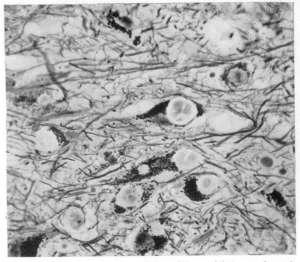

Fig. 34.152.§ Myoclonic epilepsy (Unverricht's syndrome) showing intracytoplasmic inclusion bodies of Lafora type distending the pigmented cells of the substantia nigra. *Haematoxylin–eosin.* × 400.

found free in the tissues after the death of the nerve cell in which they were formed.[807] They must not be confused with the Lewy bodies of paralysis agitans (see page 2267): both these distinctive types of body occur with particular frequency in the substantia nigra. Lafora bodies may also be found in the liver and in the myocardium.[808]

DEFICIENCY DISEASES AND THE CENTRAL NERVOUS SYSTEM[809]

Since the central nervous system is so dependent upon carbohydrates for its metabolism, it is particularly vulnerable to lack of a sufficient supply of those members of the B group of vitamins that are essential for normal carbohydrate utilization. When some of these vitamins are deficient in the diet, or are insufficiently absorbed, certain types of neurological disorder are apt to develop. The progress of these deficiency diseases can often be halted by prompt administration of the appropriate vitamins: failure of such therapy to restore the nervous system to its normal condition is to be attributed to irreversible effects of damage, such as loss of neurons or myelin. In parts of the world where the diet is deficient in this group of vitamins, these diseases are common; in occidental countries they are now rare, with the exception of subacute combined degeneration of the spinal cord.

Subacute Combined Degeneration of the Spinal Cord (Posterolateral Sclerosis)

The first full clinical and pathological account of this disease was published by Risien Russell, Frederick Batten and James Collier at the National Hospital, Queen Square, London, in 1900:[810] although the association of severe neurological disturbances with Addisonian anaemia (pernicious anaemia) had previously been recognized, the pathological changes had scarcely been observed. The anaemia is seldom severe; indeed, the haemoglobin concentration may be within normal limits, especially if the patient has been under treatment, but there is always some increase in the mean diameter of the erythrocytes and in the mean corpuscular haemoglobin concentration. In doubtful cases, cytological examination of the bone marrow may prove helpful. The most reliable evidence of the specific deficiency that is responsible for subacute combined degeneration of the spinal cord is obtained by estimation of the amount of vitamin B_{12} in the blood: its mean normal concentration in serum is from 160 to 925 pg/l (approximately 120 to 685 pmol/l when expressed in SI units [*Système international d'unités*]). The progress of the disease is arrested by the administration of vitamin B_{12} (which has the pharmaceutical name of cyanocobalamin).

In the majority of cases of subacute combined degeneration of the spinal cord, there is complete absence of pepsin and hydrochloric acid in the gastric secretion: this state is not affected by the administration of histamine. Addisonian anaemia (see page 454, Volume 2) and subacute combined degeneration of the spinal cord may occur alone or together. The anaemia responds to treatment with folic acid, but this substance does not influence the course of the degeneration in the spinal cord and is in fact contraindicated in the presence of the neurological disorder. In contrast, both conditions respond to the administration of cyanocobalamin.

In the spinal cord, there is loss of myelin, particularly in the posterior and lateral columns (Fig. 34.153): the changes are severest in the thoracic region. In the cervical part of the cord the posterior columns are mainly affected whereas in the lumbar part the pyramidal tracts are mainly involved: in other words, the midthoracic region of the cord is damaged first and most severely, and this is followed by ascending degeneration of the sensory tracts and descending degeneration of the motor tracts. The spinocerebellar tracts may be involved. In early cases there is patchy demyelination of the posterior funiculi in the midthoracic segments. The demyelinated areas have a spongy appearance in histological sections that is very characteristic (spongiform degeneration). There is a tendency for gliosis to occur in severe lesions, particularly after the progress of the disease has been halted by treatment.[811]

In addition to the cord lesions, foci of demyelination and loss of axons are not infrequently found in the cerebral white matter, and this may account for the symptoms of cerebral involvement that are occasionally observed clinically.[812] Peripheral neuropathy accounts for numbness and tingling in the hands and feet, which are among the earliest symptoms of the disease (see page 2324).[813]

Little is yet known about the biochemical changes that result from the deficiency of vitamin B_{12}: high concentrations of pyruvic acid in the blood have been observed, with reversion to a normal level after treatment with cyanocobalamin.[814] Methyl malonic acid accumulates in the tissues and is excreted in excess in the urine when there is a deficiency of vitamin B_{12}: it has been suggested that this metabolite may be toxic to neural tissues and therefore the cause of the lesions.[815] Another suggestion is that there is a reciprocal relation between cyanide and vitamin B_{12} in the plasma, and that detoxication of cyanide may be dependent on this vitamin.[816] If this is so, some of the pathological effects of vitamin B_{12} deficiency may result from cyanide intoxication. Thiocyanate oxidase, present in erythrocytes, probably acts on thiocyanate derived from the diet to form a small, metabolically active cyanide pool. Cyanide accumulation may thus depend on red cell mass and thiocyanate concentration: paradoxically, severe anaemia may therefore protect against cyanide intoxication. The adverse effect of folic acid therapy on subacute combined degeneration of the spinal cord might be explained by a rise in the amount of red cell thiocyanate oxidase consequent on the haematological remission. Vitamin B_{12} deficiency accompanied by neurological lesions similar to those that occur in man has been induced in monkeys fed on vegetarian diets.[817]

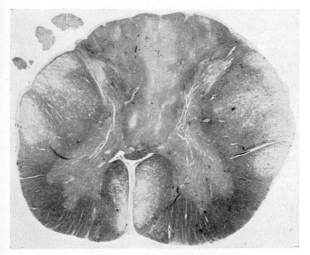

Fig. 34.153. Subacute combined degeneration of the cord (level of the second cervical segment). There is patchy demyelination of the posterior funiculi (particularly of the fasciculi graciles) and of the lateral and anterior corticospinal tracts. *Celloidin section. Heidenhain's stain.* ×9.

Pellagra

Pellagra is characterized clinically by cutaneous, gastrointestinal and neurological disturbances. The most typical skin lesions are the erythematous, scaly patches that develop at the wrists and ankles, particularly on their dorsal aspect. There is also a general roughening of the skin, and increased pigmentation of the exposed parts of the body. The cutaneous changes are accompanied by glossitis. In the later stages of the disease, which usually runs a long course, achylia, diarrhoea and anaemia develop. The neurological disorders that occur in the advanced disease include spastic paraplegia, extrapyramidal disturbances, ataxia, visual disturbances and mental deterioration.

The association of pellagra with subsistence on a predominantly maize diet had been known for many years before its cause was recognized to be specifically a deficiency of nicotinic acid.[818] Maize contains no tryptophan, and this amino acid is believed to be the main source from which bacteria synthetize nicotinic acid in the intestines. People whose diet is based almost wholly on this grain are, therefore, liable to suffer, *inter alia*, from nicotinic acid deficiency. Similarly, circumstances that greatly modify the normal bacterial flora of the intestines, such as chronic diarrhoea, or prolonged treatment with certain antibiotics or other drugs, may result in deficient synthesis of nicotinic acid and the consequent development of pellagra.

It has to be remembered, in connexion with all deficiency diseases, that shortages of essential factors are seldom confined to a single substance. For this reason it may be difficult to ascribe any particular symptom or lesion to a particular deficiency. Pellagra, for instance, is not a clearly defined clinical entity, and there are some who believe that a deficiency of nicotinic acid—despite its undoubted efficacy in treatment—is not the sole cause of all the clinical features of the pellagra syndrome.

In fatal cases of pellagra, degenerative changes are found in the posterolateral columns of the spinal cord and are often associated with a demyelinating peripheral neuropathy.[819] However, the most constant neuropathological finding is central chromatolysis of the Betz cells of the motor cortex and of the neurons of the anterior grey columns of the spinal cord, and of many nerve cells in the basal ganglia and in the brainstem.[820]

Beri-Beri

Beri-beri is a form of malnutrition endemic among rice-eating peoples; it is due to deficiency of thiamin (vitamin B_1). The form that is known as wet beri-beri is characterized by the development of heart failure and oedema, which result from changes in the myocardium that are specifically due to lack of thiamin (see page 44, Volume 1). Dry beri-beri is characterized by a peripheral and central neuropathy, which develops in the absence of oedema. Indeed, it is widely believed that the wet and dry forms of beri-beri are different diseases. This may well be so, in view of the multiple dietetic deficiencies prevalent among rice-eating people.[821]

In dry beri-beri, the peripheral neuropathy (see page 2317) is associated with demyelination that begins in the distal portion of the nerves and appears to precede any detectable changes in their axons. Occasionally, demyelination is also present in the dorsal tracts of the spinal cord. A cerebral form of beri-beri occurred in prisoners of war in Japanese labour camps.[822]

A neuropathy that bears a striking resemblance to dry beri-beri can be produced in pigeons by feeding them on polished rice; the affected birds recover rapidly when given thiamin. The disease of horses known as 'the staggers' is due to thiamin deficiency caused by the presence of an enzyme, thiaminase, in fodder that contains bracken; it, too, is quickly cured by treatment with thiamin.[823]

Wernicke's Encephalopathy[824]

In 1881, Wernicke described a condition that he named acute superior haemorrhagic polioencephalitis;[824a] his patient had pyloric stenosis, but in most subsequent instances of the disease the patients have been alcoholics. Wernicke's disease is a manifestation of a deficiency of thiamin, and its development in association with chronic alcoholism is the result of the gastric mucosal dysfunction that follows prolonged consumption of spirits. The same deficiency syndrome may complicate atrophic gastritis, whatever its cause. It may also develop in association with carcinoma of the stomach or with persistent vomiting, as in hyperemesis gravidarum.

The symptoms include ataxia, nystagmus, visual disturbances and stupor. The distinctive psychotic state that is known as Korsakov's syndrome[824b] is now believed to be a chronic form of Wernicke's disease.[825, 826]

Wernicke's disease is characterized structurally by the presence of petechial haemorrhages in the region of the third and fourth ventricles and round the aqueduct. The heaviest involvement is in the mamillary bodies (Fig. 34.154), where there may also be marked proliferation of capillaries.[827] Similar vascular changes may be found elsewhere—for instance, in the chiasma and optic nerves, the

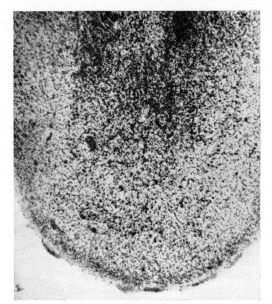

Fig. 34.154. Wernicke's encephalopathy induced by chronic alcoholism. This mamillary body, which appeared shrunken to the naked eye, shows marked proliferation of blood vessels and an almost complete loss of neurons. *Celloidin section. Haematoxylin–Van Gieson.* × 40.

nuclei of the vestibular nerves, the dorsal nuclei of the vagus nerves, and the inferior olivary nuclei. In the more chronic forms of the disease there may be degeneration of the dorsomedial thalamic nuclei and of the Purkyně cells, and also sclerosis of Ammon's horn. Coexisting disease of the liver may give rise to alterations in the astrocytes (see page 2249).

Neurological Complications of Steatorrhoea and Related Gastrointestinal Disorders

Gluten-Sensitive Enteropathy ('Adult Coeliac Disease')

The neurological complications of gluten-sensitive enteropathy (which is known also as non-tropical sprue) (see page 1084, Volume 3) include peripheral neuropathy, cerebellar dysfunction and unexplained episodes of unconsciousness.[828] Mental disturbance may also occur.[829]

The neuropathological changes are numerous and widespread: degeneration of the white matter of the spinal cord (mainly in the posterior funiculi); demyelination of nerve roots; hypothalamic lesions similar to those of Wernicke's encephalopathy (see above); proliferation of Alzheimer type II astrocytes (see page 2240) in the basal ganglia; cerebellar cortical degeneration; and atrophy and loss of neurons in the cerebral cortex and in the anterior grey columns of the spinal cord. There is a resemblance, both clinical and pathological, to 'carcinomatous neuropathy' (see page 2326).

Muscle biopsy shows neural abnormalities, particularly collateral branching and diffuse swelling of terminal axons, with electron microscopical evidence of severe changes in the internal structure of the terminal axonic expansions.[830]

Post-Gastrectomy States

The neuropathy that occasionally follows gastrectomy may not appear until many years after the operation.[831] The legs are affected predominantly, the signs including weakness and wasting, difficulty in walking, paraesthesiae, and evidence of degeneration in the posterior funiculi of the spinal cord. Pathological studies of this condition have been conspicuously few. In the one case in our personal experience there was demyelination of the posterior funiculi and dorsal nerve roots and atrophy of neurons in the dorsal root ganglia and in the anterior grey columns of the spinal cord; spongiform degeneration of the posterior and lateral funiculi of the cord, characteristic of vitamin B_{12} deficiency (page 2243), was not present.[832]

Whipple's Disease (Intestinal Lipodystrophy)

Cerebral complications, especially mental disturbances, may occur in Whipple's disease.[833, 834] Material that gives a positive periodic-acid/Schiff reaction, and apparently identical with that present in the intestinal tract (see page 1084, Volume 3), is found in microscopical aggregates in the brain. As in the bowel, this material includes structures that in electron micrographs resemble bacteria:[834, 835] their identity and significance are debatable.

Amylodosis Involving Ganglia and Nerves

Amyloid infiltration, particularly in cases of 'primary' amyloidosis, may cause degeneration of axons and myelin in the autonomic ganglia and nerve plexuses of the bowel when these structures are involved: severe diarrhoea and steatorrhoea may result.[836] Amyloid deposits may similarly affect spinal nerve roots and ganglia, peripheral nerves (see page 2314) and the main autonomic nerves and ganglia: peripheral sensory and motor disturbances, postural hypotension and anhidrosis are among the clinical consequences.

INTOXICATIONS AND THE CENTRAL NERVOUS SYSTEM

Intoxication with Metals and Metalloids[837]

Lead

Plumbism generally develops as a cumulative intoxication, which results from repeated and sometimes unsuspected exposure to this element, either by inhalation or ingestion. Formerly, it was a common hazard in many trades in Britain, but legislation has almost eliminated it as an occupational disease, in spite of the steadily increasing use of lead in industry.[838] Lead poisoning, however, still remains a danger for children, because compounds of the metal continue to be employed in paints and for other domestic purposes.[839]

Lead poisoning may be acute or chronic, and its symptomatology is very diverse. Apart from the nervous system, the parts most affected in chronic plumbism are the bone marrow (anaemia), kidneys (chronic renal failure and hypertension), skeletal muscles (weakness) and bowel (colic).

Neurological disorders may result from the effects of lead on the central nervous system and on peripheral nerves (see page 2329). In acute lead poisoning, delirium, convulsions and coma develop; they are often associated with papilloedema. In chronic lead poisoning, which is usually the result of exposure over a period of many years, dementia and convulsions are the commonest neurological manifestations. Narrowing of the smaller cerebral blood vessels by proliferation of their endothelium causes ischaemia and it is to this that the symptoms are due. There is nothing specific about the pathological findings.

When intoxication follows the inhalation of substances in which lead is combined with some organic compound, the nervous lesions may be partly or mainly due to the organic constituent of the material. In cases of poisoning with tetraethyl lead, for example, which can cause lesions like those of Wernicke's encephalopathy (see page 2244), no lead is demonstrable at necropsy in the central nervous system.

Mercury

Poisoning by mercury, like poisoning by lead, may cause a wide variety of clinical manifestations, and may be acute or chronic (see also page 2318). The technical uses of mercury in industry are now very numerous and varied, and each carries its own dangers.[840, 841]

Neurological manifestations are among the earliest and most prominent symptoms of chronic mercury poisoning. An initial phase of fatigue, irritability and emotional instability (erethism) soon gives place to depression. Coarse tremor is a characteristic symptom, and these clinical findings, associated with the typical profuse salivation, clearly indicate the diagnosis. This is the picture of mercury poisoning that was familiar in the days when mercury, applied by inunction, was extensively used in the treatment of syphilis.

Organic compounds of mercury are the usual causes of mercury poisoning today, and they are generally absorbed by inhalation. The early signs are ataxia and contraction of the visual fields. In one case that came to necropsy 15 years after exposure to methyl mercury, degenerative changes were present in the granular layer of the cerebellar cortex, particularly in the depths of the sulci, and there were peculiar argyrophile bodies in the molecular layer that were thought to be altered dendritic processes of Purkyně cells.[842] There was also severe atrophy of the calcarine cortex and of the underlying white matter; patchy areas of atrophy were present elsewhere in the cerebral cortex. When death occurs a few weeks after exposure to an organic mercurial compound selective damage to the cerebral cortex, especially the calcarine cortex (Fig. 34.155), may be found, with, in addition, degeneration of Purkyně and granule cells in the cerebellum. In a case of short duration, in which chemical studies of the brain were made, the content of mercury was highest in the corpus callosum.[843]

Pink Disease.—Young children seem to be particularly susceptible to poisoning by mercury. Some babies who were given powders containing calomel (mercurous chloride)—for instance, as a household remedy for teething troubles or intestinal disturbances—developed the condition known as pink disease ('erythroedema polyneuriticum'), a peculiar syndrome of anorexia, irritability and erythematous swelling of the extremities.[844] This condition was accompanied by fever and profuse sweating. The affected child commonly developed a distinctive patch of thinning of the hair on the back of the head, due to constantly rubbing it against the pillow. At necropsy, demyelination was found in some peripheral nerves.[845] It is not certain that all cases of pink disease were associated with mercury.

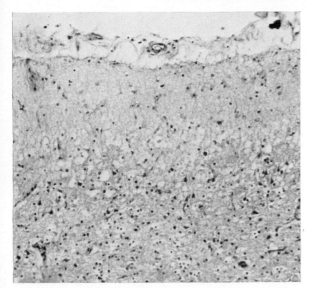

Fig. 34.155. Mercurial intoxication. The calcarine cortex has a spongy appearance because of the considerable loss of nerve cells: the few remaining cells show ischaemic change. The glial response is slight. Note the thickened capillaries in the leptomeninges. *Haematoxylin–eosin.* × 90.

However, the condition has disappeared following a campaign to stop the marketing of teething powders containing calomel (see also page 2318).

Minamata Disease.—A peculiar disease that was prevalent from 1953 to 1956 among the people who lived on the shore of Minamata Bay, in Kyushu, Japan, was found to be due to eating fish from the local waters, which were heavily contaminated with an organic mercurial compound in the effluent from a chemical factory. The signs were progressive numbness of the extremities and often of the lips and tongue, ataxia, choreoathetosis, blurring of vision and contraction of the visual fields.[846, 847] The fish in the bay were noted to be thin and to swim erratically, and cats feeding on them developed a disease that resembled the disease in man.

Thirty-five (40 per cent) of 88 affected people died. Necropsy revealed cerebral oedema, degenerative changes in the cerebellum (especially in its granular layer), and loss of neurons in the cerebral cortex, particularly in the calcarine, precentral and postcentral areas. The hypothalmus and basal ganglia were often involved. The spinal cord was unaffected. Sensory neurons were also involved (see page 2319).

A congenital palsy has been described in the Minamata area, similar in pathology to Minamata disease in adults.[848] It is believed that the lesions develop *in utero*; the mothers of the affected children have not shown evidence of the disease.

Mercurial Content of Fish.—Since the recognition of Minamata disease (see above), it has been found that there may be high levels of methyl mercury in fish taken from fresh and sea waters in various parts of the world not known to be artificially contaminated. For instance, fresh water fish in Sweden and canned tunny (tuna) on sale in Britain have been found to contain potentially harmful amounts of such compounds.[849] Not all the hazardous mercurial content of water originates in industrial and other artificial effluents. Natural waters contain inorganic mercury compounds that may act as receptors for methyl groups of organic metabolites formed by micro-organisms.

All fishing waters should be monitored for evidence of contamination by heavy metals.

Manganese

Manganese poisoning is usually the result of inhalation of dust containing salts of this metal. Its most striking neurological manifestation is a tremor that, while coarse in type, has been likened to the tremor of Parkinson's disease because it is associated with extrapyramidal rigidity.[850, 851] The nature of the neurological lesions underlying these signs is obscure, although loss of neurons in the cerebral cortex, basal ganglia and cerebellum has been described.[852] In addition to the changes in the brain, multilobular cirrhosis of the liver and interstitial fibrosis of the kidneys have been found.

Experimentally, it has proved possible to produce degeneration of the Purkyně and granule cells of the cerebellum and of the cells of the dentate nuclei in a monkey by causing it to inhale finely pulverized manganese metal; no lesions were found in the liver or kidneys.[853] These findings have been regarded as evidence that manganese in comparable amounts may cause neuronal damage in man.

Tin

Interest in the toxic action of the organic compounds of tin was renewed after fatalities in France caused by a medicament that contained diethyl tin diiodide.[854] Such compounds cause one of the most striking forms of cerebral oedema yet recognized; similar changes, which are reversible, appear when triethyl tin is given to animals.[855] The oedema is accompanied by conspicuous accumulation of fluid within the oligodendrocytes, as in acute renal failure (see page 2250), although there is no evidence of injury to the kidneys by these compounds.[856]

Arsenic

An encephalopathy was an occasional complication of treatment with organic arsenical compounds such as neoarsphenamine and tryparsamide (see pages 2183 and 2252). It was characterized by congestion and oedema of the brain, with petechial haemorrhages scattered abundantly throughout the white matter.[857] The condition can be reproduced experimentally in monkeys.[858]

Intoxication with Organic Substances

Ethyl Alcohol (Ethanol*)

After absorption into the blood, ethyl alcohol is rapidly distributed to every tissue in the body, accumulating in each roughly in proportion to the water content of the part. Eventually, most of the alcohol is oxidized in the liver to acetic acid; a small proportion—less than 10 per cent—is excreted unchanged through the lungs, kidneys and skin. An average adult can metabolize about 10 ml of pure ethyl alcohol hourly—roughly the amount present in a 'small whisky' (which, in England, is $\frac{5}{6}$ fl oz—23·68 ml). If this amount or more is taken at once, and absorbed quickly from the fasting stomach, the concentration of alcohol in the blood reaches its peak half an hour to an hour later. The impairment of brain function that results from acute alcoholic intoxication is manifested by loss of normal inhibitions, prolongation of reaction time, dysarthria and lack of muscular coordination: these effects point to the functional impairment of a wide range of nerve cells. Ability to drive a motor car safely has been found to deteriorate significantly when the concentration of alcohol in the blood exceeds about 17·5 mmol/l (80 mg/dl).[859]

Once the alcohol has disappeared from the blood, the functions of the central nervous system quickly return to normal; however, repeated episodes of acute alcoholism or sustained bouts of drinking undoubtedly damage nerve and glial cells, and lead, over the years, to progressive mental deterioration. In advanced chronic alcoholism, there may be persistent symptoms of cerebellar incoordination, involving especially the lower limbs and trunk (the *drunkards' paraplegia* described in 1868 by Samuel Wilks[860]). This is associated with degeneration of the Purkyně cells (Fig. 34.156) and, to a lesser extent, of the granule cells of the anterior and upper parts of the vermis (the central lobule,

* The terms *ethanol* and *ethanolic*, although preferred by biochemists, are in general less familiar in medical usage than *ethyl alcohol* and *alcoholic* (the latter implying 'ethyl-alcoholic'). In this chapter contemporary medical usage is followed.

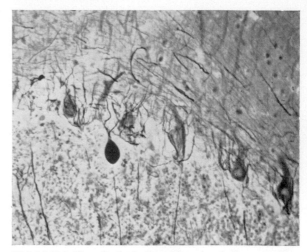

Fig. 34.156. Chronic alcoholism. There is a bulbous swelling ('torpedo') on the axon of a degenerating Purkyně cell. The processes of the 'basket cells' can be seen enveloping the Purkyně cells. *Celloidin section. Davenport's stain.* × 140.

the culmen and the declive).[861] A decrease in the number of the highly distinctive Purkyně cells is readily recognizable; in contrast, loss of neurons from the cerebral cortex may be difficult to assess, even when the number destroyed is large. That such a loss does take place is borne out by examination of the cerebral cortex, especially of the frontal lobes, where proliferation of astrocytes is associated with a disappearance of neurons in all laminae, and particularly in the third lamina. It must be emphasized that the alcoholic patient may be liable not only to this toxic damage to cells in the cerebellum and cerebrum, but also to the consequences of a deficiency of vitamins of the B group, for malnutrition is common, and often aggravated by chronic gastritis and impairment of absorption from the intestine. Therefore, in advanced cases, there are likely to be extensive degenerative changes in the mamillary bodies, as a manifestation of Wernicke's encephalopathy (see page 2244).

Central Necrosis of the Corpus Callosum.—Central necrosis of the corpus callosum (Marchiafava–Bignami disease[861a]) is an uncommon manifestation of chronic alcoholism. Loss of myelin in the corpus callosum is accompanied with disappearance of some of the axons. Sometimes there are also foci of demyelination in the white matter of the cerebral hemispheres, not far from the principal lesions in the corpus callosum. Similar areas may also be present in the cerebellar peduncles.

For many years, Marchiafava–Bignami disease was regarded as exclusively a disease of Italians resident in Italy and heavily addicted to drinking Chianti. It is now known that similar cases may be seen in other parts of the world, particularly in those of Latin stock, but exceptionally in others.[862–864] Also, it is now realized that the disease may occur, although comparatively rarely, in spirit and beer drinkers,[865] and even in people who are believed not to be alcoholic. A few of the patients have been women. The disease has seldom, if ever, been diagnosed during life. The symptoms that might result from a callosal defect (loss of the finer shades of awareness of right-sidedness and left-sidedness, and of the coordination of movements dependent on them) are obscured by the mild dementia and loss of coordination that characterize the drunkard. Other neurological manifestations of alcoholism may coexist with this disease, especially those of Wernicke's encephalopathy. Malnutrition is usual, and death occurs from intercurrent infection. Cirrhosis of the liver has been found at necropsy in several instances.

The pathogenesis of this curiously selective form of degeneration of the white matter is not known. Toxic factors other than alcohol have been considered, but none has been found. It has not been possible to reproduce the condition in animals, although experimental chronic cyanide poisoning has provoked comparable changes in the corpus callosum in rats.[866]

Central Pontine Myelinolysis.[867]—This rare disease, which is also known as central pontine myelinoclasis, is characterized by very extensive demyelination of the pons. It was originally described as a complication of alcoholism[868] but has since been recognized in cases of malnutrition not associated with alcoholism[869] and in patients dying after renal transplantation.[870] Its pathogenesis is obscure.

Methyl Alcohol

The drinking of methyl alcohol, which is sometimes added as an adulterant to cheap spirits, is attended by all the dangers of ordinary alcoholism, with the further grave liability to blindness caused by degeneration of the ganglion cells of the retina.[871]

Morphine

Respiratory failure is the main hazard of acute morphine poisoning. In fatal cases, in which there has been a terminal period of hypoxia of several hours' duration, early degenerative changes can be found in the cortical neurons, and there may be reactive changes in the glial cells. The brain is oedematous. Petechial haemorrhages may develop in the central nervous system and other organs as a non-specific manifestation of the hypoxia.

Intoxication Due to Metabolic Disturbances
Hepatic Coma[872]

In patients with chronic hepatic failure, the accumulation in the blood of toxic metabolites, among them ammonia, may give rise to an encephalopathy.[873] Often there is an associated hypoglycaemia. In those patients who survive the coma for a few days there is widespread loss of nerve cells, especially in the deeper layers of the cerebral cortex and in the basal ganglia and cerebellum. This loss of nerve cells is accompanied by proliferation of astrocytes, which present an appearance identical with that of the astrocytes in the putamina in Wilson's disease (Alzheimer's type II astrocytes—see page 2240). Glycogen-containing intranuclear inclusions have also been found in the astrocytes in these cases. An occasional feature is microcavitation of the deeper layers of the cerebral cortex, the immediately subcortical zone of the white matter and the basal ganglia.

The biochemical disturbances underlying the development of hepatic encephalopathy are not fully understood. There is a close correlation between the depth of coma and the blood ammonium level but the explanation of such an association has proved difficult. It has been thought that the disturbance might be due to accumulation in the brain of glutamine derived from the combination of ammonium with glutamate:[874] evidence in support of this includes the facts that some of the ammonium in the blood, particularly when its concentration is high, is removed as the blood circulates through the brain, and that hepatic coma is accompanied by a significant rise in the concentration of glutamine both in the blood and in the brain, as indicated by its level in the cerebrospinal fluid.[875] Further, glutamine accumulates in the brain after portocaval anastomosis in rats:[876] in these experiments Alzheimer type II astrocytes are regularly found if the plasma ammonium nitrogen levels remain raised for more than five weeks. It may be that the astrocytes make up the compartment of the brain in which glutamine is synthetized from endogenous ammonium ions released from neurons: the appearance of the Alzheimer type II cells may indicate the expansion of this compartment in relation to the increased glutamine storage.

Uraemia

In cases of acute renal failure, the brain may be slightly swollen, the extra fluid appearing to have collected inside distended oligodendrocytes, especially those of the white matter. In chronic uraemia, there may be some neuronal degeneration, with regressive changes in the astrocytes, amounting in some instances to clasmatodendrosis (see page 2083).

PRIMARY DEMYELINATING DISEASES

Demyelination and myelinoclasis are synonymous terms that are employed to indicate that the myelin sheath of the nerve fibre has been lost. Demyelination in the central nervous system may be primary or secondary: in the former case, the axons remain intact, at least initially, whereas in the latter the demyelination is a consequence of the destruction of the axons themselves. Secondary demyelination in the brain and spinal cord may be the result of trauma, certain intoxications and certain nutritional deficiencies: it may be regarded as analogous to the Wallerian degeneration that takes place in peripheral nerves distal to the level of a lesion that separates part of an axon from its perikaryon (see page 2305).

Our knowledge of the causation of the primary demyelinating diseases remains fragmentary. In one group—the post-infective encephalomyelopathies—something is known of the aetiology of the conditions although their pathogenesis remains problematical. However, neither aetiology nor pathogenesis is known in the majority of these diseases, including multiple sclerosis, which is by far the most important. No truly comparable, naturally-occurring disease of animals is known that might provide the basis for experimental investigations.

POST-INFECTIVE ENCEPHALOMYELOPATHIES

Several common viral diseases may be complicated by a demyelinating encephalomyelopathy.[877, 878] Among them are measles, varicella, rubella, mumps and, more rarely, influenza (Fig. 34.157). Occasionally, a comparable condition complicates vaccination against smallpox (post-vaccinial encephalomyelopathy). Such inflammatory changes as may be found in cases of post-infective encephalopathy may be regarded as attributable—in part, at least—to an injury to the myelin sheaths, for local demyelination is one of the earliest changes to be recognized. A descriptive expression, *post-infective*

perivenous myelinoclasis, is favoured by some pathologists; we find the non-committal term *post-infective encephalopathy* to be preferable. The name acute disseminated encephalomyelitis is still widely used, especially by clinicians.

Encephalomyelopathy Complicating the Acute Infectious Exanthems and Mumps

Of all the acute infectious fevers, *measles* is the one most frequently associated with encephalomyelopathy: the complication develops once in about 10 000 cases—in some epidemics oftener—and it is least rare in older children. It manifests itself in the form of convulsions, meningism or coma, usually beginning about four or five days after the appearance of the rash, although it may develop concurrently with the rash or up to 24 days after it. The case fatality rate is from ten to twenty per cent; the patients who recover have little or no residual disability. Occasional reports of finding the virus in the spinal fluid suggest that some instances of measles encephalomyelopathy may be due to spread of the virus to the central nervous system. The relation of persistent infection with measles virus to subacute sclerosing panencephalitis is discussed on page 2160.

Encephalomyelopathy is less frequent as a complication of *chickenpox* and *rubella*; the clinical features and prognosis are much the same as in the disease that complicates measles. The mild form of smallpox known as *alastrim* was also sometimes followed by encephalomyelopathy. A comparable, but usually milder, form of encephalopathy may complicate *mumps*: it must be distinguished from the much commoner mumps meningitis and meningoencephalitis, which are directly due to infection of the central nervous system by the virus, which in these cases can be isolated from the brain and from the cerebrospinal fluid.

In these encephalomyelopathies, lesions are found round veins and venules (Fig. 34.157), mainly in the ventral parts of the pons and in the

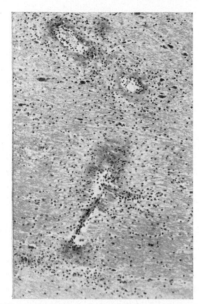

Fig. 34.157. Post-influenzal encephalopathy. An acute inflammatory reaction involves the white matter, especially round the blood vessels. The cells surrounding the latter are lymphocytes and Hortega cells. *Haematoxylin–eosin.* × 70.

white matter of the cerebral hemispheres and cerebellum. Lesions may also be found in the deeper layers of the cerebral cortex, in the thalami and substantia nigra, and in the white matter of the spinal cord.[879] In most cases, the walls of the veins in the affected areas undergo necrosis, and this is accompanied by a local accumulation of Hortega cells, and sometimes also of neutrophils; collections of lymphocytes and small focal haemorrhages are occasionally found. In sections stained for myelin there is a distinct zone of pallor round the affected veins (Fig. 34.158): this pallor is the result partly of local oedema, and partly, in those patients who have survived for a few days, of demyelination.

Post-Vaccinial Encephalomyelopathy

Although encephalomyelopathy had long been recognized as an occasional sequel of vaccination against smallpox, it was the occurrence of an unprecedentedly large number of cases in the Netherlands and in Britain in the years from 1922 to 1930 that first attracted particular attention to the condition.[880] In the period 1951–60 the incidence of neurological complications of primary vaccination at all ages in England and Wales was 12·5 per million with a mortality of 4·4 per million: for the first year of life the corresponding figures were 13·3 and 5·7 respectively.[881]

Post-vaccinial encephalomyelopathy is particularly likely to develop in older children or young adults who have not been vaccinated before. Revaccination does not seem to carry the same risk. The clinical signs usually appear on about the tenth or twelfth day after vaccination, and the patient passes quickly through a phase of drowsiness into coma. The case fatality rate ranges from about 35 to about 50 per cent.

In most cases, histological examination shows that the affected vessels in the brain are cuffed with lymphocytes and Hortega cells.[882] When the disease occurs in children under two years of age, there is no such cellular reaction: in these cases, the findings in the brain are mainly those of acute oedema and are, perhaps, indicative of a generalized viraemic infection. Save for the absence of a cellular reaction in the infant's brain, the changes in the central nervous system in post-vaccinial encephalomyelitis seem to be identical with those of the post-infective encephalomyelopathies described above.

Pathogenesis of the Post-Infective Encephalomyelopathies

The part played by viruses in the causation of these lesions is still obscure. In some forms, and notably in post-vaccinial encephalomyelopathy, the virus may be recovered from other organs, although not from the brain and cerebrospinal fluid.

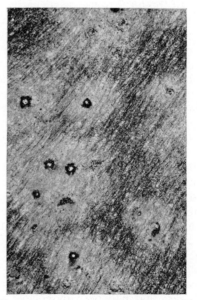

Fig. 34.158. Post-measles encephalopathy. White matter showing circumvenous myelinoclasis. *Heidenhain's stain.* × 70.

It is significant that there is a close similarity of incubation period, clinical course and pathology in cases of post-infective encephalomyelopathy, irrespective of the identity of the particular and distincive viral disease—measles, chickenpox, rubella or vaccinia—that precedes the neurological illness. This suggests that the latter may not be caused directly by the virus of the antecedent infection, but by activation of another virus already latent in the brain. This explanation could account for a remarkable, and otherwise apparently inexplicable, clinical observation: a single batch of calf lymph was widely employed in vaccination against smallpox both in the Netherlands and in Spain—its use was followed by many cases of encephalomyelopathy in the former country but by only one in the latter.[883] However, the attempts that have been made to isolate the latent virus have been so regularly unsuccessful that activation of such an agent seems unlikely to be the correct explanation.[884] Alternative theories are that the encephalopathy is caused by a myelinolytic substance (produced or released as a result of the infection), and that it is the outcome of an allergic reaction akin to that seen in experimental allergic encephalopathy (see page 2258).

Acute Haemorrhagic Leucoencephalitis[885–887]

This is a fatal disease with a fulminating course. It was first described by Weston Hurst in 1941.[885] Necrosis of blood vessels, particularly venules, results in multiple petechial haemorrhages in the white matter, with accumulation of neutrophils round the vessels and local oedema. Circumvascular demyelination is a feature.

On clinical and pathological grounds the disease is usually regarded as a form of post-infective encephalopathy or as an 'allergic' encephalopathy. Pathological findings identical with those in acute haemorrhagic leucoencephalitis have been associated with allergy to drugs, particularly arsenical preparations (see page 2183). In one reported case, in which allergy to an organic arsenical preparation appeared to be the cause, the typical changes of acute haemorrhagic leucoencephalitis were associated with the classic clinical and pathological picture of thrombotic thrombocytopenic purpura (see page 2182).[887]

Pathological changes comparable with those of acute haemorrhagic leucoencephalitis have been found in rats that had been inoculated intraperitoneally or in a footpad with a mixture of homogenate of spinal cord and pertussis vaccine.[888]

Nothing is certain about the aetiology and pathogenesis of multiple sclerosis, yet it causes as much chronic disability as any other disease of the nervous system. It has been estimated that there are between 40 000 and 50 000 people with multiple sclerosis in Britain.[889] In 1976, the number of deaths from multiple sclerosis notified in England and Wales was 764 (278 in males and 486 in females);[890] these figures vary little from year to year.

The clinical picture, in its classic form, is distinctive. Pathologically, however, there is no clear distinction between this disease and several other less common conditions that have less well defined clinical features: these diseases include diffuse cerebral sclerosis (Schilder's disease) (see page 2259), Baló's disease (see page 2260) and optic neuromyelopathy (Devic's disease) (see page 2260). Some authorities group them with multiple sclerosis on the grounds that all are manifestations of primary demyelination.

Multiple Sclerosis (Disseminated Sclerosis)[891, 892]

Clinical Features

Multiple sclerosis is mainly a disease of young adults. It is rare before puberty. Women are more liable to be affected than men. The disease is recognized in a few patients after the age of 50 years: however, bearing in mind its relapsing nature and that an interval of many years may separate attacks, it is always possible that in these seemingly late cases the disease began much earlier, with symptoms so trivial that their significance was not appreciated at the time. The symptoms may appear for the first time after a mild infection, a dental extraction, an accident, the administration of an anaesthetic, or an emotional shock: such circumstances may also precipitate relapses, but whether they have any real aetiological importance is debatable. It has been widely considered that the disease is aggravated by pregnancy and lactation, but some contemporary neurologists discount this belief.[893]

Many of the early symptoms of multiple sclerosis, such as dysaesthesiae in the limbs and transient paralyses, are referable to lesions in the spinal cord, particularly the cervical and lumbar enlargements. The classic syndrome that is known as Charcot's triad[894]—nystagmus, intention tremor and slurring speech—is due to the presence of sharply defined and irregularly shaped plaques of demyelination and gliosis in the pons and medulla oblongata. Occasionally, the disease may present with perplexing symptoms: for instance, the initial manifestations may simulate a tumour in the cerebellopontine angle or take the form of tic douloureux.

Classically, multiple sclerosis is a chronic disease with intervals of remission between successive relapses, each of which is accompanied by further deterioration. A relapse may begin with the same symptoms as the preceding attack, suggesting that the same lesion has been reactivated or has extended.[895] Sometimes, however, there are long periods of freedom from exacerbations, and then the prognosis both for life and for work may be favourable. When a plaque forms in the pons or medulla oblongata, the vital centres may be affected and death may soon follow. In such cases there may or may not be plaques elsewhere in the brain or in the spinal cord; the lesion that has proved fatal will be found to be of recent development, with little or no gliosis. In fact, lesions in which gliosis is minimal cannot properly be described as plaques of sclerosis.

Epidemiology

Multiple sclerosis occurs mainly in temperate climates. It is particularly liable to affect people of northern European origin.[896] It is rare in Africans and Asians. In tropical and subtropical lands even Europeans are seldom affected. The disease is uncommon in Japan,[897] although more frequent there than was formerly believed; it is also uncommon in Australia, where both diffuse cerebral sclerosis (see page 2259) and optic neuromyelopathy (see page 2260) occur more frequently.[898] It must be emphasized, however, that comparisons of the morbidity and mortality statistics of different countries are not always straightforward: in official returns in some countries deaths from multiple sclerosis and from cerebral sclerosis of vascular origin are combined.

In the United Kingdom, familial cases account for about 7 per cent of all cases of the disease;[899, 900] in the Shetland Islands the proportion is even higher.[901] Such familial cases may be attributable to genetical factors; alternatively, they may be the result of an aetiological factor in the environment that is common to the household. A genetical element in the aetiology of the disease is possibly indicated by the observation that in western Europe, Canada and the United States of America the incidence of the disease in the general population ranges from 1·3 to 6·7 per 10 000 but is as high as 62 per 10 000 among the relatives of patients with the disease.[902, 903] Over one per cent of patients with multiple sclerosis are the offspring of marriages between first cousins.[902, 903] Studies on the incidence of multiple sclerosis in monozygotic and dizygotic twins also indicate a genetical influence; they also suggest that exogenous factors play an important part in the pathogenesis of the disease.[904]

Structural Changes[905, 906]

While plaques may be found anywhere in the central nervous system (Figs 34.159 and 34.160) they form most characteristically in the white matter round the lateral ventricles, and especially in relation to their posterior horns. Many of these lesions are symptomless. Occasionally, indeed, typical plaques are found in the brain of people who have died from other diseases, and who have had no neurological symptoms of any sort.[907] The plaques in clinically recognized cases may be few in number, although careful search of the brain and spinal cord after fixation will usually disclose more numerous lesions than was at first suspected. In a minority, the lesions appear to be confined either to the brain or to the spinal cord. The optic nerves, optic tracts and chiasma are commonly involved: this accounts for the frequency of visual disturbances, including optic atrophy, which occur especially in the early stages of the disease.

Old plaques have a grey, translucent appearance and are firm. Plaques of more recent origin are softer, and yellowish or very slightly pink. They vary greatly in size and shape; the larger ones look as if they have been formed by confluence of smaller plaques. Preparations stained for myelin almost always show lesions that are overlooked when the brain is first examined after fixation (Fig. 34.161).

The plaques are commonest in the white matter, for it is here that myelin is present in greatest amount. Some plaques, especially those in the juxtaventricular parts of the occipital lobes, are sharply limited to the white matter (Fig. 34.159): the cortex and the arcuate fibres between the cortex and the main mass of the white matter are then spared. Sometimes, however, the plaques involve grey matter and white matter indiscriminately and more or less equally. Because there are fewer myelinated axons in the cortex than in the white matter, demyelination in the former is less conspicuous; for this reason, when examining preparations stained for myelin, particular atten-

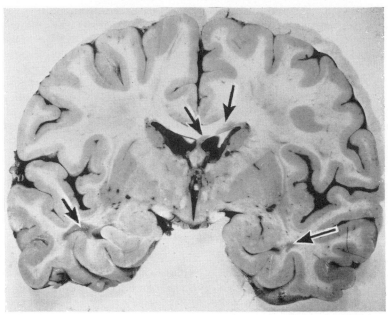

Fig. 34.159. Multiple sclerosis. Several plaques are seen (arrows). The one in the white matter of the right temporal lobe (left of picture) impinges on but has not extended into the overlying cortex. [The darkened area in the left centrum semiovale is not a plaque but the grey matter at the base of a sulcus.]

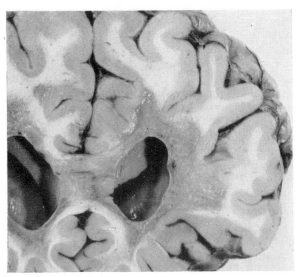

Fig. 34.160. Multiple sclerosis. The plaques are commonly situated in the white matter round the ventricles and especially in the occipital lobes. In this old-standing case there is diffuse demyelination round the dilated anterior horns of the lateral ventricles and spreading over the genu of the corpus callosum.

plaque of sclerosis (Fig. 34.159). Similarly, it has to be remembered that the distinct appearance of the normally well-defined visual pathway in the occipital white matter is likely to be accentuated in specimens that have been well fixed in formalin.

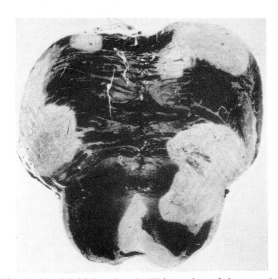

Fig. 34.161. Multiple sclerosis. This section of the pons has been stained for myelin: the plaques appear white because of the complete absence of myelin in them. Note the irregular but sharply-defined contours of the plaques. *Celloidin section. Weigert–Pal stain.* × 2.

tion should be paid to the cortex, lest plaques there be overlooked.

Care is needed when examining the fixed brain to avoid mistaking a transversely cut gyrus for a

Sometimes the cerebral lesions of multiple sclerosis seem to be most numerous at the junction of the cortex with the white matter. It is noteworthy that this zone is a particularly common location of metastatic lesions, both cancerous and pyaemic, as well as of blood-borne parasitic infestation (see page 2138). It is here that the pial arterioles, having penetrated the cortex, break up into branches, thus favouring the impaction of small emboli. However, this does not indicate that an embolic process accounts for the lesions of multiple sclerosis.

If the smaller plaques of sclerosis are carefully studied, especially with the aid of serial sections, a venule can often be seen in or near the centre of the lesion.[908] There is commonly, but not invariably, cuffing of the vessel by lymphocytes, and this may attract attention to the presence of the plaque. Macrophages, distended with the lipid breakdown products of myelin, and swollen astrocytes are often present in freshly demyelinated areas (Fig. 34.162).[909] When there is much cuffing of vessels the lesions will be readily seen in haematoxylin–eosin preparations, but in its absence the plaques may be overlooked: this is especially so in the grey matter, because the neurons in a demyelinated area appear to be unaffected and the fat-laden cells may be inconspicuous. In haematoxylin–eosin preparations, too, the extraordinary proliferation of the astrocytic fibres will be noticeable. When the plaque involves white matter, its recognition may be

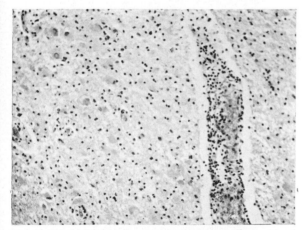

Fig. 34.162. Multiple sclerosis: lymphocytes cuffing a blood vessel within a young plaque in the white matter. The cell bodies of the astrocytes are swollen, and their nuclei are both prominent and of varied appearance. Glial fibres, which are not evident with this stain, are being formed. The small pyknotic nuclei mostly belong to histiocytes, some of which surround small blood vessels; others belong to the scanty oligodendrocytes that remain in the affected part. *Celloidin section. Nissl's stain.* × 150.

facilitated by the empty appearance of the myelin sheaths and the naked aspect of the axons. Recognition of older plaques may be even more difficult, because after a few months the fat-laden phagocytes disappear and the astrocytes become fewer.

It is important to stress that the two most characteristic features of the plaque—the loss of myelin and the great proliferation of glial fibres—are seen to advantage only when use is made of special stains. Demyelination may be demonstrated by various staining methods, most of which are based on iron haematoxylin or luxol fast blue: these stain the myelin and leave unstained the areas in which it has been lost (Fig. 34.163A). The best results are obtained by applying the myelin techniques to thick celloidin sections. Proliferation of glial fibres may be shown by Holzer's crystal violet stain (Fig. 34.163B) or phosphotungstic acid haematoxylin: these give satisfactory results on paraffin wax sections or celloidin-embedded material, especially if thick sections are cut.

A striking feature of the plaque is the sharpness of its outline. There is no gradual merging of the demyelinated area into the adjacent area of normal myelination. Usually, there is complete demyelination throughout the plaque, but sometimes so-called 'shadow plaques' are seen, in which the loss of myelin, although uniform, is only partial. A completely demyelinated plaque may partly overlap a shadow plaque. Almost as clear cut as the area of demyelination is the gliosis, which is surprisingly dense (Fig. 34.164). Indeed, the development of glial fibres is so remarkable that some authors have doubted if it is a secondary phenomenon, and have suggested the possibility that the primary lesion of multiple sclerosis may be a pathological change in the astrocytes. Although this view seems to be untenable, it is true that there is no other condition in which the glial scar is so striking. It is probable that whatever causes the disintegration of the myelin also stimulates the astrocytes in the affected part to form fibres.

It is remarkable how little discernible alteration is to be found in any neurons that may lie within a plaque. A virtual absence of oligodendrocytes from the plaques is a common feature: it is not possible to say whether this results from the demyelination or contributes in some way to its development. It has been suggested that the lesions are due to a failure of the oligodendrocytes to maintain the myelin sheaths in a normal state, but no explanation has been advanced to account for this hypothetical failure or to relate it to the sharpness of the outline of the plaques. Moreover, it is difficult to reconcile

sively, sometimes over years, and fresh lesions may arise at any time during the course of the disease. Their histological appearances suggest that their evolution is slow, and that the pattern that they follow is fairly constant. It is possible that the early phase of exudation and myelin disruption

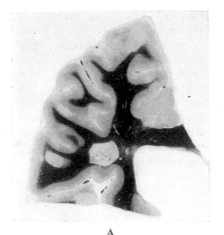

A

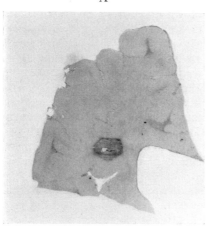

B

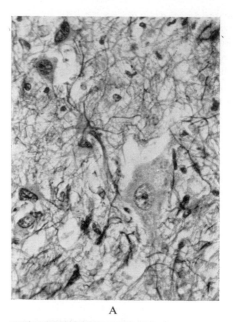

A

Fig. 34.163. Multiple sclerosis. Contiguous sections from a celloidin block, stained (A) for myelin by Heidenhain's method, and (B) for glial fibres by Holzer's method. There is one markedly gliotic plaque that is well seen in both sections. A study of the Holzer preparation permits recognition of plaques that are not at first sight obvious in the myelin preparation because they have encroached on the grey matter. The age of a plaque can be assessed by the density of the gliosis: one that is about six weeks old is usually faintly Holzer-positive to the naked eye.

this suggestion with the fact that oligodendrocytes are plentiful at the periphery of a plaque, where they may be responsible for the demonstrably increased local enzyme activity noted (Fig. 34.165).[910] Although the function of the axons that pass through the plaque is impaired by demyelination, as is clearly shown by the symptomatology of the disease, neither the loss of myelin nor the local disappearance of oligodendrocytes results in axon destruction. It is only later, when gliosis is advanced, that the axons disappear (Fig. 34.166).

The plaques of multiple sclerosis appear succes-

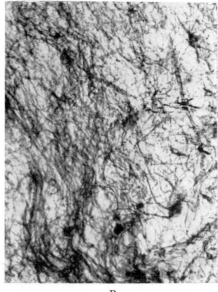

B

Fig. 34.164. Multiple sclerosis. A: Proliferating astrocytes with fibre formation in the vicinity of a nerve cell in a young plaque. *Celloidin section. Mallory's phosphotungstic acid haematoxylin.* × 360.
B: Dense gliosis in an old plaque situated in white matter. *Celloidin section. Holzer's stain.* × 160.

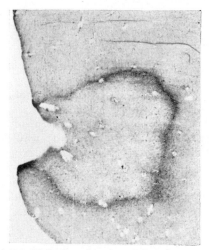

Fig. 34.165.§ Multiple sclerosis: active plaque stained to show the concentration of adenosine triphosphatase at its periphery. This illustrates the extent to which oligodendrocytes are found round the plaques, for the adenosine triphosphatase activity is located in the mitochondria of these cells.

takes place quickly, for fresh lesions are sometimes found to be outlined by a zone of fat-laden histiocytes that, during the ensuing few months, migrate into the circumvascular space of the blood vessels in the vicinity. In fact, the age of a plaque is best indicated by the use of stains for lipids;[909] stains for glial fibres provide valuable supplementary evidence. The axons within the plaques may look irregular and tortuous, but long remain preserved. Demyelination and the local disappearance of the oligodendrocytes may be responsible for the onset of symptoms; however, the progressive clinical manifestations may well result from the dense gliosis and consequent distortion of the axons. Acute and fleeting symptoms, and exacerbation of existing symptoms, may, however, be due to temporary vascular engorgement in or near the plaque. These evanescent symptoms may last only for minutes; they may appear during bouts of exertion—on the tennis court, for instance —and not infrequently they are bilateral.[911]

The Cerebrospinal Fluid in Multiple Sclerosis

The total amount of protein and the amount of gammaglobulin in the cerebrospinal fluid are usually increased, particularly when the disease is active. The increase in gamma globulin may be demonstrated in the form of a first-zone Lange curve (see footnote on page 2121); it is more precisely studied by electrophoresis. It is usually

accompanied by an increase in the number of lymphocytes.

Pathogenesis

There have been many hypotheses about the causation of multiple sclerosis: none has received general acceptance. Many investigators have thought that the lesions may be the result of an allergic response to some antigen that is normally present in the central nervous system or that is immunologically akin to a normal constituent of the system. This possibility and others will be reviewed briefly.

Infection.—No infective agent has been demonstrated in the central nervous system in multiple sclerosis. Various investigators reported finding spirochaetes in the plaques, but efforts to confirm these claims failed, and they are no longer seriously considered.

Attempts to recover a virus have been unsuccessful: however, in judging these results it must be realized that most of the procedures employed in the past would not be acceptable to virologists today.[912] Infection of the skin by the virus of herpes simplex provides an analogue of a lifelong infection characterized by alternation of remission and relapse. The hypothesis that multiple sclerosis is an infective disease has been revived by the recognition of the occurrence of latent viral infections (page 2156) and slow viral infections

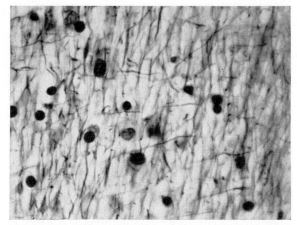

Fig. 34.166. Multiple sclerosis. An old plaque involving white matter, stained to show the paucity of axons. The smaller and darker nuclei are those of oligodendrocytes: they can at times be confused with bulbous processes on axons. The larger and more vesicular nuclei of astrocytes can also be seen. *Celloidin section. Glees' silver impregnation.* × 280.

(page 2161) of the central nervous system. It has been shown that the titre of antibody to measles virus is higher in the serum of patients with multiple sclerosis than in other people.[913, 914] However, no correlation has been shown between the occurrence of clinical attacks of measles and the eventual development of multiple sclerosis. It has been reported that paramyxoviruses can be isolated from cerebral tissue in cases of multiple sclerosis by co-cultivation techniques and that electron microscopy revealed structures that could be measles virus in one such case.[915, 916] As it has been suggested that the presence of paramyxoviruses may facilitate the capacity of constituents of the brain to become antigenic,[917] and as there is a temporary increase in lymphocyte response to the encephalitogenic factor of brain tissue during the course of clinical measles, it is possible that multiple sclerosis results from persistence of measles virus in the central nervous system, with consequently raised, but local, sensitivity to encephalitogenic factors, leading to demyelination on the basis of an auto-immune reaction. Alternatively, other viruses may be concerned, and in this context it is relevant that conventional viruses, among which the paramyxoviruses are numbered, have been thought to facilitate infection by slow viruses.[918] These possibilities are far from substantiated: for the moment they are little more than an indication of what may prove to be factors in the aetiology and pathogenesis of this common, serious disease.

Hypoxia.—It has long been known that oligodendrocytes are sensitive to deprivation of oxygen (see page 2084) and that when they die the nearby myelin sheaths disintegrate quickly. Local hypoxia may be caused by vascular obstruction, and some authors have been impressed by the frequency with which thrombi may be present in the vessels inside plaques;[919] this observation gave rise to a vogue for anticoagulant therapy. Others have suggested that vascular obstruction may result from the agglomeration of fat droplets in the lumen of the arterioles:[920] although this view has not found favour, it is noteworthy that multiple, irregular foci of demyelination in a case of fat embolism could be likened to the lesions of multiple sclerosis.[921]

Demyelination may occur in the white matter in some cases of cyanide poisoning. This is believed to result from the action of the poison on the cytochrome oxidase system within the cytoplasm of the oligodendrocytes.[922] Demyelination may also occur in cases of poisoning by carbon monoxide or nitrous oxide. It has also been observed as a

consequence of high altitude hypoxia, which suggests that the intracellular enzymes may be rendered ineffective by simple hypoxia.

Allergy.—The possibility that an encephalopathy might arise as a manifestation of allergy was first suggested by findings in the occasional cases of paralysis complicating Pasteur's method of rabies prophylaxis, in which an emulsion of rabbit's spinal cord was injected subcutaneously daily for about 10 days (see page 2151). Much experimental work has been done in this field.[923-926] A demyelinating disease can be produced in monkeys by parenteral injection of emulsions of rabbit brain.[923] Later workers used the Freund technique, in which a suspension of dead tubercle bacilli in liquid paraffin acts as an adjuvant to enhance the antigenic action of the heterologous brain emulsion. In more recent experiments, specific constituents of brain tissue, from the same or a different species, have been used as antigens.

In general, the pathological picture in experimentally-induced allergic encephalomyelitis has been more akin to that of the post-infective type of encephalomyelopathy (see page 2250) than to multiple sclerosis: sometimes, however, it has shown features recalling the latter. For instance, an experimentally induced, relapsing, demyelinating disease in monkeys was shown to be caused by an agent present in the brain of man, monkey, rabbit and chicken, but not in that of frog or fish.[927] In the rabbit, the agent was present in the spinal cord at birth but in the cerebrum only after the eleventh day—an interesting correlation with the time-sequence of myelination in these two parts of the central nervous system in this species.

Reports of encephalopathy following Pasteur's rabies prophylaxis,[928] and of encephalomyelopathy following treatment of Parkinsonism by injection of calf brain extracts,[929] somewhat reduced the gap between experimental allergic encephalomyelopathy and multiple sclerosis: the lesions of these iatrogenic diseases have some resemblance to rapidly developing lesions in cases of multiple sclerosis. A review of the resemblances between the demyelinating diseases of man and the experimental allergic diseases in animals led to the conclusion that the human diseases, including the chronic forms, should be regarded as allergic in character.[930-932]

Naturally Occurring Demyelinating Diseases of Animals

There are no known demyelinating diseases of animals that have any close resemblance to multiple sclerosis in man, although in the past some parallels were drawn that are now seen to have been fallacious. For instance, the lesions of encephalomyelopathy accompanying *canine distemper*,[933] while predominantly affecting the white matter and characterized by conspicuous demyelination, are frankly inflammatory and altogether different from those of multiple sclerosis.[934] Similarly, *visna*, a disease of sheep in Iceland (see page 2161), is not a demyelinating disease but a form of granulomatous encephalomyelitis with no features to support the former supposition of a similarity to multiple sclerosis.

The condition of monkeys that is known as *cage paralysis*[935] has also been likened to multiple sclerosis, with little reason. Cage paralysis is probably not an entity but a heterogeneous group of diseases, the common factor being disturbed mobility. The group includes not only various degenerative and inflammatory encephalomyelopathies but possibly also such nutritional disorders as vitamin B_{12} deficiency (see page 2242)[936] and scurvy rickets, the latter essentially affecting bones and joints without any accompanying neurological disturbance.

RARER PRIMARY DEMYELINATING DISEASES

Diffuse Cerebral Sclerosis

Diffuse cerebral sclerosis (Schilder's disease, or Sudanophile cerebral sclerosis) is a condition in which a gradually progressive neurological illness, extending over a period of many months or years, is associated with diffuse demyelination of the white matter of the cerebral hemispheres. Usually, both hemispheres are affected, but the lesions may be unilateral. The white matter of the cerebellum may also be involved.

Although generally known as Schilder's disease, the condition was first described by Heubner in 1897.[937] Schilder's account appeared in 1912:[937a] he regarded the disease as a variant of multiple sclerosis.* The occipital lobe is most frequently affected, and blindness due to demyelination of the optic radiation is, therefore, a common symptom. The frontal lobes are also often involved. A feature

---

* It should be noted that of three cases reported by Schilder, only the first (1912—reference 937a on page 2292) was an example of the condition that now goes by his name. Case 2 (Schilder, P., *Z. ges. Neurol. Psychiat.*, 1913, **15**, 358) was clearly an instance of familial leucodystrophy, while Case 3 (Schilder, P., *Arch. Psychiat. Nervenkr.*, 1924, **71**, 327) seems to have been a case of subacute sclerosing leucoencephalitis (Lumsden, C., *Brit. med. J.*, 1951, **1**, 1035).

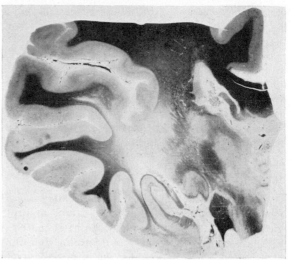

Fig. 34.167. Diffuse cerebral sclerosis (Schilder's disease). Diffuse demyelination in the temporal lobe is shown. The subcortical arcuate fibres ('U-fibres') are preserved in places —for instance, round the hippocampal gyrus (below, to right of centre)—but the upper part of the area of demyelination has extended through these fibres to involve the grey matter of the superior temporal gyrus and the anterior part of the insula. Diffuse demyelination was present in the temporal and occipital lobes of both hemispheres; there was also a solitary plaque in the cerebellum. The patient was a girl of 14. *Celloidin section. Heidenhain's stain.*

of Schilder's disease is that the arcuate fibres—immediately deep to the cortical grey matter—are spared, as in some cases of multiple sclerosis (Fig. 34.167). When the greater part of the cerebral white matter is affected, and gliosis is well established, there is a notable shrinkage of the centrum semiovale of the side or sides involved, with consequent ventricular dilatation. The scarred areas are greyish and translucent, and their consistence is firmer than that of normal white matter. In contrast, the more recently affected parts are softer than normal and faintly yellowish. Histologically, the findings resemble those of multiple sclerosis. As well as the sparing of the arcuate fibres there are, occasionally, narrow zones of normally myelinated fibres round some of the blood vessels. Because of the great severity of the demyelination in diffuse sclerosis, there is more destruction of axons than in multiple sclerosis, and Sudanophile lipids are present in larger amounts.

The disease occurs rather more frequently in children than in adults.

Sometimes it develops rapidly, and death occurs within a few weeks, or even days. In a case in which the clinical illness had lasted less than seven weeks, degeneration of the interfascicular oligodendroglia was found;[938] it was suggested that a lipolytic enzyme might have been liberated from these cells.

In many examples of Schilder's disease, especially in adults, plaques identical with those of multiple sclerosis may be found, either elsewhere in the brain or in the spinal cord. The name *transitional sclerosis** has been given to these mixed cases.[939] Many now believe that there is no true distinction between the two diseases.

Baló's Disease (Concentric Sclerosis)

This disease is a rare, chronic demyelinating condition, clinically indistinguishable from multiple sclerosis.[940] Pathologically, it is characterized by a series of concentric zones of demyelination that alternate with bands in which the myelin is intact: the appearance has been compared to the concentric pattern of Liesegang rings. This appearance suggests a series of demyelinating episodes that originate from a central focus, possibly a blood vessel. The concentric pattern of the demyelination has been likened to that of the changes that give ring-spot virus disease of plants its name.[941] Although Baló's disease usually runs a chronic course there are occasional exceptions—for instance, in the case of one young adult the illness lasted for only five days.[942]

Baló's disease may occur in association with the classic lesions of multiple sclerosis.

Optic Neuromyelopathy

Optic neuromyelopathy ('neuromyelitis optica') was first recognized by Allbutt in 1870.[943] It was described in France by Devic,[944, 944a] in 1894, and it is often known as Devic's disease. It is characterized by demyelination of the optic nerves and of parts of the spinal cord. The condition is not inflammatory, and the designation 'neuromyelitis' is inappropriate. The symptoms of optic nerve disease and the involvement of the spinal cord commonly develop together, or within a few days of each other, but either may precede the other by several weeks. The prognosis is generally serious, although in some cases there is partial or complete recovery; in a few cases, apparent recovery is followed by relapse, and the further course of the illness is then typical of multiple sclerosis. The disease has been seen in identical twins; it was rapidly fatal in both patients.[945]

* This term is inappropriate as it implies a change from one type to the other rather than a mixture of the two.

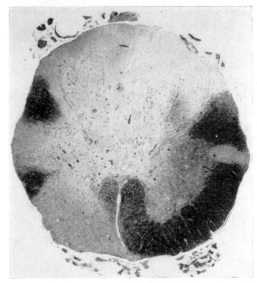

Fig. 34.168. Optic neuromyelopathy. Mid-thoracic region of the spinal cord. Demyelination has involved large areas of the white and grey matter, mostly on the left. On the right a small peripherally placed plaque has impinged on the posterolateral part of the anterior grey column. See also Fig. 34.169. *Celloidin section. Heidenhain's stain.* × 7.

In fatal cases, there is extensive breakdown of myelin in the optic nerves and in the spinal cord (Figs 34.168 and 34.169); this is accompanied by an abundant accumulation of fat-laden phagocytes and some proliferation of astrocytes. The picture, in fact, resembles that of infarction after vascular occlusion, but the smaller blood vessels show no abnormality apart from some swelling of the endothelial cells. Gliosis is found only in those cases that pass into the chronic stage.

The protein content of the cerebrospinal fluid is usually from 1·5 to 2·0 g/l (150 to 200 mg/dl), which is much higher than in multiple sclerosis, but there is no relative increase in the gamma globulin fraction. The cell count in the fluid is raised; most of the cells are lymphocytes.

The pattern of myelin destruction in the spinal cord varies considerably. In general, there are multiple foci of demyelination that quickly coalesce, so that substantial areas of softening develop. Identical changes are seen in the spinal cord in cases of diffuse demyelinating myelopathy (see below); there is no involvement of the optic nerve in the latter.

The condition has sometimes been associated with diffuse demyelinating lesions in the occipital white matter, reminiscent of the changes seen in cases of diffuse cerebral sclerosis (Schilder's dis-

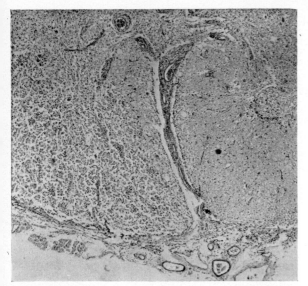

Fig. 34.169. Optic neuromyelopathy. Section adjoining that illustrated in Fig. 34.168. There is cellular infiltration in the leptomeninges covering the cord and in the anterior fissure. The demyelination is associated with necrosis that involves the white matter to the left of the fissure and the left anterior grey column. *Celloidin section. Nissl's stain.* × 30.

ease). The distinctively rapid loss of vision, and the seemingly greater frequency of the disease in particular geographical regions—Australia and the Orient—are sufficient reason for regarding optic neuromyelopathy as a clinical entity.

Diffuse Demyelinating Myelopathy

The findings in this condition are identical with those of the spinal component of optic neuromyelopathy. As in the latter, any part of the cord may be affected, and there may be one or several foci. The affected part is markedly softened, and oozes a soft, pasty material when cut in the fresh state.

Histological examination shows severe myelin destruction, with Sudanophile fat scattered throughout the necrotic areas, both free and in Hortega cells. Inflammatory changes are usually inconspicuous or absent. In one case, a plaque of the type seen in multiple sclerosis was present in the brainstem, indicative of a previous phase of the demyelinating process.

Both clinically and pathologically, this condition must be distinguished from softening of the spinal cord due to thrombosis of the anterior spinal artery or of the spinal veins.

Progressive Multifocal Leucoencephalopathy

This progressive demyelinating disease, which occurs as a terminal complication of some systemic diseases of the lymphoreticular system, is now generally recognized to be an 'opportunistic' viral infection. It is discussed accordingly on page 2161.

DEGENERATIVE DISEASES

The diseases considered in this section are of obscure nature and pathogenesis. Some of them appear to be determined genetically, but it must be emphasized that the occurrence of a disease in more than one sibling does not necessarily indicate a genetical origin.

It has sometimes been said that the brain and spinal cord together comprise a series of related nervous systems—motor, sensory, cerebellar and extra-pyramidal—grouped in the form of a single organ. The sensory system itself may be divided into several distinct units, of which the exteroceptive and proprioceptive divisions are the most important. There is a large group of neurological diseases in which, for reasons yet unknown, degenerative changes appear in the neurons of only one of these systems. Many patterns of such distinctive cell and tract degenerations have been recognized; occasionally more than one system may be affected in the

one patient. These degenerative system diseases are sometimes familial, and often hereditary: they are often referred to as the *heredodegenerations*.

In order to bring together in one group the various diseases characterized pathologically by unexplained degeneration of the affected tissues, Gowers,[946] early in this century, advanced the concept of 'abiotrophy', by which he implied an innate 'defect of vital endurance'[946a]—that is, premature senescence—of a particular tissue. As examples of abiotrophic diseases of the nervous system Gowers instanced spastic paraplegia, Parkinson's disease, Friedreich's ataxia, tabes dorsalis, general paresis, 'simple mental failure', myopathy, peroneal muscular atrophy, and arsenical neuropathy. He postulated that an inherent but latent defect in a particular system was brought to light by the action of an exogenous factor, such as an infection: in this way he accounted for the well-known, but otherwise inexplicable, observation that only a proportion of those who contract syphilis develop tabes dorsalis or general paresis. Although more is known nowadays about the pathogenesis of some of the diseases listed by Gowers, the term abiotrophy has persisted in neurological terminology and is still sometimes used.

Many, but not all, of the diseases described in the following pages can be regarded as system diseases, in the sense indicated above. Their manifestations are seemingly the outcome of a primary neuronal degeneration. It is possible that some of them will turn out to be biochemical disorders, due perhaps to failure of an enzyme system or its inactivation by some toxic substance. Others may prove to be slow viral infections (see page 2165).

Motor Neuron Diseases

Amyotrophic Lateral Sclerosis (Progressive Muscular Atrophy; Myatrophic Lateral Sclerosis)

This is a chronic disorder with its greatest incidence in the fifth and sixth decades. It is characterized by selective degeneration of the neurons of the anterior grey columns of the spinal cord, especially of the cervical enlargement, and of the Betz cells of the motor cortex. In most cases, the primary degeneration is confined to these cells: their disappearance gives rise to spastic paraplegia accompanied by 'amyotrophy' (wasting of the muscles) of the upper limbs. The spastic paraplegia is due to upper motor neuron degeneration (involvement of the Betz cells); the neurons in the anterior grey columns of the segments of the spinal cord that supply the paraplegic parts remain intact. The amyotrophy is the expression of denervation due to degeneration of the lower motor neurons in the cervical enlargement of the spinal cord.

Occasionally, the neurons of the anterior grey columns throughout a larger number of segments of the spinal cord may be affected; the neurons of the motor centres of the brainstem may also be lost, leading to lower motor neuron paralysis of—for instance—the masseter muscles (trigeminal nerves) or the tongue (hypoglossal nerves). When the muscular atrophy is more generalized, because of more extensive involvement of the lower motor neurons, the syndrome is known as *progressive muscular atrophy*, and spasticity of the lower limbs may not be much in evidence. Occasionally, the motor neurons of the brainstem may be first and most severely affected, and the patient may die from

bulbar palsy before degenerative changes affect other muscles. The centres concerned with eye movements are almost invariably spared.

At necropsy, the ventral spinal roots, especially those of the cervical enlargement, may be notably shrunken. Histologically, the nerve cells of the anterior grey columns are reduced in number (Fig. 34.170), and the glial cells increased. Some of the surviving anterior column neurons in the affected segments of the cord lose their usual triangular shape and become oval and shrunken. The changes in the Betz cells and other neurons of the precentral gyrus resemble those in the affected neurons of the anterior grey columns. Exceptionally, neuronophagia may be seen.

Examination of the spinal cord characteristically shows degeneration of the lateral and anterior corticospinal tracts (Fig. 34.171). In myelin preparations these show as pale areas that contrast markedly with the darkly stained, intact, posterior funiculi. The degeneration is clearly visible in the pyramids of the medulla oblongata; above that level it becomes less evident, although pallor may be noted as high as the precentral gyrus. However, if the Marchi technique is employed, degenerating fibres may be seen even in the cortex, and not only in the precentral gyrus: they may for instance be found in the postcentral gyrus and in the adjacent parietal and frontal gyri and the paracentral lobule.[946b]

Amyotrophic lateral sclerosis is occasionally a familial disease. It is of interest, therefore, that in the Marianas Islands in the Pacific Ocean, and particularly in Guam, where the disease is some thousand times commoner among the indigenous Chamarros than among Americans and Europeans, familial cases are frequent.[947] Familial cases also occur, although less frequently, in the Kii Peninsula (in the south of Honshu, in Japan)[948] and in western regions of the island of New Guinea. Extrapyramidal involvement, particularly Parkinsonism, and dementia are found in some 10 per cent of the patients in the Pacific regions (see also page 2270—*Parkinsonism–Dementia Complex of Guam*). Some familial cases in Europe and North America have shown degeneration of the posterior funiculi of the spinal cord and of the spinocerebellar tracts, with loss of neurons in the nuclei dorsales (Clarke's columns); there have been lesions in the cerebral cortex and basal ganglia in a proportion of these cases, and it is then difficult to distinguish the condition from the variety of Creutzfeldt–Jakob disease that is known as corticostriatospinal degeneration (see page 2163). The Pacific cases are distinguished

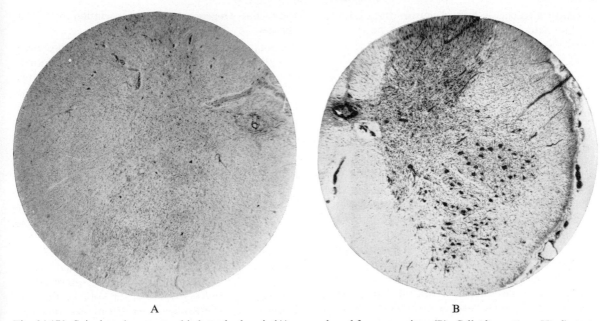

A   B

Fig. 34.170. Spinal cord: amyotrophic lateral sclerosis (A); normal cord for comparison (B). *Celloidin sections. Nissl's stain.* × 25.

A. Anterior grey column of left side, at lumbar enlargement, showing considerable reduction in the number of large nerve cells.

B. Normal appearance of anterior grey column (of right side) at lumbar enlargement, for comparison with 'A': from a person of similar age (both sections are of the same thickness).

by the lack of involvement of the posterior funiculi and by the presence of widespread degeneration of neurons in the cerebral cortex, basal ganglia and midbrain; the neuronal changes include granulovacuolar degeneration (page 2275) and the formation of neurofibrillary tangles (page 2275), but there are no 'senile plaques' (see page 2274); Lewy bodies (page 2267) are often present in the substantia nigra.[949, 950]

The cause of the disease is obscure. Extensive investigations of hereditary, dietary and nutritional factors, soil and water, and other environmental conditions, have been unhelpful. Inoculation experiments in the search for persistent infective agents have been negative.

Werdnig–Hoffmann Disease[951, 951a]

This is a form of motor neuron disease that occurs in infancy (see page 2316). The changes in the neurons of the anterior grey columns are essentially the same as in amyotrophic lateral sclerosis. The condition has to be distinguished from other causes of the 'floppy baby' syndrome (see page 2362): in Werdnig–Hoffmann disease, groups of atrophic muscle fibres can usually be found among others that are normal or somewhat hypoplastic. The condition has a simple autosomal recessive inheritance.

Motor Neuron Disease Associated with Carcinoma

An atypical form of 'motor neuron disease' has been described in association with carcinoma.[952]

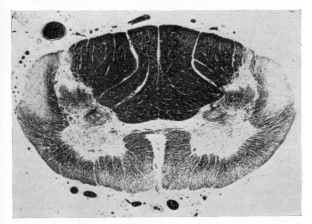

Fig. 34.171. Amyotrophic lateral sclerosis. Cervical part of the spinal cord showing demyelination of lateral corticospinal tracts, with less pronounced loss of myelin in the anterior corticospinal tracts and spinocerebellar tracts. *Celloidin section. Heidenhain's stain.* × 6.

Its relation to classic motor neuron disease (amyotrophic lateral sclerosis) has not been established.[952a]

The Cerebellar Degenerations[953]

Cerebello-Olivary Degeneration

This disease, in which the degeneration is particularly marked in the vermis, was observed by Holmes in a family in which four siblings developed ataxia during the fourth decade of life.[954] Cases have been reported in other families. Loss of Purkyně cells is associated with proliferation of Bergmann cells (see page 2082),[955] and there may be signs of damage in the granular layer of the cerebellar cortex. Degenerative changes also occur in the inferior and accessory olivary nuclei, although parts of the latter may be spared. A similar condition sometimes occurs without any familial predisposition: such cases are sometimes referred to as late *cortical cerebellar atrophy*.

A form of degeneration in which there is a great loss of cells in the granular layer of the cerebellar cortex, but no loss of Purkyně cells, is occasionally seen in children. It is sometimes referred to as Marie's cerebellar atrophy.[955a] This condition, which may be familial, is associated with mental retardation, and must be distinguished from those lipidoses in which degeneration of the cerebellar cortex sometimes occurs (see pages 2236 and 2237).

Olivopontocerebellar Degeneration (Menzel Type)

This is a distinctive variety of cerebellar degeneration that occurs in young or middle-aged patients and tends to be familial.[956, 957] There is marked atrophy of the middle cerebellar peduncles and of the ventral surface of the pons, with loss of myelin in the white matter of the cerebellum and of neurons in the olivary nuclei and the nuclei pontis, and in the Purkyně and granular cell layers of the cerebellum. The degenerative changes, which begin in the myelin, are by no means confined to the cerebello-olivary system, for there may be a loss of neurons in the nuclei of the lower part of the brainstem, including those of the hypoglossal, facial and trigeminal nerves, and also in the substantia nigra and the spinal cord, including the nuclei dorsales (Clarke's columns). Degeneration may also be seen in the spinocerebellar and corticospinal tracts and in the posterior funiculi. The corpus striatum may show loss of neurons and gliosis.[958]

Cerebellar Degeneration in Association with Carcinoma

Subacute atrophy of the cerebellar cortex occasionally develops in patients who have a carcinoma: in most of these cases the tumour is a small, slow-growing, clinically silent bronchial carcinoma. The earliest sign of the cerebellar degeneration is ataxia. The illness may last as much as two years, and even longer, and the neurological symptoms may long precede the appearance of those due to the tumour itself. Occasionally, the tumour is known to be present before the neurological signs appear. The course of the neurological disorder seems to be independent of that of the carcinoma, and it is often uninfluenced by removal of the cancerous lung.

The Purkyně cells suffer heavily (Fig. 34.172); in contrast, olivary degeneration is unusual. Occasionally, the subthalamic nuclei are involved. In some cases, the long tracts of the spinal cord show demyelination. Two features distinguish this condition from other forms of degeneration of the cerebellar cortex: first, its occasional accompaniment by peripheral neuropathy, with degeneration of neurons in the dorsal root ganglia (see page 2326); and second, lymphocytic cuffing of blood vessels in the brainstem, and, sometimes, in the central grey matter of the cerebrum, accompanied by lymphocytosis in the cerebrospinal fluid.

The nature of the relationship between the cerebellar degeneration and the carcinoma is unknown, but it is noteworthy that the cerebrospinal fluid usually contains an excess of gamma globulin. This has suggested to some writers that the tumour has in some way provoked an immunological response; others interpret it as indicating the possibility of an associated viral infection. It is possible also that some metabolic activity of the tumour deprives the neurons of an essential metabolite, or interferes with an essential enzyme system.

Spinal Cord Degeneration

Friedreich's Ataxia

This hereditary disease, which was first described by Friedreich,* in 1861,[959] usually becomes manifest in childhood or adolescence.[959a] It is accompanied by pes cavus. The degeneration characteristically involves the spinocerebellar tracts, the

---

* Both Friedreich's ataxia and paramyoclonus multiplex (myoclonia) are known as Friedreich's disease. Friedreich described paramyoclonus multiplex in 1881 (Friedreich, N., *Virchows Arch. path. Anat.*, 1881, **86**, 421).

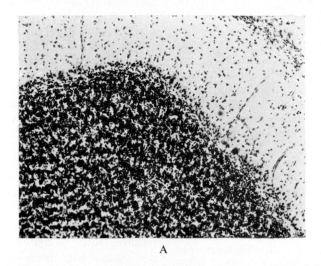

A

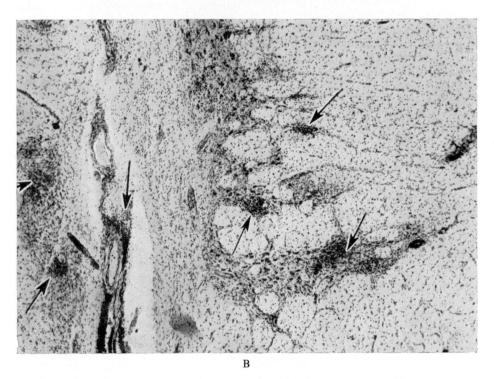

B

Fig. 34.172. Carcinomatous encephalopathy. A man, aged 62, died suddenly. There was six months' history of unsteadiness of gait, diplopia and dysarthria, followed by paraesthesiae in the hands. Necropsy disclosed a small primary carcinoma in a bronchus.

A. Cerebellum: very few Purkyně cells remain. The Bergmann astrocytes are increased in number. *Celloidin section. Nissl's stain.* × 90.

B. Medulla: there are inflammatory lesions (arrows) in relation to the arcuate nuclei. Lymphocytes (vertical arrow) are seen in the subarachnoid space in the anterior median fissure. *Celloidin section. Nissl's stain.* × 50.

posterior funiculi, and, especially terminally, the corticospinal tracts within the spinal cord. The nuclei dorsales are also atrophied. Because of the widespread loss of myelin and axons, the spinal cord has a shrunken appearance. Tract degenerations may also be evident in the brainstem and in the middle cerebellar peduncles; the neurons of the lower part of the brainstem (and sometimes those of the dentate nuclei) and the Purkyně cells are reduced in number. Extensive gliosis follows degeneration of the tracts.

The neurological changes are sometimes accompanied by enlargement of the heart, with hypertrophy of the myocardial cells and progressive interstitial fibrosis (see page 48, Volume 1).[960] Atrophy of the peroneal muscles has been noted in some affected families:[961] a form of the disease in which this feature is marked and the Friedreich component relatively inconspicuous has been called *hereditary areflexic dystasis*.[962]

As in cerebellar cortical atrophy and olivopontocerebellar degeneration, both of which are referred to above, ataxia is a conspicuous feature, but the structural changes tend to be more marked in the tracts of the spinal cord than in the cerebellum itself.

Variants.—Other forms of degeneration of the spinal cord include *familial spastic paraplegia*, in which, as in Friedreich's disease, the changes in the corticospinal tracts are most marked in the lumbar enlargement. There is also a *familial posterior funicular ataxia*, and a *hereditary spastic ataxia*. These conditions are degenerative and peculiar to certain families; they may be regarded as variant forms of Friedreich's disease. *Strümpell's spastic paraplegia*[962a] is another of these disorders: it is important because it may be confused with multiple sclerosis in siblings.

Relation to Other System Diseases.—The cerebellar and spinal cord degenerations discussed above may be related to other forms of system disease. For instance, in some families with Friedreich's ataxia the degeneration of the spinal cord is accompanied by optic atrophy.

The association of ataxic neuropathy with retinopathy (see Chapter 40, Volume 6), acanthocytosis*

* Acanthocytes, in this context, are red blood cells that appear abnormally crenated, due to an anomaly of their envelope. The supposedly spine-like protrusions from their surface are the reason for naming them 'acanthocytes'—cells with prickles, or spines.

and steatorrhoea[963-965] suggests that hereditary degeneration of the central nervous system may be a manifestation of a biochemical anomaly the effects of which are not necessarily restricted to the nervous system. There is evidence that this anomaly, which is sometimes known as Bassen–Kornzweig disease,[963, 965] is connected with an absence of betalipoprotein (abetalipoproteinaemia) and exceptionally low concentrations of cholesterol and phospholipid in the blood.[966]

Peroneal Muscular Atrophy (Charcot–Marie–Tooth Disease[966a, 966b])

In the few recorded necropsies of this rare and localized form of muscular atrophy, degeneration has occasionally been noted in the dorsal root ganglia and posterior funiculi in addition to the changes in peripheral nerves (see pages 2315 and 2330). Loss of neurons from the anterior columns has been observed in the lumbar enlargement. Further studies on this aspect of the pathology of the disease are needed. In some families peroneal atrophy coexists with Friedreich's ataxia, and so involvement of the spinal cord is not unexpected.

The atrophy commonly begins in the peroneal muscles, usually in childhood or adolescence; the muscles of the lower third of the thighs and the small muscles of the hand become involved later.

Myelopathy Associated with Carcinoma[952, 967]

Changes may be found in the spinal cord in cases of peripheral neuropathy accompanying carcinoma (see page 2367). Sensory neuropathy is characterized by degeneration of neurons in the posterior root ganglia, with consecutive changes in the posterior roots and posterior funiculi. Motor neuropathy is the result of degeneration of neurons in the anterior grey columns. Mixed forms probably account for most cases. The findings described under carcinomatous degeneration of the cerebellum (page 2264) may be associated with them in some degree.

Subacute necrotizing myelopathy, a condition that otherwise is usually attributable to thrombophlebitis of the spinal veins,[968] has been described also as an accompaniment of carcinoma.[969] It has to be distinguished from necrosis following X-irradiation and from the presence of a metastatic deposit within the cord.

Changes in the Nervous System Associated with Cancer Elsewhere in the Body[970]

The nervous system may be affected in many ways by the presence of a cancer elsewhere in the body. The most frequent, of course, is the development of metastatic deposits in its substance (see page 2225). These may be macroscopically evident or they may be found only on microscopical examination. Microscopical dissemination of tumour may result in widespread infiltration of the spinal cord, brain or meninges (page 2227). Occasionally, small emboli formed of tumour tissue cause focal ischaemic lesions. Infarcts in the brain and spinal cord may also result from embolism originating from the lesions of non-infective thrombotic endocardiopathy (see page 56, Volume 1) or from sites of venous or arterial thrombosis developing in the course of the disseminated thrombotic syndrome that is one of the rare accompaniments of carcinoma.

The nervous system may also be damaged in the course of metabolic disturbances caused by tumours. Primary growths or metastatic deposits may interfere with the function of the liver or kidneys; this may lead to development of a metabolic encephalomyelopathy. Similarly, tumours may be responsible for such metabolic disturbances as hypercalcaemia, hyponatraemia, hypoglycaemia and macroglobulinaemia, and for the wide range of effects of overproduction or underproduction of hormones that govern other aspects of homoeostasis: any of these disorders may affect the nervous system adversely.

Gastrointestinal tumours are recognized causes of deficiency states that may result in such conditions as Wernicke's encephalopathy (see page 2244).

Resistance to infection may be lowered by cancer, either as an unspecific effect of the general deterioration in health or because of specific interference with the functions of those systems of the body that subserve protection against infections. Leukaemia and the malignant diseases of the lymphoreticular system, particularly Hodgkin's disease, are the most familiar cancers that are prone to such complications. Again, treatment of cancer with drugs or irradiation may lower resistance to infection. The 'opportunistic' infections that arise in such circumstances commonly have a particular liability to involve the central nervous system (see footnote on page 2127).

When a patient with known cancer develops evidence of disease of the nervous system the factors mentioned above should be considered. However, there is a series of degenerative disorders of the nervous system that may complicate cancer

and that cannot, with present knowledge, be attributed to recognized effects of the tumour. In such cases the tumour may still be small and clinically silent at the time when the neurological disorder begins to appear. It is difficult to classify these neurological effects, for many levels of the nervous system may be involved, singly or in combination. The effects may be manifested mainly or exclusively in the peripheral nervous system or in the central nervous system. Sometimes the skeletal muscles are directly affected as well: the ambiguous term neuromyopathy is sometimes used in such cases. These conditions may be grouped as follows:

Encephalomyelopathy[952, 971] (the degeneration may affect various levels in the brain and spinal cord, with predominant or apparently exclusive involvement of, say, the limbic lobes, the brainstem, the spinal cord itself, the spinal roots or the root ganglia; 'encephalitic variants' are seen in which there is an infiltration by inflammatory cells, of variable intensity and distribution)

Progressive Multifocal Leucoencephalopathy (page 2161)

Cerebellar Degeneration (page 2264)

Myelopathy (see opposite)

Motor Neuron Disease (page 2263)

Peripheral Neuropathy (page 2326)

Myopathy (including polymyositis and a myasthenic syndrome) (see page 2367).

Paralysis Agitans (Parkinson's Disease)

Paralysis agitans (Parkinson's disease,[972] or 'shaking palsy') is ordinarily a disease of the elderly, although exceptionally it may develop as early as the fourth decade. It usually begins in one hand, appearing as a tremor that is present while the part is at rest and that lessens or temporarily disappears during volitional movements. The tremor soon appears in the other hand, and finally affects the arms and legs. In addition to the tremor, the muscles, particularly those of the face and trunk, develop a characteristic rigidity: the typical, mask-like facies is a manifestation of this.

Lewy noted that in paralysis agitans the cytoplasm of some of the neurons in the midbrain is vacuolate and that the vacuoles may contain round, concentrically laminate bodies (Figs 34.173 and 34.174).[972a] These Lewy bodies are most typically present in the pigmented cells of the substantia nigra and the substantia ferruginea.[972b] They also occur in the cells of the oculomotor,

7*

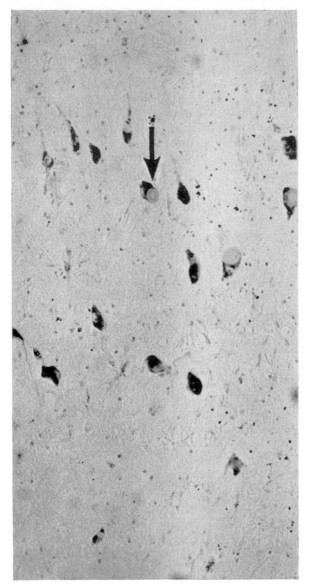

Fig. 34.173. Parkinson's disease. Pigmented cells in the substantia nigra showing intracytoplasmic bodies of the Lewy type (see also Fig. 34.174). The one below the arrow is laminated. The cells are reduced in number. *Nissl's stain.* × 120.

dorsal vagal and facial nuclei and in the substantia innominata, and, outside the central nervous system, in sympathetic ganglia.[973, 974] Being acidophile, they are well displayed by Mallory's tri-chrome stains and by Lendrum's phloxine-tartrazine method; they are less well seen in Nissl preparations. They may grow to such a size that they dwarf and almost obscure what remains of the cells in which they are formed. Indeed, they often lie free,

together with granules of pigment released from cell bodies that have disintegrated. Occasionally, several Lewy bodies are found inside a single cell. Their number seems to bear little relation to the duration of the illness. Moreover, although characteristic of Parkinson's disease, they are occasionally found in small numbers in senile brains and in some other conditions (page 2263). They should be distinguished from the morphologically somewhat similar Lafora bodies of Unverricht's disease (see page 2242) and from corpora amylacea (see page 2085).

As the disease advances, the number of neurons in the substantia nigra decreases considerably, but because of proliferation of glial cells there may be an overall increase in the number of nuclei. In advanced cases, the loss of pigmentation is evident to the naked eye. A small number of binucleate neurons may be seen (Fig. 34.174C): their significance is unknown (see page 2092).

It is generally agreed that in Parkinson's disease the pathological changes are most conspicuous in the substantia nigra. The function of this distinctive group of cells is obscure. It receives afferent fibres from the subthalamic nuclei and elsewhere; its efferent fibres pass to the ipsilateral globus pallidus and other parts of the corpus

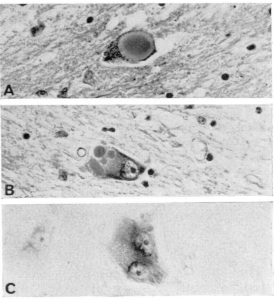

Fig. 34.174. Parkinson's disease. A: Massive Lewy body in a pigmented cell of the locus caeruleus. Note the thin layer of pigment-containing cytoplasm stretched over the inclusion. *Haematoxylin–eosin.* × 280.
B: Cell in substantia nigra that has lost most of its pigment and contains five Lewy bodies. The nucleus is well preserved. *Haematoxylin–eosin.* × 280.
C: Binucleate neuron in substantia nigra. *Nissl's stain.* × 280.

striatum; it may well have additional connexions. The loss of cells sometimes noted in the pallidum in Parkinson's disease has been regarded as a trans-synaptic degeneration. Destruction of the pallidum or of the dorsolateral part of the thalami abolishes the troublesome tremors of the disease; the same result follows destruction of the fibres of the anterior part of the posterior limb of the internal capsule.[975] The subthalamic nuclei, the substantia nigra and the corpora striata appear to operate through the pallidum.[976] In Parkinson's disease, there is little or no change in the caudate nuclei, the putamina, the thalami and the subthalamic nuclei. Although the frontal lobes may be atrophic, impairment of mental activity is not a feature of the disease.[977]

Parkinsonism

Tremor and rigidity may occur in various other diseases: it is usual to refer to this syndrome as Parkinsonism. Postencephalitic Parkinsonism is a formerly well known example (see page 2165 and below). The condition also occurs in cases of chronic manganese poisoning, in patients who have survived severe carbon monoxide or nitrous oxide intoxication, in striatonigral degeneration (see page 2271) and in boxers (see page 2193). At necropsy in cases of Parkinsonism following poisoning it is usual to find softening of the pallidum; this is associated with degeneration of the elastic lamina of the small central branches of the middle cerebral arteries, which supply these nuclei. These branches are specially liable to senile changes: it is possible that ischaemia of the neurons in the pallidum may contribute to the development of Parkinsonism.

Functional Basis of Parkinson's Disease[977a–977d]

The major efferent fibres from the substantia nigra run to the ipsilateral corpus striatum. These are dopaminergic fibres: dopamine has an inhibitory effect on the neurons of the corpus striatum, particularly those of the caudate nucleus and putamen. Progressive loss of the dopaminergic nigrostriatal fibres in consequence of atrophy of the substantia nigra is thought to promote the excitatory effect of the intact cholinergic fibres that also terminate round the striatal neurons. The clinical manifestations of Parkinsonism (tremor, rigidity and akinesia) are believed to result from the loss of dopaminergic predominance. The dopamine depletion of the caudate nuclei and putamina is accompanied by a variable reduction in the amount of the principal excretion products of dopamine,

particularly 3-methoxy-4-hydroxyphenylacetic acid (homovanillic acid, or HVA), in the cerebrospinal fluid.

Administration of dopamine to patients with Parkinson's disease is ineffectual as it does not cross the blood–brain barrier. In contrast, racemic dopa and its less toxic and more effective isomer levodopa (L-dihydroxyphenylalanine) readily enter the central nervous system. Levodopa is used therapeutically and has proved valuable, especially to patients with severe akinesia, for whom surgical interruption of the feedback pathways is usually unsuitable. Levodopa is decarboxylated to dopamine in the substantia nigra and corpus striatum and thus provides a supply of the missing transmitter and so restores at least some measure of functional capacity to the system.

A recent hypothesis is that the primary defect in the substantia nigra is a failure of tyrosine hydroxylase activity with consequent impairment of the conversion of tyrosine to dopa. The early depletion of neuromelanin in the substantia nigra may be a compensatory phenomenon as this pigment is a potential source of both dopamine and dopa when these are not otherwise available.

The Relation between Encephalitis Lethargica and Paralysis Agitans

During the pandemic of encephalitis lethargica of 1917 to 1924 (see page 2165) it was not doubted that the Parkinsonian state that developed as a complication within weeks or months of the acute illness was distinct from paralysis agitans (Parkinson's disease). Once the pandemic had subsided physicians took it for granted that the development of Parkinsonism in a patient who had no history of encephalitis lethargica, and in whom the syndrome could not be attributed to some other known cause of Parkinsonism (see above), was diagnostic of paralysis agitans. More recently, the distinction between paralysis agitans and postencephalitic Parkinsonism has again become uncertain, particularly in the light of epidemiological evidence. Some of the patients who were recognized to have encephalitis lethargica during the pandemic did not begin to show signs of Parkinsonism until as long as 20 years afterwards; other patients whose Parkinsonism was clinically of the type characteristic of the postencephalitic disease had no history of encephalitis or even of any illness during the period of the pandemic; further, by the middle of the 1950s new cases classifiable on clinical grounds as of postencephalitic type had ceased to appear. A study of patients with Parkinsonism seen in Massachusetts in the period 1915–61 showed an increasing mean age at the time of onset of their symptoms during the succession of years following the pandemic: this suggested that most of the patients presenting with Parkinsonism during this time belonged to a group of people who were ageing together.[978] A comparative analysis indicated that this group aged at a rate remarkably similar to the ageing of a population comparable to that involved in the pandemic of encephalitis lethargica. A deduction from these observations was that by 1970 or thereabouts cases of Parkinsonism occurring as a sequel of the pandemic should have ceased to appear, and that the Parkinsonian syndrome developing thenceforth would be symptomatic of the disease described in 1817 by James Parkinson[972]—a less frequent and therefore a relatively less important neurological problem.

The evidence considered above suggested that the majority of cases of Parkinsonism, including both those considered to be postencephalitic and those diagnosed as Parkinson's disease (paralysis agitans) might be regarded as sequelae of encephalitis lethargica acquired during the pandemic. If this is so, the clinical and pathological distinctions between postencephalitic Parkinsonism and paralysis agitans have been based on false premises. This view is not universally accepted: other explanations of the relevant observations require consideration, including the improved diagnostic standards that result from the wider availability and use of specialist medical services for older people.[979] The correct interpretation is likely to become evident during the next decade or so.

Parkinsonism–Dementia Complex of Guam[980]

This condition is characterized by a gradually progressive Parkinsonian state and progressive dementia. It occurs particularly in Guam, in the Marianas Islands, where it affects the Chamorro population: it is sometimes associated with familial amyotrophic lateral sclerosis (see page 2262). Clinically, the disease bears some resemblance to Creutzfeldt–Jakob disease (see page 2163). Pathologically, however, there is widespread neurofibrillary degeneration of the neurons of the thalami, hypothalamus, substantia nigra, substantia ferruginea and amygdaloid bodies and of the pallidum, and also of the cortical neurons of the frontal and temporal lobes: the changes in the cells are identical with those in 'Alzheimer nerve cells' (see page 2275). There is gliosis of the corpora mamillaria. Argyrophile plaques are not found in the Parkinsonism–dementia complex: this is the

main point of pathological distinction from Alzheimer's disease (see page 2275). Electron microscopy has shown inclusions similar to those found in Pick's disease (page 2273).[981]

It is currently believed that the Parkinsonism–dementia complex of Guam and amyotrophic lateral sclerosis among the same population are manifestations of a single entity. Searches for environmental factors have been unsuccessful.[949]

Progressive Supranuclear Palsy[982]

The clinical manifestations of this rare condition are ophthalmoplegia (particularly affecting vertical eye movements), dysarthria, rigidity of the neck and of the upper parts of the trunk, pseudobulbar palsy and dementia. It is a disease of late middle age, and its evolution is slow. Neuronal changes are found in the pallidum, subthalamic and red nuclei, substantia nigra and superior colliculi, and in the circumaqueductal grey matter and the tegmental region of the pons. Some nerve cells are lost and others show neurofibrillary degeneration or a form of granular cytoplasmic degeneration that is seen in no other condition. There may be secondary demyelination in the cerebellum, basal ganglia and brainstem. The disease in some ways resembles the Parkinsonism–dementia complex of Guam (see above), but the cerebral cortex is not involved. There is also a resemblance between the lesions in the substantia nigra and substantia ferruginea in this condition and the changes in these parts in postencephalitic Parkinsonism (see page 2166), but there have been no inflammatory features and no history of encephalitis in any of the reported cases.

Huntington's Chorea*

Huntington's chorea is a progressive disease that becomes apparent in about the fourth decade. Its course is very long and may last for up to 30 years. The symptoms are choreoathetosis, affecting

---

* Huntington's chorea is, of course, distinct from Sydenham's chorea. The latter is a manifestation of acute rheumatic fever (Sydenham, T., *Schedula monitoria de novae febris ingressu*, page 25; Londini, 1686 [reprinted in: *Med. Classics*, 1939, **4**, 327]). Traditionally it is said to be a rheumatic form of meningoencephalitis, although specific histological features appear not to be present. The neuropathology of rheumatic fever has not been extensively studied (but see: Bruetsch, W. L., *Proceedings of the 4th International Congress on Neurology, Paris, 1949*, vol. 3, page 297 [Paris, 1949]; Buchanan, D. N., Walker, A. E., Case, T. J., *J. Pediat.*, 1942, **20**, 555; Costero, I., *Arch. Neurol. Psychiat.* [*Chic.*], 1949, **62**, 48).

especially the upper limbs and head, and mental deterioration. The disease is transmitted by simple dominant inheritance: it is a classic example of a very severe dominant defect that is transmissible over many generations because it does not manifest itself until comparatively late in life, when the affected individual has already had children.[983] Half the offspring of an affected parent will be affected.[983a] Dementia, which usually develops *pari passu* with the abnormal movements, occasionally precedes their appearance.

Huntington wrote his classic paper in 1872, a year after completing his medical training.[983b] The patients whose cases he described had long been under observation by his grandfather and his father before he joined the family practice in Long Island, New York. There are reports of the condition in the literature before Huntington's account of it:[983c] indeed, the disease, which is now world-wide in its distribution, appears to have been well known in the English county of Suffolk in the seventeenth century. It was carried to America by emigrants from that county.[984, 985]

The brain in this disease is rather smaller than normal, due to atrophy that affects particularly the frontal and central gyri. There is secondary dilatation of the ventricular system and thinning of the corpus callosum.[986] The caudate nuclei and the putamina appear shrunken (Fig. 34.175) and often brownish. The loss of small nerve cells in the corpus striatum is so striking that the large neurons, which are unaffected, and the proliferating astrocytes are conspicuous. A spongy appearance may result if the astrocytes have produced abundant glial fibres; this is particularly likely to be found in the atrophic corpus striatum (Fig. 34.176). There is a diffuse loss of neurons in the outer laminae of the cerebral cortex, but the astrocytic proliferation makes it difficult to evaluate the extent of the cell loss. The blood vessels are not significantly affected.

Dopamine Activity.—The amounts of dopamine and its excretory products, particularly homovanillic acid, in the brain and cerebrospinal fluid respectively are normal or slightly reduced in cases of Huntington's chorea. In contrast to Parkinson's disease (see page 2269), administration of levodopa aggravates the manifestations of Huntington's disease; drugs such as the phenothiazine tranquillizers and reserpine, which aggravate the symptoms and signs of Parkinson's disease, have sometimes been found to ameliorate those of Huntington's disease, possibly by reducing the amount of dopa in the corpus striatum.[977b]

Striatonigral Degeneration

This condition is characterized by atrophy and discoloration of the putamina, with depigmentation of the substantia nigra. It occurs in middle-aged patients and causes Parkinsonism, with rigidity. The pallidum and the caudate and subthalamic nuclei are also affected, but to a smaller degree.[987, 988]

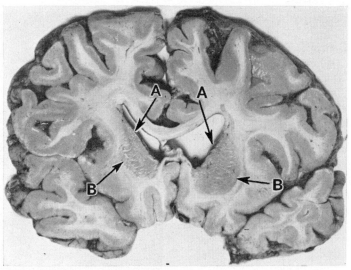

Fig. 34.175. Huntington's chorea. There is marked atrophy of the caudate nuclei (A, A) and the putamina (B, B). In addition, there is atrophy of the frontal and parietal cortex.

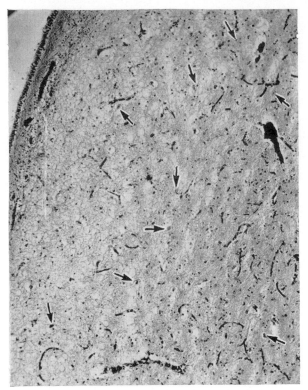

Fig. 34.176. Huntington's chorea. The section shows an atrophied caudate nucleus, with status spongiosus and complete absence of small neurons. A few large neurons have survived (arrows) but the majority of the nuclei belong to astrocytes. *Celloidin section. Haematoxylin–eosin.* × 120.

Pick's Disease

Pick's disease is a peculiarly localized form of atrophy of the brain, first described by Arnold Pick, in Prague, at the turn of the century.[989, 989a] It is a rare condition, which occurs mainly in the later years of life, although ordinarily before the usual age of senility. The oldest patient on record was 91 and the youngest 21. Women are affected oftener than men; familial cases have been recognized. The range of symptoms depends on the parts of the brain affected; gradual mental deterioration is the rule. The dementia is progressive, and the course of the illness covers from 2 to 10 years.

The brain is remarkably shrunken, and may weigh as little as 900 g and even less (Figs 34.177 and 34.178). The atrophy, which is usually symmetrical, involves the frontal and temporal lobes, either separately or, more frequently, together. Occasionally, the parietal lobes share in the atrophy; rarely, they are affected alone. The sensory and motor cortex, the parahippocampal

gyrus and the occipital lobe generally escape. Particularly characteristic is involvement of the anterior third of the superior temporal gyrus, together with the middle and inferior temporal gyri and the medial occipitotemporal gyrus while the posterior two thirds of the superior temporal gyrus are spared (Fig. 34.178). The degree of atrophy may be extreme: when the meninges are stripped off, the convolutions are found to be so narrow that the term 'knife blade' atrophy has been used to describe their appearance. Sometimes, the corpus striatum, the cerebellum, the brainstem nuclei and the spinal cord are involved.

Histologically, the neurons of the outer three laminae of the cerebral cortex are found to have disappeared; their place is taken by astrocytes (Fig. 34.179). The brain, in histological sections, has a spongy appearance, not unlike that of the caudate nuclei and putamina in Huntington's chorea (page 2271). If death occurs early, however, when there is less macroscopical evidence of atrophy, some neurons show swelling of the cytoplasm and peripheral displacement of the nucleus. The cytoplasm contains material that is both Sudanophile and argyrophile: these abnormal neurons are usually referred to as Pick cells (Fig. 34.180). In later stages of the disease nerve cells in the atrophied parts of the brain may show neurofibrillary degeneration, and there may be argyrophile plaques (see page 2274).

There is fragmentation of axons, and sometimes the myelin is lost. The Hortega cells, however,

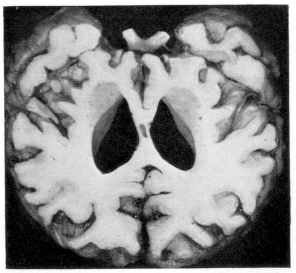

Fig. 34.177. Pick's disease. Coronal section of brain showing gross cortical atrophy and ventricular dilatation.

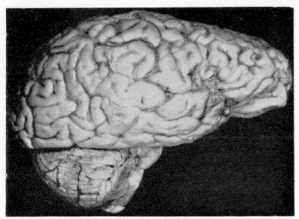

Fig. 34.178. Pick's disease. There is a moderate degree of atrophy of the parietal lobe and gross atrophy of the frontal and temporal lobes but notable preservation of two thirds of the superior temporal gyrus and also of the precentral and postcentral gyri and the occipital lobe.

seem inactive and contain no ingested fat. Typically, there is intense gliosis of the white matter of the affected parts of the brain, and it is for this reason that the condition is sometimes called lobar sclerosis. The gliosis is not a consequence of the loss of myelin.

It is the projection areas in the cerebrum that are chiefly involved in Pick's disease; these are, in general, the parts of the brain that have developed

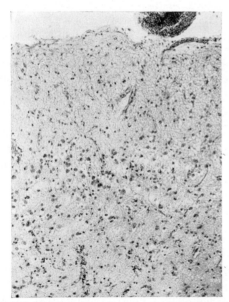

Fig. 34.179. Pick's disease. Superior frontal gyrus showing loss of nerve cells and proliferation of astrocytes, which together give rise to the status spongiosus. *Celloidin section. Haematoxylin–eosin.* × 100.

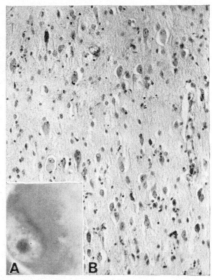

Fig. 34.180. Pick's disease. Cingulate gyrus, showing many of the characteristic ballooned nerve cells with displacement of the nucleus to the periphery (Pick cells). Part of the swollen cytoplasm and displaced nucleus of a Pick cell is shown in the inset. *Celloidin section. Haematoxylin–eosin.* × 150 (inset × 750).

last in phylogenesis. Spatz regarded the disease as a system disorder and suggested that the primary lesion is in the axon.[989b] This belief is supported by the peculiar swelling of the perikaryon of the neurons, which has been likened to that associated with axonal retrograde degeneration (see page 2087).

Electron microscopical studies in Pick's disease have shown inclusions in neurons and peculiar juxtaneuronal rod-like bodies (Hirano bodies).[981] The inclusions and the rod-like bodies appear to be related. They are also found in cases of the Parkinsonism–dementia complex of Guam and in the associated indigenous cases of amyotrophic lateral sclerosis (see page 2270).

Progressive Subcortical Gliosis.[990]—This condition is characterized by severe gliosis of the white matter of the subcortical zone of the cerebral hemispheres and in the basal ganglia, brainstem and spinal cord. There is no accompanying demyelination. Clinically, it is difficult to distinguish from Pick's and Alzheimer's diseases. The possibility that it is a variant of Pick's disease remains under consideration.

Alpers' Disease

Alpers' disease,[991] or poliodystrophia cerebri, is a rare disease of young children, characterized by degeneration of the neurons in the cerebral cortex and elsewhere.[992, 992a] Its cause is unknown. It has been described in siblings. Epilepsy is a frequent symptom but it is generally held that hypoxia, such as may complicate epilepsy (see page 2104), cannot account for all of the findings. Chemical studies on cerebral biopsy specimens indicate some damage to the white matter, and there may be an increased excretion of amino acids.[993]

The possibility that Alpers' disease is the childhood equivalent of Creutzfeldt–Jakob disease (page 2163) has often been raised,[994, 995] since both conditions in their advanced stages show spongiform transformation. The validity of this concept will be confirmed if a persistent infective agent is found in the former as it has been in the latter.

Infantile Subacute Necrotizing Encephalitis

This disease of infancy, which is often familial, has attracted increasing attention since it was first described by Leigh.[996, 997] The illness is progressive and of only a few months' duration. Multiple foci of degeneration of neurons, proliferation of Hortega cells and astrocytes, and overgrowth of capillaries are found in the thalami, subthalamic nuclei and substantia nigra, and in the grey matter of the pons and medulla. There are comparable changes in the posterior columns of the spinal cord. Occasionally, there may be involvement of the corpus striatum, the cerebral cortex and the white matter of the cerebral and cerebellar hemispheres. The proliferation of capillaries that is so characteristic of the condition suggested the possibility that it might be a chronic form of Wernicke's disease (see page 2244), but the mamillary bodies have been involved only exceptionally. Two instances of what appears pathologically to be the same disease have been reported in siblings:[998] the clinical manifestations were hyperpnoea, progressive ataxia and convulsions, and these were associated with acidosis (due to excessive glycolytic formation of lactic acid), renal aminoaciduria and hypophosphataemia. It has been suggested that an increase in the ratio of phosphorylated hexoses to free glucose in the blood may account in part for the increased rate of glycolysis: this has not yet been confirmed.

The Brain in Old Age

Some degree of what may be regarded as a physiological form of atrophy occurs in the brain in old age: this is manifest in narrowing of the gyri, the presence of excess fluid in the subarachnoid space, and slight enlargement of the ventricles. The neurons tend to shrink, and there is little doubt that there is a fall in their number. As they age their lipochrome content increases and—in the larger nerve cells particularly—may become very conspicuous. It should be noted, however, that many normal nerve cells contain lipid pigment, even in early life—for instance, the cells of sympathetic ganglia, of the inferior olivary nuclei and of the lateral geniculate bodies; assessment of the significance of intracellular lipid must, therefore, be made with caution. In old age, fatty droplets appear in the cytoplasm of the astrocytes also, and their processes tend to become coarser.

Occasionally, in haematoxylin–eosin preparations of the brain of old people, faintly staining, amorphous masses, from 40 to 80 μm in diameter, may be found between the neurons, particularly in the frontal cortex and the hippocampus. When impregnated with silver, these bodies become more conspicuous, and are seen to consist of a halo of argyrophile filaments and particles, with a less densely stained aggregate of particles in the centre. Lipid can sometimes be identified in this central zone. When these *argyrophile plaques*, as they are called, are stained with Congo red and examined under polarized light they are often seen to be doubly refractile. They were first described in the brain of elderly epileptic patients.[999] It was soon realized, however, that they are not necessarily a pathological feature but may be an occasional manifestation of the ordinary processes of ageing: they are therefore also known as 'senile plaques'.

Corpora amylacea are a frequent finding in the ageing brain (see page 2085).

Attention has recently been drawn to similarities between certain diseases caused by slow viruses—kuru (page 2163) and scrapie (page 2162)—and natural ageing in animals and man.[1000] Gliosis, spongiform change, neuronal degeneration and amyloid-containing deposits occur in all: it may be said that kuru and scrapie are characterized by changes that represent the changes of ageing, but in exaggerated form. The theoretical implications of this speculation are intriguing.

Alzheimer's Disease

In 1906, Alzheimer described a subacute form of dementia associated with agnosia, apraxia and focal paralysis.[1001, 1001a] His patient was a middle-aged woman whose illness lasted $4\frac{1}{2}$ years. Familial and hereditary cases have since been described, and the disease has been recognized in those born of first-cousin marriages. The disease is not uncom-

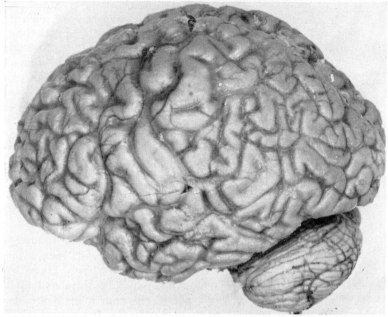

Fig. 34.181. Alzheimer's disease. There is generalized atrophy of the brain. This may be contrasted with the lobar atrophy seen in Pick's disease (see Fig. 34.178).

mon. Although its incidence is greatest in older patients, it may be seen in the fifth and fourth decades (for instance, in cases of Down's syndrome —see page 2205) and, exceptionally, even earlier. Its cause is not known.

At necropsy, the brain is uniformly shrunken, owing to a loss of nerve cells (Fig. 34.181). There is a peculiar abnormality of many of the remaining cortical neurons: these so-called 'Alzheimer nerve cells' are characterized by thickening and clumping together of the neurofibrils ('neurofibrillary degeneration': the alternative descriptive name, 'neurofibrillary tangle', is particularly apt for this appearance). The change can be recognized with certainty only by the use of silver techniques (Figs 34.182 and 34.183). These cells may give the staining reactions of amyloid, and they may then be doubly refractile.[1001b] The neurons of the hippocampus may show a cytoplasmic degeneration that is characterized by the presence of discrete argyrophile granules inside small vacuoles (Fig. 34.184). This granulovacuolar degeneration is found in fewer than 10 per cent of hippocampal neurons of people over 60 years of age who had not been affected with dementia: in cases of Alzheimer's disease the proportion of affected hippocampal neurons is much larger (up to 50 per cent).[1002]

In addition to the changes just described, argyro-

phile plaques (see opposite) are found in large numbers, particularly in the cerebral cortex, hippocampi and amygdaloid bodies, and occasionally in the caudate nuclei and putamina. The

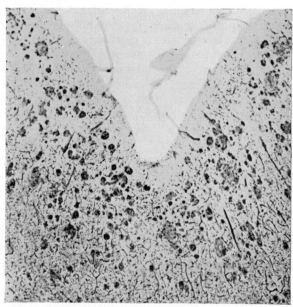

Fig. 34.182. Alzheimer's disease. Greatly atrophied cortex of superior temporal gyrus showing abundance of 'argyrophile plaques'. *Frozen section. Von Braunmühl's method.* × 100.

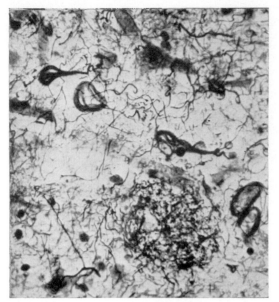

Fig. 34.183. Alzheimer's disease. Occipital cortex showing an argyrophile plaque and several foci of neurofibrillary degeneration. *Frozen section. Bielschowsky's method.* × 280.

plaques are rarely, if ever, absent in Alzheimer's disease; their number is related to the duration of the disease rather than to its severity. They probably originate in axons and dendrites. Their presence is, in general, a more striking feature of the disease than the neurofibrillary degeneration.

Electron microscopy[1003-1006] has confirmed the presence of extracellular amyloid in the core of the 'senile plaques'; there are also fibril-filled dendrites, axons and axon terminals that correspond to the argyrophile fibres seen on light microscopy. Hortega cells that infiltrate the plaques may be the source of the amyloid material. The neurofibrillary degeneration represents the accumulation of large numbers of fibrils that resemble those seen in normal neurons: these fibrils are predominantly small neurofilaments (10 nm in diameter—see page 2088). The filaments displace the organelles and are not in continuity with them.

Senile Dementia

The term senile dementia is a clinical one and is best reserved for the familiar clinical entity of progressive mental deterioration in elderly people. Women are affected oftener than men. Various pathological changes may be found in such cases. The brain of an elderly patient who has been demented for some years may show the histological features of Alzheimer's disease (see above): such cases are properly regarded as instances of that disease. In other cases of senile dementia there may be marked atrophy of the brain associated with conspicuous loss of neurons and abundant lipochrome in those that remain: neurofibrillary degeneration and argyrophile plaques are absent in this condition, which has been named '*atrophia cerebri senilis simplex*'. In yet other cases, atrophy of the neurons is associated with some features of Alzheimer's disease (see above). Cerebral atherosclerosis may complicate the picture and sometimes is the major pathological feature (see page 2171).

Encephalopathy and Fatty Degeneration of the Viscera[1007]

It is not yet possible to give this condition an appropriate, concise name: the heading of this section is accordingly taken from the title of a classic paper by Reye and his colleagues[1008] (the disease is often known now as *Reye's syndrome*, although it was first reported by others many years earlier[1009]). The patients are children—the recorded ages range from two months to 15 years. The onset is acute, with vomiting, convulsions, disorientation and coma. The liver and spleen are enlarged on clinical examination in about half the cases. The mortality has ranged from 20 to 80 per cent in different series, death usually occurring within a few days of the first signs of illness. Many of the patients who survive have permanent neurological sequelae, including mental impairment, fits, and hemiplegia or other paretic signs.

The brain is very oedematous. There is evidence

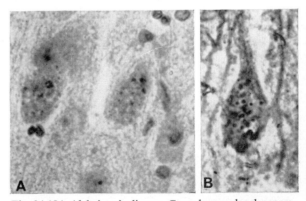

Fig. 34.184. Alzheimer's disease. Granulovacuolar degeneration in pyramidal cells of the hippocampus. This change (which may coexist with neurofibrillary degeneration) is best demonstrated by silver impregnation but can be recognized in haematoxylin–eosin preparations. *Celloidin sections.* × 420. A: *Haematoxylin–eosin.* B: *Davenport's method.*

of hypoxic neuronal damage but neither inflammatory infiltration nor demyelination has been found. The liver is enlarged and shows severe fatty change; in fatal cases there is often hepatic necrosis. Similar changes may be present in other organs, particularly the kidneys.

The cause of the disease is not known. Infective agents, exogenous poisons and toxic metabolites have not been recognized. The occurrence of small outbreaks of the condition has suggested that there may be an environmental factor, but if this is so its nature remains unidentified.

REFERENCES

THE CYTOLOGY OF THE CENTRAL NERVOUS SYSTEM

1. Ketty, S. S., Schmidt, C. F., *J. clin. Invest.*, 1948, **27**, 476.
2. Nylin, G., Silfverskiöld, B. P., Löfstedt, S., Regnström, O., Hedlund, S., *Brain*, 1960, **83**, 293.
3. Sholl, D. A., *The Organization of the Cerebral Cortex*, chap. 3. London, 1956.
4. Burns, B. D., *The Mammalian Cerebral Cortex*. London, 1958.
5. Nurnberger, J. I., Gordon, M. W., in *Ultrastructure and Cellular Chemistry of Neural Tissue*, edited by H. Waelsch, page 100. London, 1957.
6. Korey, S. R., Orchen, M., *J. Neurochem.*, 1959, **3**, 277.
7. Penfield, W. G., in *Cytology and Cellular Pathology of the Nervous System*, edited by W. G. Penfield, vol. 2, page 423. Philadelphia, 1932.
8. Blackwood, W., in *Greenfield's Neuropathology*, 3rd edn, edited by W. Blackwood and J. A. N. Corsellis, page 21. London, 1976.
9. Lumsden, C. E., *Acta neurol. psychiat. belg.*, 1957, **57**, 472.
10. Peters, A., Palay, S. L., Webster, H. de F., *The Fine Structure of the Nervous System*. Philadelphia, 1976.
11. Del Río Hortega, P., *Trab. Lab. Invest. biol., Univ. Madr.*, 1916, **14**, 269.
11a. Fañanás, J., *Trab. Lab. Invest. biol. Univ. Madr.*, 1916, **14**, 163.
12. Del Río Hortega, P., Penfield, W. G., *Bull. Johns Hopk. Hosp.*, 1927, **41**, 278.
13. Brewer, D. B., *Proc. roy. Soc. Med.*, 1967, **60**, 778.
13a. Golgi, C., *Sulla anatomia degli organi centrali del sistema nervoso*. Milano, 1886.
14. Woollam, D. H. M., Millan, J. W., in *Pathology of the Nervous System*, edited by J. Minckler, vol. 1, chap. 41. New York, 1968.
15. Dempsey, E. W., Luse, S. A., in *Biology of Neuroglia*, edited by W. F. Windle, page 101. Springfield, Illinois, 1958.
16. Schultz, R. L., Maynard, E. A., Pease, D. C., *Amer. J. Anat.*, 1957, **100**, 369.
17. Luse, S. A., in *Pathology of the Nervous System*, edited by J. Minckler, vol. 1, chap. 45. New York 1968.
18. Hudspeth, E. R., Swann, H. G., Pomerat, C. M., *Texas Rep. Biol. Med.*, 1950, **8**, 341.
19. Cavanagh, J. B., in *Modern Trends in Neurology—5*, edited by D. Williams, chap. 8. London, 1970.
20. Madge, E., Scheibel, A. B., in *Biology of Neuroglia*, edited by W. F. Windle, page 5. Springfield, Illinois, 1958.
21. Del Río Hortega, P., *Bol. Soc. esp. Biol.*, 1919, **9**, 154.

22. Bornstein, M. B., Murray, M. R., *J. biophys. biochem. Cytol.*, 1958, **4**, 449.
23. Causey, G., *The Cell of Schwann*, page 77. London, 1960.
24. Cammermeyer, J., *Amer. J. Anat.*, 1960, **106**, 197; 1960, **107**, 107.
25. Palay, S. L., in *Biology of Neuroglia*, edited by W. F. Windle, page 24. Springfield, Illinois, 1958.
26. Scheibel, A. B., in *Biology of Neuroglia*, edited by W. F. Windle, page 39. Springfield, Illinois, 1958.
27. Bunge, R., *Physiol. Rev.*, 1968, **48**, 197.
28. Bunge, R., Bunge, M. B., Ris, H., *J. biophys. biochen. Cytol.*, 1961, **7**, 685.
29. Levine, S., Hirano, A., Zimmerman, H. M., *J. Neuropath. exp. Neurol.*, 1967, **26**, 200.
30. Cramer, F., Alpers, B. J., *Arch. Path. (Chic.)*, 1932, **13**, 23.
31. Robertson, W. F., *J. ment. Sci.*, 1900, **46**, 724.
32. Robertson, W. F., *Scot. med. surg. J.*, 1899, **4**, 23.
33. Ramón y Cajal, S., *Trab. Lab. Invest. biol.*, 1913, **11**, 255.
34. Del Río Hortega, P., *Mem. real. Soc. esp. Hist. nat.*, 1921, **11**, 213 [reprinted in: *Arch. Histol. (Buenos Aires)*, 1954, **5**, 105].
35. Del Río Hortega, P., in *Cytology and Cellular Pathology of the Nervous System*, edited by W. G. Penfield, vol. 2, page 483. Philadelphia, 1932.
36. Tennyson, V. M., Pappas, G. D., in *Pathology of the Nervous System*, edited by J. Minckler, vol. 1, chaps 42 and 43. New York, 1968.
37. Ramsey, H. J., *J. Neuropath. exp. Neurol.*, 1965, **24**, 25.
38. *The Neuron*, edited by H. Hydén. Amsterdam, 1967.
39. Luse, S. A., in *Pathology of the Nervous System*, edited by J. Minckler, vol. 1, chap. 46. New York, 1968.
39a. Corsellis, J. A. N., *personal communication*, 1976.
39b. Tomlinson, B. E., *personal communication*, 1976.
40. Crick, F. H. C., Nirenberg, M. W., in *The Molecular Basis of Life, Readings from Scientific American*, pages 198–223, papers 20–22. San Francisco, 1970.
41. Nissl, F., *Cbl. Nervenheilk.*, 1894, **17**, 337.
42. Hydén, H., Hartelius, H., *Acta psychiat. (Kbh.)*, 1948, suppl. 48.
43. Deitch, A. D., Murray, M. R., *J. biophys. biochem. Cytol.*, 1956, **2**, 433.
44. Deitch, A. D., Moses, M. J., *J. biophys. biochem. Cytol.*, 1957, **3**, 449.
45. Hamberger, C. A., Hydén, H., *Acta oto-laryng. (Stockh.)*, 1949, suppl. 82, 75.
46. Tureen, L. L., *Arch. Neurol. Psychiat. (Chic.)*, 1936, **35**, 789.
47. Einarson, L., *Amer. J. Anat.*, 1933, **53**, 141.

48. Hydén, H., in *Genetic Neurology*, edited by P. Weiss, page 177. Chicago, 1950.

49. Koenig, H., *J. biophys. biochem. Cytol.*, 1958, **4**, 785.

50. Glees, P., Soler, J., Bailey, R. A., *J. Neurol. Neurosurg. Psychiat.*, 1951, **14**, 281.

50a. Torvik, A., *J. Neuropath. appl. Neurobiol.*, 1976, **2**, 423.

51. Clarke, J. A. Lockhart, *Phil. Trans.*, 1851, **142**, 607.

52. *Mitochondria and Other Cytoplasmic Inclusions: Symposia of the Society for Experimental Biology, No. 10.* Cambridge, 1957.

53. Cameron, G. R., *New Pathways in Cellular Pathology*, chap. 5. London, 1956.

54. Schmitt, F. O., *Proc. nat. Acad. Sci.*, 1968, **60**, 1092.

55. Wuercker, R. B., Palay, S. L., *Tissue and Cell*, 1969, **1**, 387.

56. Yamada, K. M., Spooner, B. S., Wessells, N. K., *J. Cell Biol.*, 1970, **66**, 1206.

57. Terry, R. D., *J. Neuropath. exp. Neurol.*, 1971, **30**, 8.

58. Gray, E. G., Guillery, R. W., *J. Physiol. (Lond.)*, 1961, **157**, 581.

59. Moses, H. L., Beavor, D. L., Ganote, C. E., *Anat. Rec.*, 1966, **155**, 167.

60. Foley, J. M., Baxter, D., *J. Neuropath. exp. Neurol.*, 1958, **17**, 586.

61. Warren, P. J., Earl, C. J., Thompson, R. H. S., *Brain*, 1960, **83**, 709.

62. Marsden, C. D., *J. Anat. (Lond.)*, 1961, **95**, 256.

63. Pearce, A. G. E., *Histochemistry—Theoretical and Applied*, 3rd edn, vol. 2, page 1076. Edinburgh and London, 1972.

64. Leading Article, *Lancet*, 1970, **2**, 451.

65. Dayan, A. D., Trickey, R. J., *Lancet*, 1970, **2**, 296.

66. Harris, G. W., *Neural Control of the Pituitary Gland*. London, 1955.

67. Gray, E. G., *J. Anat. (Lond.)*, 1959, **93**, 420.

68. *The Biology of Myelin*, edited by S. R. Korey. New York, 1959.

69. Hild, W., in *The Biology of Myelin*, edited by S. R. Korey, page 229. New York, 1959.

70. Finean, J. B., Robertson, J. D., *Brit. med. Bull.*, 1958, **14**, 267.

71. Geren, B., *Exp. Cell Res.*, 1954, **7**, 558.

72. Murray, M. R., in *The Biology of Myelin*, edited by S. R. Korey, page 210. New York, 1959.

73. Luse, S. A., in *The Biology of Myelin*, edited by S. R. Korey, page 59. New York, 1959.

74. Bunge, M. B., Bunge, R. P., Ris, H., *J. biophys. biochem. Cytol.*, 1961, **10**, 67.

75. Bunge, R. P., *Physiol. Rev.*, 1968, **48**, 197.

76. Davison, A. N., Dobbing, J., Morgan, R. S., Wright, G. Payling, *Lancet*, 1959, **1**, 658.

77. Davison, A. N., Morgan, R. S., Wajda, M., Wright, G. Payling, *J. Neurochem.*, 1959, **4**, 360.

78. Waelsch, H., in *Biochemistry of the Developing Nervous System*, edited by H. Waelsch, page 190. New York, 1955.

79. Davison, A. N., Gregson, N. A., *Biochem. J.*, 1966, **96**, 915.

80. Drabkin, D. L., *Thudichum, Chemist of the Brain*. London, 1958.

81. Tomasch, J., *Anat. Rec.*, 1954, **119**, 119.

82. Waller, A., *Phil. Trans. roy. Soc.*, 1850, **140**, 423.

83. Johnson, A. C., McNabb, A. R., Rossiter, R. J., *Arch. Neurol. Psychiat. (Chic.)*, 1950, **64**, 105.

83a. Cavanagh, J. B., Webster, G. R., *Quart. J. exp. Physiol.*, 1955, **40**, 12.

84. Castro, F. de, *Arch. int. Physiol.*, 1951, **59**, 479.

85. Scheibel, M. E., Scheibel, A. B., in *Biology of Neuroglia*, edited by W. F. Windle, pages 5 and 45. Springfield, Illinois, 1958.

85a. Grossman, R. G., in *Scientific Foundations of Neurology*, edited by M. Critchley, J. L. O'Leary and B. Jennet, page 9. London, 1972.

86. Korey, S. R., in *The Biology of Myelin*, edited by S. R. Korey, page 253. New York, 1959.

87. Lumsden, C. E., *J. Neurol. Neurosurg. Psychiat.*, 1950, **13**, 1.

88. Hess, A., *J. comp. Neurol.*, 1953, **98**, 69.

89. Dempsey, E. W., Luse, S. A., in *Biology of Neuroglia*, edited by W. F. Windle, page 107. Springfield, Illinois, 1958.

90. Lumsden, C. E., in *Biology of Neuroglia*, edited by W. F. Windle, page 157. Springfield, Illinois, 1958.

91. Feigin, I., in *Pathology of the Nervous System*, edited by J. Minckler, vol. 1, chap. 35. New York, 1968.

92. Hager, H., in *Pathology of the Nervous System*, edited by J. Minckler, vol. 1, chap. 11. New York, 1968.

93. Klatzo, I., Miquel, J., Otenasek, R., *Acta neuropath. (Berl.)*, 1962, **2**, 144.

94. Long, D. M., Hartmann, J. F., French, L. A., *J. Neuropath. exp. Neurol.*, 1966, **25**, 373.

95. Klatzo, I., *J. Neuropath. exp. Neurol.*, 1967, **26**, 1.

96. Dobbing, J., *Guy's Hosp. Rep.*, 1963, **112**, 267.

97. Bairati, A., in *Biology of Neuroglia*, edited by W. F. Windle, page 85. Springfield, Illinois, 1958.

98. Dewey, W. C., *Amer. J. Physiol.*, 1959, **197**, 43.

99. Dobbing, J., *Physiol. Rev.*, 1961, **41**, 130.

100. Rowe, G. G., Maxwell, G. M., Castillo, C. A., Freeman, D. J., Crumpton, C. W., *J. clin. Invest.*, 1959, **38**, 2154.

101. Wislocki, G. B., Leduc, E. H., *J. comp. Neurol.*, 1952, **96**, 37.

102. Brierley, J. B., *Acta psychiat. (Kbh.)*, 1955, **30**, 553.

103. Russell, D. S., *Amer. J. Path.*, 1929, **5**, 451.

HYPOXIA

104. Hoff, E. C., Grenfell, R. G., Fulton, J. F., *Medicine (Baltimore)*, 1945, **24**, 161.

105. Brierley, J. B., in *Greenfield's Neuropathology*, 3rd edn, edited by W. Blackwood and J. A. N. Corsellis, chap. 2. London, 1976.

106. *Selective Vulnerability of the Brain in Hypoxaemia*, edited by J. P. Schadé and W. H. McMenemey. Oxford, 1963.

107. *Brain Hypoxia*, edited by J. B. Brierley and B. S. Meldrum. London, 1971.

108. Weinberger, L. M., Gibbon, M. H., Gibbon, J. H., Jr, *Arch. Neurol. Psychiat. (Chic.)*, 1940, **43**, 615, 971.

109. Meessen, H., *Beitr. path. Anat.*, 1944, **109**, 352.

110. Cope, D. H. P., Argent, D. E., Buxton, P. H., *Proc. roy. Soc. Med.*, 1960, **53**, 678.

111. Strughold, H., *J. Aviat. Med.*, 1954, **25**, 113.

112. Spielmeyer, W., *Histopathologie des Nervensystems*. Berlin, 1922.

113. Wertham, R., Wertham, F. L., *The Brain as an Organ*. New York, 1934.

114. Greenfield, J. G., Meyer, A., in *Greenfield's Neuropathology*, 2nd edn, by W. Blackwood, W. H.

McMenemey, A. Meyer, R. M. Norman and D. S. Russell, chap. 1 [pages 29–34]. London, 1963.

115. Cammermeyer, J., *Acta neuropath. (Berl.)*, 1961, **1**, 245.

116. Brown, A. W., Brierley, J. B., in *Brain Hypoxia*, edited by J. B. Brierley and B. S. Meldrum, chap. 6. London, 1971.

117. Jacob, H., in *Selective Vulnerability of the Brain in Hypoxaemia*, edited by J. P. Schadé and W. H. McMenemey, page 160. Oxford, 1963.

118. Brown, A. W., Brierley, J. B., *J. neurol. Sci.*, 1972, **16**, 59.

118a. Chaslin, P., *C.R. Soc. Biol. (Paris)*, 1889, **1**, 169.

119. Hurst, E. Weston, *J. Path. Bact.*, 1926, **29**, 65.

120. Hadfield, G., *J. Path. Bact.*, 1929, **32**, 135.

121. Courville, C. B., *Contributions to the Study of Cerebral Anoxia*. Los Angeles, 1953.

122. Környey, S., in *Selective Vulnerability of the Brain in Hypoxaemia*, edited by J. P. Schadé and W. H. McMenemey, page 165. Oxford, 1963.

123. Richter, R. B., *J. Neuropath. exp. Neurol.*, 1945, **4**, 324.

124. Scholz, W., Schmidt, H., *Arch. Psychiat. Nervenkr.*, 1952, **189**, 231.

125. Meyer, A., *Z. ges. Neurol. Psychiat.*, 1932, **139**, 422.

126. Meyer, A., in *Greenfield's Neuropathology*, 2nd edn, by W. Blackwood, W. H. McMenemey, A. Meyer, R. M. Norman and D. S. Russell, pages 255–261. London, 1963.

127. Eros, G., Priestman, N. Y., *J. Neuropath. exp. Neurol.*, 1942, **1**, 158.

128. Schwedenberg, T. H., *J. Neuropath. exp. Neurol.*, 1959, **18**, 597.

129. Dawes, G. S., Mott, J. C., Shelley, H. J., *J. Physiol. (Lond.)*, 1959, **146**, 516.

130. Little, W. J., *On the Nature and Treatment of the Deformities of the Human Frame*, page 114. London, 1953.

131. Schwartz, P., *Birth Injuries of the Newborn*. Basel, 1961.

132. Norman, R. M., Urich, H., McMenemey, W. H., *Brain*, 1957, **80**, 49.

133. Urich, H., in *Greenfield's Neuropathology*, 3rd edn, edited by W. Blackwood and J. A. N. Corsellis, chap. 10. London, 1976.

134. Haymaker, W., Margoles, C., Pentschew, A., Jacob, H., Lindenberg, R., Arroyo, L. S., Stockdorph, O., Stowens, D., *Kernicterus and Its Importance in Cerebral Palsy*, page 21. Springfield, Illinois, 1961.

135. Arias, I. M., *Advanc. clin. Chem.*, 1960, **3**, 35.

136. Osterberg, K., in *Pathology of the Nervous System*, edited by J. Minckler, vol. 2, chap. 95. New York, 1971.

137. Schmorl, G., *Verh. Dtsch. path. Ges.*, 1903, **6**, 109.

138. Fitzgerald, G. M., Greenfield, J. G., Kounine, D., *Brain*, 1939, **62**, 292.

139. Odell, G. B., *J. clin. Invest.*, 1959, **38**, 823.

140. Aidin, R., Corner, B., Tovey, G., *Lancet*, 1950, **1**, 1153.

141. Zuelzer, W. W., Mudgett, R. T., *Pediatrics*, 1950, **6**, 452.

142. Crigler, J. F., Najjar, V. A., *Pediatrics*, 1952, **10**, 169.

143. Lucey, J. F., Behrman, R. E., Esquivel de Gallardo, F. O., Windle, W. F., *Trans. Amer. neurol. Ass.*, 1963, **88**, 165.

144. Freytag, E., Lindenberg, R., *Arch. Path. (Chic.)*, 1964, **78**, 274.

145. Corsellis, J. A. N., in *Modern Trends in Neurology (Series 5)*, edited by D. Williams, chap. 15. London, 1970.

146. Earle, K. M., Baldwin, M., Penfield, W. G., *A.M.A. Arch. Neurol. Psychiat.*, 1953, **69**, 27.

147. Cavanagh, J. B., *Brain*, 1958, **81**, 389.

148. Taylor, D. C., Falconer, M. A., Bruton, C. J., Corsellis, J. A. N., *J. Neurol. Neurosurg. Psychiat.*, 1971, **34**, 369.

149. Rowe, G. G., Maxwell, G. M., Castillo, C. A., Freeman, D. J., Crumpton, C. W., *J. clin. Invest.*, 1959, **38**, 2154.

150. Lawrence, R. D., Meyer, A., Nevin, S., *Quart. J. Med.*, 1942, N.S. **35**, 181.

151. Meyer, A., in *Greenfield's Neuropathology*, 2nd edn, by W. Blackwood, W. H. McMenemey, A. Meyer, R. M. Norman and D. S. Russell, page 252. London, 1963.

151a. Brierley, J. B., in *Greenfield's Neuropathology*, 3rd edn, edited by W. Blackwood and J. A. N. Corsellis, page 74. London, 1976.

152. Kahn, K. J., Myers, R. E., in *Brain Hypoxia*, edited by J. B. Brierley and B. S. Meldrum, chaps. 19 and 20. London, 1971.

153. Meldrum, B. S., Horton, R. W., Brown, A. W., Brierley, J. B., in *Brain Hypoxia*, edited by J. B. Brierley and B. S. Meldrum, chaps 21 and 22. London, 1971.

154. Jones, E. L., Smith, W. T., in *Brain Hypoxia*, edited by J. B. Brierley and B. S. Meldrum, chap. 23. London, 1971.

155. Scholz, W., in *Selective Vulnerability of the Brain in Hypoxaemia*, edited by J. P. Schadé and W. H. McMenemey, page 259. Oxford, 1963.

156. Vogt, C., Vogt, O., *J. Psychol. Neurol. (Lpz.)*, 1922, **28**, 39.

157. Brown, R. J. K., Wallis, P. G., *Lancet*, 1963, **1**, 1278.

158. Haworth, J. C., McRae, K. N., *Canad. med. Ass. J.*, 1965, **92**, 861.

159. Anderson, J. M., Milner, R. D. G., Strich, S. J., *Lancet*, 1966, **2**, 372.

PYOGENIC INFECTIONS

160. *Statistics of Infectious Diseases: Notifications of Infectious Diseases in England and Wales, 1976* (Series MB2, No. 3). London, 1978.

160a. *On the State of the Public Health—The Annual Report of the Chief Medical Officer of the Department of Health and Social Security for the Year 1973*, page 42. London, 1974.

161. Dickson, W. E. Carnegie, *Brit. med. J.*, 1917, **1**, 454.

162. Gee, S., Barlow, T., *St Bart.'s Hosp. Rep.*, 1878, **14**, 23.

163. Smith, M. V., Norman, R. M., Urich, H., *J. Neurol. Neurosurg. Psychiat.*, 1957, **20**, 250.

164. Smith, J. F., Landing, B. H., *J. Neuropath. exp. Neurol.*, 1960, **19**, 248.

165. Dungal, N., *Lancet*, 1961, **2**, 513.

166. Flewett, T. H., in *The Pathological Basis of Medicine*, edited by R. C. Curran and D. G. Harnden, chap. 39. London, 1972.

167. Alston, J. M., Broom, J. C., *Leptospirosis in Man and Animals*, page 172. Edinburgh and London, 1958.

168. Randall, K. J., *J. clin. Path.*, 1948, **1**, 150.

168a. Rabinowitz, S. G., MacLeod, N. R., *Amer. J. Dis. Child.*, 1972, **123**, 259.

168b. Denis, F., Badiane, S., Chiron, J. P., Sow, A., Diop Mar, I., *Lancet*, 1977, **1**, 910.

169. Greenfield, J. G., Carmichael, E. A., *The Cerebro-Spinal Fluid and Clinical Diagnosis*, page 183. London, 1925.
170. Noran, H. H., Baker, A. B., Larson, W. P., *Arch. Neurol. Psychiat.* (*Chic.*), 1947, **58**, 653.
171. Newton, E. J., *Quart. J. Med.*, 1956, N.S. **25**, 201.
172. Berry, R. G., Alpers, B. J., in *Pathology of the Nervous System*, edited by J. Minckler, vol. 3, page 2362. New York, 1972.

TUBERCULOSIS

173. Whytt, R., *Observations on the Dropsy in the Brain*. Edinburgh, 1768.
174. Bayle, A. L. J., *Recherches sur l'arachnitis chronique*. Thesis, Paris, 1822. [English translation in: *Arch. Neurol. Psychiat.* (*Chic.*), 1934, **32**, 84.]
174a. *The Registrar General's Statistical Reviews of England and Wales for the Years 1946 to 1973*. London, 1947–75.
174b. *Mortality Statistics—Cause: Review of the Registrar General on Deaths by Cause, Sex and Age, in England and Wales, 1976* (Series DH2, No. 3). London, 1978.
175. Udani, P. M., Parekh, U. C., Dastur, D. K., *J. neurol. Sci.*, 1971, **14**, 341.
176. Rich, A. R., *The Pathogenesis of Tuberculosis*, 2nd edn, page 886. Springfield, Illinois, 1951.
177. Rich, A. R., McCordock, H. A., *Bull. Johns Hopk. Hosp.*, 1933, **52**, 5.
178. MacGregor, A. R., Green, C. A., *J. Path. Bact.*, 1937, **45**, 613.
179. Evans, H. S., Courville, C. B., *Arch. Surg.*, 1938, **36**, 637.
180. Doniach, I., *J. Path. Bact.*, 1949, **61**, 253.
181. Voljavec, B. F., Orton, S. P., Corpe, R. F., *Amer. Rev. resp. Dis.*, 1959, **80**, 388.
182. Nickerson, G., Morgante, O., MacDermot, P. N., Ross, S. G., *Amer. Rev. Tuberc.*, 1957, **76**, 832.
183. Ashby, M. G. C., Grant, H. C., *Lancet*, 1955, **1**, 65.
184. Miller, F. J. W., Seal, R. M. E., Taylor, M. D., *Tuberculosis in Children*. London, 1963.
185. Brain, Walton, J. N., *Diseases of the Nervous System*, 7th edn, page 373. London, 1969.
186. Arseni, C., Samitca, D. C.-T., *Brain*, 1960, **83**, 285.
187. Dastur, D. K., in *Pathology of the Nervous System*, edited by J. Minckler, vol. 3, chap. 174. New York, 1972.

SYPHILIS

188. Merritt, H. H., Adams, R. D., Solomon, H. C., *Neurosyphilis*. New York, 1946.
189. *Annual Reports of the Chief Medical Officer of the Ministry of Health/Department of Health and Social Security for the Years 1962 to 1970*. London, 1963–1972.
189a. *On the State of the Public Health—The Annual Report of the Chief Medical Officer of the Department of Health and Social Security for the Year 1976*, page 63, table 4.1. London, 1977.
189b. *On the State of the Public Health—The Annual Report of the Chief Medical Officer of the Department of Health and Social Security for the Year 1974*, page 78. London, 1975.
189c. Obersteiner, H., Redlich, E., *Arb. Inst. Anat. Physiol. Zentr.-Nervensyst. Univ. Wien*, 1894, **2**, 158; 1895, **3**, 192.

190. Robertson, A., *Edinb. med. J.*, 1868, **14**, 696.
190a. Noguchi, H., Moore, J. W., *J. exp. Med.*, 1913, **17**, 232.
191. Lissauer, H., *posthumous case study, published by:* Storch, E., *Mschr. Psychiat. Neurol.*, 1901, **9**, 401.
191a. Galbraith, A. J., Meyer, A., *J. Neurol. Psychiat.*, 1942, **5**, 22.
192. Greenfield, J. G., in *Greenfield's Neuropathology*, 2nd edn, by W. Blackwood, W. H. McMenemey, A. Meyer, R. M. Norman, and D. S. Russell, page 166. London, 1963.
192a. Erb, W. H., *Neurol. Zbl.*, 1892, **11**, 161.
193. Moore, J. E., *The Modern Treatment of Syphilis*, 2nd edn, page 41. Springfield, Illinois, 1943.
194. Turner, T. B., *Bull. Johns Hopk. Hosp.*, 1930, **46**, 159.

WEST INDIAN AND SIMILAR NEUROPATHIES

195. Montgomery, R. D., Cruickshank, E. K., Robertson, W. B., McMenemey, W. H., *Brain*, 1964, **87**, 425.
196. Robertson, W. B., Cruickshank, E. K., in *Pathology of the Nervous System*, edited by J. Minckler, vol. 3, chap. 178. New York, 1972.
197. Main, K. S., Main, J. A., Montgomery, R. D., *J. neurol. Sci.*, 1969, **9**, 179.
198. Haddock, D. R. W., Ebrahim, G. J., Kapur, B. B., *Brit. med. J.*, 1962, **2**, 1442.
199. Money, G. L., *W. Afr. med. J.*, 1959, **8**, 13.
200. Osuntokun, B. O., Monekosso, G. L., Wilson, J., *Brit. med. J.*, 1969, **1**, 547.
201. Osuntokun, B. O., Langman, M. J. S., Wilson, J., Aladetoyinbo, A., *J. Neurol. Neurosurg. Psychiat.*, 1970, **33**, 663.

RICKETTSIAL ENCEPHALITIS

202. Zinsser, H., *Rats, Lice and History*. Boston [and London], 1935.
203. Woodward, T. E., Jackson, E. B., in *Viral and Rickettsial Infections of Man*, 4th edn, edited by F. L. Horsfall, Jr, and I. Tamm, page 1905. Philadelphia and London, 1965.

FUNGAL INFECTIONS

204. Symmers, W. St C., *Vie méd.*, 1966, **47**, 353.
205. Fetter, B. F., Klintworth, G. K., Hendry, W. S., *Mycoses of the Central Nervous System*. Baltimore, 1967.
206. Cope, Z., *Actinomycosis*, page 170. London, 1938.
207. Stevens, H., *Neurology* (*Minneap.*), 1953, **3**, 761.
208. Welsh, J. D., Rhoades, E. R., Jaques, W., *Arch. intern. Med.*, 1961, **108**, 73.
209. Straatsma, B. R., Zimmerman, L. E., Gass, J. D. M., *Lab. Invest.*, 1962, **11**, 963.
210. Gregory, J. E., Golden, A., Haymaker, W., *Bull. Johns Hopk. Hosp.*, 1943, **73**, 405.
211. Rose, F. C., Grant, H. C., Jeanes, A. L., *Brain*, 1958, **81**, 542.
212. Symmers, W. St C., *Rev. lyon. Méd.*, 1963, **12**, 979.
212a. Middleton, F. G., Jurgenson, P. F., Utz, J. P., Shadomy, S., Shadomy, H. J., *Arch. intern. Med.*, 1976, **136**, 444.
213. Cooper, R. A., Jr, Goldstein, E., *Amer. J. Med.* 1963, **35**, 45.
214. Shapiro, J. L., Lux, J. J., Sprofkin, B. E., *Amer. J Path.*, 1955, **31**, 319.

215. Fiese, M. J., *Coccidioidomycosis*, page 117. Springfield, Illinois, 1958.
215a. *Coccidioidomycosis*, edited by L. Ajello, sect. 1. Tucson, Arizona, 1967.
216. Baum, G. L., Schwarz, J., *Amer. J. med. Sci.*, 1959, **238**, 661.

ARACHNOIDITIS
217. Hurst, E. Weston, *J. Path. Bact.*, 1955, **70**, 167.

PROTOZOAL INFECTIONS
218. Lombardo, L., Alonso, P., Saenz, A. L., Brandt, H., Mateos, J. H., *J. Neurosurg.*, 1964, **8**, 704.
218a. Pérez-Tamayo, R., Brandt, H., in *Pathology of Protozoal and Helminthic Diseases with Clinical Correlation*, edited by R. A. Marcial-Rojas and E. Moreno, chap. 8 [page 174]. Baltimore, 1971.
219. Carter, R. F., *Trans. roy. Soc. trop. Med. Hyg.*, 1972, **66**, 193.
220. Culbertson, C. G., *Ann. Rev. Microbiol.*, 1971, **25**, 231.
221. Symmers, W. St C., *Brit. med. J.*, 1969, **4**, 449.
222. Carter, R. F., *J. Path.*, 1970, **100**, 217.
223. Fowler, M., Carter, R. F., *Brit. med. J.*, 1965, **2**, 740.
224. *Human Toxoplasmosis*, edited by J. C. Siim. Copenhagen, 1960.
224a. Frenkel, J. K., in *Pathology of Protozoal and Helminthic Diseases with Clinical Correlation*, edited by R. A. Marcial-Rojas and E. Moreno, chap. 13. Baltimore, 1971.
225. Beverley, J. K. A., in *Recent Advances in Clinical Pathology*, series 3, edited by S. C. Dyke, M. Barber, E. N. Allott, R. Biggs and A. H. T. Robb-Smith, chap. 4. London, 1960.
226. Beattie, C. P., in *Recent Advances in Medical Microbiology*, edited by A. P. Waterson, chap. 9. London, 1967.
227. Wolf, A., Cowen, D., *Bull. neurol. Inst. N.Y.*, 1937, **6**, 306.
227a. Wolf, A., Cowen, D., Paige, B., *Science*, 1939, **89**, 226.
227b. Janků, J., *Čas. Lék. čes.*, 1923, **62**, 1021.
228. Wolf, A., Cowan, D., *J. Neuropath. exp. Neurol.*, 1959, **18**, 191.
229. Beattie, C. P., *Trans. ophthal. Soc. U.K.*, 1958, **78**, 99.
230. *Malariology*, edited by M. F. Boyd, vol. 2, page 882. Philadelphia, 1949.
230a. Dürck, H., *Arch. Schiffs- u. Tropenhyg.*, 1925, **29**, Beiheft 1, 43.
231. Scheiddeger, S., in *Handbuch der speziellen pathologischen Anatomie und Histologie*, vol. 13, edited by W. Scholz, part 2, book A, page 1113. Berlin, Göttingen and Heidelberg, 1958.
232. Bogaert, L. van, in *Handbuch der speziellen pathologischen Anatomie und Histologie*, vol. 13, edited by W. Scholz, part 2, book A, page 1086. Berlin, Göttingen and Heidelberg, 1958.
233. Chagas, C., *Mem. Inst. Oswaldo Cruz*, 1909, **1**, 159.
234. Alençar, A., in *Pathology of the Nervous System*, edited by J. Minckler, vol. 3, chap. 184. New York, 1972.
235. Köberle, F., *Virchows Arch. path. Anat.*, 1957, **330**, 267.
236. Köberle, F., *Zbl. allg. Path. path. Anat.*, 1957, **96**, 244.

METAZOAL INFESTATIONS
237. Dixon, H. B. F., Lipscomb, F. M., *Spec. Rep. Ser. med. Res. Coun. (Lond.)*, No. 299, 1961.

238. Bickerstaff, E. R., Cloake, P. C. P., Hughes, B., Smith, W. T., *Brain*, 1951, **74**, 1.
239. Bickerstaff, E. R., Small, J. M., Woolf, A. L., *Brain*, 1956, **79**, 622.
240. Becker, B. J. P., Jacobson, S., *Lancet*, 1951, **2**, 198.
241. Kuper, S., Mendelow, H., *Brain*, 1958, **81**, 235.
242. Greenfield, J. G., Pritchard, E. A. B., *Brain*, 1947, **60**, 361.
242a. Marcial-Rojas, R. A., in *Pathology of Protozoal and Helminthic Diseases with Clinical Correlation*, edited by R. A. Marcial-Rojas and E. Moreno, chap. 16 [page 404]. Baltimore, 1971.
242b. Cohen, J., Capildeo, R., Rose, F. C., Pallis, C., *Brit. med. J.*, 1977, **2**, 1258.
243. Brain, Allan, B., *Lancet*, 1964, **1**, 1355.
244. Ashton, N., *Brit. J. Ophthal.*, 1960, **64**, 129.
245. Bogaert, L. van, Dubois, A., Janssens, P. G., Radermecker, J., Tverdy, G., Wanson, M., *J. Neurol. Neurosurg. Psychiat.*, 1955, **18**, 103.
245a. Toussaint, D., Danis, P., *Arch. Ophthal.*, 1965, **74**, 470.
245b. Mya, T., *Indian med. Gaz.*, 1928, **63**, 636.

VIRAL DISEASES: INTRODUCTION
246. Nieberg, K. C., Blumberg, J. M., in *Pathology of the Nervous System*, edited by J. Minckler, vol. 3, chap. 169. New York, 1972.
247. *Host-Virus Reactions with Special Reference to Persistent Agents*, edited by G. Dick, *J. clin. Path.*, 1972, **25**, suppl. 6 (Roy. Coll. Path.).

CONVENTIONAL VIRAL DISEASES
248. Beale, A. J., in: Rhodes, A. J., Rooyen, C. E. van, *Textbook of Virology*, 5th edn, sect. 5, chap. 3. Baltimore, 1968.
248a. Heine, J., *Beobachtungen über Lähmungszustände der untern Extremitäten und deren Behandlung*. Stuttgart, 1840.
248b. Medin, O., *Hygiea (Stockh.)*, 1890, **52**, 657.
249. Landsteiner, K., Popper, E., *Z. Immun.-Forsch.*, 1909, **2**, 377.
250. Landsteiner, K., Levaditi, C., *C.R. Soc. Biol. (Paris)*, 1909, **67**, 592.
251. Sabin, A. B., Olitsky, P. K., *Proc. Soc. exp. Biol. (N.Y.)*, 1936, **34**, 357.
252. Elford, W. J., Galloway, I. A., Perdrau, J. R., *J. Path. Bact.*, 1935, **40**, 135.
253. Taylor, A. R., McCormick, M. J., *Yale J. Biol. Med.*, 1956, **28**, 589.
254. Hill, A. Bradford, *Proc. roy. Soc. Med.*, 1954, **47**, 795.
255. Faber, H. K., *The Pathogenesis of Poliomyelitis*, page 117. Springfield, Illinois, 1955.
256. Melnick, J. L., Penner, L. R., *Proc. Soc. exp. Biol. (N.Y.)*, 1947, **65**, 342.
257. Sabin, A. B., *Wld Hlth Org. Monogr. Ser.*, No. 26, 1955, 301.
258. Gear, J. H. S., *Wld Hlth Org. Monogr. Ser.*, No. 26, 1955, 31.
259. Gard, S., in *Die Infektionskrankheiten des Menschen und ihre Erreger*, edited by A. Grumbach and W. Kikuth, vol. 2, page 1423. Stuttgart, 1958.
260. Bodian, D., *Amer. J. Hyg.*, 1949, **49**, 200.
261. Schabel, F. M., Smith, H. T., Fishbein, W. I., Casey, A. E., *J. infect. Dis.*, 1950, **86**, 214.
262. Enders, J. F., Weller, T. H., Robbins, F. C., *Science*, 1949, **109**, 85.

263. Public Health Laboratory Service, Report on Immunization against Poliomyelitis, *Brit. med. J.*, 1961, **2**, 1037.

264. Lennartz, H., Valenciano, L., *Dtsch. med. Wschr.*, 1961, **86**, 1497.

265. Geffen, T. J., *Mth. Bull. Minist. Hlth Lab. Serv.*, 1960, **19**, 196.

266. Salk, F. J., *Lancet*, 1960, **2**, 715.

267. Teelock, B., *Brit. med. J.*, 1960, **2**, 1272.

268. Horstmann, D. M., *Amer. J. Med.*, 1949, **6**, 535.

269. Brierley, J. B., *Acta psychiat. (Kbh.)*, 1955, **30**, 553.

270. Waksman, B. H., *J. Neuropath. exp. Neurol.*, 1961, **20**, 35.

271. Russell, W. Ritchie, *Brit. med. J.*, 1947, **2**, 1023.

272. Medical Research Council: Poliomyelitis and Prophylactic Inoculation against Diphtheria, Whooping Cough and Smallpox, *Lancet*, 1956, **2**, 1223.

273. Faber, H. K., *The Pathogenesis of Poliomyelitis*, page 118. Springfield, Illinois, 1955.

274. Bower, A. G., *Diagnosis and Treatment of the Acute Phase of Poliomyelitis and Its Complications*, page 2. London, 1954.

275. Sharrard, W. J. W., in *Proceedings of the Second International Congress of Neuropathology, London, 1955*, part 1, page 437. Amsterdam, 1955.

276. Howe, H. A., Bodian, D., *Neural Mechanisms in Poliomyelitis*, page 168. London, 1942.

277. Sharrard, W. J. W., *J. Bone Jt Surg.*, 1955, **37B**, 540.

278. Bodian, D., *Bull. Johns Hopk. Hosp.*, 1948, **83**, 1.

279. Bodian, D., in *Poliomyelitis* (Second International Poliomyelitis Congress, Copenhagen, 1951), page 61. Philadelphia, 1952.

280. Einarson, L., *Acta orthop. scand.*, 1949, **19**, 27.

281. Flewett, T. H., in *The Pathological Basis of Medicine*, edited by R. C. Curran and D. G. Harnden, chap. 36. London, 1972.

282. Sharrard, W. J. W., *British Surgical Practice: Surgical Progress*, page 83. London, 1956.

283. Pette, H., in *Fifth Symposium, European Association against Poliomyelitis*, page 154. Madrid, 1958.

284. Galpine, J. F., Wilson, W. C. MacC., *Brit. med. J.*, 1959, **2**, 1379.

285. O'Leary, J. L., King, R. B., Meagher, J. N., *A.M.A. Arch. Neurol. Psychiat.*, 1955, **74**, 611.

286. Denny-Brown, D., Foley, J. M., *Arch. Neurol. Psychiat. (Chic.)*, 1950, **61**, 141.

287. Wohlfart, G., Hoffman, H., *Acta psychiat. scand.*, 1956, **31**, 345.

288. Dalldorf, G., *Bull. N.Y. Acad. Med.*, 1950, **26**, 329.

289. Beeson, P. B., Scott, T. F. McNair, *Proc. roy. Soc. Med.*, 1942, **35**, 733.

290. Moossy, J., Geer, J. C., *A.M.A. Arch. Path.*, 1960, **70**, 614.

291. Giunchi, G., in *Virus Meningo-Encephalitis*, edited by G. E. W. Wolstenholme and M. P. Cameron, page 40. London, 1961.

292. Vernon, E., *Mth. Bull. Minist. Hlth Lab. Serv.*, 1964, **23**, 210.

293. Heathfield, K. W. G., Pilsworth, R., Wall, B. J., Corsellis, J. A. N., *Quart. J. Med.*, 1967, N.S. **36**, 571.

294. Olderhausen, H. F., in *Virus Meningo-Encephalitis*, edited by G. E. W. Wolstenholme and M. P. Cameron, page 34. London, 1961.

295. Duncan, I. B. R., *Lancet*, 1960, **2**, 470.

295a. Peckham, C. S., *Mth. Bull. Minist. Hlth Lab. Serv.*, 1964, **23**, 217.

296. *Rabies—The Facts*, edited by C. Kaplan. Oxford, 1977.

297. Hurst, E. Weston, *J. Path. Bact.*, 1932, **35**, 301.

298. West, G., *Rabies in Animal and Man*. London, 1972.

298a. Macdonald, J., *Hlth Trends*, 1977, **9**, 33.

299. Constantine, D. G., *Publ. Hlth Rep. (Wash.)*, 1962, **77**, 287.

300. Babès, V., *Ann. Inst. Pasteur*, 1892, **6**, 209.

301. Schaffer, K., *Z. ges. Neurol. Psychiat.*, 1931, **136**, 547.

302. Wright, G. Payling, in *Modern Trends in Pathology*, edited by D. Collins, chap. 11. London, 1959.

302a. Negri, A., *Boll. Soc. med.-chir. Pavia*, 1903, 88, 229; 1904, 22; 1905, 321.

302b. Negri, A., *Z. Hyg. Infekt.-Kr.*, 1903, **43**, 507.

303. Ditchfield, W. J. B., in: Rhodes, A. J., Rooyen, C. E. van, *Textbook of Virology*, 5th edn, page 497. Baltimore, 1968.

304. Miyamoto, K., Matsumoto, S., *J. Cell Biol.*, 1965, **27**, 677.

304a. Pasteur, L., *C.R. Acad. Sci. (Paris)*, 1885, **101**, 765; 1886, **102**, 459, 835; 1886, **103**, 777.

305. Shiraki, K., Otani, S., in '*Allergic*' *Encephalomyelitis*, edited by M. W. Kies and E. C. Alvord, page 58. Springfield, Illinois, 1959.

306. Expert Committee on Rabies (4th Report), *Wld Hlth Org. techn. Rep. Ser.*, No. 201, 1960.

307. Expert Committee on Rabies (5th Report), *Wld Hlth Org. techn. Rep. Ser.*, No. 321, 1966.

308. Sabin, A. B., Wright, A. M., *J. exp. Med.*, 1934, **59**, 115.

309. Breen, G. E., Lamb, S. G., Otaki, A. T., *Brit. med. J.*, 1958, **2**, 22.

310. Davidson, W. L., Hummler, K., *Ann. N.Y. Acad. Sci.*, 1960, **85**, 970.

311. Keeble, S. A., Christofinis, G. J., Wood, W., *J. Path. Bact.*, 1958, **76**, 189.

312. Thomas, E., Henschel, E., *Dtsch. Z. Nervenheilk.*, 1960, **18**, 494.

313. Keeble, S. A., *Ann. N.Y. Acad. Sci.*, 1960, **85**, 960.

314. Pierce, E. C., Pierce, J. D., Hull, R. N., *Amer. J. Hyg.*, 1958, **68**, 242.

315. Wallgren, A., *Acta paediat. (Uppsala)*, 1925, **4**, 158.

316. Wallgren, A., *Acta med. scand.*, 1927, **65**, 722.

317. Armstrong, C., Lillie, R. D., *Publ. Hlth Rep. (Wash.)*, 1934, **49**, 1019.

318. Syverton, J. T., Berry, G. P., *Science*, 1935, **82**, 596.

319. Wooley, J. G., Armstrong, C., *Publ. Hlth Rep. (Wash.)*, 1934, **49**, 1495.

320. Irvine, R. A., Grant, L. S., Belle, E. A., *Amer. J. trop. Med. Hyg.*, 1963, **12**, 916.

321. Feemster, R. F., *Amer. J. publ. Hlth*, 1938, **28**, 1403.

322. Meyer, K. F., Haring, C. M., Howitt, B. F., *Science*, 1931, **74**, 227.

323. Casals, J., Reeves, W. C., in *Viral and Rickettsial Infections of Man*, 4th edn, edited by F. L. Horsfall, Jr, and I. Tamm, page 590. Philadelphia and London, 1965.

324. Hart, K. L., Keen, D., Belle, E. A., *Amer. J. trop. Med. Hyg.*, 1964, **13**, 331.

325. Belle, E. A., Grant, L. S., Thorburn, M. J., *Amer. J. trop. Med. Hyg.*, 1964, **13**, 335.

326. Beck, C. E., Wyckoff, R. W. G., *Science*, 1938, **88**, 530.

327. Hammon, W. M., Reeves, W. C., *Amer. J. Hyg.*, 1947, **46**, 326.

328. Grascenkov, N. I., *Bull. Wld Hlth Org.*, 1964, **30**, 161.

329. Kawakita, Y., *Jap. J. exp. Med.*, 1939, **17**, 211.

330. Gresser, I., Hardy, J. L., Hu, S. M., Scherer, W. F., *Amer. J. trop. Med. Hyg.*, 1958, **7**, 365.
331. Haymaker, W., *personal communication*, 1959.
332. Pond, W. L., Russ, S. B., Rogers, N. G., Smadel, J. E., *J. Immunol.*, 1955, **75**, 78.
333. Robertson, E. G., *Med. J. Aust.*, 1952, **1**, 107.
334. Innes, J. R. M., Saunders, L. Z., *Comparative Neuropathology*, page 345. New York, 1962.
335. Pool, W. A., *Vet. J.*, 1931, **87**, 177, 222.
336. Casals, J., Reeves, W. C., in *Viral and Rickettsial Infections of Man*, 4th edn, edited by F. L. Horsfall and I. Tamm, page 641. London, 1965.
337. Likar, M., Dane, D. S., *Lancet*, 1958, **1**, 456.
338. McLean, D. M., Donohue, W. L., *Canad. med. Ass. J.*, 1959, **80**, 708.
339. McLean, D. M., Larke, R. P. B., *Canad. med. Ass. J.*, 1963, **88**, 182.
340. Rooyen, C. E. van, Rhodes, A. J., *Virus Diseases of Man*, 2nd edn, page 800. New York, 1948.
341. McLean, D. M., in: Rhodes, A. J., Rooyen, C. E. van, *Textbook of Virology*, 5th edn, sec. 6, chap. 1. Baltimore, 1968.
341a. Cowdry, E. V., *Arch. Path. (Chic.)*, 1934, **18**, 527.
342. Oseasohn, R., Adelson, L., Kaji, M., *New Engl. J. Med.*, 1959, **260**, 509.
343. Greenfield, J. G., *J. Path. Bact.*, 1930, **33**, 453.
344. Hoult, J. J., Flewett, T. H., *Brit. med. J.*, 1960, **1**, 1187.
345. McGill, R. J., Goodbody, R. A., *Lancet*, 1958, **1**, 320.
346. Flewett, T. H., Hoult, J. J., *Lancet*, 1958, **2**, 11.
347. Warren, J., in *Viral and Rickettsial Infections of Man*, 4th edn, edited by F. L. Horsfall and I. Tamm, chap. 23. London, 1965.
348. Innes, J. R. M., Saunders, L. Z., *Comparative Neuropathology*, page 443. London, 1965.
348a. Aujesky, A., *Zbl. Bakt.*, 1902, **32**, 353.
349. Hurst, E. W., *J. exp. Med.*, 1933, **58**, 415.
350. Martini, G. A., Siegert, R., *Marburg Virus Disease*. Berlin, 1971.
351. Smith, C. E. G., *Sci. Basis Med.*, 1971, 58.
352. Siegert, R., in *Modern Trends in Medical Virology—2*, edited by R. B. Heath and A. P. Waterson, page 204. London, 1970.
353. Jacob, H., Solcher, H., *Acta neuropath.*, 1968, **11**, 29.

LATENT (PERSISTENT) VIRAL DISEASES
354. *Host–Virus Reactions with Special Reference to Persistent Agents*, edited by G. Dick, *J. clin. Path.*, 1972, **25**, suppl. 6 (Roy. Coll. Path.).
355. Waterson, A. P., *J. clin. Path.*, 1972, **25**, suppl. 6 (Roy. Coll. Path.), 1.
356. Allison, A. C., *J. clin. Path.*, 1972, **25**, suppl. 6 (Roy. Coll. Path.), 121.
357. Downie, A. W., *Brit. med. Bull.*, 1959, **15**, 197.
358. McCarthy, K., *J. clin. Path.*, 1972, **25**, suppl. 6 (Roy. Coll. Path.), 46.
359. Goodbody, R. A., *J. Path. Bact.*, 1953, **65**, 221.
360. Thalimer, W., *Arch. Neurol. Psychiat. (Chic.)*, 1924, **12**, 73.
361. Schiff, C. I., Brain, W. R., *Lancet*, 1930, **2**, 70.
362. Biggart, J. H., Fisher, J. A., *Lancet*, 1938, **2**, 944.
363. Dudgeon, J. A., in *Modern Trends in Medical Virology —2*, edited by R. B. Heath and A. P. Waterson, chap. 4. London, 1970.
364. Leading Article, *Brit. med. J.*, 1973, **3**, 124.
365. Adams, J. H., Jennet, W. B., *J. Neurol. Neurosurg. Psychiat.*, 1967, **30**, 248.

366. Marshall, W. J. S., *Lancet*, 1967, **2**, 579.
367. Harland, W. A., Adams, J. H., McSeveney, D., *Lancet*, 1967, **2**, 581.
367a. Becker, W. B., Kipps, A., McKenzie, D., *Amer. J. Dis. Child.*, 1968, **115**, 1.
368. Wolf, A., Cowen, D., in *Pathology of the Nervous System*, edited by J. Minckler, vol. 3, chap. 185. New York, 1972.
369. Banatvala, J. E., in *Modern Trends in Medical Virology—2*, edited by R. B. Heath and A. P. Waterson, chap. 5. London, 1970.
370. Rorke, L. B., Spiro, A. J., *J. Pediat.*, 1967, **70**, 243.
371. Wolf, A., Cowen, D., in *Pathology of the Nervous System*, edited by J. Minckler, vol. 3, page 2575. New York, 1972.
372. Stern, H., *J. clin. Path.*, 1972, **25**, suppl. 6 (Roy. Coll. Path.), 34.
373. Dawson, J. R., Jr, *Amer. J. Path.*, 1933, **9**, 7.
374. Dawson, J. R., Jr, *Arch. Neurol. Psychiat. (Chic.)*, 1934, **31**, 685.
375. Bogaert, L. van, *J. Neurol. Neurosurg. Psychiat.*, 1945, **8**, 107.
376. Greenfield, J. G., *Brain*, 1950, **73**, 141.
377. Cobb, W. A., Morgan-Hughes, J. A., *J. Neurol. Neurosurg. Psychiat.*, 1968, **31**, 115.
378. Kennedy, C., *Neurology (Minneap.)*, 1968, **18**, 58.
379. Malamud, N., Haymaker, W., Pinkerton, H., *Amer. J. Path.*, 1950, **26**, 113.
380. Corsellis, J. A. N., *J. ment. Sci.*, 1951, **97**, 570.
381. Pette, H., Döring, G., *Dtsch. Z. Nervenheilk.*, 1939, **149**, 7.
382. Bonhoff, G., *Arch. Psychiat. Nervenkr.*, 1948, **181**, 421.
383. Connolly, J. H., Allen, I. V., Hurwitz, L. J., Millar, J. H. D., *Quart. J. Med.*, 1968, N.S. **37**, 625.
384. Herndon, R. M., Rubinstein, L. J., *Neurology (Minneap.)*, 1968, **18**, 8.
385. Paine, F. E., Baublis, J. E., *Perspect. med. Virol.*, 1971, **7**, 179.
386. Meulen, V. ter, Katz, M., Muller, D., *Curr. Topics Microbiol. Immunol.*, 1972, **57**, 1.
387. Barbanti Brodano, G., Oyanagi, S., Katz, M., Koprowski, H., *Proc. Soc. exp. Biol. (N.Y.)*, 1970, **134**, 230.
388. Dayan, A. D., *J. neurol. Sci.*, 1971, **14**, 315.
389. Brody, J. A., Detels, R., Sever, J. L., *Lancet*, 1972, **1**, 177.
390. Brody, J. A., Detels, R., *Lancet*, 1970, **2**, 500.
391. Connolly, J. C., *J. clin. Path.*, 1972, **25**, suppl. 6 (Roy. Coll. Path.), 73.

'OPPORTUNISTIC' VIRAL INFECTIONS
392. Waterson, A. P., *J. clin. Path.*, 1972, **25**, suppl. 6 (Roy. Coll. Path.), 1.
393. Schober, R., Herman, M., *Lancet*, 1973, **1**, 962.
394. Aström, K. E., Mancall, E. L., Richardson, E. P., *Brain*, 1958, **81**, 93.
395. Richardson, E. P., Jr, *New Engl. J. Med.*, 1961, **265**, 815.
396. ZuRhein, G. M., Chou, S. M., *Science*, 1968, **148**, 1477.
397. Howatson, A. F., Nagai, M., ZuRhein, G. M., *Canad. med. Ass. J.*, 1965, **93**, 379.
398. Silverman, L., Rubinstein, L. J., *Acta neuropath. (Berl.)*, 1965, **5**, 215.
399. Woodhouse, M. A., Dayan, A. D., Bruston, J., Caldwell, I., Adams, J. H., Melcher, D., Urich, H., *Brain*, 1967, **90**, 863.

400. Padgett, B. L., Walker, D. L., ZuRhein, G., Eckroade, R. J., Dessel, B. H., *Lancet*, 1971, **1**, 1257.

SLOW VIRAL DISEASES

401. Field, E. J., *Int. Rev. exp. Path.*, 1969, **8**, 130.
402. *Host–Virus Reactions with Special Reference to Persistent Agents*, edited by G. Dick, *J. clin. Path.*, 1972, **25**, suppl. 6 (Roy. Coll. Path.).
403. Sigurdsson, B., *Brit. vet. J.*, 1954, **110**, 255, 307, 341.
404. Sigurdsson, B., Palsson, P. A., Bogaert, L. van, *Acta neuropath. (Berl.)*, 1962, **1**, 343.
405. Palsson, P. A., *J. clin. Path.*, 1972, **25**, suppl. 6 (Roy. Coll. Path.), 115.
406. Daniel, P. M., *Proc. roy. Soc. Med.*, 1971, **64**, 787.
407. Gordon, W. S., *Vet. Rec.*, 1946, **58**, 516.
408. Alper, T., *J. clin. Path.*, 1972, **25**, suppl. 6 (Roy. Coll. Path.), 154.
409. Barlow, R. M., *J. clin. Path.*, 1972, **25**, suppl. 6 (Roy. Coll. Path.), 102.
410. Hornabrook, R. W., *Brain*, 1968, **91**, 53.
411. Beck, E., Daniel, P. M., Alpers, M., Gajdusek, D. C., Gibbs, C. J., *Lancet*, 1966, **2**, 1056.
412. Gajdusek, D. C., *J. clin. Path.*, 1972, **25**, suppl. 6 (Roy. Coll. Path.), 78.
413. Hadlow, W. J., *Lancet*, 1959, **2**, 289.
414. Gibbs, C. J., Gajdusek, D. C., *J. clin. Path.*, 1972, **25**, suppl. 6 (Roy. Coll. Path.), 84.
415. Mathews, J. D., Glasse, R., Lindenbaum, *Lancet*, 1968, **2**, 449.
416. Kirschbaum, W. R., *Jakob–Creutzfeldt Disease*. New York, 1968.
416a. Creutzfeldt, H. G., *Z. ges. Neurol. Psychiat.*, 1920, **57**, 1.
416b. Jakob, A., *Z. ges. Neurol. Psychiat.*, 1921, **64**, 147.
417. Jacob, H., Eicher, W., Orthner, H., *Dtsch. Z. Nervenheilk*, 1958, **178**, 330.
418. Nevin, S., McMenemey, W. H., Behrman, S., Jones, D. P., *Brain*, 1960, **83**, 519.
418a. Heidenhain, A., *Z. ges. Neurol. Psychiat.*, 1929, **118**, 49.
419. Beck, E., Daniel, P. M., Mathews, W. B., Stevens, D. L., Alpers, M. P., Asher, D. M., Gajdusek, D. C., Gibbs, C. J., *Brain*, 1969, **92**, 699.
420. Klatzo, I., Gajdusek, D. C., Zigas, V., *Lab. Invest.*, 1959, **8**, 799.
420a. Bernoulli, C., Siegfried, J., Baumgartner, G., Regli, F., Rabinowicz, T., Gajdusek, D. C., Gibbs, C. J., Jr, *Lancet*, 1977, **1**, 478.
420b. Duffy, P., Wolf, J., Collins, G., De Voe, A. G., Streeten, B., Cowen, D., *New Engl. J. Med.*, 1974, **290**, 692.
421. Crompton, M. R., *Acta neuropath. (Berl.)*, 1968, **10**, 99.
422. Smith, W. T., in *Modern Trends in Neurology—5*, edited by D. Williams, page 111. London, 1970.
423. Gibbs, C. J., Gajdusek, D. C., *J. clin. Path.*, 1972, **25**, suppl. 6 (Roy. Coll. Path.), 132.
424. Hotchin, J., *Curr. Topics Microbiol. Immunol.*, 1967, **40**, 33.

DISEASES PRESUMPTIVELY OR POSSIBLY CAUSED BY VIRUSES

425. Economo, C. von, *Encephalitis Lethargica—Its Sequelae and Treatment*. London, 1931.
426. Buzzard, E. F., Greenfield, J. G., *Brain*, 1919, **13**, 305.
427. Medical Research Council: *The Sheffield Outbreak of Epidemic Encephalitis in 1924*, Spec. Rep. Ser. med. Res. Coun. (*Lond.*), No. 108, 1926.

428. Hall, A. J., *Epidemic Encephalitis*, page 3. Bristol, 1924.
429. Brown, E. L., Knox, E. G., *Lancet*, 1972, **1**, 974.
430. Hallervorden, J., *Dtsch. Z. Nervenheilk.*, 1935, **136**, 68.
431. Greenfield, J. G., Bosanquet, F. D., *J. Neurol. Neurosurg. Psychiat.*, 1953, **16**, 213.
432. McIntosh, J., *Brit. J. exp. Path.*, 1920, **1**, 257.
433. Levaditi, C., *L'Herpes et le zona*. Paris, 1926.
434. Bogaert, L. van, Radermecker, J., Devos, *Rev. neurol.*, 1955, **92**, 329.
435. Crawford, A. R., Robinson, F. L. J., *Brain*, 1957, **80**, 209.
436. Greenfield, J. G., *Brain*, 1950, **73**, 141.
437. Behçet, H., *Derm. Wschr.*, 1937, **105**, 1152.
437a. Rubinstein, L. J., Urich, H., *Brain*, 1963, **86**, 151.
438. Medical Staff of the Royal Free Hospital, *Brit. med. J.*, 1957, **2**, 895.
439. Geffen, D. H., Tracy, S. M., *Brit. med. J.*, 1957, **2**, 904.
440. Rhodes, A. J., Rooyen, C. E. van, *Textbook of Virology*, 5th edn, sect. 2, chap. 6. Baltimore, 1968.
441-450. *References revoked*.
451. Henle, W., Henle, G., in *Perspectives in Virology—VI*, edited by M. Pollard, chap. 7. New York, 1968.
452. Chanarin, I., Walford, D. M., *Lancet*, 1973, **2**, 238.
453. Dolgopol, V. B., Husson, G. S., *Arch. intern. Med.*, 1949, **83**, 179.
454. Bergin, J. D., *J. Neurol. Neurosurg. Psychiat.*, 1960, **23**, 69.
455. Mollaret, P., Reilly, J., Bastin, R., Tournier, P., *Presse méd.*, 1951, **59**, 681, 701.
456. Kalter, S. S., Kim, C. S., Heberling, R. L., *Nature (Lond.)*, 1969, **224**, 190.
457. Nieberg, K. C., Blumberg, J. M., in *Pathology of the Nervous System*, edited by J. Minckler, vol. 3, page 2308. New York, 1972.

CHLAMYDIAL INFECTIONS

458. Rhodes, A. J., Rooyen, C. E. van, *Textbook of Virology*, 5th edn, sect. 8, chap. 4. Baltimore, 1968.
459. Bedson, S. P., Western, G. T., Simpson, S. L., *Lancet*, 1930, **1**, 235, 345.
460. Walton, K. W., *J. Path. Bact.*, 1954, **68**, 565.
461. Yow, E. M., Brennan, J. C., Preston, J., Levy, S., *Amer. J. Med.*, 1959, **27**, 739.
462. D'Aunoy, R., Von Haam, E., *Arch. Path. (Chic.)*, 1939, **27**, 1032.

VASCULAR DISEASES OF THE CENTRAL NERVOUS SYSTEM

463. Batson, O. V., *Fed. Proc.*, 1944, **3**, 139.
464. Hutchinson, E. C., Yates, P. O., *Brain*, 1956, **79**, 319.
465. Brain, W. R., *Lancet*, 1957, **2**, 857.
466. Eecken, H. M. van der, *Anastomoses between the Leptomeningeal Arteries of the Brain: Their Morphological, Pathological and Clinical Significance*. Springfield, Illinois, 1959.
467. Meyer, J. S., Fang, H. C., Denny-Brown, D., *A.M.A. Arch. Neurol. Psychiat.*, 1954, **72**, 296.
468. Grashchenkov, N. I., Klosovskii, B. N., Kosmarskaia, E. N., Siskin, L. N., *A.M.A. Arch. intern. Med.*, 1960, **106**, 532.
469. Yates, P. O., Hutchinson, E. C., *Spec. Rep. Ser. med. Res. Coun. (Lond.)*, No. 300, 1961.
470. Carmichael, R., *J. Path. Bact.*, 1950, **62**, 1.
471. Garland, H., Greenberg, J., Harriman, D. G. F., *Brain*, 1966, **89**, 645.

472. Henson, R. A., Parsons, M., *Quart. J. Med.*, 1967, N.S. **36**, 205.

473. Leading Article, *Lancet*, 1967, **2**, 143.

474. Gillilan, L. A., *J. comp. Neurol.*, 1958, **110**, 75.

475. Moossy, J., *Neurology* (*Minneap.*), 1959, **9**, 569.

476. Young, W., Gofman, J. W., Malamud, N., Simon, A., Waters, E. S. G., *Geriatrics*, 1956, **11**, 413.

477. Moore, R. Foster, *Quart. J. Med.*, 1917, **10**, 29.

478. *Reference revoked.*

479. Brain, *Brit. med. J.*, 1963, **1**, 771.

480. Mitchell, J. R. A., Schwarz, C. J., *Arterial Disease*. Oxford, 1965.

481. Battacharji, S. K., Hutchinson, E. C., *Brain*, 1967, **90**, 747.

482. Ross Russell, R. W., in *Modern Trends in Neurology*—5, edited by D. Williams, chap. 10. London, 1970.

483. Maroon, J. C., Campbell, R. L., *J. Neurol. Neurosurg. Psychiat.*, 1969, **32**, 129.

484. Yates, P. O., *Lancet*, 1964, **1**, 65.

485. Bickerstaff, E. R., Holmes, J. M., *Brit. med. J.*, 1967, **1**, 726.

486. Altshuler, H. G., McLaughlin, R. A., Neubuerger, K. T., *Arch. Neurol.* (*Chic.*), 1968, **19**, 264.

487. Masi, A. T., Dugdale, M., *Ann. intern. Med.*, 1970, **72**, 111.

488. Jennett, W. B., Cross, J. N., *Lancet*, 1967, **1**, 1019.

489. Collaborative Group for the Study of Stroke in Young Women, *New Engl. J. Med.*, 1973, **288**, 871.

490. Kalbag, R. M., Woolf, A. L., *Cerebral Venous Thrombosis: with Special Reference to Primary Aseptic Thrombosis*. London, 1967.

491. Atkinson, E. A., Fairburn, B., Heathfield, K. W. G., *Lancet*, 1970, **1**, 914.

492. Poltera, A. A., *J. Path.*, 1972, **106**, 209.

493. Olszewski, J., *Wld Neurol.*, 1962, **3**, 359.

494. Smith, W. T., Whittaker, S. R. F., *J. clin. Path.*, 1963, **16**, 419.

495. Mair, W. G. P., Folkerts, J. F., *Brain*, 1953, **76**, 563.

496. Wildi, E., *Bull. schweiz. Akad. med. Wiss.*, 1959, **15**, 18.

496a. Charcot, J. M., Bouchard, C., *Arch. Physiol. norm. path.*, 1868, **1**, 110. 163.

497. Green, F. H. K., *J. Path. Bact.*, 1930, **33**, 71.

498. Zimmerman, H. M., *N.Y. St. J. Med.*, 1949, **49**, 2153.

499. Russell, R. W. Ross, *Brain*, 1963, **86**, 425.

500. Cole, F. M., Yates, P. O., *J. Neurol. Neurosurg. Psychiat.*, 1967, **30**, 61.

501. Cole, F. M., Yates, P. O., *Brain*, 1967, **90**, 759.

502. Cole, F. M., Yates, P. O., *J. Path. Bact.*, 1967, **93**, 393.

503. Cole, F. M., Yates, P. O., *Neurology* (*Minneap.*), 1968, **18**, 255.

504. Cooke, T. A., Yates, P. O., *J. Path.*, 1972, **108**, 119, 129.

505. Russell, D. S., *Proc. roy. Soc. Med.*, 1954, **47**, 689.

506. Okinaka, S., Kameyama, M., *Trans. Amer. neurol. Ass.*, 1960, **85**, 114.

507. Hassler, O., *Acta neurol. scand.*, 1962, **38**, 29.

508. De Villiers, J. C., *Brit. J. Psychiat.*, 1966, **112**, 109.

509. *Side Effects of Drugs—A Survey of Unwanted Effects of Drugs Reported in 1965–67*, edited by L. Meyler and A. Herxheimer, vol. 6, page 22. Amsterdam, 1968.

510. Eppinger, H., *Arch. klin. Chir.*, 1887, **35**, Suppl.-Heft, 1.

510a. Turnbull, H. M., *Brain*, 1918, **41**, 50.

511. Glynn, L. E., *J. Path. Bact.*, 1940, **51**, 213.

512. Meadows S. P., in *Modern Trends in Neurology*, edited by A. Feiling, page 391. London, 1951.

513. Stehbens, W. E., *Arch. Neurol.* (*Chic.*), 1963, **8**, 272.

514. Stehbens, W. E., *Arch. Path.*, 1963, **75**, 45.

515. Crawford, T., *J. Neurol. Neurosurg. Psychiat.*, 1959, **22**, 259.

516. Fearnsides, E. G., *Brain*, 1916, **39**, 224.

517. Ask-Upmark, E., Ingvar, D., *Acta med. scand.*, 1950, **138**, 15.

518. Hyland, H. H., *Arch. Neurol. Psychiat.* (*Chic.*), 1950, **63**, 61.

519. Walton, J. N., *Subarachnoid Haemorrhage*. Edinburgh and London, 1956.

520. Tomlinson, B. E., *J. clin. Path.*, 1959, **12**, 391.

521. Crompton, M. R., *J. Neurol. Neurosurg. Psychiat.*, 1962, **25**, 378.

522. Smith, B., *J. Neurol. Neurosurg. Psychiat.*, 1963, **26**, 535.

523. Schneck, S. A., *Neurology* (*Minneap.*), 1964, **14**, 691.

524. Crompton, M. R., *Brain*, 1964, **87**, 263.

525. Crompton, M. R., *Brain*, 1964, **87**, 491.

526. Buckell, M., *J. Neurol. Neurosurg. Psychiat.*, 1964, **27**, 198.

527. Raynor, R. B., McMurtry, J. G., Pool, J. L., *J. Neurosurg.*, 1963, **20**, 1.

528. Wolman, L., *Brain*, 1959, **82**, 276.

529. Scott, G. E., Neubuerger, K. T., Denst, J., *Neurology* (*Minneap.*), 1960, **10**, 22.

530. Spudis, E. V., Scharyj, M., Alexander, E., Martin, J. F., *Neurology* (*Minneap.*), 1962, **12**, 862.

531. Alexander, G. L., Norman, R. M., *The Sturge–Weber Syndrome*. Bristol, 1960.

531a. Weber, F. Parkes, *Rare Diseases and Some Debatable Subjects*, 2nd edn, page 9. London and New York, 1948.

531b. Sturge, W. A., *Trans. clin. Soc. Lond.*, 1879, **12**, 162.

531c. Kalischer, S., *Arch. Psychiat. Nervenheilk.*, 1901, **34**, 171.

532. Weber, F. Parkes, *Proc. roy. Soc. Med.*, 1928–29, **22**, 431.

533. Cobb, S., *Ann. Surg.*, 1915, **62**, 641.

534. Bruetsch, W. L., in *Pathology of the Nervous System*, edited by J. Minckler, vol. 2, chap. 109. New York, 1971.

535. Crompton, M. R., *Brain*, 1959, **82**, 377.

536. Foster, D. B., Malamud, N., *Univ. Mich. med. Bull.*, 1941, **7**, 102.

537. Lindenberg, R., Spatz, H., *Virchows Arch. path. Anat.*, 1939, **305**, 531.

538. Symmers, W. St C., *Brain*, 1956, **79**, 511.

539. Adams, R. D., Cammermeyer, J., Fitzgerald, P. J., *J. Neurol. Neurosurg. Psychiat.*, 1948, **11**, 27.

540. Byrom, F. B., *Lancet*, 1954, **2**, 20.

541. Byrom, F. B., *Lect. sci. Basis Med.*, 1958/59, **8**, 256.

542. Impastato, D. J., *Dis. nerv. Syst.*, 1957, **18**, suppl., 34.

543. Allen, I. M., *N.Z. med. J.*, 1959, **58**, 369.

EFFECTS OF TRAUMA

544. Courville, C. B., *Pathology of the Central Nervous System*, 3rd edn, page 248. Mountain View, California, 1950.

545. Tomlinson, B. E., in *Acute Injuries of the Head*, 4th edn, edited by G. F. Rowbotham, page 93. Edinburgh and London, 1964.

546. Sevitt, S., Stoner, H. B., *J. clin. Path.*, 1970, **23**, suppl. 4 (Roy. Coll. Path.), 150.

547. Strich, S. J., in *The Late Effects of Head Injury*, edited by A. E. Walker, W. F. Caveness and M. Critchley, page 501. Springfield, Illinois, 1969.
548. Adams, H., Graham, D. I., in *Scientific Foundations of Neurology*, edited by M. Critchley, J. L. O'Leary and B. Jennett, sect. 10, chap. 6. London, 1972.
549. Gurdjian, E. S., Webster, J. E., *Ass. Res. nerv. Dis. Proc.*, 1945, **24**, 48.
550. Russell, W. R., *Brain*, 1932, **55**, 549.
551. Denny-Brown, D., Russell, W. R., *Brain*, 1941, **64**, 93.
552. Gurdjian, E. S., Webster, J. E., Lissner, H. R., *Surg. Gynec. Obstet.*, 1945, **81**, 679.
553. Windle, W. F., Groat, R. A., Fox, C. A., *Surg. Gynec. Obstet.*, 1944, **79**, 561.
554. Strich, S. J., *J. Neurol. Neurosurg. Psychiat.*, 1956, **19**, 163.
555. Strich, S. J., *Lancet*, 1961, **2**, 443.
556. Oppenheimer, D. R., *J. Neurol. Neurosurg. Psychiat.*, 1968, **31**, 299.
557. Strich, S. J., *J. clin. Path.*, 1970, **23**, suppl. 4 (Roy. Coll. Path.), 166.
558. Pudenz, R. H., Shelden, C. H., *J. Neurosurg.*, 1946, **3**, 487.
559. Holbourn, A. H. S., *Lancet*, 1943, **2**, 438.
560. Holbourn, A. H. S., *Lancet*, 1944, **1**, 483.
561. Ommaya, A. K., Faas, F., Yarnell, P., *J. Amer. med. Ass.*, 1968, **204**, 285.
562. Unterharnscheidt, F., Higgins, L. S., *Tex. Rep. Biol. Med.*, 1969, **27**, 127.
563. Lindenberg, R., Freytag, E., *A.M.A. Arch. Path.*, 1960, **69**, 440.
564. Jefferson, G., *Glasg. med. J.*, 1942, **20**, 77.
565. Del Río Hortega, P., Penfield, W. G., *Bull. Johns Hopk. Hosp.*, 1927, **41**, 278.
566. Nevin, N. C., *J. Neuropath. exp. Neurol.*, 1967, **26**, 77.
567. Peerless, S. J., Rewcastle, N. B., *J. Canad. med. Ass.*, 1967, **96**, 577.
568. Daniel, P. M., Strich, S. J., *Acta neuropath. (Berl.)*, 1969, **12**, 314.
569. Bignami, A., Ralston, J. H., *Brain Res.*, 1969, **13**, 444.
570. Gurdjian, E. S., Webster, J. E., Arnkoff, H., *Surgery*, 1943, **13**, 333.
571. Naffziger, H. C., *J. Amer. med. Ass.*, 1924, **82**, 1751.
572. Abbott, W. D., Due, F. O., Nosik, W. A., *J. Amer. med. Ass.*, 1943, **121**, 664.
573. Tomlinson, B. E., *J. clin. Path.*, 1970, **23**, suppl. 4 (Roy. Coll. Path.), 154.
574. Lund, O. E., *Dtsch. med. Wschr.*, 1956, **81**, 968.
575. Benda, C. E., Hoessly, G.-F., in *Proceedings of the Second International Congress of Neuropathology, London, 1955*, part 1, page 455. Amsterdam, 1955.
576. Corsellis, J. A. N., Bruton, C. J., Freeman-Browne, D., *Psychol. Med.*, 1973, **3**, 270.
577. Klatzo, I., Piraux, A., Laskowski, E. J., *J. Neuropath. exp. Neurol.*, 1958, **17**, 548.
578. Klatzo, I., *J. Neuropath. exp. Neurol.*, 1967, **26**, 1.
579. Emery, J. L., Reid, D. A. C., *Brit. J. Surg.*, 1962–63, **50**, 53.
580. Haynes, B. W., Bright, R., *J. Trauma*, 1967, **7**, 464.
581. Treip, C. S., *J. clin. Path.*, 1970, **23**, suppl. 4 (Roy. Coll. Path.), 178.
582. Sevitt, S., *Fat Embolism*. London, 1962.
583. *Pathology of Injury—The Report of a Working Party of the Royal College of Pathologists*, edited by A. C. Hunt. London, 1972.
584. Scott, G. B. D., Gracey, L. R. H., *Arch. Path.*, 1969, **87**, 643.
585. Sevitt, S., *Lancet*, 1960, **2**, 825.
586. Szabo, Gy., *J. clin. Path.*, 1970, **23**, suppl. 4 (Roy. Coll. Path.), 123.
587. Hansen, O. H., *Acta chir. scand.*, 1969, **136**, 161.
588. Jennett, W. G., *J. clin. Path.*, 1970, **23**, suppl. 4 (Roy. Coll. Path.), 172.
589. Graham, D. I., Adams, J. H., *Lancet*, 1971, **1**, 265.
590. Zeman, W., in *Pathology of the Nervous System*, edited by J. Minckler, vol. 1, chap. 65. New York, 1968.
591. Pennybacker, J., Russell, D. S., *J. Neurol. Neurosurg. Psychiat.*, 1948, **11**, 183.
592. Russell, D. S., Wilson, C. W., Tansley, K., *J. Neurol. Neurosurg. Psychiat.*, 1949, **12**, 187.
593. Zeman, W., in *Pathology of the Nervous System*, edited by J. Minckler, vol. 1, chap. 66. New York, 1968.
594. Malamud, N., Haymaker, W., Custer, R. P., *Milit. Surg.*, 1946, **99**, 397.
595. Sevitt, S., *Burns—Pathology and Therapeutic Applications*. London, 1957.
596. Warlow, C. P., Hinton, P., *Lancet*, 1969, **2**, 978.
597. Zeman, W., in *Pathology of the Nervous System*, edited by J. Minckler, vol. 1, chap. 68. New York, 1968.
598. Nelson, E., Lindstrom, P. A., Haymaker, W., *J. Neuropath. exp. Neurol.*, 1959, **18**, 489.
599. *Pathology of Injury—The Report of a Working Party of the Royal College of Pathologists*, edited by A. C. Hunt, chap. 5. London, 1972.
600. Hughes, J. T., *Pathology of the Spinal Cord*. London, 1966.
601. Wilkinson, M., *Cervical Spondylosis*, 2nd edn. London, 1971.
602. Clarke, E., Robinson, P. K., *Brain*, 1956, **79**, 483.
603. Mair, W. G. P., Druckman, R., *Brain*, 1953, **76**, 70.

DEVELOPMENTAL ANOMALIES
604. Urich, H., in *Greenfield's Neuropathology*, 3rd edn, edited by W. Blackwood and J. A. N. Corsellis, chap. 10. London, 1976.
605. *Congenital Malformations*, edited by G. E. W. Wolstenholme and C. M. O'Connor. London, 1960.
606. Crome, L., Stern, J., *The Pathology of Mental Retardation*, 2nd edn. London, 1972.
607. Towbin, A., in *Pathology of the Nervous System*, edited by J. Minckler, vol. 2, chap. 139. New York, 1971.
608. Willis, R. A., *The Borderland of Embryology and Pathology*, 2nd edn, chap. 6. London, 1962.
609. Hicks, S. P., *Physiol. Rev.*, 1958, **38**, 337.
610. Fritz-Niggli, H., *Strahlenbiologie*, chap. 6. Stuttgart, 1959.
611. Crome, L. I., *Wld Neurol.*, 1961, **2**, 447.
612. Diezel, P. B., *Virchows Arch. path. Anat.*, 1954, **325**, 109.
613. Crome, L., France, N. E., *J. clin. Path.*, 1959, **12**, 427.
614. Lenz, W., *Amer. J. Dis. Child.*, 1966, **112**, 99.
614a. *Deformities Caused by Thalidomide*, *Rep. publ. Hlth med. Subj.*, No. 112. London, 1964.
615. Symmers, W. St C., *personal communication*, 1974.
616. Yakovlev, P. I., Wadsworth, R. C., *J. Neuropath. exp. Neurol.*, 1946, **5**, 116, 169.
617. Dandy, W. E., Blackfan, K. D., *J. Amer. med. Ass.*, 1913, **61**, 2216.

618. Dandy, W. E., Blackfan, K. D., *Amer. J. Dis. Child.*, 1914, **8**, 406.

619. Russell, D. S., *Spec. Rep. Ser. med. Res. Coun.* (*Lond.*), No. 265. London, 1949.

620. Davson, H., *Physiology of the Cerebrospinal Fluid.* Boston, 1967.

620a. Millen, J. W., Woollam, D. H. M., *The Anatomy of the Cerebrospinal Fluid*, page 116. London, New York and Toronto, 1962.

620b. Pacchioni, A., *Dissertatio epistolaris ad Lucam Schroekium de glandulis conglobatis durae meningis humanae.* Romae, 1705.

621. Urich, H., in *Greenfield's Neuropathology*, edited by W. Blackwood and J. A. N. Corsellis, 3rd edn, page 372. London, 1976.

622. Cameron, A. H., *J. Path. Bact.*, 1957, **73**, 213.

623. Daniel, P. M., Strich, S. J., *J. Neuropath. exp. Neurol.*, 1958, **17**, 255.

624. Russell, D. S., Donald, C., *Brain*, 1935, **58**, 203.

625. Daniel, P. M., Strich, S. J., *J. Neuropath. exp. Neurol.*, 1958, **17**, 255.

626. Ingraham, F. D., Scott, H. W., *New Engl. J. Med.*, 1943, **229**, 108.

627. Russell, D. S., *Spec. Rep. Ser. med. Res. Coun.* (*Lond.*), No. 265, page 14. London, 1949.

628. Bickers, D. S., Adams, R. D., *Brain*, 1949, **72**, 246.

629. Ariëns Kappers, J., in *The Cerebrospinal Fluid*, edited by G. E. W. Wolstenholme and C. M. O'Connor, page 29. London, 1958.

630. Woolam, D. H. M., Millen, J .W., *Brain*, 1953, **76**, 104.

631. Taggart, J. K., Walker, A. E., *Arch. Neurol. Psychiat.* (*Chic.*), 1942, **48**, 583.

632. Maloney, A. F. J., *J. Neurol. Neurosurg. Psychiat.*, 1954, **17**, 134.

633. Sutton, J. B., *Brain*, 1887, **9**, 352.

634. Schmidt, H., Fischer, E., *Die okzipitale Dysplasie.* Stuttgart, 1960.

634a. Klippel, M., Feil, A., *Nouv. Iconogr. Salpêt.*, 1912, **25**, 223.

635. Willis, R. A., *The Borderland of Embryology and Pathology*, 2nd edn, page 156. London, 1962.

635a. Rokos, J., *J. Path.*, 1975, **117**, 155.

635b. Rokos, J., *J. Neuropath. appl. Neurobiol.*, 1976, **2**, 111.

636. Renwick, J. H., *Brit. J. prev. soc. Med.*, 1972, **26**, 67.

637. Bournville, D. M., *Arch. Neurol.* (*Paris*), 1880, **1**, 69.

638. Critchley, M., Earl, C. J. C., *Brain*, 1932, **55**, 311.

638a. Stewart, R. M., *Brit. med. J.*, 1935, **2**, 60.

639. Moolten, S. E., *Arch. intern. Med.*, 1942, **69**, 589.

640. Willis, R. A., *The Borderland between Embryology and Pathology*, 2nd edn, page 365. London, 1962.

641. Wishart, J. H., *Edinb. med. surg. J.*, 1822, **18**, 393.

641a. Krishnan, K. R., Smith, W. T., *J. Neurol. Neurosurg. Psychiat.*, 1961, **24**, 350.

642. Gardner, W. J., *J. Neurol. Neurosurg. Psychiat.*, 1965, **28**, 247.

643. Hankinson, J., in *Modern Trends in Neurology—5*, edited by D. Williams, chap. 7. London, 1970.

644. Down, J. L., *Lond. Hosp. clin. Lect. Rep.*, 1866, **3**, 224, 259.

644a. Benda, C. E., in *Pathology of the Nervous System*, edited by J. Minckler, vol. 2, chap. 97. New York, 1971.

644b. Hamerton, J. L., Giannelli, F., Polani, P. E., *Cytogenetics*, 1965, **4**, 171.

644c. Giannelli, F., Hamerton, J. L., Carter, C. O., *Cytogenetics*, 1965, **4**, 186.

644d. Polani, P. E., Hamerton, J. L., Giannelli, F., Carter, C. O., *Cytogenetics*, 1965, **4**, 193.

645. Carter, C. O., Hamerton, J. L., Polani, P. E., Gunalp, A., Weller, S. D. G., *Lancet*, 1960, **2**, 678.

646. Penrose, L. S., *Proc. roy. Soc. Med.*, 1961, **54**, 671.

647. Hamerton, J. L., Briggs, S. M., Giannelli, F., Carter, C. O., *Lancet*, 1961, **2**, 788.

648. Hall, B., *Lancet*, 1962, **2**, 1026.

649. Urich, H., in *Greenfield's Neuropathology*, 3rd edn, edited by W. Blackwood and J. A. N. Corsellis, page 420. London, 1976.

650. Smith, W. T., in *Modern Trends in Neurology—5*, edited by D. Williams, page 98. London, 1970.

651. Olson, M., Shaw, Cheng-Mei, *Brain*, 1969, **92**, 147.

652. Malamud, N., in *Mental Retardation*, edited by H. A. Stevens and R. Lever. Chicago, 1964.

653. Levinson, A., Friedman, A., Stamps, F., *Pediatrics*, 1955, **16**, 43.

654. Crome, L., Stern, J., *The Pathology of Mental Retardation*, 2nd edn. London, 1972.

PRIMARY TUMOURS

655. Russell, D. S., Rubinstein, L. J., *Pathology of Tumours of the Nervous System*, 4th edn. London, 1977.

656. Zülch, K. J., *Brain Tumours*, 2nd edn. New York, 1965.

657. Rubinstein, L. J., quoted in *Pathology of Tumours of the Nervous System*, by D. S. Russell and L. J. Rubinstein, 4th edn, page 227. London, 1977.

658. Rosenthal, W., *Beitr. path. Anat.*, 1898, **23**, 111.

658a. Herndon, R. M., Rubinstein, L. J., Freeman, J. M., Mathieson, G., *J. Neuropath. exp. Neurol.*, 1970, **29**, 524.

659. Russell, D. S., Bland, J. O. W., *J. Path. Bact.*, 1934, **39**, 375.

660. Kernohan, J. W., Mabon, R. F., Svien, H. J., Adson, A. W., *Proc. Mayo Clin.*, 1949, **24**, 71.

661. Bailey, P., Cushing, H., *A Classification of Tumors of the Glioma Group.* Philadelphia, 1926.

662. Russell, D. S., Rubinstein, L. J., *Pathology of Tumours of the Nervous System*, 4th edn, page 191. London, 1977.

663. Russell, S. D., in *Proceedings of the Second International Congress of Neuropathology, London, 1955*, part 1, page 259. Amsterdam, 1955.

664. Barnard, R. O., *J. Path. Bact.*, 1968, **96**, 113.

665. Russell, D. S., Rubinstein, L. J., *Pathology of Tumours of the Nervous System*, 4th edn, page 204. London, 1977.

666. Chason, J. L., *J. Neuropath. exp. Neurol.*, 1956, **15**, 461.

667. Kernohan, J. W., Mabon, R. F., Svien, H. J., Adson, A. W., *Proc. Mayo Clin.*, 1949, **24**, 71.

667a. Svien, H. J., Mabon, R. F., Kernohan, J. W., Adson, A. W., *Proc. Mayo Clin.*, 1949, **24**, 54.

668. Seligman, A. M., Shear, M. J., Alexander, L., *Amer. J. Cancer*, 1939, **37**, 364.

669. Zimmerman, H. M., *Amer. J. Path.*, 1955, **31**, 1.

670. Willis, R. A., *Pathology of Tumours*, 4th edn, page 38. London, 1967.

671. Oberling, C., Guérin, M., Guérin, P., *C.R. Soc. Biol.* (*Paris*), 1936, **123**, 1152.

672. Druckrey, H., Ivanković, S., Preussmann, R., *Z. Krebsforsch.*, 1965, **66**, 389.

673. Jones, E. L., Searle, C. E., Smith, W. T., *J. Path.*, 1973, **109**, 123.

674. Oppenheimer, D. C., *J. Neurol. Neurosurg. Psychiat.*, 1955, **18**, 199.

675. Courville, C. B., *Arch. Neurol. Psychiat. (Chic.)*, 1930, **24**, 439.

676. Christensen, E., in *Proceedings of the Second International Congress of Neuropathology, London, 1955*, part 1, page 243. Amsterdam, 1955.

677. Kadin, M. E., Rubinstein, L. J., Nelson, J. S., *J. Neuropath. exp. Neurol.*, 1970, **29**, 583.

677a. Jones, E. L., Searle, C. E., Smith, W. T., *Acta neuropath. (Berl.)*, 1976, **36**, 57.

678. Bratton, A. B., Robinson, S. H. G., *J. Path. Bact.*, 1946, **58**, 643.

679. Russell, D. S., Rubinstein, L. J., *Pathology of Tumours of the Nervous System*, 4th edn, page 255. London, 1977.

680. Makeever, L. C., King, J. D., *Amer. J. clin. Path.*, 1966, **46**, 245.

681. Bickerstaff, E. R., Small, J. M., Guest, I. A., *J. Neurol. Neurosurg. Psychiat.*, 1958, **21**, 89.

682. Rosendo, A. G., Oliveras, C., Ley, A., in *Proceedings of the Second International Congress of Neuropathology, London, 1955*, part 1, page 113. Amsterdam, 1955.

683. Lindau, A., *Acta path. microbiol. scand.*, 1926, suppl. 1.

684. Hippel, E. von, *Albrecht v. Graefes Arch. Ophthal.*, 1904, **59**, 83.

685. Russell, D. S., Marshall, A. H. E., Smith, F. B., *Brain*, 1948, **71**, 1.

686. Adams, J. H., Jackson, J. M., *J. Path. Bact.*, 1966, **91**, 369.

687. Russell, D. S., Rubinstein, L. J., *Pathology of Tumours of the Nervous System*, 4th edn, page 106. London, 1977.

687a. Schneck, S. A., Penn, I., *Lancet*, 1971, **1**, 983.

687b. Marshall, G., Roessmann, U., Noort, S. van den, *Cancer (Philad.)*, 1968, **22**, 621.

687c. Brazinsky, J. H., *J. Neurosurg.*, 1973, **38**, 635.

687d. John, H. T., Nabarro, J. D. N., *Brit. J. Cancer*, 1955, **9**, 386.

METASTATIC TUMOURS

688. Willis, R. A., *The Spread of Tumours in the Human Body*, 2nd edn, chap. 25. London, 1952.

689. Halpert, B., Erickson, E. E., Fields, W. S., *A.M.A. Arch. Path.*, 1960, **69**, 93.

690. Kernohan, J. W., Sayre, G. P., in *Cancer*, edited by R. W. Raven, vol. 2, chap. 27. London, 1958.

691. Meyer, P. C., Reah, T. G., *Brit. J. Cancer*, 1953, **7**, 438.

692. Symmers, W. St C., *personal communication*, 1960.

693. Fischer-Williams, M., Bosanquet, F. D., Daniel, P. M., *Brain*, 1955, **78**, 42.

694. Madow, L., Alpers, B. J., *Arch. Neurol. Psychiat. (Chic.)*, 1951, **65**, 161.

MISCELLANEOUS NEOPLASMS AND CYSTS OF DEVELOPMENTAL ORIGIN

695. Ariëns Kappers, J., *J. comp. Neurol.*, 1955, **102**, 425.

696. Müller, H., *Z. rat. Med.*, 1858, **2**, 202.

696a. Schmorl, C. G., *Verh. dtsch. orthop. Ges.*, 1926, **21**, 3.

697. Cappell, D. F., *J. Path. Bact.*, 1928, **31**, 797.

697a. Harvey, W. F., Dawson, E. K., *Edinb. med. J.*, 1941, **48**, 713.

697b. Virchow, R., *Untersuchungen ueber die Entwickelung des Schädelgrundes*. Berlin, 1857.

698. Crawford, T., *J. clin. Path.*, 1958, **11**, 110.

699. Smith, W. T., in *The Pathological Basis of Medicine*, edited by R. C. Curran and D. G. Harnden, chap. 55. London, 1972.

700. Miller, D., Adams, H., in *Scientific Foundations of Neurology*, edited by M. Critchley, J. L. O'Leary and B. Jennett, sect. 8, chap. 5. London, 1972.

701. Kernohan, J. W., Woltman, H. W., *Arch. Neurol. Psychiat. (Chic.)*, 1929, **21**, 274.

702. Corsellis, J. A. N., *J. Neurol. Neurosurg. Psychiat.*, 1958, **21**, 279.

703. Yates, P. O., in *Greenfield's Neuropathology*, 3rd edn, edited by W. Blackwood and J. A. N. Corsellis, page 121. London, 1976.

704. Wolman, L., *J. Path. Bact.*, 1956, **72**, 575.

INBORN ERRORS OF METABOLISM

705. Garrod, A. E., *Lancet*, 1908, **2**, 1, 73, 142, 214.

706. Garrod, A. E., *Inborn Errors of Metabolism*, 2nd edn, page 193. London, 1923.

707. Meckel, J. F., *Handbuch der pathologischen Anatomie*, vol. 2, part 2, page 3. Leipzig, 1816.

708. Mansfeldt, H., *Arch. Anat. Physiol.*, 1826, **1**, 96.

709. Poser, C. M., in *Pathology of the Nervous System*, edited by J. Minckler, vol. 1, chap. 60. New York, 1968.

709a. Bielschowsky, M., Henneberg, R., *J. Psychol. Neurol. (Lpz.)*, 1928, **36**, 131.

710. Seitelberger, F., in *Modern Scientific Aspects of Neurology*, edited by J. N. Cumings, page 178. London, 1960.

710a. Merzbacher, L., *Med. Klin.*, 1908, **4**, 1952.

710b. Pelizaeus, F., *Arch. Psychiat. Nervenkr.*, 1885, **16**, 698.

711. Tyler, H. R., *A.M.A. Arch. Neurol. Psychiat.*, 1958, **80**, 162.

712. Krabbe, K. H., *Brain*, 1916, **39**, 74.

713. Austin, J. H., in *Pathology of the Nervous System*, edited by J. Minckler, vol. 1, chap. 62. New York, 1968.

714. Blackwood, W., in *Proceedings of the First International Congress of Neuropathology, Rome, 1952*, page 265. Amsterdam, 1952.

715. Crome, L., Stern, J., in *Greenfield's Neuropathology*, 3rd edn, edited by W. Blackwood and J. A. N. Corsellis, page 547. London, 1976.

716. Diezel, P. B., in *Cerebral Lipidoses*, edited by J. N. Cumings, page 63. Oxford, 1957.

717. Hager, H., Oehlert, W., *Méd. et Hyg. (Genève)*, 1958, **16**, 84.

718. Lichtenstein, B. W., Rosenbluth, P. R., *J. Neuropath. exp. Neurol.*, 1959, **18**, 384.

719. Menkes, J. H., Duncan, C., Moossy, J., *Neurology (Minneap.)*, 1966, **16**, 581.

720. Bachhawat, B. K., Austin, J., Armstrong, D., *Biochem. J.*, 1967, **104**, 15C.

721. Suzuki, Y., Suzuki, K., *J. biol. Chem.*, 1974, **249**, 2105.

721a. Austin, J. H., in *Proceedings of the Fourth International Congress of Neuropathology, Stuttgart, 1962*, edited by H. Jacob, vol. 1, page 35. Stuttgart, 1962.

722. Scholz, W., *Z. Neurol. Psychiat.*, 1925, **99**, 651.

723. Hirsch, T. von, Peiffer, J., *Arch. Psychiat. Nervenkr.*, 1955, **194**, 88.

724. Thomas, G. H., Howell, R. R., *Selected Screening Tests for Genetic Metabolic Diseases.* Chicago, 1973.

725. Bogaert, L. van, Scholz, W., *Z. ges. Neurol. Psychiat.*, 1932, **141**, 510.

726. Greenfield, J. G., *J. Neurol. Psychopath.*, 1933, **13**, 292.

727. Bertrand, I., Thieffry, S., Bargeton, E., *Rev. neurol.*, 1954, **91**, 161.

728. Hagberg, B., Sourander, P., Svennerholm, L., Voss, H., *Acta paediat. (Uppsala)*, 1960, **49**, 135.

729. Brain, W. R., Greenfield, J. G., *Brain*, 1950, **73**, 291.

730. Hagberg, B., Sourander, P., Thoren, L., *Acta paediat. (Uppsala)*, 1962, suppl. 135, 63.

731. Austin, J. H., *Neurology (Minneap.)*, 1957, **7**, 415.

732. Norman, R. M., *Brain*, 1947, **70**, 234.

733. Pfeiffer, J., *Arch. Psychiat. Nervenkr.*, 1959, **199**, 386.

734. Alexander, W. S., *Brain*, 1949, **72**, 373.

735. Friede, R. L., *Arch. Neurol. (Chic.)*, 1964, **11**, 414.

736. Canavan, M. M., *Arch. Neurol. Psychiat. (Chic.)*, 1931, **25**, 299.

737. Cumings, J. N., in *Cerebral Lipidoses*, edited by J. N. Cumings, page 115. Oxford, 1957.

738. Bogaert, L. van, *Proceedings of the London Conference for the Scientific Study of Mental Deficiency*, vol. 2, page 444. London, 1962.

739. Brain, W. R., in *Proceedings of the Fifth International Congress of Neurology, Lisbon, 1953*, vol. 1, page 263. Amsterdam, 1953.

739a. *Lysosomes and Storage Diseases*, edited by H. G. Hers and F. van Hoof. New York and London, 1973.

739b. Crome, L., Stern, J., in *Greenfield's Neuropathology*, 3rd edn, edited by W. Blackwood and J. A. N. Corsellis, chap. 12. London, 1976.

739c. Hug, G., in *The Liver*, edited by E. A. Gall and F. K. Mostofi, page 48. Baltimore, 1973.

740. Diezel, P. B., in *Modern Scientific Aspects of Neurology*, edited by J. N. Cumings, page 99. London, 1960.

741. Tay, W., *Trans. ophthal. Soc. U.K.*, 1881, **1**, 55.

742. Sachs, B., *J. nerv. ment. Dis.*, 1887, **14**, 566.

743. Greenfield, J. G., *Proc. roy. Soc. Med.*, 1951, **44**, 686.

744. Steegman, T., Karnosh, L. J., *Amer. J. Psychiat.*, 1936, **92**, 1413.

745. Klenk, E., *Wien. Z. Nervenheilk.*, 1957, **13**, 309.

746. Svennerholm, L., in *Cerebral Lipidoses*, edited by J. N. Cumings, page 144. Oxford, 1957.

747. Norman, R. M., Wood, N., *J. Neurol. Psychiat.*, 1941, **4**, 175.

748. Bielschowsky, M., *Z. ges. Neurol. Psychiat., Orig.*, 1914, **26**, 133.

749. Batten, F. E., *Brain*, 1903, **26**, 147.

749a. Mayou, M. S., *Trans. ophthal. Soc. U.K.*, 1904, **24**, 142.

749b. Vogt, H., *Mschr. Psychiat. Neurol.*, 1905, **18**, 161, 310.

749c. Spielmeyer, W., *Neurol. Cbl.*, 1905, **24**, 51.

750. Kufs, H., *Z. ges. Neurol. Psychiat.*, 1925, **95**, 169.

750a. Zeman, W., *J. Neuropath. exp. Neurol.*, 1974, **33**, 1.

750b. Zeman, W., Siakotos, A. N., in *Lysosomes and Storage Diseases*, edited by H. G. Hers and F. van Hoof, page 519. New York and London, 1973.

751. Eastham, R. D., Jancar, J., *Clinical Pathology in Mental Retardation*, page 113. Bristol, 1968.

752. Aronson, S. M., Perle, G., Saifer, A., Volk, B. W., *Proc. Soc. exp. Biol. (N.Y.)*, 1962, **111**, 664.

753. Niemann, A., *Jb. Kinderheilk.*, 1914, **79**, 1.

753a. Pick, L., *Ergebn. inn. Med. Kinderheilk.*, 1926, **29**, 520.

753b. Crocker, A. C., Farber, S., *Medicine (Baltimore)*, 1958, **37**, 1.

754. Diezel, P. B., in *Modern Aspects of Neurology*, edited by J. N. Cumings, page 117. London, 1960.

755. Diezel, P. B., in *Cerebral Lipidoses*, edited by J. N. Cumings, page 11. Oxford, 1957.

756. Hsia, D. Y.-Y., Naylor, J., Bigler, J. A., in *Cerebral Sphingolipidosis*, edited by S. M. Aronson and B. W. Volk, page 327. New York and London, 1962.

757. Hunter, C., *Proc. roy. Soc. Med.*, 1917, **10**, 104.

758. Hurler, G., *Z. Kinderheilk.*, 1919, **24**, 222.

759. Brante, G., in *Cerebral Lipidoses*, edited by J. N. Cumings, page 164. Oxford, 1957.

759a. Pfaundler, M., *Jb. Kinderheilk.*, 1920, **92**, 421.

759b. Ellis, R. W., Sheldon, W., Capon, N. B., *Quart. J. Med.*, 1936, N. S. **5**, 119.

760. Dawson, I. M. P., *J. Path. Bact.*, 1954, **67**, 587.

761. Eastham, R. D., Jancar, J., *Clinical Pathology in Mental Retardation*, page 184. Bristol, 1968.

762. Diezel, P. B., in *Modern Scientific Aspects of Neurology*, edited by J. N. Cumings, page 130. London, 1960.

763. Crome, L., Stern, J., in *Greenfield's Neuropathology*, 3rd edn, edited by W. Blackwood and J. A. N. Corsellis, page 523. London, 1976.

764. Feigin, I., *J. Neuropath. exp. Neurol.*, 1956, **15**, 400.

765. Fabry, J., *Arch. Derm. Syph. (Wien u. Lpz.)*, 1898, **43**, 187.

765a. Anderson, W., *Brit. J. Derm.*, 1898, **10**, 113.

766. Scriba, K., *Verh. dtsch. ges. Path.*, 1951, **34**, 221.

767. Wise, D., Wallace, H. J., Jellinek, E. H., *Quart. J. Med.*, 1962, N.S. **31**, 177.

767a. Rahman, A. N., Lindenberg, R., *Arch. Neurol. (Chic.)*, 1963, **9**, 373.

768. Pompe, J.-C., *Ann. Anat. path.*, 1933, **10**, 23.

769. Hers, H. G., *Biochem. J.*, 1963, **86**, 11.

770. Fölling, A., *Hoppe-Seylers Z. physiol. Chem.*, 1934, **227**, 169.

771. Harris, H., *Human Biochemical Genetics*, page 36. Cambridge, 1959.

772. Woolf, L. I., Griffiths, R., Moncrieff, A., *Brit. med. J.*, 1955, **1**, 57.

773. Jepson, J. B., in *The Metabolic Basis of Inherited Disease*, 2nd edn, edited by J. B. Stanbury, J. B. Wyngaarden and D. S. Frederickson, page 1283. New York, 1966.

774. Baron, D. N., Dent, C. E., Harris, H., Hart, E. W., Jepson, J. B., *Lancet*, 1956, **2**, 421.

775. Milne, M. D., Crawford, M. A., Girão, C. B., Loughridge, L. W., *Quart. J. Med.*, 1960, N.S. **29**, 407.

776. Milne, M. D., in *Biochemical Disorders in Human Disease*, 3rd edn, edited by R. H. S. Thompson and I. D. P. Wootton, page 594. London, 1970.

777. Jonxis, J. H. P., *Ned. T. Geneesk.*, 1957, **101**, 569.

778. Lowe, C. U., Terrey, M., MacLachlan, E. A., *A.M.A. Amer. J. Dis. Child.*, 1952, **83**, 164.

779. Lowe, C. U., *Maandschr. Kindergeneesk.*, 1960, **28**, 77.

780. Crome, L., Duckett, S., Franklin, A. W., *Arch. Dis. Childh.*, 1963, **38**, 505.

781. Snyderman, S. E., *Amer. J. Dis. Child.*, 1967, **113**, 68.

782. Crome, L., Dutton, G., Ross, C. F., *J. Path. Bact.*, 1961, **81**, 379.

783. Menkes, J. H., in *Pathology of the Nervous System*, edited by J. Minckler, vol. 2, chap. 90. New York, 1971.

784. Eastham, R. D., Jancar, J., *Clinical Pathology in Mental Retardation*, chap. 3. Bristol, 1968.

785. Levin, B., *Amer. J. Dis. Child.*, 1967, **113**, 162.

786. Ghadimi, H., Partington, M. W., *Amer. J. Dis. Child.*, 1967, **113**, 93.

787. McKusick, V. A., *Heritable Disorders of Connective Tissue*, 3rd edn, chap. 4. St Louis, 1966.

788. Mudd, S. H., Finkelstein, J. D., Irreverre, F., Laster, L., *Science*, 1964, **143**, 1443.

789. Wilson, S. A. Kinnier, *Brain*, 1912, **34**, 295.

789a. Kayser, B., *Klin. Mbl. Augenheilk.*, 1902, **40**, 22.

789b. Fleischer, B., *Klin. Mbl. Augenheilk.*, 1903, **41**, 489.

790. Bearn, A. G., *Ann. hum. Genet.*, 1960, **24**, 33.

791. Hösslin, C. von, Alzheimer, A., *Z. ges. Neurol. Psychiat.*, 1912, **8**, 183.

792. Opalski, A., *Z. ges. Neurol. Psychiat.*, 1930, **124**, 140.

793. Smith, W. T., in *Greenfield's Neuropathology*, 3rd edn, edited by W. Blackwood and J. A. N. Corsellis, page 172. London, 1976.

794. Holmberg, C. G., Laurell, C. B., *Acta chem. scand.*, 1948, **2**, 550.

795. Walshe, J. M., *A.M.A. Arch. intern. Med.*, 1959, **103**, 155.

796. Harris, H., *Human Biochemical Genetics*, page 108. Cambridge, 1959.

797. Crome, L., *Arch. Dis. Childh.*, 1962, **37**, 415.

798. Günther, H., *Dtsch. Arch. klin. Med.*, 1912, **105**, 89.

798a. Waldenström, J., *Amer. J. Med.*, 1957, **22**, 758.

799. Goldberg, A., Rimington, C., *The Diseases of Porphyrin Metabolism*, page 14. Springfield, Illinois, 1962.

799a. Barnes, H. D., *S. Afr. med. J.*, 1959, **33**, 274.

800. Eales, L., *S. Afr. J. Lab. clin. Med.*, 1963, **9**, 143.

801. Hallervorden, J., Spatz, H., *Z. ges. Neurol. Psychiat.*, 1922, **79**, 254.

802. Seitelberger, F., in *Pathology of the Nervous System*, edited by J. Minckler, vol. 2, chap. 94. New York, 1971.

803. Jellinger, K., in *Progress in Neuropathology*, edited by H. M. Zimmerman, vol. 2, chap. 6. New York, 1973.

804. Seitelberger, F., in *Cerebral Lipidoses*, edited by J. N. Cumings, page 44. Oxford, 1957.

805. Rubinowicz, T., Wildi, E., in *Cerebral Lipidoses*, edited by J. N. Cumings, page 34. Oxford, 1957.

806. Unverricht, J., *Die Myoklonie*, Leipzig, 1891. [A clinical account of five affected siblings in a family of ten. No pathological studies were included.]

806a. Lafora, G. R., *Virchows Arch. path. Anat.*, 1911, **205**, 295.

806b. Lafora, G., *Rev. neurol.*, 1923, **2**, 399.

807. Lafora, G. R., *Trab. Lab. Invest. biol. Univ. Madrid*, 1913, **11**, 29, 43.

808. Harriman, D. G. F., Millar, J. H. D., Stevenson, A. C., *Brain*, 1955, **78**, 325.

DEFICIENCY DISEASES

809. Smith, W. T., in *Greenfield's Neuropathology*, 3rd edn, edited by W. Blackwood and J. A. N. Corsellis, chap. 5. London, 1976.

810. Russell, J. S. Risien, Batten, F. E., Collier, J., *Brain*, 1900, **23**, 39.

811. Biggart, J. H., *Pathology of the Nervous System*, 3rd edn, page 216. Edinburgh, 1961.

812. Ferraro, A., Arieti, S., English, W. H., *J. Neuropath. exp. Neurol.*, 1945, **4**, 217.

813. Greenfield, J. G., Carmichael, E. A., *Brain*, 1935, **58**, 483.

814. Earl, C. J., El Hawary, M. F. S., Thompson, R. H. S., Webster, G. R., *Lancet*, 1953, **1**, 115.

815. Cox, E. V., White, A. M., *Lancet*, 1962, **2**, 853.

816. Wilson, J., Matthews, D. M., *Clin. Sci.*, 1966, **31**, 1.

817. Torres, I., Smith, W. T., Oxnard, C. E., *J. Path.*, 1971, **105**, 125.

818. Passmore, R., Meiklejohn, A. P., in *Biochemical Disorders in Human Disease*, 1st edn, edited by E. J. King and R. H. S. Thompson, page 570. London, 1957.

819. Greenfield, J. G., Holmes, J. M., *Brit. med. J.*, 1939, **1**, 815.

820. Leigh, D., *J. ment. Sci.*, 1952, **98**, 130.

821. Passmore, R., Meiklejohn, A. P., in *Biochemical Disorders in Human Disease*, 1st edn, edited by E. J. King and R. H. S. Thompson, page 567. London, 1957.

822. De Wardener, H. E., Lennox, B., *Lancet*, 1947, **1**, 11.

823. Evans, E. T. R., Evans, W. C., Roberts, H. E., *Brit. vet. J.*, 1951, **107**, 364.

824. Victor, M., Adams, R. D., Collins, G. H., *The Wernicke–Korsakoff Syndrome*. Oxford, 1971.

824a. Wernicke, C., *Lehrbuch der Gehirnkrankheiten für Ärzte und Studierende*, vol. 2, page 229. Kassel and Berlin, 1881.

824b. Korsakov, S. S., *Ob alkogolnom paraliche* [On Alcohol Paralysis]. Moscow, 1887.

825. Malamud, N., Skillicorn, S. A., *A.M.A. Arch. Neurol. Psychiat.*, 1956, **76**, 585.

826. Delay, J., Brion, S., Elissalde, B., *Presse méd.*, 1958, **66**, 1965.

827. Campbell, A. C. P., Biggart, J. H., *J. Path. Bact.*, 1939, **48**, 245.

828. Cooke, W. T., Smith, W. T., *Brain*, 1966, **89**, 683.

829. Binder, H. J., Solitaire, G. B., Spiro, H. M., *Gut*, 1967, **8**, 605.

830. Cooke, W. T., Johnson, A. G., Woolf, A. L., *Brain*, 1966, **89**, 663.

831. Williams, J. A., Hall, G. S., Thompson, A. G., Cooke, W. T., *Brit. med. J.*, 1969, **3**, 210.

832. Smith, W. T., *unpublished observation*.

833. Badenoch, J., Richards, W. C. D., Oppenheimer, D. R., *J. Neurol. Neurosurg. Psychiat.*, 1963, **26**, 203.

834. Smith, W. T., French, J. M., Gottsman, M., Smith, A. J., Wakes-Miller, J. A., *Brain*, 1965, **88**, 137.

835. Groodt-Lasseel, M., Martin, J. J., *Path. et Biol.*, 1969, **17**, 21.

836. French, J. M., Hall, G., Parish, D. J., Smith, W. T., *Amer. J. Med.*, 1965, **39**, 277.

INTOXICATIONS

837. Cumings, J. N., *Heavy Metals and the Brain*. Oxford, 1959.

838. Hunter, D., *The Diseases of Occupations*, 6th edn, page 249. London, Sydney, Auckland and Toronto, 1978.

839. Millichap, J. G., Llewellin, K. R., Roxburgh, R. C., *Lancet*, 1952, **2**, 360.

840. Brown, I. A., *A.M.A. Arch. Neurol. Psychiat.*, 1954, **72**, 674.

841. Hunter, D., *The Diseases of Occupations*, 6th edn, page 305. London, Sydney, Auckland and Toronto, 1978.

842. Hunter, D., Russell, D. S., *J. Neurol. Neurosurg. Psychiat.*, 1954, **17**, 235.

843. Hay, W. J., Rickards, A. G., McMenemey, W. H., Cumings, J. N., *J. Neurol. Neurosurg. Psychiat.*, 1963, **26**, 199.

844. Barrett, F. R., *Med. J. Aust.*, 1957, **2**, 242.

845. Wyllie, W. G., Stern, R. O., *Arch. Dis. Childh.*, 1931, **6**, 137.

846. McAlpine, D., Araki, S., *A.M.A. Arch. Neurol.*, 1959, **81**, 522.

847. Kurland, L. T., Faro, S. N., Siedler, H., *Wld Neurol.*, 1960, **1**, 370.

848. Matsumoto, H., Koya, G., Takeuchi, T., *J. Neuropath. exp. Neurol.*, 1965, **24**, 563.

849. Leading Article, *Brit. med. J.*, 1971, **1**, 126.

850. Fairhall, L. T., *Physiol. Rev.*, 1945, **25**, 182.

851. Turner, J. W. Aldren, *Lancet*, 1955, **1**, 661.

852. Canavan, M. M., Cobb, S., Drinker, C. K., *Arch. Neurol. Psychiat. (Chic.)*, 1934, **32**, 512.

853. Bogaert, L. van, Dallemagne, M. J., *Mschr. Psychiat. Neurol.*, 1945–46, **111**, 60.

854. Stoner, H. B., Barnes, J. M., Duff, J. I., *Brit. J. Pharmacol.*, 1955, **10**, 16.

855. Magee, P. N., Stoner, H. B., Barnes, J. M., *J. Path. Bact.*, 1957, **73**, 107.

856. Torack, R. M., Terry, R. D., Zimmerman, H. M., *Amer. J. Path.*, 1960, **36**, 273.

857. Russell, D. S., *J. Path. Bact.*, 1937, **45**, 357.

858. Hurst, E. Weston, *J. Path. Bact.*, 1959, **77**, 523.

859. Drew, G. C., Colquhoun, W. P., Long, H. A., *Memor. med. Res. Coun. (Lond.)*, No. 38, 1959.

860. Wilks, S., *Med. Times Gaz.*, 1868, **2**, 470.

861. Victor, M., Adams, R. D., Mancall, E. L., *A.M.A. Arch. Neurol.*, 1959, **81**, 579.

861a. Marchiafava, E., Bignami, A., *Riv. Pat. nerv. ment.*, 1903, **8**, 544.

862. McLardy, T., *Proc. roy. Soc. Med.*, 1951, **44**, 685.

863. Nielsen, J. M., Courville, C. B., *Bull. Los Angeles neurol. Soc.*, 1943, **8**, 81.

864. Riese, W., Jones, G. L., Beamer-Maxwell, E., Davis, H. E., *J. Neuropath. exp. Neurol.*, 1954, **13**, 501.

865. Ironside, R., Bosanquet, F. D., McMenemey, W. H., *Brain*, 1961, **84**, 212.

866. Lumsden, C. E., *J. Neurol. Neurosurg. Psychiat.*, 1950, **13**, 1.

867. Schneck, S. A., in *Pathology of the Nervous System*, edited by J. Minckler, vol. 1, chap. 63. New York, 1968.

868. Adams, R. D., Victor, M., Mancall, E. L., *A.M.A. Arch. Neurol. Psychiat.*, 1959, **81**, 154.

869. Adams, J. H., in *Proceedings of the Fourth International Congress of Neuropathology, Stuttgart, 1962*, vol. 3, page 303. Stuttgart, 1962.

870. Schneck, S. A., *J. Neuropath. exp. Neurol.*, 1966, **25**, 18.

871. Bennett, I. L., Cary, F. H., Mitchell, G. L., Cooper, M. N., *Medicine (Baltimore)*, 1953, **32**, 431.

872. Victor, M., Adams, R. D., Cole, M., *Medicine (Baltimore)*, 1965, **44**, 345.

873. Phear, E. A., Sherlock, S., Summerskill, W. H., *Lancet*, 1955, **1**, 836.

874. Walshe, J. M., *Quart. J. Med.*, 1951, N.S. **20**, 421.

875. Whitehead, T. P., Whittaker, S. R. F., *J. clin. Path.*, 1955, **8**, 81.

876. Cavanagh, J. B., Kyu, M. H., *J. neurol. Sci.*, 1971, **12**, 63.

POST-INFECTION ENCEPHALOMYELOPATHIES

877. Brewis, E. G., *Brit. med. J.*, 1954, **1**, 1298.

878. Miller, H., Stanton, J. B., Gibbons, J. L., *Quart. J. Med.*, 1956, N.S. **25**, 427.

879. Blackwood, W., *Proc. roy. Soc. Med.*, 1956, **49**, 146.

880. Turnbull, H. M., McIntosh, J., *Brit. J. exp. Path.*, 1926, **7**, 181.

881. Conybeare, E. T., *Mth. Bull. Minist. Hlth Lab. Serv.*, 1964, **23**, 150.

882. De Vries, E., *Postvaccinial Perivenous Encephalitis*. Amsterdam, 1960.

883. Paschen, E., *Dtsch. med. Wschr.*, 1930, **56**, 219.

884. Pette, H., *Die akuten entzündlichen Erkrankungen des Nervensystems*. Leipzig, 1942.

885. Hurst, E. W., *Med. J. Aust.*, 1941, **2**, 1.

886. Crawford, T., *J. clin. Path.*, 1954, **7**, 1.

887. Symmers, W. St C., *Brain*, 1956, **79**, 511.

888. Levine, S., Wenke, E. J., *Amer. J. Path.*, 1965, **47**, 61.

MULTIPLE SCLEROSIS AND RELATED DISEASES

889. Vaughan-Morgan, J. K., *Hansard*, 1957, page 1671.

890. *Mortality Statistics—Cause: Review of the Registrar General on Deaths by Cause, Sex and Age, in England and Wales, 1976* (Series DH2, No. 3). London, 1978.

891. McAlpine, D., Compston, N. D., Lumsden, C. E., *Multiple Sclerosis*. Edinburgh and London, 1955.

892. McAlpine, D., Acheson, E. D., Lumsden, C. E., *Multiple Sclerosis: A Reappraisal*. Edinburgh and London, 1965.

893. Millar, J. H. D., *Proc. roy. Soc. Med.*, 1961, **54**, 4.

894. Charcot, J. M., *Gaz. Hôp. (Paris)*, 1868, 405, 409, 554, 557, 566.

895. McAlpine, D., Acheson, E. D., Lumsden, C. E., *Multiple Sclerosis: A Reappraisal*, page 179. Edinburgh and London, 1965.

896. McAlpine, D., Acheson, E. D., Lumsden, C. E., *Multiple Sclerosis: A Reappraisal*, page 3. Edinburgh and London, 1965.

897. Okinaka, S., McAlpine, D., Miyagawa, K., Suwa, N., Kuroiwa, Y., Shiraki, H., Araki, S., Kurland, L. T., *Wld Neurol.*, 1960, **1**, 22.

898. Hurst, E. Weston, in *'Allergic' Encephalomyelitis*, edited by M. W. Kies and E. C. Alvord, Jr, page 216. Springfield, Illinois, 1959.

899. Pratt, R. T. C., Compston, N. D., McAlpine, D., *Brain*, 1951, **74**, 191.

900. Allison, R. S., Millar, J. H. D., *Ulster med. J.*, 1954, **23**, suppl. 2.

901. Sutherland, J. M., *Brain*, 1956, **79**, 635.

902. Curtius, F., *Multiple Sklerose und Erbanlage*. Leipzig, 1933.

903. Curtius, F., *Fortschr. Neurol. Psychiat.*, 1959, **27**, 161.

904. Schapiro, K., Poskanzer, D. C., Miller, H., *Brain*, 1963, **86**, 315.

905. Dawson, J. W., *Trans. roy. Soc. Edinb.*, 1916, **50**, 517.

906. McAlpine, D., Compston, N. D., Lumsden, C. E., *Multiple Sclerosis*, page 211. Edinburgh and London, 1955.

907. Georgi, W., *Schweiz. med. Wschr.*, 1961, **91**, 605.

908. McAlpine, D., Compston, N. D., Lumsden, C. E., *Multiple Sclerosis*, page 231. Edinburgh and London, 1955.

909. Greenfield, J. G., King, L. S., *Brain*, 1936, **52**, 445.

910. Ibrahim, M. Z. N., Adams, C. W. M., *J. Neurol. Neurosurg. Psychiat.*, 1963, **26**, 101.

911. McAlpine, D., *Lancet*, 1955, **1**, 1033.
912. Innes, J. R. M., Kurland, L. T., *Amer. J. Med.*, 1952, **12**, 574.
913. Adams, J. M., Imagawa, D. T., *Proc. Soc. exp. Biol.* (*N.Y.*), 1962, **111**, 562.
914. Cendrowski, W., Polna, I., Niedzielska, K., *J. Neurol. Neurosurg. Psychiat.*, 1973, **36**, 57.
915. Field, E. J., Cowshall, S., Narang, H. K., Bell, T. M., *Lancet*, 1972, **2**, 280.
916. Field, E. J., *Lancet*, 1973, **1**, 295.
917. Isacson, P., *Progr. Allergy*, 1967, **10**, 256.
918. Caspary, E. A., Chambers, M. E., Field, E. J., *Neurology* (*Minneap.*), 1969, **19**, 1038.
919. Putnam, T. J., Alexander, L., *Arch. Neurol. Psychiat.* (*Chic.*), 1939, **41**, 1087.
920. Swank, R. L., *Amer. J. med. Sci.*, 1950, **220**, 421.
921. Courville, C. B., *Bull. Los Angeles neurol. Soc.*, 1959, **24**, 60.
922. Hurst, E. Weston, *Aust. J. exp. Biol. med. Sci.*, 1940, **18**, 201.
923. Rivers, T. M., Schwentker, F. F., *J. exp. Med.*, 1935, **61**, 689.
924. Cavanagh, J. B., *Guy's Hosp. Rep.*, 1956, **105**, 39.
925. Waksman, B. H., *Int. Arch. Allergy*, 1959, **14**, suppl., 3.
926. '*Allergic' Encephalomyelitis*, edited by M. W. Kies and E. C. Alvord, Jr. Springfield, Illinois, 1959.
927. Kabat, E. A., Wolf, A., Bezer, A. E., *J. exp. Med.*, 1947, **85**, 117; 1948, **88**, 417; 1949, **89**, 395.
928. Uchimura, I., Shiraki, H., *J. Neuropath. exp. Neurol.*, 1957, **16**, 139.
929. Seitelberger, F., Jellinger, K., Tschabitschev, H., *Wien. klin. Wschr.*, 1958, **70**, 453.
930. Adams, R. D., in '*Allergic' Encephalomyelitis*, edited by M. W. Kies and E. C. Alvord, Jr, page 183. Springfield, Illinois, 1959.
931. Ferraro, A., *Arch. Neurol. Psychiat.* (*Chic.*), 1944, **52**, 433.
932. Wolf, A., in *Proceedings of the Third International Congress of Neuropathology, Brussels, 1957*, page 119. Amsterdam, 1957.
933. Jubb, K. V. F., Kennedy, P. C., *Pathology of Domestic Animals*, 2nd edn, vol. 1, page 215. New York and London, 1970.
934. Innes, J. R. M., Saunders, L. Z., *Comparative Neuropathology*, page 373. New York and London, 1962.
935. Bogaert, L. van, in *Comparative Neuropathology*, edited by J. R. M. Innes and L. Z. Saunders, page 67. New York, 1962.
936. Torres, I., Smith, W. T., Oxnard, C. E., *J. Path.*, 1971, **105**, 125.
937. Heubner, O., *Charité-Ann.*, 1897, **22**, 298.
937a. Schilder, P., *Z. ges. Neurol. Psychiat.*, 1912, **10**, 1.
938. Einarson, L., Neel, A. V., *Acta jutlandica*, 1942, **14**, 2.
939. Poser, C. M., Bogaert, L. van, *Acta psychiat. scand.*, 1956, **31**, 285.
940. Baló, J., *Arch. Neurol. Psychiat.* (*Chic.*), 1928, **19**, 242.
941. Hallervorden, J., *Nervenarzt*, 1952, **23**, 1.
942. Mage, J., Kleyntjens, A., Brihaye, J., Bogaert, L. van, *Rev. neurol.*, 1958, **98**, 723.
943. Allbutt, C., *Lancet*, 1870, **1**, 76.
944. Devic, *Bull. méd.* (*Paris*), 1894, **8**, 1033.
944a. Devic, E., *Congrés français de médicine interne, 1894, Paris*, vol. 1, page 431. Paris, 1895.
945. McAlpine, D., *Brain*, 1938, **61**, 430.

DEGENERATIVE DISEASES

946. Gowers, W. R., *Lancet*, 1902, **1**, 1003.
946a. Gowers, W. R., *Lancet*, 1899, **2**, 1591.
946b. Smith, M. C., *J. Neurol. Neurosurg. Psychiat.*, 1960, **23**, 269.
947. Kurland, L. T., Mulder, D. W., *Neurology*, 1954, **4**, 356.
948. Hirano, A., in *Progress in Neuropathology*, edited by H. M. Zimmerman, vol. 2, chap. 7. New York, 1973.
949. Hirano, A., Malamud, N., Elizan, T. S., Kurland, L. T., *Arch. Neurol.* (*Chic.*), 1966, **15**, 35.
950. Hirano, A., Dembitzer, H. M., Kurland, L. T., Zimmerman, H. M., *J. Neuropath. exp. Neurol.*, 1968, **27**, 167.
951. Werdnig, G., *Arch. Psychiat. Nervenkr.*, 1891, **22**, 437.
951a. Hoffmann, J., *Dtsch. Z. Nervenheilk.*, 1891, **1**, 95; 1893, **3**, 427.
952. Brain, W. R., Croft, P. B., Wilkinson, M., *Brain*, 1965, **88**, 479.
952a. Henson, R. A., in *Modern Trends in Neurology—5*, edited by D. Williams, chap. 12. London, 1970.
953. Greenfield, J. G., *The Spino-Cerebellar Degenerations*. Oxford, 1954.
954. Holmes, G., *Brain*, 1907, **30**, 466.
955. Hall, B., Noad, K. B., Latham, O., *Brain*, 1941, **64**, 178.
955a. Marie, P., *Sem. méd.* (*Paris*), 1893, **13**, 444, 447.
956. Menzel, P., *Arch. Psychiat. Nervenkr.*, 1891, **22**, 160.
957. Schut, J. W., Book, J. A., *A.M.A. Arch. Neurol. Psychiat.*, 1953, **70**, 169.
958. Brain, W. R., Daniel, P. M., Greenfield, J. G., *J. Neurol. Neurosurg. Psychiat.*, 1951, **14**, 59.
959. Friedreich, N., *Virchows Arch. path. Anat.*, 1863, **26**, 391, 433; 1863, **27**, 1; 1876, **68**, 145; 1877, **70**, 140.
959a. Bell, J., Carmichael, E. A., *Treas. hum. Inherit.*, 1939, **4**, part 3.
960. Russell, D. S., *J. Path. Bact.*, 1946, **58**, 739.
961. Spillane, J. D., *Brain*, 1940, **63**, 275.
962. Roussy, G., Levy, G., *Rev. neurol.*, 1926, **1**, 427.
962a. Strümpell, A., *Arch. Psychiat. Nervenkr.*, 1886, **17**, 217.
963. Bassen, F. A., Kornzweig, A. L., *Blood*, 1950, **5**, 381.
964. Singer, K., Fisher, B., Perlstein, M. A., *Blood*, 1952, **7**, 577.
965. Kornzweig, A. L., Bassen, F. A., *A.M.A. Arch. Ophthal.*, 1957, **58**, 183.
966. Salt, H. B., Wolff, O. H., Lloyd, J. K., Fosbrooke, A. S., Cameron, A. H., Hubble, D. V., *Lancet*, 1960, **2**, 325.
966a. Charcot, J. M., Marie, P., *Rev. Méd.* (*Paris*), 1886, **6**, 97.
966b. Tooth, H. H., *The Peroneal Type of Progressive Muscular Atrophy*. London, 1886.
967. Brain, W. R., Henson, R. A., *Lancet*, 1958, **2**, 971.
968. Mair, W. G. P., Folkerts, J. F., *Brain*, 1953, **76**, 563.
969. Hoffman, H. L., *Brain*, 1955, **78**, 377.
970. Brain, W. R., Norris, F. H., *Remote Effects of Cancer on the Nervous System*. New York, 1965.
971. Corsellis, J. A. N., Goldberg, G. J., Norton, A. R., *Brain*, 1968, **91**, 487.
972. Parkinson, J., *An Essay on the Shaking Palsy*. London, 1817.
972a. Lewy, F. H., *Dtsch. Z. Nervenheilk.*, 1914, **50**, 50.
972b. Greenfield, J. G., Bosanquet, F. D., *J. Neurol. Neurosurg. Psychiat.*, 1953, **16**, 213.

973. Bethlem, J., Jager, W. A. D. H., *J. Neurol. Neurosurg. Psychiat.*, 1960, **23**, 74.
974. Jager, W. A. D. H., Bethlem, J., *J. Neurol. Neurosurg. Psychiat.*, 1960, **23**, 283.
975. Gillingham, F. J., Watson, W. S., Donaldson, A. A., Naughton, J. A. L., *Brit. med. J.*, 1960, **2**, 1395.
976. Martin, J. P., *Lancet*, 1959, **1**, 999.
977. Denny-Brown, D., *Lancet*, 1960, **2**, 1099, 1155.
977a. Alvord, E. C., Jr, in *Pathology of the Nervous System*, edited by J. Minckler, vol. 1, page 1152. New York, 1968.
977b. Bernheimer, H., Birkmayer, W., Hornykiewicz, O., Jellinger, K., Seitelberger, F., *J. neurol. Sci.*, 1973, **20**, 415.
977c. Fahn, S., Libsch, L. R., Cutler, R. W., *J. neurol. Sci.*, 1971, **14**, 421.
977d. Hornykiewicz, O., in *The Structure and Function of Nervous Tissue*, edited by G. H. Bourne, vol. 6, page 367. New York, 1972.
978. Poskanzer, D. C., Schwab, R. S., *J. chron. Dis.*, 1963, **16**, 961.
979. Kurland, L. T., Hauser, W. A., Okazaki, H., Nobrega, F. T., in *Proceedings of the Third Symposium on Parkinson's Disease*, edited by F. J. Gillingham and I. M. L. Donaldson, page 12. Edinburgh, 1969.
980. Hirano, A., Malamud, N., Kurland, L. T., *Brain*, 1961, **84**, 662.
981. Schochet, S. S., Jr, Lampert, P. W., Lindenberg, R., *Acta neuropath. (Berl.)*, 1968, **11**, 330.
982. Steele, J. C., Richardson, J. C., Olszewski, J., *Neurology (Minneap.)*, 1964, **10**, 333.
983. Roberts, J. A. Fraser, *An Introduction to Medical Genetics*, 6th edn, page 32. London, New York and Toronto, 1973.
983a. Bell, J., *Treas. hum. Inherit.*, 1934, **4**, part 1.
983b. Huntington, G., *Med. surg. Reporter*, 1872, **26**, 317.
983c. Waters, C. O., in *Practice of Medicine*, by R. Dunglison, vol. 2, page 321. Philadelphia, 1842.
984. Vessie, P. R., *J. nerv. ment. Dis.*, 1932, **76**, 553.
985. Critchley, M., *J. State Med.*, 1934, **42**, 575.
986. Dunlop, C. B., *Arch. Neurol. Psychiat. (Chic.)*, 1927, **18**, 867.
987. Adams, R. D., Bogaert, L. van, Eecken, N. V., *J. Neuropath. exp. Neurol.*, 1964, **23**, 584.
988. Takei, Y., Mirra, S. S., in *Progress in Neuropathology*, edited by H. M. Zimmerman, vol. 2, chap. 8. New York, 1973.
989. Pick, A., *Prag. med. Wschr.*, 1892, **17**, 165.
989a. Pick, A., *Wien. klin. Wschr.*, 1901, **14**, 403.
989b. Spatz, H., in *Proceedings of the First International Congress of Neuropathology, Rome, 1952*, vol. 2, page 375. Rome, 1952.
990. Neumann, M. A., Cohn, R., *Brain*, 1967, **90**, 405.
991. Alpers, B. J., *Arch. Neurol. Psychiat. (Chic.)*, 1931, **25**, 469.
992. Christiansen, E., Krabbe, K. H., *Arch. Neurol. Psychiat. (Chic.)*, 1949, **61**, 28.
992a. Sandbank, U., Lerman, P., *J. Neurol. Neurosurg. Psychiat.*, 1973, **35**, 749.
993. Blackwood, W., Buxton, P. H., Cumings, J. N., Robertson, D. J., Tucker, S. M., *Arch. Dis. Childh.*, 1963, **38**, 193.
994. Kirschbaum, W. R., *Jakob–Creutzfeld Disease*. New York, 1968.
995. Crompton, M. R., *Acta neuropath. (Berl.)*, 1968, **10**, 99.
996. Leigh, D., *J. Neurol. Neurosurg. Psychiat.*, 1951, **14**, 216.
997. Dayan, A. D., Ockenden, B. G., Crome, L., *Arch. Dis. Childh.*, 1970, **45**, 39.
998. Worsley, H. E., Brookfield, R. W., Elwood, J. S., Noble, R. L., Taylor, W. H., *Arch. Dis. Childh.*, 1965, **40**, 492.
999. Blocq, P., Marinesco, G., *Sem. méd. (Paris)*, 1892, **12**, 445.
1000. Field, E. J., *Int. Rev. exp. Path.*, 1969, **8**, 218.
1001. Alzheimer, A., *Neurol. Zbl.*, 1906, **25**, 1134.
1001a. Alzheimer, A., *Allg. Z. Psychiat.*, 1907, **64**, 146.
1001b. Margolis, G., *Lab. Invest.*, 1959, **8**, 335.
1002. Tomlinson, B. E., Kitchener, D., *J. Path.*, 1972, **106**, 165.
1003. Terry, R. D., Gonatas, N. K., Weiss, M., *Amer. J. Path.*, 1964, **44**, 269.
1004. Kidd, M., *Brain*, 1964, **87**, 307.
1005. Krigman, M. R., Feldman, R. G., Bensch, K., *Lab. Invest.*, 1965, **14**, 381.
1006. Wisniewski, H. M., Terry, R. D., in *Progress in Neuropathology*, edited by H. M. Zimmerman, vol. 2, chap. 1. New York, 1973.
1007. Mowat, A. P., *Arch. Dis. Childh.*, 1973, **48**, 411.
1008. Reye, R. D., Morgan, G., Baral, J., *Lancet*, 1963, **2**, 749.
1009. Brain, W. R., Hunter, D., Turnbull, H. M., *Lancet*, 1929, **1**, 221.

ACKNOWLEDGEMENTS FOR ILLUSTRATIONS

The photographs, except for those acknowledged below, were made by Mr G. Cox, Department of Pathology, Maida Vale Hospital (The National Hospitals for Nervous Diseases), London.

Fig. 34.1. Section prepared and photographed by Dr S. Duckett.

Figs 34.5, 6. Electron micrographs provided by Dr P. L. Lantos, The Middlesex Hospital Medical School, London.

Fig. 34.11. Electron micrograph provided by Dr J. F. Knowles, University of Birmingham Medical School, Birmingham.

Figs 34.26, 46A–C, 51, 54, 55B, 57A, 58. Photomicrographs provided by W. St C. Symmers.

Fig. 34.38A. Preparation provided by Dr R. O. Barnard, Maida Vale Hospital (The National Hospitals for Nervous Diseases), London, and St Thomas's Hospital Medical School, London; photomicrograph by Mr R. S. Barnett, Department of Histopathology, Charing Cross Hospital Medical School, London.

Fig. 34.38B. Photographic print—from negative in Professor W. H. McMenemy's files—provided by Dr R. O. Barnard, Maida Vale Hospital (The National Hospitals for Nervous Diseases), London.

Fig. 34.46D. Specimen presented to Charing Cross Hospital Medical School, London, by Dr D. G. F. Harriman, University of Leeds and the General Infirmary, Leeds;

photograph by Miss P. M. Turnbull, Charing Cross Hospital Medical School. Reproduced by permission of the editor from: Symmers, W. St C., *Vie méd.*, 1966, **47,** 353.

Figs 34.46E, 46F. Reproduced by permission of the editor from: Symmers, W. St C., *Vie méd.*, 1966, **47**, 353.

Fig. 34.48. Specimen presented to Charing Cross Hospital Medical School, London, by Dr A. H. Cruickshank and Dr M. D. Readett, University of Liverpool; photograph by Miss P. M. Turnbull, Charing Cross Hospital Medical School. Reproduced by permission of the editor from: Symmers, W. St C., *Vie méd.*, 1966, **47**, 353.

Fig. 34.53. Preparation provided by Professor Dorothy S. Russell, The London Hospital Medical College, London.

Fig. 34.55. Preparation provided by Professor G. B. D. Scott, Royal Free Hospital School of Medicine, London.

Fig. 34.65. Preparation provided by Dr Erna Christensen, Rigshospital, Copenhagen.

Fig. 34.69. Electron micrographs provided by Dr Anne M. Field, Virus Reference Laboratory, Public Health Laboratory Service, Colindale, London.

Fig. 34.79. Preparation provided by Dr C. W. Taylor, Birmingham and Midlands Hospital for Women, Birmingham.

Figs 34.89, 127. Specimens provided by Dr R. D. Clay, Portsmouth and Isle of Wight Pathological Laboratories, Portsmouth.

Fig. 34.94. Specimen provided by Dr H. R. R. Mavor, Lincoln County Hospital, Lincoln.

Fig. 34.99. Specimen provided by Dr F. Hampson, Royal Berkshire Hospital, Reading.

Fig. 34.102. Specimen provided by Dr P. C. Meyer, Whittington Hospital, London.

Fig. 34.151. Preparation provided by Professor G. Payling Wright, Guy's Hospital Medical School, London.

Fig. 34.152. Preparation provided by Dr D. G. F. Harriman, University of Leeds and the General Infirmary, Leeds.

Fig. 34.165. Reproduced by permission of the authors and editor from: Ibrahim, M. Z. N., Adams, C. W. M., *J. Neurol. Neurosurg. Psychiat.*, 1963, **26**, 101.

35: *The Peripheral Nervous System*

by J. B. CAVANAGH

with a section on tumours by the editor

CONTENTS

35: *The Peripheral Nervous System*

by J. B. C<small>AVANAGH</small>

with a section on tumours by the editor

In spite of the accessibility of peripheral nerve trunks both to electrical stimulation and to biopsy, the neuropathies have long been a neglected field of study. In recent decades, interest has been awakened in these problems for two reasons: the first was the practical need during the second world war for better ways of treating injuries to nerve trunks; the second is the increasing frequency with which damage to nerves follows from exposure to toxic chemicals. The war-time investigations produced some brilliant anatomical studies, particularly by workers in Oxford, but it is only recently that their quantitative anatomical approach, so valuable in unravelling the complexities of normal developmental and reparative processes, have been applied to either experimental or human disease. The impetus for these recent studies has been the realization by clinical neurologists that electrical methods can be of greater value for the investiga-tion of neurological disease if they are related to anatomical, particularly quantitative anatomical, findings. It is, of course, only in the experimental animal that the information value of electro-physiological techniques can be accurately judged. As a result of such studies there has been a steady growth of new and valuable information about the peripheral nerves in health and disease.

It is not intended here to provide detailed morphological descriptions of the various clinically defined neuropathies; such information is available in specialized texts.[1, 1a] Instead, a more general account will be given of the ways in which the normal structure and function of nerves, their cell bodies, their peripheral terminations and their covering layers can become disturbed in the course of experimental and natural disease processes. By so doing, it is hoped that a basis for an understanding of human neuropathies may best be provided.

NORMAL STRUCTURE OF PERIPHERAL NERVES

We owe to Ramón y Cajal[1b] our knowledge that both the central and peripheral nervous systems are composed of discrete units, the neurons, and that there is no syncytial continuity, only cellular contiguity, in the nervous system. This basic concept must be constantly in mind when contemplating disease processes in peripheral nerves. We must not forget that sensory nerves differ both in origin and arrangement from motor nerves; that the Schwann cells* that cover every nerve fibre outside the central nervous system lead an existence that is independent of, though interrelated with, that of the nerve axon; that myelin, although part of the Schwann cell, is distinct from the axon it surrounds; and that to separate a part of a neuron from its controlling nucleus inevitably leads to a series of changes both in the distal part of the divided axon (Wallerian degeneration) and in the structures that it normally innervates (denervation atrophy).

The Nerve Cell Body or Perikaryon

There is a general belief, now becoming better substantiated, that the perikaryon, in addition to

---

* The neurolemmal sheath (sheath of Schwann) was described by Theodor Schwann in 1839, while working in Berlin. The account is in his book on the correspondence of structure and growth in animals and plants (*Mikroscopische Untersuchungen über die Uebereinstimmung in der Struktur und dem Wachsthum der Thiere und Pflanzen*, page 174; Berlin, 1839). Electron microscopy has shown that the distinction between the 'neurolemmal sheath' and 'neurolemmal cells', formerly insisted on by some neurohistologists, is non-existent: these terms are synonymous. The generally acceptable name 'Schwann cell' will be used throughout this chapter when referring to the neurolemmal cell. In conformity with the practice adopted in other chapters, the spelling 'neurolemma' is used rather than 'neurilemma' and 'neurilema' (see footnote on page 2221).

being essential for the vitality of its axon, is also concerned with its nutrition. Assuming this to be true, the metabolic load imposed on their perikarya by the longest and largest fibres must be unequalled by that on any other type of cell in the body, for measurements have shown that the volume ratio of axon to perikaryon may be as great as a thousand to one. The neuron has all the cytological appearances usually associated with a cell that is highly active in protein synthesis—its chief morphological feature is a high content of ribonucleic acid arranged in conspicuous clumps (Nissl substance) throughout its cytoplasm (Fig. 35.1).[2] Electron

meter, also occur, especially in the axon: they are chemically different from microtubules; their function is unknown. The neuronal nucleus is large: its size is probably related to the volume of the cytoplasm. It has one or two prominent nucleoli. Female sex chromatin, the 'Barr body',[4a] can usually be seen adjacent to the nucleolus in most species (Fig. 35.4).

The cell membrane of neurons other than those in sensory ganglia is thickened at its point of contact with the 'boutons terminaux' forming the postsynaptic areas. These boutons contain not only numerous mitochondria (Fig. 35.2) but also large numbers of 'synaptic vesicles', which are some 35 to 45 nm in diameter.[5, 6] These vesicles are believed to contain protein-bound humoral transmitter agent: release of this agent effects transmission of the nervous impulse across the synapse.[7] The post-synaptic zone of thickening, like the myoneural junction (see page 2302), contains acetylcholinesterase (true cholinesterase) (Fig. 35.3).[8] Where it is not covered by boutons, the surface of the spinal

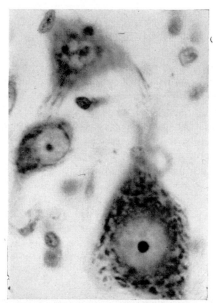

Fig. 35.1. Neurons (motor cells) of an anterior grey column of the spinal cord of a cat. The nucleolus is characteristically large and the large clumps of Nissl substance (ribonucleic acid) are evenly distributed through the perikaryon. *Cresyl violet.* × 700.

microscopy has shown that these clumps are composed of endoplasmic reticulum, a structure that is typically found in abundance in the cytoplasm of all cells that actively synthetize protein. Between the clumps lie numerous mitochondria. Running through the cytoplasm and into the dendrites and axon are numerous microtubules, 25 nm in diameter, that appear to be concerned in some way with the rapid transport of materials over long distances within the cell[3] and that may also form some kind of internal cytoskeleton.[4] The microtubules are well seen only when aldehyde fixatives have been used. Neurofibrils, 8 to 10 nm in dia-

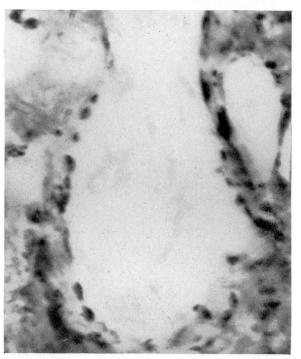

Fig. 35.2.§ 'Boutons terminaux' on body and dendrites of spinal neurons of the cat. Each bouton consists of a cluster of dark bodies, each about 1μm in diameter, which are probably mitochondria. *Method of Armstrong and Stephens* (Armstrong, J., Stephens, P. R., *Stain Technol.*, 1960, **35**, 71). × 1750.

§ See *Acknowledgements*, page 2348.

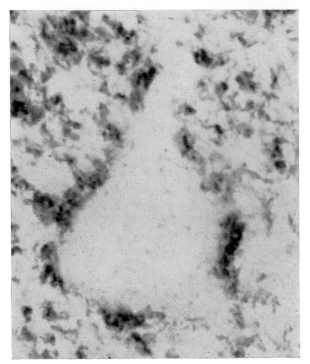

Fig. 35.3. Localization of acetylcholinesterase in the ventro-lateral region of the spinal cord of a cat. It is sharply confined to cell and dendrite surfaces, corresponding to the distribution of *boutons. Gömöri method.* × 970.

neurons is in close contact with neuroglia—a gap of only about 20 nm separates them: this gap would seem to constitute the true extracellular space of the central nervous system.

In the dorsal root ganglia, the membrane of the perikaryon is in close contact with perineuronal satellite cells (Fig. 35.4).* These are modified Schwann cells, and members of the system of cells derived from the neural crest that invest nerve fibres and neurons situated outside the central nervous system.[9] Electron micrographs show that the peri-neuronal satellite cells are in very intimate contact with one another, their surface membranes inter-digitating closely along areas of contact; however, no such features distinguish their surfaces of contact with the neuron, and their role in the life of the latter is obscure. These satellite cells show con-siderable pseudocholinesterase activity, and they contain an abundance of alkaline phosphatase.[10] They do not normally form myelin round the

* The accumulation of oligodendrocytes round a neuronal cell body in the central nervous system is also known as satellitosis (see page 2084); the term 'satellite cell' has sometimes been applied in this context also.

neuron they enclose. Immediately outside the capsule of satellite cells there is a thin layer of reticulin that is continuous with the Plenk–Laidlaw sheath[10a, 10b] of the Schwann cells.

The Nerve Fibre and Nerve Trunk

Nerve fibres, except near their terminals, are gathered into bundles (funiculi). Each bundle is enclosed by its own connective tissue sheath, the *perineurium*. The collection of bundles that forms the nerve is invested and held together by the *epineurium*, which thus constitutes both the covering of the nerve as a whole and the interfunicular connective tissue. The epineurium is continuous with the perineurial sheath of each bundle. The perineurium in its turn is continuous with the delicate connective tissue—the endoneurium—that encloses and supports the individual fibres within the bundle. The endoneurial space accommodates the nerve fibres, a few fibroblasts, mucopoly-saccharide and collagen (Figs 35.5 and 35.6). Any material that gains access to the nerve trunk may pass readily along this space.

Electron microscopy has shown that all myelin-ated and unmyelinated fibres are invested by the cytoplasm of an ensheathing cell, and that during development each of these cells may enclose as many as 15 unmyelinated axons; in fact, each fold round a nerve fibre—the so-called mesaxon—can be traced back to the surface of a sheath cell (Fig. 35.7). It is better to refer to the cells

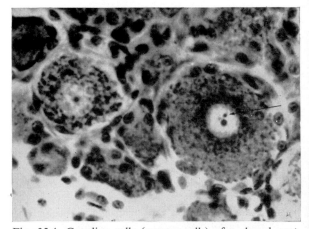

Fig. 35.4. Ganglion cells (sensory cells) of a dorsal root ganglion of a spinal nerve of a female cat. Variations in size and arrangement of Nissl substance normally occur. A Barr body (female sex chromatin) is present in the larger cell (arrow). Satellite cells (modified Schwann cells) surround each neuron. *Cresyl violet.* × 535.

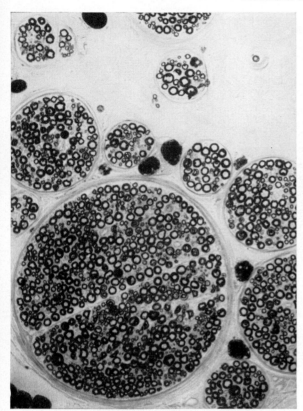

Fig. 35.5. Myelinated fibres of a normal peripheral nerve of a cat. The specimen was prepared for the purpose of measuring the diameter of the nerve fibres. Perineurium surrounds each bundle; endoneurium separates the fibres. *Osmium fixation. Iron haematoxylin.* × 15.

The Axon

The best electron micrographs show that the axonal membrane, like that of other cells, is composed of three layers, 7·5 nm thick in all, with two osmiophile components.[11] Its structure appears only slightly changed at the nodes of Ranvier. The axoplasm contains elongated mitochondria, neurofilaments (10 nm in diameter), neurotubules or microtubules (20 to 25 nm in diameter) and lengths of smooth endoplasmic reticulum. It is viscous and contains what seems to be stainable mucopolysaccharide, but nonetheless time-lapse cinephotomicrography shows that there is active movement of particles in both directions within it. This axoplasmic flow, its purpose and its mechanisms are under active study at the present: different classes of materials vary widely in the rate of their flow within axons, the distance covered by those studied ranging from 1 mm in a day to more than 500 mm in a day.[12] The microtubules play some part in this movement

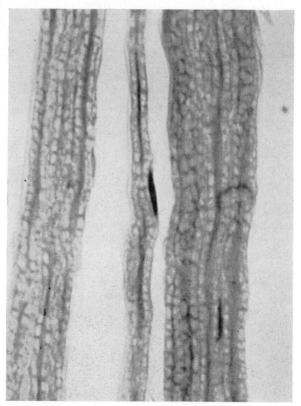

Fig. 35.6. Longitudinal section of a sciatic nerve of a normal adult rabbit. Darkly stained axon (in the separate central fibre) is ensheathed by myelin, outside which lies an elongated Schwann cell nucleus. The apparent reticulation of the myelin is an artefact. *Haematoxylin–eosin.* × 1000.

that ensheathe the unmyelinated fibres by the older name, *Remak cells*:[10c, 10d] this term, properly used, indicates both the unmyelinated nature of the fibre concerned and that the sheath may invest more than one axon. Considered from the standpoint of development, the fact that more than one axon may be enveloped by the Remak cell might be thought to indicate immaturity, for in rats axonal segregation becomes progressively more marked during development, with the result that Remak cells come to contain fewer and fewer axons. What stimulus prompts the Remak cell to reduce its load of axons is unknown, but since the shedding appears to proceed uniformly along individual axons it must presumably arise in the latter. It may be a similar influence that operates in the subsequent development of the myelin sheath and determines the sheath thickness appropriate for the function of the fibre.

8*

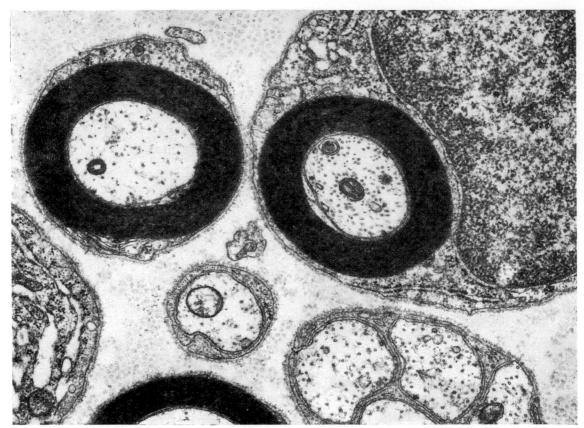

Fig. 35.7.§ Electron micrograph of a nerve of an adult rat, showing two small myelinated fibres. That on the right shows a Schwann cell nucleus and inner and outer mesaxons. That on the left shows myelin lamellae opening out at the beginning of a Schmidt–Lantermann incisure. Below, two Remak cells enclose unmyelinated fibres. Note the microtubules in the axons. × 30 000.

for it ceases or becomes slowed if they are depolymerized by the local introduction of colchicine.[13] It may be that some such transport system is essential to the development and survival of such enormously long cells as neurons may become, with the sites of enzyme and metabolite synthesis in the perikaryon far removed from the points of utilization at the nerve terminals. Breakdown of such a system of transport may be the basis of certain pathological changes in long fibre systems. Although there must be some centripetal movement, axoplasmic flow is largely centrifugal, since constriction of a nerve leads to swelling of the proximal portion of the axon, beginning about one week after the compression is applied and subsiding after it is removed.[14] It is natural to ask whither this fluid is passing, since the axon, like every other cell, is enclosed by a well-defined membrane. It may be that there is constant loss of water and consumption of other substances in the metabolically active parts of the fibre, both at the nodes of Ranvier and at the terminals.

The Schwann Cell and the Myelin Sheath

In peripheral nerves, the *myelin sheath* is modified portion of the cell membrane and cytoplasm of the Schwann cell (see footnote on page 2296). One Schwann cell is responsible for one internodal length of myelin, and the minute gap in the myelin sheath where one Schwann cell abuts on its neighbour is the node of Ranvier.[14a] During myelination, the infolded portion of the Schwann cell membrane, termed the mesaxon, comes to enclose a single axon; in time this infolding grows progressively to form a spiral layer round the fibre. The spiral arrangement is almost certainly not produced by rotation of the cell and consequent drawing out of the mesaxon. It probably develops through elongation of the membrane as a whole by insertion of 'units' into it at all points. Even when the coils have packed down and tightened after their first loose arrangement, and the opposing surfaces, both internal and external, have fused to form the repeating pattern of 12 nm found in adult peripheral myelin, there must still be an increase in thickness and in internal diameter (axon diameter) during growth to the adult state. The coils must both slip and increase in their circumference so that this may happen. Moreover, increase in length of the coils must also take place at all levels to allow for growth of the internode from between 200 and 300 μm at the onset of myelination to between 1000 and 1500 μm in the largest adult fibres. Such conformational changes must mean that the myelin can be added to at all points even when as apparently tightly packed and rigid as the ultrastructural appearances first suggest.

Elements of cytoplasm persist at intervals in the fully formed myelin sheath, both in the Schmidt–Lantermann incisures (the oblique or spiral clefts that occur at several places in the longitudinal course of each myelin segment[14b, 14c])[15] and in the paranodal 'loops' at the ends of the internodes. In both these regions, microtubules are visible which, if we assume that they have the same functions as elsewhere, would allow for the rapid passage of materials along the tortuous spiral channels.

While much information is now available on the structure of the myelin sheath, less is known about the *nodes of Ranvier* (Fig. 35.8). These nodes are of great interest in both physiology and pathology, because it is here that the nerve impulse receives the boost that, in the process known as '*saltatory conduction*', sends it to the next node. While an impulse may be able to jump two, or even three, blocked nodes, blocking of more than this number will bring conduction to a standstill. The nodes could thus become sites for a selective disease that could impede conduction in a nerve fibre or even block it altogether, although the change responsible might not be readily discernible histologically.

The nodes lie in the gaps, 0·5 to 1·0 μm wide, between successive myelin segments. The axon at this point is significantly narrowed, and may contain a few mitochondria; the lamellae of the myelin sheaths are folded back on themselves on each side of the node, and the cytoplasm of the Schwann cells is more conspicuous at this point.[16] Indeed, the amount of unmodified Schwann cell cytoplasm and the numbers of mitochondria are probably greater in this juxtanodal region than elsewhere in the internode.[17] On its inner aspect, the Schwann cell cytoplasm comes into intimate contact with the axon by means of a series of finger-like processes that occupy about 40 per cent of this short myelin-bare length of axon. Between these processes an electron-dense 'gap substance', containing acid mucoproteins, is in contact with the basement membrane[18] and the Plenk–Laidlaw reticulin layer[10a, 10b] that invests the fibre throughout its length.[19] It is in the nodal region that the ionic exchanges, on which nerve impulse conduction depends, take place across the axon membrane. It is at this site, too, that the energy needed for maintaining a high resting potential between the axon and its surroundings appears to be generated and stored. The morphological appearances suggest that the Schwann cell plays an active role in this process and is not merely a passive sheath. Specific Schwann cell diseases probably have a marked and selective effect upon conduction for this reason.

Variations in Thickness of the Myelin Sheath

Conduction velocity in an axon is directly proportional to the external diameter of the nerve fibre; it may also be directly proportional to internodal length.[20] These facts have important implications in relation to the mechanism and possible selectivity of peripheral neuropathic processes. Their significance has also to be considered when attempts are made to correlate clinical and electrical observations with anatomical lesions. While it is possible with suitably selected experimental material to ascertain fairly simply any changes in fibre diameter patterns, this is much more difficult to do under the unselected conditions pertaining to disease in man. However, attempts have been made to carry out such studies on peripheral nerves in subacute combined degeneration of the spinal cord[21] and in motor neuron disease:[22] the observations in both conditions need to be repeated and extended. That such studies are possible on human post-mortem material has been shown by work on the sciatic nerve.[23] Normally, the sciatic nerve has 13 000 or more myelinated fibres per square millimetre of cross section: changes in fibre diameter patterns can be demonstrated by measuring the diameter of such a number of fibres that the results indicate a consistent pattern—this usually entails measurements on about a thousand fibres. When more studies of this kind have been made, in a wide range of neuropathies, it will be feasible to assess the value of a clinical and electrophysiological appraisal of the degree of damage to motor or sensory fibres, as well as whether one modality of sensation is affected more than another. This

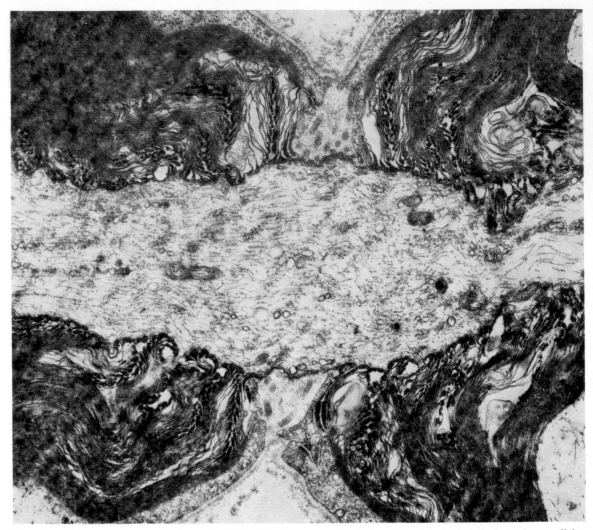

Fig. 35.8.§ Electron micrograph of a node of Ranvier in a nerve of a baboon (longitudinal section). It shows: slight constriction of axon at termination of myelin segment; myelin cytoplasmic 'loops' touching axon surface, and others folded back into a 'herring bone' pattern; 'fingers' of Schwann cell making contact with axon membrane in nodal gap; and gap-substance 'fuzz' between the Schwann cell 'fingers'. × 23 000.

statistical approach, when combined with studies on any changes in nerve terminals, would clarify thought about the pathogenetic processes that lead to the various types of peripheral neuropathy.

Nerve Terminals

Motor Terminals.—As motor fibres stream from the final nerve bundle, they splay and make contact usually with a single motor endplate (Fig. 35.9). The ratio of terminal nerve fibres to muscle fibres is the *terminal innervation ratio*, and is ordinarily 1 : 1 or 1 : 1·1.[24] At this point, the terminal fibres are still myelinated, and in frozen sections stained with Sudan black B their diameter is uniformly 2 to 3 μm. Immediately before these fibres enter the myoneural junction, they lose their sheath; they then divide into fine branches and lie closely within the folds of the subneural apparatus—the *post-synaptic gutter*. On their outer aspect they continue to have an investment of cells, known as the *teloglia*, which are probably modified Schwann cells. The neural membrane is separated by a gap only 20 nm wide from the highly folded, specialized muscle-cell membrane or *subneural apparatus*. The neural endings contain mitochondria and many synaptic vesicles, which are the carriers of the protein-bound transmitter substance; on the muscle

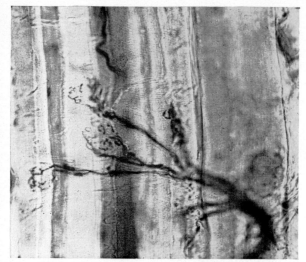

Fig. 35.9.§ Terminal motor arborization in normal cat muscle. The branched endings lie in the postsynaptic gutter of the subneural apparatus. *Intravital methylene blue.* × 180.

side of the gap, the muscle-cell membrane is much modified and contains abundant true cholinesterase (Fig. 35.10).

Many biopsy studies of normal and pathological muscles have employed an intravital methylene blue technique to obtain information about the terminal arborization of motor fibres in disease states. When combined with parallel histochemical studies on cholinesterase in the subneural apparatus, this approach has been singularly informative about changes in nerve terminations during life. The necessary cutting of the muscle into thin strips, however, disturbs its architectural relationships; moreover, the technique is not applicable to necropsy material. Despite these drawbacks, the method is valuable, especially for assessing the extent of any compensatory collateral sprouting (see Figs 36.29A and 36.29B, page 2374).

Sensory Terminals.—The sensory endings in muscle and elsewhere have been well described,[25] and a common pattern is recognizable in all but the least specialized. Where the myelin sheath ends, the axon may continue into a specialized structure composed of non-neural elements, such as the pressure-sensitive lamellate corpuscles (of Pacini), the tactile corpuscles (of Meissner) and the neurotendinous endings (Golgi tendon organs). In muscle the axon enters the muscle spindle, where it lies between the intrafusal muscle fibre and the Schwann cell sheath. The fine structure of the mammalian muscle

spindle and its relation to the sensory and motor endings have been described by Landon.[26]

Sensory endings in muscle are well displayed by the simple method of staining frozen sections, 50 to 80 μm thick, with Sudan black B.[27] By this means the endings (Fig. 35.11) are demonstrated sufficiently clearly for any pathological change involving a large number of muscles to be surveyed. The myelinated fibres to the sensory endings can be recognized by their relatively large size (Fig. 35.12), for, unlike the repeatedly branching motor nerve fibres, they do not become much attenuated before reaching their terminations.

Blood Vessels, Lymphatics and Other Channels in Nerve Trunks

The blood vessels and lymphatic channels of nerve trunks, and the connexions, especially within the spinal canal, of the potential (endoneurial) spaces that separate individual nerve fibres, are of great importance in the pathogenesis of certain toxic and viral diseases of the spinal cord. They are equally important in the understanding of immunological mechanisms that may underlie certain diseases in peripheral nerves and ganglia.

Nerve trunks depend for their blood supply mainly on branches of the arteries in the regions through which they pass, and there is a rich inter-regional network within the trunk which is capable of preventing local ischaemia should any single

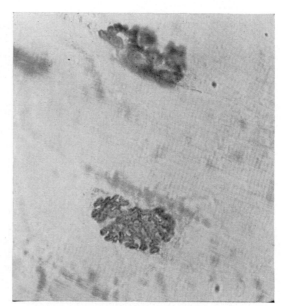

Fig. 35.10. Subneural apparatus of myoneural junction of cat muscle shown by cholinesterase staining. Compare with Fig. 35.9. *Modified Koelle technique.* × 500.

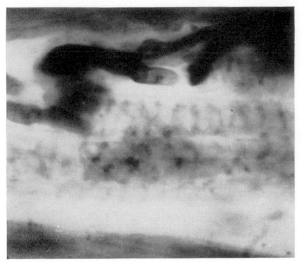

Fig. 35.11. Intramuscular spindle of a normal cat. Nuclear 'bag' (equatorial region) (unstained) is surrounded by coils of naked but Sudanophile nerve fibres. Above is the thick, myelinated, primary sensory fibre. *Sudan black B.* × 650.

vessel be obstructed.[28] The spinal root ganglia also receive vessels from the segmental arteries of the region, the branches entering their poles. The capillary network in nerve trunks and ganglia is extensive, especially in the latter. In man, monkey and rabbit the ganglia contain numerous bead-like ampullary dilatations of the capillary bed, some 8 to 20 times the diameter of the ordinary capillary.

It has been estimated that these dilatations provide a surface area for the vascular bed of the ganglia that, weight for weight, is equal to that of the parietal cerebral cortex.[29]

Little is known about the lymphatic vessels of the nerve trunks. A rich plexus of lymphatics in the epineurial connective tissue (outside the perineurium) drains to regional lymph nodes, but there are no such vessels within the nerve bundle itself. Material draining from the endoneurial space must pass through the perineurial sheath in order to gain access to the lymphatics.

Knowledge of the potential spaces within nerve trunks and their connexions with the subarachnoid space and intraspinal tissues on the one hand,[30] and with neural lymphatics on the other, has been stimulated by the observations that viruses and toxins, especially tetanus toxin, may enter the central nervous system by this route. When a small volume of dye solution or India ink is injected intraneurally, either of two results may follow.[31] One is characterized by little resistance to the injection, and a sharply defined, coloured column of fluid runs rapidly up the undistended trunk for a centimetre or more. In this, the '*cord/cerebrospinal-fluid type*' of injection, the dye lies in the spaces between the individual nerve fibres. If a radioactive phosphate solution is being used when this type of injection results, the tracer reaches and ascends the spinal cord, and also enters the cerebrospinal fluid;

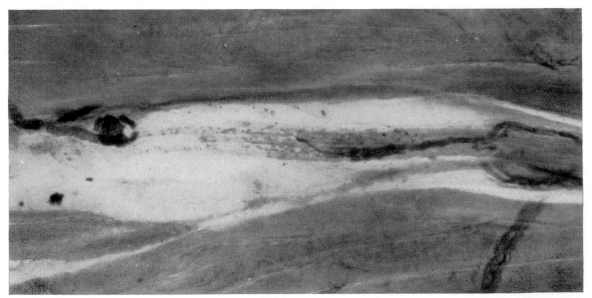

Fig. 35.12. Intramuscular spindle of cat. The thin intrafusal muscle fibres lie in a lymph space. Myelinated nerve fibres run in this space. The primary sensory fibre (left) is larger than the secondary sensory fibre (middle and right). Thin gamma-efferent fibres (motor) are present at the extreme right. *Sudan black B.* × 200.

very little escapes in the blood. In contrast, in cases in which the injection meets with resistance, the coloured solution collects in an artificial epineurial space. In this, the '*blood type*' of injection, very little tracer ascends the nerve trunk, and most passes by lymphatics to the blood stream.

The relation of the spinal nerve roots to the meninges, especially their proximity to the arachnoid granulations through which cerebrospinal fluid is returned to the circulation, and the structural aspects of the changeover from Schwann cells to oligodendroglia at the point where the fibres enter or leave the spinal cord (the so-called 'root entry zone'—see page 2120), are of special importance in the pathogenesis of lesions in these regions. Cerebrospinal fluid is passed through specialized arachnoid formations that lie adjacent to each sensory root as it runs through the meninges and are exactly comparable to the arachnoid villi and arachnoid granulations (Pacchionian bodies) elsewhere in the neuraxis (see page 2198). If India ink is injected into the subarachnoid space it collects in cuffs round each sensory root:[32] there appears, however, to be no way by which crystalloids or particulate matter can pass from the subarachnoid space to the endoneurial space, despite the possibility that such substances can travel freely in the reverse direction. It is possible that potentially toxic materials may become concentrated close to the sensory roots and cause localized damage,[29] but data in support of this suggestion are scanty.

It is still uncertain how the transition between Schwann cell investment and oligodendroglial investment of the myelin sheaths is effected at the point where the nerve fibres enter and leave the central nervous system. What happens to the endoneurial space at this point is also unknown. When so much important knowledge is still lacking, it may be wondered whether there is any justification at the present time for formulating even the most tentative hypothesis about the manner in which substances travel in these regions. Nonetheless, there is little doubt that the spaces in a motor nerve trunk do in fact provide a potential route for the ascent of particulate or soluble noxious agents, and that in the special case of local or ascending

tetanus they probably form the main route along which the toxin passes to the spinal cord.

While it can be accepted that nerve trunks offer a possible pathway from the periphery to the cerebrospinal axis, evidence is divided whether neurotropic viruses invade the central nervous system by this route.[33] In poliomyelitis (see page 2144) it now seems likelier that invasion of the brain and spinal cord follows a viraemia. How the viraemia becomes translated into an encephalomyelitis is not known, but suspicion has fallen on the spinal ganglia as one possible portal of entry for the virus. While, in the adult, acid dyes and large molecules introduced into the blood do not leave the latter in any quantity to enter the substance of the central nervous system, they can pass easily into the tissues of the dorsal root ganglia. This has been demonstrated by the intravenous injection of the dyes erythrosin and fluorescein labelled with radioactive iodine; after two hours the concentration of the dyes in the ganglia is about four times that in the brain.[29]

The problems of the blood–ganglion barrier and the blood–nerve barrier have been re-examined, particularly by Waksman,[33a] and species differences have been emphasized. With various methods, he found the former barrier to be as effective in rabbits as in guinea-pigs, while the latter is more evident in rabbits than it is in guinea-pigs. It was on the basis of differential permeability that he attempted to explain the restriction of damage to the ganglion and root regions in experimental diphtheritic and allergic neuropathy in rabbits, and the more widespread distribution of the corresponding neuropathies in guinea-pigs. While there are grounds for questioning Waksman's interpretation of his findings,[34] his work has emphasized a key problem in the pathogenesis of radiculitis and toxic neuropathy. It has also laid stress on the general neuropathological principle that if one region of a tissue of seemingly uniform structural composition is damaged selectively by a pathological process, this selectivity must contain some clue to the mechanism by which the pathogen operates. Until the selectivity is explained, no certainty about the mechanism may exist.

DISEASES OF NERVES

THE REACTIONS OF NERVE TRUNKS TO TRANSECTION

In 1850, Augustus Waller described the changes, since known as Wallerian degeneration, that

followed division of the ninth and twelfth cranial nerves of frogs.[35] He observed no alteration until the third or fourth day, when the nerves began to show a 'turbid or coagulated appearance'. By the fifth or sixth day, the 'coagulation of the medulla [as he called the myelin of the nerve trunk] had proceeded to separate particles of various sizes', and by the tenth day these particles were breaking down to form fine granules, a process that was complete by the twentieth day. This is the sequence of events in any nerve fibre that is separated from its cell body, and except for more understanding of the details of the process, little new has become known about it since Waller's investigations.

The first change apparent in a nerve fibre distal to the level at which it has been divided is fibrillation of the axon, which may be seen within as little as 12 hours.[36] The first major change is widening of the nodes of Ranvier.[37]

During the first week the myelin and axon break up into ovoid bodies and the Schwann cells begin to proliferate (Figs 35.13A to 35.13C). At this early phase the myelin lipids undergo only physicochemical alteration; there is no change in the chemical composition of the nerve, although its water content becomes greatly increased during the first four days.[38] From the eighth day onward, esterified cholesterol becomes detectable, and the amounts of cerebroside and sphingomyelin begin to decline. With the onset of cholesterol esterification, the Marchi reaction* becomes positive, and indeed this reaction seems to be a relatively specific test for cholesterol esters.[39]

In general, the changes in the myelin and axon during the first week of Wallerian degeneration are closely analogous to those in autolysis. Nerves that have been transected *in situ*, and isologous nerve grafts (that is, nerves transplanted and therefore without blood supply), continue to conduct for about 72 hours;[40] it should be realized, however, that this method of study gives information only about the conducting capacity of the nerve trunk as a whole. As Ramón y Cajal pointed out, there is great variation in the rapidity of the early disruption of nerve fibres. In general, unmyelinated fibres break down most slowly, while a few finely myelinated fibres may break down faster than those of larger diameter. It has also been shown that sensory fibres degenerate more rapidly than motor fibres, and it would therefore appear that persistent passage of impulses—which arise continuously in

* The Marchi reaction has very little place in the study of neuropathic processes. In the past it has been responsible for more misleading reports, especially in experimental work, than any other single method, partly because of its tendency to produce artefacts and partly because workers have sometimes relied upon it to the exclusion of more dependable methods. It shows nothing that cannot be demonstrated by other techniques: its use should be avoided.

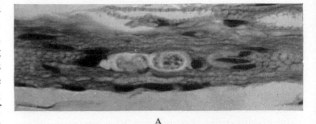

A

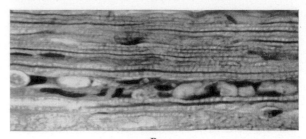

B

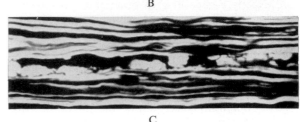

C

Fig. 35.13. Wallerian degeneration of isolated fibres in rabbit nerve. × 530.
A. Fragmenting myelin 'ovoids' in first stage of breakdown. *Haematoxylin–eosin.*
B. 'Digestion' vacuoles with increased numbers of nuclei during second week. *Haematoxylin–eosin.*
C. Axonal swelling and fragmentation. *Glees and Marsland method.*

peripheral receptors—may in some way hasten the change, possibly by causing more rapid consumption of stored metabolites that normally would be replaced by the perikaryon.

Change in the cell population of the nerve trunk begins about 48 hours after section. The number of cells steadily increases during the first 10 days and then continues to rise, but more slowly, to its peak, which is reached within three to four weeks (Fig. 35.14): thereafter it declines slowly and progressively.[41] Cytological changes indicative of increased nuclear and cytoplasmic activity may be discernible in Schwann cells as early as 24 hours after section of the nerve. Macrophages and, to a lesser extent, fibroblasts and even perineurial cells all participate in this proliferation: little is known of the cell-stimulating factors responsible. There is also an increase in the number of mast cells in the endoneurium,[42] and an increase in vascular perme-

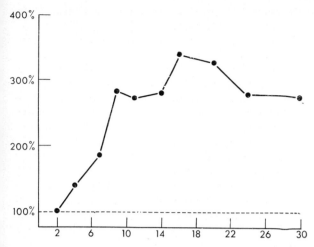

Fig. 35.14.§ Changes in nuclear population of the sciatic nerve of chickens following nerve section. *Ordinate:* percentage of initial cell numbers. *Abscissa:* time in days from nerve section. (Redrawn from: Cavanagh, J. B., Webster, G. R., *Quart. J. exp. Physiol.*, 1955, **40**, 12.)

ability.[43] However, the ultimate total cell increase is dependent upon the amount of myelin initially present in the nerve: in an unmyelinated nerve there may be only minimal proliferation of cells after section.[44]

After the first week there is a histochemically traceable degradation of myelin lipids to compounds of smaller and simpler molecules, and to neutral lipids, which stain strongly with Sudan III or IV.[45] It was this cellular degradation of myelin that Waller observed and considered to be complete after the twentieth day. The process in fact continues for much longer than this, and small quantities of lipids may still be discernible many weeks later.

The ultimate practical purpose of these changes, considering the matter teleologically, is the production of continuous cords or chains of cells within the basement membrane and Plenk–Laidlaw sheath of each nerve fibre: these are known as von Büngner's bands,[45a] and they serve for the reception, guidance and remyelination of regenerated axons. Since the length of the normal adult internode is a product of the growth of the part after myelin formation has begun, and since the original, or 'natural', length of a myelinating Schwann cell is 200 to 300 μm, this difference is made good by proliferation. Indeed, proliferation may be initiated by loss of contact of the Schwann cells with one another when the myelin breaks up.[46] Essentially, therefore, the whole process is not 'degeneration' but 'regeneration', and myelin begins to be formed

soon after the regenerating axons enter the bands of von Büngner, long before they reach their terminals. The myelinated internodes ultimately formed in this way, in mammalian nerves, have a uniform length of 200 to 300 μm, regardless of ultimate axon thickness, since in the adult there is no elongation due to growth of the part.

Regenerative Phenomena

Two distinct reparative responses are found in nerves following damage. The first is *collateral sprouting*, a reaction by healthy fibres to the loss of nearby fibres, and an immediate effort to mitigate the consequences of the damage. This is, in fact, a form of compensatory hypertrophy. The second is *regeneration*, the response of the mutilated nerve cell attempting to re-establish contact with its former terminal.

Collateral sprouting is a most important process of compensation for the casual loss of individual fibres, and its role in human disease has not yet been fully assessed. After partial denervation, whether by local division of the nerve or by section of the nerve root, sprouting begins on the third day,[47] the sprouts developing from the nodes of Ranvier of nearby fibres and pushing their way out to make contact with denervated endplates (Figs 35.15A and 35.15B). These collaterals are extremely fine, and are shown accurately only in gold impregnation preparations or in intra-vital methylene blue preparations. In chronic denervating diseases in man, the complex branching that results from such sprout formation grossly disturbs the normal 1 : 1 terminal innervation ratio. The natural factors that stimulate sprouting are unknown; the dye pyronin is a powerful stimulant, and so also are extracts of brain and nerves collectively referred to by the term *neurocletin*.[48]

The ultimate functional value and effectiveness of collateral sprouting has yet to be assessed. It would certainly be expected to prevent general atrophy of denervated skeletal muscle fibres, and thus to save them for possible later reinnervation by regenerating neurons. The extremely fine calibre of such sprouts and the fact that the majority of them are unmyel. ated make it probable that conduction in them is very slow, and that they would not be capable of mediating muscular movements that require well-controlled innervation.

Provided the nerve cell is healthy it can be relied upon to make every effort, by the *regeneration* of its axon, to re-establish contact with its former terminal organ. Many factors must be taken into

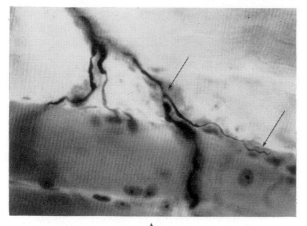

A

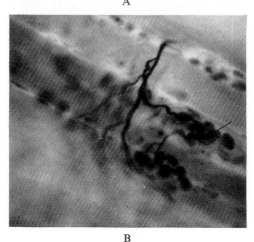

B

Fig. 35.15. Regeneration of motor nerve terminals following crushing of a muscle of a cat. *Glees and Marsland method.* × 530.

A. Collateral sprouting. A thin branch (arrows) runs from a surviving fibre to enter an empty endplate.

B. Ultraterminal sprouting. Having innervated one endplate (oblique marker near centre of right margin) the fibre continues to a second empty endplate.

account in considering the expectation of successful re-innervation;[49] under experimental conditions the factors include the age of the animal, the distance of the damage from the terminal organ, the degree of this damage, and whether the injury is crushing (axonotmesis), cutting followed by suturing (neurotmesis), or resection of a length of nerve. The initial delay in axonal growth is least when the amount of damage is smallest. Once growth has begun and the sprouting fibres have passed beyond the damaged area, the rate of the advance of the growing tips of the nerve fibres is approximately 1 to 1·5 mm per day. This rate falls off when the

distances concerned are very long, and also at the terminal arborizations.

On reaching the terminals the motor fibres may merely re-enter the somewhat shrunken, but persisting, original endplate region, or they may form ultraterminal branches that continue beyond the old endplate, either to join other endplates or to induce new endplates upon their own or other muscle fibres. The likelihood that such aberrant formations will develop increases with the distance of the muscle from the point of damage to the nerve; their occurrence is probably related to irregularity of the rate of growth in individual fibres and to an increase in the rate of failure of re-establishment of the original innervation due to the greater chance of fibres taking the wrong path when they have a longer distance to cover.[50]

Sensory reinnervation has received less attention than motor reinnervation, but it is apparent that the same principles obtain.[51] Sensory loss in the denervated area is minimized by the normal overlapping of innervation areas, by active ingrowth of sprouts from surrounding normal areas, and ultimately by the extension of regenerating fibres down the original nerve trunks. Even such highly specialized organs as the muscle spindles seem to undergo reinnervation with time, but the degree of anatomical and functional success is unknown.

Nerve Cell Changes Following Axonal Section

The change known as *central chromatolysis* is the usual reaction of the perikaryon to damage to its axon. Although so well known, this change is difficult to produce experimentally, unless certain procedures are adopted. Following section of a peripheral nerve on a single occasion, no change occurs in the perikaryon. If, after 10 days, the nerve is cut again, above the first site of section, or if it is forcibly pulled away from its roots,[52] the perikaryon will be found after a further period of about 10 days to have swollen, the nucleus to lie close to the cell membrane, and the Nissl substance to have disappeared except for a narrow ring beneath the cell membrane (Figs 35.16A and 35.16B).

Chromatolysis should certainly be regarded not as a degenerative phenomenon but rather as an index of the vitality of a cell and of its response to the challenge to synthetize new axonal protoplasm. Cytochemical studies have demonstrated clearly that there is an increase in the protein and lipid content of chromatolytic neurons during the reactionary phase after axon injury,[53] although their

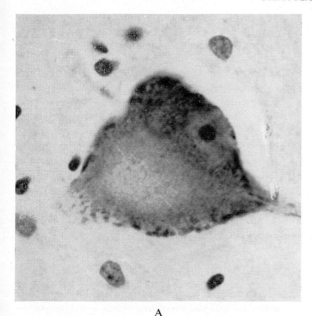

A

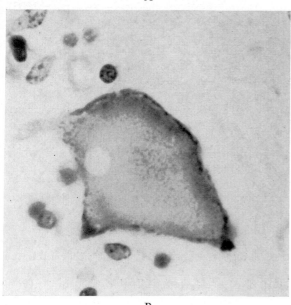

B

Fig. 35.16. Chromatolysis of neurons in an anterior grey column of the spinal cord following an attack of acute porphyria. See also Fig. 35.21C, page 2321. *Cresyl violet.* × 825.

A. Dissolution of central Nissl substance, displacement of nucleus to periphery, and swelling of the cell.

B. Severer change, only a thin rim of stainable Nissl substance remaining.

concentration falls because of an accompanying increase in the amount of water in the cells. The ribonucleic acid content of the cells rises later and slowly, although in the earlier reactionary phase

there is a change from an active to a more active stage. This superactivation of ribonucleic acid is associated with dispersion of the large orderly blocks of endoplasmic reticulum (Nissl substance) and the appearance of large numbers of discrete polyribosomes scattered throughout the cytoplasm. An autoradiographic study showed that ^{3}H-labelled ribonucleic acid precursors entered the nuclei of hypoglossal neurons and passed to the cytoplasm at a greatly increased rate 48 hours after injury to the hypoglossal nerve; later, during the axon growth phase, the nucleus–cytoplasm transfer rate fell to below normal.[54] The size of the nucleolus increased before cytoplasmic swelling occurred and this enlargement was accompanied by an increase in the amount of ribonucleic acid in the nucleolus. The shorter the distance between the site of the injury and the cell body, the sooner these responses occurred; the more distant the lesion, the larger was the response.[55] The initiating stimulus for these changes was not separation of the nerve cell from its effector organ, for they occurred as much after a second cut as after the first; similarly, the later decline in ribonucleic acid activity was not related to the establishment of contact between the regenerating neurite and an effector organ, for it occurred equally when contact was blocked. A further interesting observation was that these chromatolytic responses occurred after local injection of botulinum toxin, which blocked synaptic transmission but left the axon intact.[56] There is a marked proliferation of terminal neurites after exposure to this toxin:[57] this observation suggested that membrane expansion or synthesis might be the demand that initiates the chromatolytic response.[56] What is most interesting about reactions at a distance of this sort is that there must be a constant two-way flow of information under normal circumstances between the periphery and the centre: interruption of this feed-back control is followed within 24 hours by visible evidence of a neuronal response.[58]

Similar changes occur in the dorsal spinal root (sensory) ganglion cells, but they are less marked, and sometimes they are difficult to distinguish from the normal fine, powdery state of the Nissl substance of some of these cells. There is, moreover, a wide variety of appearances of the Nissl substance in the normal animal from one nuclear group to another, and it is probable that the blocks of ribonucleoprotein are constantly being rearranged during the responses to functional stresses.[59]

When regenerating nerves completely fail to establish functional connexions with end-organs, as inevitably occurs following amputation of a limb, the neurons concerned become smaller and finally disappear. This *retrograde atrophy* is a phenomenon common in the nervous system; it is a consequence of disuse. Since the volume of the nucleus and of the perikaryon of a nerve cell is an expression of the 'connectivity' of the cell—that is, of the extent of the field innervated by the cell—any reduction of the innervation field will lead to shrinkage of the cell body. This has been well demonstrated in a study of partial denervation of the spinocerebellar pathway.[60]

CIRCULATORY DISORDERS AND THE EFFECTS OF COMPRESSION TRAUMA

The blood supply to peripheral nerves is rich, and there is a sufficient margin of safety in the collateral anastomotic network to allow for occlusion of a large branch without noticeable disturbance of the function of the nerve. On the other hand, nerves are at least as susceptible to hypoxia as other tissues, but because of the difficulties in distinguishing the effects of direct compression from those of vascular obstruction, it has never been possible to assess properly the relative effects of each. Motor nerves and sensory nerves differ in their susceptibility to nerve compression. When paralysis and anaesthesia have been caused by compressing nerves for 45 minutes by means of a cuff round a limb, sensory function returns much more rapidly than motor function.[61] Clinical evidence suggests that it is the largest fibres that are most liable to be affected by compression of this sort.[62] With severer compression, paralysis may not recover for many weeks: the slowness of recovery is related to loss of myelin sheaths, which must be reformed before function can return. The severest damage that may result from compression is complete interruption of the fibres.[63] The fact that local myelin loss occurs before interruption of the axons is of considerable interest, for it suggests that the integrity of the myelin sheath may be metabolically more dependent on aerobic energy sources than that of the nerve fibre itself. This observation tallies with the fact that the number of mitochondria is very much greater in the juxtanodal regions of the cell than in the axon. It is also further evidence for the probability that Schwann cells have an important role in the conductive function of nerve fibres, perhaps by maintaining the appropriate ionic relations in the immediate vicinity of the axon membrane at the nodes of Ranvier.[64] Remyelination of damaged internodal myelin segments is readily effected, and is an important function of the Schwann cells. It is not uncommon to encounter internodes of reduced length, particularly in the nerves of older people (see page 2307): this may be a result of the repeated minor injuries and episodes of compression to which nerves are exposed in the course of a lifetime.

There is little doubt that the local nerve palsies, such as *tourniquet paralysis*, '*Saturday night paralysis*', and other pressure lesions, may be explained in this way. Recovery in individual cases will depend upon the duration of the pressure ischaemia and the area affected, for these factors determine the degree of damage to Schwann cells and to axons, and it is upon the regeneration of both of these that recovery ultimately depends.

Polyarteritis

The nerve lesions in polyarteritis are basically due to acute ischaemia resulting from obstruction of the nutrient vessels of the nerves (see page 2303). As many as 50 per cent of patients who have polyarteritis show some manifestation of peripheral neuropathy.[65] The changes of polyarteritic neuropathy may be described by the term *mononeuritis multiplex*, which is intended to indicate that the nerve lesions occur in an irregularly timed succession of episodes, affecting individual nerves at random. They often involve the proximal parts of the larger nerves.[66] The apparently symmetrical distribution of the resulting neurological disturbances is due to the multiplicity and widespread distribution of the vascular lesions. Motor symptoms predominate, but pain and paraesthesiae are very common. The degree of recovery varies according to the size of the vessels involved, the extensiveness of the neural involvement and the size of the nerves affected. In the nerve itself the changes are those of Wallerian degeneration, secondary to infarction (Figs 35.17A to 35.17C). Regeneration may be expected, for the nerve cells are intact and arteritic lesions of the vasculature of the central nervous system are very unusual; but, because of the widespread occurrence of the lesions and of the distance that may separate them from the perikarya, recovery may be very incomplete.

Atherosclerosis and Thromboangitis Obliterans

No one has attempted to make a full analysis of the anatomical changes that occur in nerves as a result of the chronic ischaemia produced by atherosclerosis and thromboangitis obliterans. Studies of

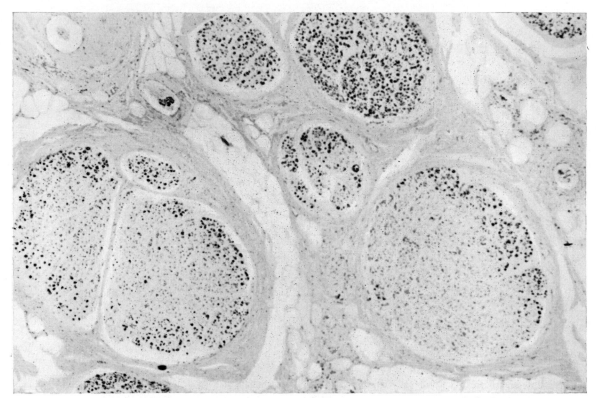

Fig. 35.17A. Polyarteritis. Transverse section of affected nerve showing severe but patchy reduction in the number of myelin sheaths. *Iron haematoxylin.* × 95.

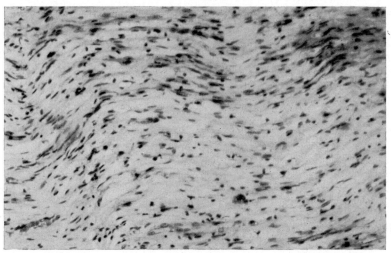

Fig. 35.17B. Polyarteritis. Wallerian degeneration of many fibres in an affected nerve. *Haematoxylin–eosin.* × 95.

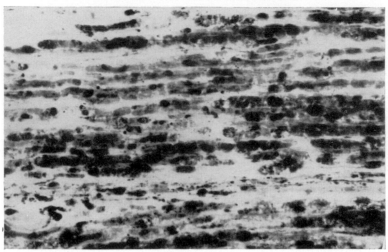

Fig. 35.17C. Polyarteritis. Fragmenting myelin sheaths in an affected nerve. *Osmium tetroxide.* × 95.

fibre diameter have been undertaken in two cases of atherosclerotic vascular disease of the legs: these showed a pronounced reduction in the total number of fibres, a change that was progressively more marked toward the distal parts of the nerve trunks.[67] There is also a pronounced reduction in the number of fibres of over 8 μm in diameter (Fig. 35.18). At first sight this might appear to be the result of selective degeneration of the large diameter, long fibres, but there is the possibility of an alternative explanation—namely, that there is an overall reduction in the number of fibres, but because regeneration and remyelination are constantly proceeding at the same time as fresh damage is being sustained by other fibres, there are many newly formed fibres that are of small diameter, in addition to any original small diameter fibres that have survived. Which of these inferences is correct could be determined by examining the terminations of the nerves in muscles.

It is noteworthy that patients with chronic occlusive vascular disease complain mainly of sensory disturbances: motor changes are often less in evidence despite severe loss of large diameter fibres. It is possible, therefore, that the compensatory effect of collateral sprouting is more efficacious on the motor side than on the sensory.

Neuropathy in Diabetes Mellitus

There is little doubt that in many cases of diabetic neuropathy, especially in the older age groups, vascular insufficiency plays an important role in producing nerve damage, but whether it is the only

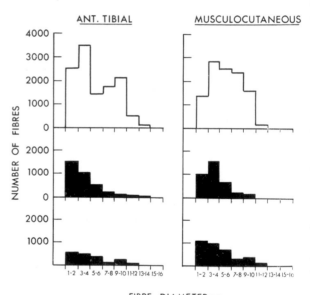

Fig. 35.18.§ Histograms of nerve fibre diameters in chronic obliterative vascular disease. *White:* normal nerves. *Black:* measurements in two cases with neuropathy. *ANT. TIBIAL:* deep peroneal nerve. *MUSCULOCUTANEOUS:* superficial peroneal nerve. (Redrawn from: Garven, H. S. D., Gairns, F. W., Smith, G., *Scot. med. J.*, 1962, **7**, 250.)

factor is another matter. The view that a vascular basis underlies much of the neurological change[68, 69] has given way to the belief that the nervous tissue itself—the Schwann cells and neurons—suffers primarily from some metabolic disturbance that may sensitize it to vascular insufficiency. While it is not thought that nerve cells are dependent upon insulin for their normal metabolism, there is no doubt that Schwann cells, like most other cells, are dependent upon it:[70] indeed, there is a substantial increase in the intracellular products of the sorbitol metabolic pathway in the peripheral nerves in diabetes.[71] While this may help to explain the Schwann cell changes about to be described, it does not clarify the neuronal degeneration that undoubtedly also occurs in diabetes.

There are several clinical types of diabetic neuropathy: their names indicate their chief features— symmetrical sensory neuropathy, autonomic neuropathy, mononeuropathy, multiple mononeuropathy, amyotrophy, and diabetic pseudotabes. The overall incidence in the diabetic population increases with age and with the duration of the diabetes, rising from about 16 per cent in the fifth decade to about 37 per cent in the seventh decade.[72, 73] Neuropathy is particularly prone to occur in patients whose diabetes is poorly controlled; occasionally it develops when control is apparently good. When the onset of neuropathy is acute the condition usually responds well to proper diabetic care; in cases with an insidious onset the outlook usually is poor, especially in the older patient. It should be noted that the prognosis is related to the type of cellular pathology underlying the manifestations: this may involve Schwann cell changes or denervation predominantly—recovery from demyelination will always be rapider and more satisfactory than recovery from a denervating process, and failure to take account of these differences in response may distort interpretation of the outcome of therapy. On the other hand, just as wound healing and other reparative processes are impaired in diabetics, it is conceivable that reparative processes in Schwann cells and neurons are also to some extent defective: only further study can help to clarify this problem.

Disturbances of Schwann cells are frequent in diabetic neuropathy but in most instances can be satisfactorily demonstrated only by studying dissociated nerve fibres.[74] This feature of diabetic neuropathy is the more relevant because of the common occurrence of marked slowing of the conduction rate of the nerve impulse in this condition. Slowing of the conduction rate is pathognomonic of Schwann cell disease, and abundant evidence of juxtanodal and segmental myelin breakdown is found in these diabetic cases, usually with more or less complete remyelination.[74] Occasionally the Schwann cell changes are sufficiently marked to produce alterations similar to those of 'hypertrophic' neuropathy (see page 2329), with concentric bundles of Schwann cells forming an 'onion bulb' appearance in transverse sections under the light microscope. These Schwann cell clusters are usually centred on an axon with or without a thin myelin sheath.

Evidence of denervation also may be present in diabetic neuropathy. Primary loss of sensory nerve cells has been observed and may be sufficiently severe to be accompanied by degeneration and gliosis in the posterior funiculi of the spinal cord (Fig. 35.19).[75] The ataxia and other features of the condition that is referred to clinically as diabetic pseudotabes can be explained in part by such changes and in part perhaps by temporal dispersion of conduction in nerves affected by multiple segmental demyelination.[76]

Motor denervation is frequent in diabetic neuropathy: occasionally it dominates the clinical picture, giving rise to the condition referred to as diabetic amyotrophy.[77] Clear-cut' bundle atrophy' of muscle fibres is seen, but whether there is a detectable loss of neurons from the anterior grey columns of the spinal cord may depend on the severity and duration of the condition. There is considerable doubt whether this process represents a true 'dying back' degeneration of the motor neurons; it is not associated with upper motor neuron degeneration, and chromatolytic changes have not been noted.

An interesting and as yet unanswered question arises in connexion with a condition such as diabetes in which both Schwann cells and nerve fibres are affected. Assuming that the sheath cell— whether round the axon or, as in the dorsal root ganglia, round the cell body—has an important role to play in the maintenance of the neuron, might it not then be the case that survival of the neuron or its axon would be prejudiced when that sheath cell is chronically disordered? Precisely the

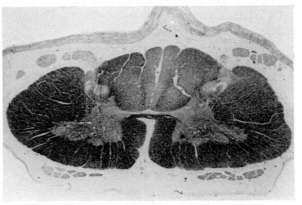

Fig. 35.19. Diabetic pseudotabes. A cervical segment of the spinal cord showing loss of fibres in the fasciculi graciles and pallor of the fasciculi cuneati. *Iron haematoxylin.* × 45.

same question poses itself in connexion with the pathogenesis of the axon degeneration in 'hypertrophic' neuropathy and the significance of the great excess of Schwann cells that cluster round surviving axons in that condition (page 2330). If it is agreed that a basic metabolic disturbance in the Schwann cells causes them to become inadequate individually to supply the requirements of the axon, it is conceivable that the 'hypertrophy' (in reality hyperplasia) is of a compensatory nature. However, this overgrowth is seen but rarely in diabetic nerves: it is therefore likely that other factors are more important in causing the neuronal degeneration.

The role of a vascular element in diabetic neuropathy has been frequently, but inconclusively, discussed. Woltman and Wilder,[68] in 1929, considered this the chief basis of the degeneration, and others have also believed that there is a close relation between arteriopathy in other organs and neuropathy.[69] More recently, these views have been contested by most workers. In view of the finding that in diabetic patients there is a localized slowing of conduction over sites that are habitually exposed to pressure,[78] it is probable that diabetics may be more sensitive to the effects of mild vascular occlusion and pressure than normal people: whether this is because their vessels are abnormal or because there is some intrinsic disturbance of the Schwann cells and axons cannot yet be decided.

Involvement of the autonomic nervous system is not uncommon in diabetics, particularly in young patients whose disease is difficult to stabilize.[73, 79] In such cases gross disturbances of vasomotor and visceral responses are not uncommonly associated with diminution of pain perception, and in this occurrence a selective loss of small unmyelinated axons may be discerned. Abnormalities in the autonomic ganglion cells—degeneration and giant cell formation—have been recorded.[80] The significance of these changes is uncertain.

Amyloid Neuropathy

The deposition of amyloid round the blood vessels of autonomic and peripheral nerves probably occurs, without symptoms, in most cases of secondary amyloidosis. In primary amyloidosis, however, it reaches proportions sufficient to cause neurological disturbances in some 13 per cent of cases.[81, 82] The onset of the neurological changes is usually insidious, and 'glove and stocking' sensory disturbances are the chief feature. Motor weakness and wasting also occur and tend to have a distal distribution. The nerves may be palpably thickened, but this is not usual. Irregularity of the pupils is often present, and there are usually other features suggesting involvement of the autonomic nervous system.

Even in the absence of peripheral neuropathy, amyloid deposits are present in the endoneurial vessels in most cases of primary amyloidosis. The amyloid deposition is essentially focal, commencing in and around the walls of medium-sized and small arteries. In severe cases it sometimes forms nodular masses, or it may extend diffusely throughout the interstices between the nerve fibres. The changes in the nerve fibres are those of Wallerian degeneration; whether there is any special susceptibility of particular fibres is unknown. The early involvement of sensory nerves may, in some cases, be due to amyloid infiltration of dorsal root ganglia.[83]

Familial cases of atypical amyloidosis with particularly striking involvement of peripheral nerves have been reported from Portugal[84] and various other parts of the world.[84a] The pattern of sensory loss in these cases is unusual and requires further investigation: apparently pain and temperature sensibility are lost first, while postural sensation is retained until later.

PARENCHYMATOUS NEUROPATHIES

Primary degeneration of the nerve cell and its fibres (the so-called 'dying-back process') has various causes. These range from hereditary inadequacies (peroneal muscular atrophy; Friedrich's ataxia and related disorders) and congenital degenerations (Werdnig–Hoffmann disease), through states in which toxic, metabolic or deficiency factors are known to be responsible (poisoning by organic phosphorus compounds; porphyria; vitamin B deficiency), to conditions of which the aetiology is still unknown (motor neuron disease). Regardless of the primary cause, all these conditions are expressions of a pathological process that can operate generally throughout the nervous system. The most important question in relation to them is not why they occur, but what factors are responsible for the development of predominantly sensory disturbances in one disease, motor disturbances in another, and mixtures of the two, with or without spinal lesions, in others.

It was realized by workers in the latter part of the last century that the distal parts of long nerve fibres may atrophy in the absence of changes in the parent cell bodies, or with notably delayed development of such changes. Gowers regarded this condition as the basis of various systemic degenerations of the central nervous system, which he referred to as the 'abiotrophies'.[85] The importance of this concept as a general expression of neuron pathology was largely forgotten until Greenfield[85a] re-emphasized its place in the pathology of spino-cerebellar disorders, and Spatz[86] grouped some primary system degenerations, including Arnold Pick's disease and amyotrophic lateral sclerosis, as examples of this type of pathological change. When peripheral nerves are affected in such disorders, certain characteristics of abiotrophic diseases will be recognized if carefully sought, whether the process affects sensory fibres or motor fibres alone, or both types together. Since the longest (and largest diameter) fibres are often most liable to be involved, the symptoms and signs frequently have a peripheral distribution. On the motor side, this implies that the rapidly conducting fibres innervating large motor units may degenerate before the small diameter fibres innervating muscle spindle fibres. On the sensory side, the fibres of larger diameter (12 to 15 μm), running from the primary anulospiral formations of the spindles, may degenerate before the medium diameter fibres from, for instance, Golgi tendon organs, Pacinian corpuscles and various skin receptors. Vibration sense and two-point discrimination sense are subserved by fibres of a diameter greater than that of the fibres that subserve thermal and pain sensation, and the former therefore often show earlier and more extensive damage. This pattern is not, however, constant for all examples of this process.

Histological studies show that the number of degenerating fibres in a nerve trunk is fewer the nearer the level examined is to the spinal cord. Extension of degeneration proximally toward the perikaryon may not even proceed beyond the point where the nerve enters the muscle. Despite severe paralysis, therefore, the nerve to the affected muscle may appear normal if it is sampled above the proximal limit of the degenerative process. Because this degeneration affects individual fibres, there is collateral sprouting from viable cells and fibres: this is a marked feature of such slowly progressive disorders as motor neuron disease. Indeed, it is probable that symptoms arise only when this compensatory process itself begins to fail.

Changes in the cell bodies in the anterior grey columns of the spinal cord and in dorsal root ganglia are predictable on the basis of this concept. Thus, if the damage to an axon is largely confined to its distal part and affects a relatively short length, the reaction of the perikaryon may be as slight as that following a distal nerve section. As the degeneration approaches the cord there is a cor-respondingly greater likelihood of a chromatolytic reaction in the perikaryon. The occurrence of chromatolysis must also depend upon the capacity of the cell to react: following temporary, exogenous intoxications or deficiency disturbances a brisk chromatolytic response occurs if the perikaryon remains essentially undamaged or is recovering from temporary intoxication. In motor neuron disease, on the other hand, degeneration is progressive and the whole neuron finally disintegrates.

The affected motor cells are characteristically most numerous in the lateral nuclei of the anterior grey column of the spinal cord—that is, where the cells supplying the most distal parts of the limbs are situated. The cells in the medial nuclei may still be normal after those in the lateral nuclei have degenerated. It is also characteristic that degeneration in the posterior funiculi of the spinal cord occurs earlier and is severer in the fasciculi graciles, which carry the longer fibres from the lumbar region, than in the shorter fasciculi cuneati. A comparable distribution of fibre degeneration is found in the spinocerebellar tracts, in which the fibres are also regionally packed; similarly, if the corticospinal tracts are involved, their lumbar and lower thoracic segments are most affected. In motor neuron disease, and in poisoning by organic phosphorus compounds, no changes may be found in the corticospinal pathways at the cervical and medullary levels. The conclusion from these general observations is that only the distal parts of the axons running to the lower spinal levels have degenerated. What ultimately happens to the perikaryon if the cause of the damage to the axon is removed seems to depend upon whether there are intact collateral branches of the affected fibres at higher levels: if the nerve cell continues to have a functioning terminal it will survive, but if no such terminal exists, retrograde degeneration will inevitably occur. This is the ultimate consequence of the lack of regenerative capacity in the central nervous system: in the peripheral nerves regenerative activity may effectively restore function, but even in them if connexion with a terminal is not established retrograde degeneration will ultimately develop.

Hereditary and Congenital Parenchymatous Neuropathies

Peroneal Muscular Atrophy (Charcot–Marie–Tooth Disease[87, 87a]) and Friedreich's Ataxia[87b]

These are hereditary disorders affecting the distal muscles of the legs and to a lesser degree those of the hands. The findings in many families are on record and it is now clear that these conditions are part of a disease complex that can affect peripheral nerves, spinal tracts and the cerebellum.[87c] What determines the form of the disease to which a particular family is liable is not known: variants and mixed forms of Friedreich's ataxia (see page 2264), of peroneal atrophy (Charcot–Marie–Tooth disease —see page 2266) and of the various conditions that have been loosely known as Marie's cerebellar atrophy (see page 2264)[87] may be peculiar to certain families. In cases of peroneal atrophy, motor and discriminative sensory fibres in the lower part of the legs are predominantly affected. The onset of symptoms is usually in adolescence and the evolution of the disease is slow, with gradual wasting of the muscles below the knees and later of those of the lower third of the thighs; the hands may also be affected. There is a mild degree of loss of the sensations of position and vibration in the distal parts of the affected limbs.

The structural changes in peroneal muscular atrophy include Wallerian degeneration of a varying number of the fibres in the distal parts of the nerve trunks, the trunks themselves showing a concomitant degree of atrophy. There may be Schwann cell hyperplasia (see page 2330). In longstanding cases, denervation of the muscles is followed by their wasting: histologically, there are many atrophic fibres and a few hypertrophic fibres in the muscles, and these changes have a patchy distribution.[88] In biopsy specimens that have been stained intravitally with methylene blue, the changes may be indistinguishable from those of motor neuron disease: collateral sprouting of nerve fibres is abundant, and ultraterminal branching, with new endplate formation, is also conspicuous. This compensatory reaction of the nerves probably assists in maintaining the strength of partially denervated muscles, and accounts for the patchiness of the muscle atrophy. The spinal cord may appear normal, or the cells of the anterior grey columns may be reduced in number; cell counts have not been made, however, and the topography of the cell loss has not been determined. Some of the neurons in the dorsal root ganglia of the lumbar segments may disappear; their loss is followed by degeneration in the fasciculi graciles.

Werdnig–Hoffmann Disease (Infantile Progressive Spinal Muscular Atrophy)[89, 89a]

This is a congenital, and often familial, disorder in which extensive and progressive degeneration of motor nerve cells occurs at an early age. Atrophy may begin in fetal life, but usually the disease becomes apparent only during the first two years. The course is steadily downhill with weakness and wasting of muscles.

The affected nerves show Wallerian degeneration; the small-sized fibres,[89b] however, apparently persist, although no quantitative data are available. The muscles contain bundles of denervated and atrophied fibres (Fig. 35.20), and there may be marked collateral sprouting of nerve fibres with only small, poorly-developed endplates. The sensory nerves in muscle spindles may appear normal, but there may be degeneration of occasional dorsal root ganglion cells; rarely, there is extensive loss of sensory cells, especially in the lumbar ganglia.[90] The question of sensory damage needs to be reinvestigated anatomically (the patients are usually too young to allow of adequate clinical appraisal).

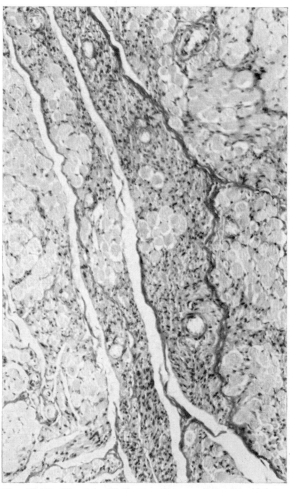

Fig. 35.20. Werdnig–Hoffmann disease. Atrophy of large groups of muscle fibres (denervation atrophy). *Van Gieson's stain.* ×175.

The neurons of the anterior grey columns of the spinal cord are reduced in number. In early cases there may be active, rapidly progressive cell degeneration, with neuronophagia. In later cases, reduction in the number of cells may alone be evident. Topographical analysis shows that the lumbar part of the spinal cord is more affected than the cervical part or the medulla, that lateral (limb) nuclei are always more depleted than medial (spinal) nuclei, and that the nuclei dorsales (Clarke's columns) are occasionally affected.[91] Some thalamic neurons and the Betz cells of the precentral gyri may also be involved.

Parenchymatous Neuropathies Resulting from Deficiencies and Intoxications

Chronic Thiamin (Vitamin B$_1$) Deficiency

It has never been proven, either in man or in animals, that the neuropathy that is generally regarded as due to thiamin deficiency is due in fact solely to lack of this vitamin;[92] however, the circumstantial evidence is very strong. Thiamin in the form of the coenzyme, thiamin pyrophosphate, is necessary for the breakdown of pyruvate in the tricarboxylic acid cycle (Krebs's cycle). Acute lack of thiamin causes Wernicke's encephalopathy (see page 2244). Chronic lack of the vitamin affects the two tissues that utilize pyruvate most actively—the myocardium (see page 44, Volume 1) and the nervous system (see page 2244). In nervous tissue, thiamin deficiency may not act simply by interfering with the energy-producing system that is essential for synthesis of synaptic transmitter, although this may be one factor in producing the symptoms. The fact that degeneration of nerves is evident at or soon after the time of onset of the neurological disturbances in pigeons experimentally deprived of thiamin strongly suggests that these effects are the result of anatomical lesions.[93]

The pattern of changes found in man and experimental animals is consistent with the concept that the lesion of the nerve fibre is an ascending or 'dying-back' process. Thus, the peripheral nerve changes are those of Wallerian degeneration, and the distal portions of the fibres are affected more markedly than those more proximal.[94] The nerve cells are intact. Changes in the long spinal tracts occur only in the posterior funiculi.

It is probable that the manifestations of human *beri-beri* are the result of multiple deficiencies, in view of the conditions of malnourishment under which it occurs. Similarly, it is probable that something more than a simple deficiency of thiamin is responsible for the *neuropathy of chronic alcoholism*. Degenerative changes occur in the nerves in these conditions and, therefore, clinical recovery must depend upon regeneration: a slight, immediate, neurological response to administration of the vitamin may be expected, but only the biochemical lesion will be reversed by such therapy. A diagnosis of thiamin deficiency can be accepted only if the level of pyruvate in the blood and cerebrospinal fluid is high and there is an abnormally low tolerance of pyruvate: the diagnosis is confirmed by the reversion of these biochemical changes to normal when thiamin is administered. Because of the uncertainty about the part played by factors other than thiamin deficiency in the aetiology of beri-beri and of the peripheral neuropathy of chronic alcoholism, studies of the state of the nerves in these conditions must be interpreted cautiously: the changes found may have causes other than a lack of thiamin. It is of interest, however, that analyses of fibre diameter have shown a loss of large diameter fibres.[95, 96]

Nitrofuran Neuropathy

The neuropathy that may complicate treatment with nitrofurans is of relevance here. Nitrofurantoin (used for the treatment of chronic urinary tract infections),[97] nitrofurazone (an antibacterial compound that is used also in the treatment of trypanosomiasis),[98] and furaltadone (an antibacterial agent now regarded as too toxic to use)[99] are all known to cause a syndrome similar to that found in avitaminosis B$_1$—polyneuritis, cardiac and other circulatory disturbances, and abnormality of pyruvate metabolism.[100] Paraesthesia is a common symptom, particularly 'burning feet', and there is motor weakness of the feet and hands. Nitrofurans act as competitive inhibitors of pyruvate metabolism,[101] and their administration results in abnormally high levels of pyruvate in the blood. With a competitive inhibitor of this type, the dose of the drug and therefore its concentration in the circulation are important in relation to the occurrence of symptoms; similarly, the presence of chronic renal failure, preventing proper excretion of the drug, is an important factor in the development of nitrofurantoin-induced neuropathy. The relatively very large doses of nitrofurazone used in treating trypanosomiasis (of the order of 1·5 g a day) in contrast to those of nitrofurantoin in cases of bacterial infection of the urinary tract (about

200 mg a day) are the probable explanation of the rapider onset and greater severity of the neuropathy associated with administration of the former. Severe degeneration of peripheral nerves and of the dorsal and ventral roots of the spinal nerves has been found at necropsy.[99,102]

Arsenical Neuropathy

Very little seems to be known about the histopathological changes in arsenical neuropathy and no experimental work has been reported. However, foot-drop and wrist-drop are common, and the weakness and wasting are distal in distribution and more marked in the legs.[103] Pain and tenderness are usually present, and loss of reflexes is common. Romberg's sign (swaying of the body when standing with the feet together and the eyes closed—a classic sign of sensory ataxia) has been a feature of many reported cases, and there may be other evidence of ataxia and incoordination. The anatomical implications of these clinical findings are that this is a 'dying-back' process affecting the longest (large diameter) fibres, and not necessarily restricted to the peripheral nerves; the presence of Rombergism and ataxia suggests that fibres in the posterior funiculi—but probably not fibres in the spinocerebellar tracts—may also be involved. Follow-up studies to elucidate this point have not yet been made; they should show whether the degenerative changes are purely peripheral, and therefore potentially capable of recovery, or whether they are accompanied by lesions of the spinal tracts, which would not be reversible.

The biochemical lesion in arsenical neuropathy is apparently due to the combination of inorganic arsenic with sulphydryl groups. Enzymes, such as succinate dehydrogenase, and the coenzyme, lipoic acid, are consequently inactivated, and this induces a partial block in the aerobic pathway of pyruvate breakdown. An abnormal pyruvate tolerance should, therefore, be detectable in cases of arsenical neuropathy, and pyruvic acid metabolism should be restored to normal when treatment with dimercaprol (BAL) is instituted.

Mercurial Neuropathy

'Erythroedema Polyneuriticum' (Pink Disease; Acrodynia)

The pathological changes in the nerves in the condition that was known as 'pink disease' are characteristic of a 'dying-back' process in the axon. In most of these cases, mercurial poisoning —specifically, poisoning by mercurous chloride (calomel)—seems to have been responsible (see also page 2246). The disease affected infants and children under the age of five years and was characterized by the pink, smooth appearance of the skin of the distal parts of the arms and legs, excessive perspiration, profound misery, insomnia, anorexia, and hypotonia of the limbs, with anaesthesia. The degenerative changes particularly affected the distal parts of the nerves, and the clinical findings suggested that sensory fibres were more liable to involvement than motor.[104, 105] Chromatolytic changes were recorded in a few cases in cells of the lumbar anterior grey columns; slight denervation atrophy was found in the muscles. An unexplained feature, present in many cases, was a striking infiltration of the meninges and spinal cord by small round cells, presumably lymphocytes. Bronchopneumonia or other complications caused the death of up to 5 per cent of the children affected: the others recovered completely. No evidence of changes in the spinal tracts was reported.

It was the finding of mercury in concentrations of more than 50 μg/l in the urine of children with pink disease that led to identification of the nature and cause of the condition.[106] In Sheffield, for instance, the withdrawal from sale of teething powders containing calomel led to an immediate fall in the incidence of the disease in that city.[107] Before 1951, when steps were taken to stop the sale of mercury-containing teething powders, almost 60 children with pink disease were admitted to the Sheffield hospitals yearly; the number fell to 45 in 1952, by 1955 it was 15 and thereafter the condition virtually disappeared. Factors other than mercury poisoning, however, must also play a part, for about a quarter of all infants in Sheffield were believed to have been given mercury-containing teething powders: only a small proportion developed polyneuropathy. There is no metabolic process with which mercury is known to be specially likely to interfere: the final solution of the problems relating to the aetiology and pathogenesis of pink disease has still to be found.

Neuropathy Caused by Organic Compounds of Mercury

While pink disease is happily a thing of the past, a new and more sinister form of mercury poisoning has become established during the last 20 years: this is due to alkyl mercury compounds. The role of methyl mercury as an agent capable of producing a distinctive pattern of degeneration in the central nervous system was established by Hunter and Russell.[108, 109] Alkyl mercury compounds have been widely used as fungicidal seed dressings and thus have caused neuropathy either during their manufacture, as in Hunter's cases, or through consumption of seed corn thus treated, as in outbreaks in Iraq in 1960 and 1972.[109a] In the outbreak in Iraq in 1972 more than 6000 people were admitted to hospital and more than 500 died. Unfortunately, this is not the only cause of this type of poisoning: it is now realized that inorganic mercury wastes from wood pulp and other industries, such as the plastics industry, may undergo methylation through the activity of bacteria in estuarine and sea deposits and so are converted into methyl mercury. Because of its lipid solubility and stable chemical bonding, methyl mercury persists in the organisms that take it up: it thus passes up the food chain, becoming more concentrated at each stage. Consequently, fish sometimes contain dangerously high quantities of methyl mercury and indeed may themselves show changes in the central nervous system. It was this train of events that led to the outbreaks of paralysis in Japan among the predominantly fish-eating communities on Minamata Bay, Kyushu, from 1953 to 1956, and in the city of Niigata, Honshu, in 1964 (see page 2247).[110, 110a]

Because of the stability of methyl mercury compounds in the tissues—their half life is about 40 days—poisoning is cumulative and of slow onset. The symptomatology is quite characteristic, involving principally the visual system, the cerebellum and the primary sensory neurons. Extrapyramidal and other symptoms also occur, but less regularly. Since the visual disturbances are due to widespread degeneration of the small neurons of the calcarine cortex there is gross constriction of the visual fields that may lead to complete blindness. In the cerebellum there are multiple, often confluent, foci of degeneration of the granule cells, usually most marked in the depths of the cerebellar sulci. Purkyně cells are not greatly affected; in severe cases they may be reduced in number.[109]

The primary sensory neurons in the ganglia of the dorsal roots of the spinal nerves and the corresponding neurons of the cranial nerves, including the vestibulocochlear nerve, are invariably affected to some degree. While in the original cases sensory involvement was overshadowed by the grosser cerebral and cerebellar disturbances, all patients with 'Minamata disease' showed early sensory disturbances, usually including nerve deafness. In rats poisoned experimentally with these compounds it is the sensory neurons that

constitute the major area of neuronal degeneration, while the cerebral cortex, probably due to its simpler organization in this species, is not seriously affected. The experimental degeneration may involve the whole cell, or at least the whole fibre, so that even at the onset of ataxia there is extensive degeneration of all sensory nerves, of sensory roots and of the fibres within the ganglia.[111] Nerve cells in the ganglia may also show degeneration, although this is less in evidence than the changes in their fibres. By comparison, motor nerve cells are almost completely unaffected, and no changes are found in long spinal tracts other than the degeneration of the posterior funiculi.

Methyl mercury is present in the organs of the affected patients. The site of the action of the poison within the cells is not certain. It has been found in mitochondria and microsomes in experimentally poisoned animals,[112] but whether these are its real sites of concentration is not known. There is as yet no information about its mode of action on any metabolic system. No interference with oxidative and glycolytic mechanisms of the brain in poisoned animals has been found;[113] however, it has been demonstrated *in vitro* that the uptake of amino acids by brain slices is inadequate, and this has been confirmed *in vivo*.[113] It is of interest that all the tissues studied, including liver, were affected in this way, suggesting that the reason for selective damage to certain neurons may be their greater structural dependence upon the disordered metabolic system.

Neuropathy Complicating Acute Porphyria

Neuropathy ('polyneuritis') may occur in acute intermittent porphyria ('Swedish' porphyria) and in variegate porphyria ('South African' porphyria). It is commoner in the former, but by no means all attacks of acute porphyria are complicated by clinically evident neurological disease. There is a close association between taking certain hypnotic drugs, particularly barbiturates (malonylurea derivatives), and the occurrence of the neuropathy: it is interesting in this context that the manifestation of paralysis in porphyria was first recognized as a consequence of the introduction of sulphonal, or 2,2-di(ethylsulphonyl)propane,[114] a synthetic hypnotic developed some years before the first of the hypnotic barbiturates was produced (1903) and chemically quite different from the latter. Apronal ('Sedormid'), the sedative that caused thrombocytopenia by an allergic mechanism (see page 493, Volume 2), was also among the drugs that led to porphyriac neuropathy.

Analysis of the sequence of events leading to paralysis shows that the neurological disturbance always follows an episode of abdominal pain and constipation that is itself symptomatic of the porphyria.[115] Persistent tachycardia is an important prognostic sign in this disease: it has been suggested that both this and the abdominal symptoms are due to involvement of autonomic nerves in the degenerative process.[116] This is an important observation, for—if it is correct—it implies that there may be involvement of the nervous system, subclinical if not overt, in the course of almost every porphyriac attack.

There is no doubt that the entire nervous system may be affected in porphyria. Coma and convulsions may occur. Mental symptoms are often so obtrusive that the condition leads to admission to a mental hospital before its nature is recognized.

At some stage of the attack the urine may assume the classic dark red, port or burgundy, colour on exposure to air. More constant is the finding in the urine of an increased amount of porphobilinogen and of the intermediate metabolite, delta-aminolaevulic acid.

An analysis of 26 cases[115] showed that the onset of subjective weakness and sensory disturbances usually preceded objective signs by several days: this suggests that subjective weakness after a known attack of porphyria, even in the absence of overt neurological signs, indicates that some degree of denervation has taken place. The neurological signs are principally motor, but sensory disturbances will be found in a high proportion of cases if carefully sought.[117] Usually it is either the legs or the arms that are affected; the signs may be predominantly proximal or, less often, distal in distribution. It is not yet clear what determines the pattern of paralysis in individual cases. Recovery from the paralysis may be comparatively rapid, taking a few weeks, but more usually is spread over many months; its rate is determined by the length of the nerve fibres involved in the degeneration.

Structural changes in the nerves have been variously described. In some cases no abnormality has been found; in others patchy demyelination of the fibres has been noted. In fact, the microscopical picture varies greatly, depending upon the duration of the paralysis and its extent, and whether there has been a previous attack or not. The position of the nerve examined in relation to the distribution of the paralysis may be conducive or otherwise to the demonstration of the abnormalities; similarly, the presence of naked regenerating fibres can give a false impression of demyelination. Segmental demyelination can be demonstrated with certainty only by the examination of teased nerves, not histological sections. Failure to take account of these various factors has led to misinterpretation.

In appropriate samples of nerves it is possible to demonstrate Wallerian degeneration (Figs 35.21A and 35.21B): it may be possible to show that there is less degeneration in proximal samples than in distal ones. The degeneration is a typical 'dying back' process: in some cases it may go back as far as the spinal roots.[118] Both sensory and motor fibres are affected, but whether any particular fibre size is implicated has not been determined.

Nerve cells are not usually lost. If the disease has been severe they show marked chromatolysis (Figs 35.16 and 35.21C), provided death has not taken place so quickly that there has not been time for this to occur. Spinal tracts are rarely affected, but the fasciculi graciles, which have their cell bodies in the lumbosacral ganglia, and therefore have the longest course in the posterior funiculi, may in severe cases show degeneration in their upper regions.[119] This is in keeping with the 'dying back' nature of the process. There is no evidence that a vascular factor is involved[120] or that there is a primary demyelinating process.[121] There may be degenerative changes in nerve fibres in the autonomic ganglia:[121] this is pertinent to the suggestion, noted above, that involvement of the autonomic system is regularly part of the pathological picture of the disease—further studies on this aspect of porphyria would be of interest.

Much is known about the general biochemical disorder in acute intermittent porphyria.[122] It is clear that at the root of the disturbance is a marked increase in activity of the hepatic enzyme, delta-aminolaevulic acid synthetase, the conjugating enzyme involved in the first, and rate-limiting, step in the synthesis of porphyrins. An excess of this enzyme can be induced artificially in animals by a number of substances, including allylisopropylacetamide, griseofulvin and barbiturates. The metabolic step, an amino decarboxylation, requires the co-factor, pyridoxidine phosphate (pyridoxal phosphate). It appears that the excess enzyme activity may be so great as to precipitate a general tissue depletion of pyridoxine phosphate: if a testing load of L-tryptophan is given to the patient during an acute attack, large quantities of intermediates—xanthurenic acid, kynurenic acid and others—that require pyridoxine for their further metabolism may be excreted in the urine.[123] The possible relevance of this observation to the mech-

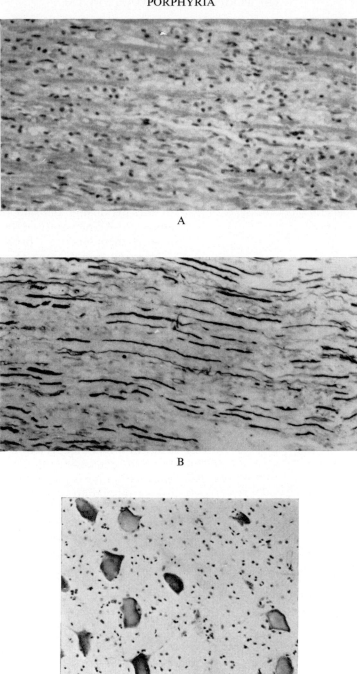

Fig. 35.21. Polyneuritis of acute porphyria: a severe and late example. See also Figs 35.16A and 35.16B, page 2309.

A. Massive Wallerian degeneration in the distal end of a lumbar nerve root. *Haematoxylin–eosin.* × 175.
B. Equivalent severe loss of nerve fibres in section adjacent to (A) above. *Glees and Marsland method.* × 175.
C. Numerous chromatolytic neurons in lumbar spinal cord. *Cresyl violet.* × 100.

anism of the neuropathy of porphyria became apparent when it was observed that the pattern of denervation produced by isoniazid in animals (see below) was very similar to that occurring in porphyria:[124] isoniazid blocks the phosphorylation of pyridoxine (vitamin B_6) and thus causes a tissue depletion of the co-factor pyridoxine phosphate. It has been suggested, therefore, that the mechanism of porphyriac neuropathy is the same:[125] confirmation is necessary, for if the suggestion is substantiated the need to give vitamin B_6 from the outset of the acute attack of porphyria will be clearly evident—such treatment might prevent paralysis. How the metabolic lesion leads to degeneration of the nerve fibres is a still unanswered question.

Isoniazid Neuropathy

Isoniazid neuropathy begins with burning sensations and sensory loss, particularly in the legs. If the drug is not stopped, motor weakness and ataxia may also appear, but sensory disturbances predominate.[126, 127] Recovery is slow, particularly when there are motor signs, which indicate severe denervation; in the milder cases, with sensory disturbances only, recovery may be virtually complete.

Experimental studies show that in rats the denervation of isoniazid neuropathy is more marked in motor fibres than in sensory fibres, and that, while the latter may be affected only in their distal parts, the former degenerate back to the spinal roots.[124, 128] Degeneration of the dorsal funiculi may also be present. The fact that the pattern of denervation is so similar led to the suggestion that porphyriac neuropathy is likely to be due to excessive consumption and consequent deficiency of pyridoxine phosphate (see above).[125]

There is an interesting feature about isoniazid neuropathy that may have relevance to other toxic conditions in man. Most drugs are detoxicated, usually in the liver: in the case of isoniazid this is by an acetylation process. About 50 per cent of people are 'rapid inactivators'—acetylation is rapid and most of the drug is very soon excreted in this form. The rest are 'slow inactivators', most of the drug being excreted unchanged: because inactivation is slower, there is longer persistence of relatively high levels of the drug in plasma. It is the slow inactivators who are particularly liable to toxic complications.[129, 130] In relation to the various neuropathies the possibility must therefore be considered that some people, for genetic or nutritional reasons, or because of the presence of some disease of the liver, may be less capable than most of detoxicating drugs or other foreign substances. It is well established that hepatic microsomal enzymes, which are often concerned with drug detoxication, may be depressed by malnutrition:[131] poorer communities may be thereby rendered more susceptible to untoward effects of drugs.

The mode of action of isoniazid in the context of pyridoxine (vitamin B_6) deficiency is twofold. First, it prevents the phosphorylation of pyridoxine by the enzyme pyridoxine phosphokinase; second, it chelates with pyridoxine phosphate to form a Schiff base. This conjugate is even more inhibitory to the pyridoxine phosphokinase than isoniazid alone.[132] Administration of excess pyridoxine reverses these inhibitory processes.

Isoniazid is not alone in interfering with pyridoxine metabolism: other chelating agents, such as L-penicillamine[133] (but not D-penicillamine) and hydrallazine,[134] have the same effects and are thus also able to induce peripheral neuropathy similar in general pattern to that caused by isoniazid. Tests for vitamin B_6 deficiency, such as the L-tryptophan load test, are helpful in determining the type of metabolic lesion that may be responsible.

Poisoning with Organic Compounds of Phosphorus

Phosphorylated phenols are widely used as high temperature lubricants and in the plastics industry. From the clinical standpoint, tri-*ortho*-cresyl phosphate poisoning is the best documented representative of this group of intoxications, because of the occasional explosive epidemics that result from contamination of drink or food. The outbreak in 1930 of 'ginger jake' paralysis in the southern states of the United States of America involved some 30 000 people, and the more recent outbreak in Morocco paralysed about 10 000 people. The potential hazard of other related compounds is far greater, for tri-*ortho*-cresyl phosphate is among the least toxic members of the group.

The general formula of these compounds is:

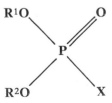

In the *aryl phosphates*, the substituent groups (R^1, R^2 and X) are phenols, and the presence of one *ortho*-substituted phenol in the molecule confers neurotoxicity. In the *alkyl phosphates*, which are widely used as insecticides, the side chains R¹O and R²O appear to be less important from the neurotoxic standpoint, although they affect the character of the anticholinesterase action of the compounds, as well as the general physicochemical properties of the molecule; by contrast, the substituent X is highly important, for all such compounds with a fluorine radicle in this position are neurotoxic, regardless of the nature of the alkyl side chains.[135] Other substituents of the radicle X are also known to be toxic.

There is no evidence that true cholinesterase and pseudocholinesterase, although sensitive to the inhibitory action of these poisons, play a part in the neurotoxic process. However, inhibition of true cholinesterase is certainly the cause of the acute toxic effects, which are in fact the manifestations of acetylcholine poisoning. There is a possibility that neurotoxic chemicals selectively inhibit an as yet unidentified esterase in nervous tissue.[136]

One of the most constant features of this form of poisoning, both in man and in all animals so far tested, is the delay period of about eight to ten days before the onset of symptoms. What metabolic disturbance is taking place inside the nerve cell during this period is not known, but the cholinesterase levels in the blood and in the brain are well on their ascent toward normal by the time paralysis develops.

In man there are premonitory gastrointestinal and subjective sensory disturbances. However, the neurological lesion appears to be severest on the motor side.[137] The feet and lower parts of the legs are affected first and most severely. A few days later the hands may be involved. Foot-drop with a high-stepping gait is a characteristic feature. Objective sensory disturbances may be found later.

The great majority of patients recover from the disability during the ensuing weeks or months, as the damaged nerves regenerate back to their end-organs. About 5 per cent of severely poisoned patients have residual disabilities, probably due in part to incomplete regeneration of peripheral nerve fibres and in part to the effects of spinal tract degeneration.

The effects of tri-*ortho*-cresyl phosphate on cats have been analysed in detail. It has been found that there is a selective susceptibility of large diameter fibres in peripheral nerves and that the degeneration affects the sensory fibres as well as motor fibres (Fig. 35.22).[138] Because the large diameter sensory fibres come from the anulospiral

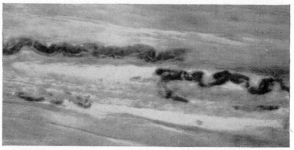

Fig. 35.22. Tri-*ortho*-cresyl phosphate poisoning in a cat. Muscle spindle showing loss of the anulospiral ending and early Wallerian fragmentation of myelinated sensory fibres. The 'dying-back' process has not advanced to the apparently normal large diameter sensory fibre above. *Sudan black B.* × 195.

formations of muscle spindles, and because there is no satisfactory clinical test for spindle function, the appearance of a predominantly motor lesion is thus produced. Damage to medium-sized fibres may be relatively unimportant: even in the moderately severely poisoned animal, the medium-sized fibres (8 to 10 μm in diameter), which subserve all but the least and the most discriminative sensory modalities, may be little affected.

The process of dying back from the extremity of the axon toward the perikaryon is also evident in the spinal cord, for the posterior funiculi and the spinocerebellar tracts show changes only in their most rostral parts, while the corticospinal pathways show changes in their caudal parts.[139] The nerve cells show little change except for slight chromatolysis during the recovery phase.

Motor Neuron Disease

There has been little progress toward understanding this disease since its earliest thorough description, nearly a century ago.[140] The condition is not strictly a neuropathy but—like the other abiotrophies—part of a disorder in which a large number of nerve cells is likely to be affected although only a few overtly show disease (see page 2262). The term 'motor neuron disease' is frequently used in two senses. As a generic term, it is used to include all forms of the disease and thus implies disease of both upper and lower motor nerve cells. In the more restricted sense, it is applied to the form of the disease that manifests itself as a disorder of the lower motor neuron. In fact, however, it is rare not to be able to disclose changes in the upper motor neuron *post mortem*, even when there has been no clinical evidence of such changes.[141]

The most frequent form of the disease is *amyotrophic lateral sclerosis* (Fig. 35.23), and often this term is applied to the whole group. Another form is known as *chronic bulbar palsy*, in which the brunt of the disease is borne by the motor cranial nerves in the lower part of the brainstem.

It is probably true to say that in this condition the number of pathways found to be involved is largely determined by the thoroughness of the methods of examination. It is doubtful whether we are dealing with a single disease entity, for, while most of the cases are sporadic, a few (probably 10 per cent or less) may have a familial background, and these may show slight variations in the pattern of affected neurons.[142] A condition very like motor neuron disease is found among the inhabitants of the Marianas Islands (see page 2262).[143] In symptomatology and course, and even in the microscopical changes, the similarity between this condition and motor neuron disease is close. However, its high incidence (10 per cent of the population of the islands are affected, and even more in some districts) and the frequent association with a syndrome of Parkinsonism and dementia (see page 2270), characterized by neurofibrillary degeneration of nerve cells in the brain and elsewhere, suggest that it and motor neuron disease are of different aetiology.

Clinical descriptions of the classic forms of motor neuron disease particularly emphasize that their initial and severest manifestations are usually in the distal parts of the limbs. Sometimes the arms or the cranial nerves are affected first. Weakness, wasting and fasciculation of the muscles begin in the lower parts of the legs and in the hands, thence advancing proximally. There are no sensory disturbances, and changes can very rarely be demonstrated in the sensory neurons, even

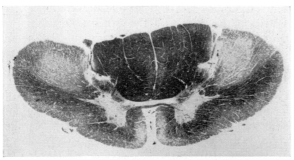

Fig. 35.23. Amyotrophic lateral sclerosis (motor neuron disease). Degeneration (pallor) of the lateral and anterior corticospinal tracts and to a less extent (general lightening of myelin staining) of the lateral and anterior funiculi. The posterior funiculi are normal. *Weigert's myelin stain.* × 8.

microscopically. It is a disease of late middle life and men are affected twice as often as women. The course is inexorable and death is to be expected within about three years from the onset. However, many patients die sooner, and a very few survive many years. Studies of motor terminals by biopsy and at necropsy show that one of the most conspicuous changes apart from Wallerian degeneration is increased terminal branching and the development of ultraterminal sprouts.[144] This appears to be a compensatory outgrowth from surviving nerve fibres, and accounts for the marked variation in the size of the atrophic bundles of denervated muscle fibres in this disease. It implies, too, that the symptoms of the disease come on when the compensatory mechanism fails. It also accounts for the relative rapidity with which the final stages of motor weakness and wasting develop, because degeneration of nerve fibres late in the disease will lead to denervation not only of the motor unit originally supplied by the fibre, but also of the large number of additional muscle fibres that its collaterals have come to support.

In few, if any, cases of motor neuron disease are changes strictly confined to the final common pathway neurons. Changes consistently occur in the crossed and uncrossed pyramidal tracts: these may be traceable to the motor cortex and may disappear at the level of the medulla oblongata or of the cervical part of the spinal cord. Pallor of myelin staining has been observed in the posterior funiculi only in familial cases.

Besides the pre-eminent susceptibility of long motor fibres, fibre size is also an important factor in determining degeneration in motor neuron disease. Measurements of the diameter of the fibres in motor and sensory roots in this disease show normal proportions of fibres of various diameters in the latter but a striking loss of fibres of 8 μm in diameter and upward in the former (Fig. 35.24). Small diameter fibres are spared, thus explaining the integrity of the muscle spindles, the fibres to which are of the order of 5 μm in diameter. Whatever the primary reason for the degeneration of nerve cells in this condition, those with large fibres seem most liable to involvement.

Other Parenchymatous Neuropathies

Vitamin B$_{12}$ Deficiency

The pathogenesis of the peripheral neuropathy associated with deficiency of vitamin B$_{12}$ differs from that of the lesions in the spinal cord and

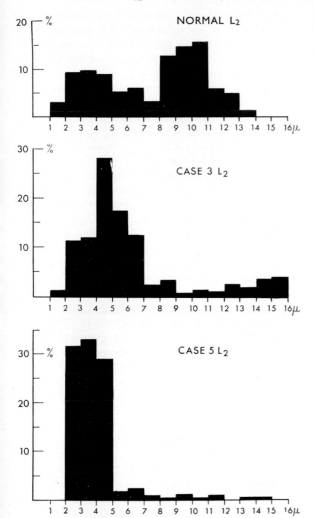

Fig. 35.24.§ Histograms of fibre diameters of ventral spinal roots (level of second lumbar roots—'L$_2$') of two cases of motor neuron disease. Compared with the normal there is profound reduction in numbers of large diameter fibres and persistence of small diameter (gamma-efferent) fibres. (Redrawn from the originals in: Wohlfart, G., Swank, R. L., *Arch. Neurol. Psychiat.* [*Chic.*], 1941, **46**, 783.)

elsewhere in the central nervous system (see page 2242).

In the central nervous system the condition begins with vacuolation and degeneration of the myelin sheaths of the fibres round veins.[145] This process involves progressively more fibres, and eventually secondary degeneration occurs in the axons in the damaged areas.[146] The changes are detected earliest in the thoracic segments of the spinal cord.

By contrast, the changes in the peripheral nerves have the character of a distal degeneration of nerve fibres. Fibre measurements in one case showed a severe reduction in the number of large diameter fibres.[96] Inferences from these measurements cannot be accepted without reserve, because the investigation was confined to the terminal portion of the medial terminal branch of the deep peroneal nerve: it is very probable that this branch, because of its position in the first interosseous space of the foot, is ordinarily subjected to repeated trauma and may become abnormal in consequence. However, in other cases of this disease biopsy studies have shown that the nerves in distal muscles show marked collateral sprouting, a disturbed terminal innervation ratio, and remarkable ovoid swellings on many of the finer branches.[147] It will not be possible to come to any final conclusion about the nature and origins of these changes until more detailed anatomical information is available.

Miscellaneous Metabolic, Deficiency and Toxic Disorders

Various vitamin deficiencies and chemical intoxications may produce parenchymatous neuropathies in man and in laboratory animals.[148] Among them may be listed nicotinic acid deficiency (pellagra) and deficiencies of other members of the vitamin B group (pyridoxine, riboflavin and pantothenic acid). Isoniazid neuropathy should also be noted here, since its effects are mainly peripheral in distribution, and the compound is believed to act by blocking the proper utilization of pyridoxine (see page 2322). Thalidomide (see page 2197) is said to have produced a sensory peripheral neuropathy in a proportion of patients for whom it was prescribed as a sedative.[148a] Many other chemical substances used in industry and in the home have been incriminated from time to time: for instance, the insecticides dinitro-*ortho*-cresol (DNOC) and dicophane (chlorophenothane; DDT).

No useful purpose would be served by critically analysing nutritional causes of neuropathies, for it is rare in man to get a dietary deficiency that is pure, and it is rarer still to obtain anatomical confirmation of the disturbances produced. Experimental deficiency states in animals, while of much theoretical interest, are of doubtful relevance to human conditions because, for instance, the importance of the various co-factors in their metabolism differs from one species to another.

Again, in considering intoxications that cause peripheral neuropathies, it is rare to get anatomical confirmation of functional disturbances, and the results of clinical neurological examination cannot be regarded as giving a complete picture of the damage to individual neuron systems. In animals, too, studies have often been too incomplete to be of much value in identifying the nature of the process.

Peripheral Neuropathy Associated with Malignant Neoplasia

This section is concerned principally with the development of peripheral neuropathy as one of those effects of carcinoma that are not directly due to the presence of tumour tissue in the affected structures. This development is part of a wider involvement of nervous tissue by a process that we do not understand.[149] Among the first to describe the occurrence of neuronal degeneration as a non-metastatic complication of carcinoma was Denny-Brown, who observed it in a case of sensory neuropathy.[150] Originally it was considered that about 2 per cent of cases of carcinoma of the lung showed evidence of neuropathy,[151] but more detailed studies[152] have shown that as many as 16 per cent of these tumours are accompanied by some evidence of a neuromyopathy. Similarly, just over 4 per cent of women with carcinoma of the breast develop this condition.

The pattern of neurological disease associated with tumours is by no means simple, and peripheral neuropathy is only part of a complex spectrum of neuronal degeneration. Thus, in a series of 162 cases of neuropathy,[152] mixed (motor and sensory) neuropathy was present in 22 per cent, cerebellar disturbances associated with Purkyně cell loss occurred in 9 per cent, myelopathy with spinal tract degeneration in 9 per cent, and pure sensory neuropathy in 5 per cent. However, the largest group in the series (48 per cent of the cases) showed involvement of both nerve and muscle tissue (neuromyopathy); 16 per cent showed pure myopathic features. It is clear from these findings that there may be a wide range of presenting symptoms, and in the absence of an obvious aetiological mechanism it is difficult to analyse these satisfactorily. The associated tumour, which may be quite small, arises in a lung in about half the cases, in a breast in about 11 per cent and in the stomach in about 10 per cent.

The pathological features differ according to the symptomatology.[153] Sensory neuropathy is associated with loss of nerve fibres both peripherally and in the posterior funiculi (Fig. 35.25), and nerve cell degeneration with clusters of satellite cells—Nageotte's residual nodules[153a]—is commonly seen in the ganglia. Schwann cell disease must also be considered to be present as well as neuronal disease, since segmental demyelination may be extensive. This can be confirmed by teasing and is associated with reduced conduction velocity. Even though the main changes may occur in the primary sensory cells, other neurons may show degeneration, such as Purkyně cells of the cerebellum, and long tract degeneration may be found also. Indeed, cases of carcinoma associated with extensive cerebellar cortical atrophy due to loss of Purkyně cells and granule cells are well documented.[154] To add to the complexity of the situation, seemingly pure myopathic conditions, such as a myasthenic syndrome,[155, 156] occur, with or without a neural component.

At present we do not know the basis of this widely ranging and varied affection of nervous and muscular tissues that leads to specific cellular degeneration in one part or another of the locomotor apparatus. The degenerative patterns do not

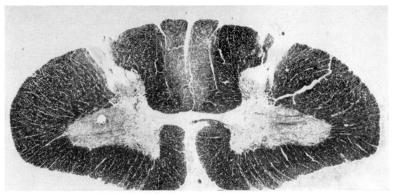

Fig. 35.25. Carcinomatous sensory neuropathy. Cervical part of spinal cord: degeneration of fasciculi graciles but not of fasciculi cuneati. *Iron haematoxylin.* × 8.

follow the course of any known nutritional or biochemical defects. The possibility that the tumour competes for—or produces an anti-metabolite active against—a known co-factor or enzyme may be largely discounted. A problem is posed, however, by the neuropathic complications of intestinal malabsorption ('adult coeliac disease'): it is evident that most of the syndromes that may be associated with carcinoma may also accompany this form of steatorrhoea, in the absence of cancer.[157] Whether this means that viral[158] or immunological[159] agencies may be discounted is an open question.

DISORDERS OF THE SCHWANN CELLS*

Segmental Demyelination

Primary damage to Schwann cells was well known to students of peripheral nerve disorders before the end of the last century (Fig. 35.26): it had been observed both in man and in experiments on diphtherial paralysis and lead paralysis in guinea-pigs.[160-162] However, the condition was virtually forgotten by neurologists during the first half of this century, and, while it is much better studied now, the underlying mechanisms are still not understood. One of the chief reasons for such neglect in the past was the almost compulsive tendency for

* Schwann cell tumours are considered on page 2334.

neuropathologists to depend on thin paraffin wax sections of nerves, and to neglect the earlier and far more informative method of examination by the teasing apart of the fibres, now again being widely used. Indeed, it is only by using this technique that quantitative data can be obtained.

Two features of the process of segmental demyelination require to be particularly studied. The first is the significance of the finding, common to all the natural and experimental conditions in which this kind of change occurs, that only part of the myelin related to the affected Schwann cell undergoes degeneration. Thus, it is often found that the juxtanodal regions are damaged over a length of 50 μm or so on each side of a node of Ranvier while the remainder of the internode is intact. The damaged region is in fact the part of the cell with the greatest amount of cytoplasm and abundance of mitochondria, and with specialized functional relations to the axon at the node and to the myelin at the cytoplasmic loops. In consequence of the breakdown of the relation with the axon, the ionic mechanisms concerned with saltatory impulse conduction at the node break down also. The relative ease with which the juxtanodal myelin degenerates suggests that it may be more unstable than the rest of the internode myelin and, therefore, that it may have a higher energy requirement. The second feature that should be

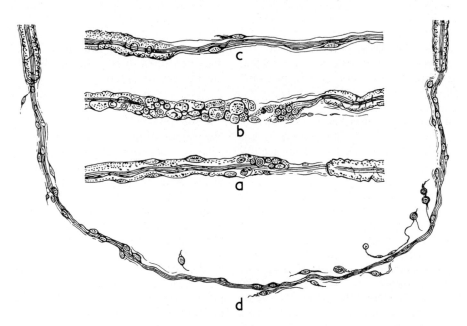

Fig. 35.26.§ Changes in the myelin internode in diphtherial neuropathy. The change apparently begins in the juxtanodal region (a) and may extend to destroy the whole internode (b, c, d). (Redrawn from: Meyer, P., *Virchows Arch. path. Anat.*, 1881, **85**, 181.)

investigated is the mechanism of remyelination. It has been found in animals that if the gap formed by segmental demyelination is greater than about 15 μm—that is, rather greater than the length of a Schwann nucleus—a new cell finds its way into the space and spins a new myelin sheath.[163] This begins to happen within a few days of the myelin breakdown, and within two to three weeks new myelin can be plainly seen. The new cell apparently forms from the damaged one by an unequal division. In contrast, if the gap is less than 15 μm the broken ends of the myelin may grow into it, by a process that is not yet understood.[164] After a single episode of demyelination, as in experimental diphtheria intoxication, restoration of function occurs within three to four weeks. In diseases in man, other than lesions due simply to local pressure, recovery may be slower, presumably because of continuing cell damage.

Diphtherial Paralysis

Paralysis and heart block as complications of faucial diphtheria were common causes of death in childhood before the era of prophylactic immunization. The onset of paralysis is slow, and it advances from one neural territory to another in a curious and still unexplained manner. With faucial diphtheria, the common palatal paralysis follows some 6 to 36 days after the infection, and in most cases it is accompanied by paralysis of accommodation.[165] As the palatal paralysis passes off, a symmetrical neuropathy, which affects both sensory and motor fibres, appears in the limbs. Provided that the respiratory muscles are not extensively affected, and that the patient does not die from some cardiac lesion (see page 45, Volume 1), recovery, though slow, is always functionally complete.[166]

In cases of cutaneous diphtheria,[166a] which is a relatively common form of the disease in hot climates, palatal paralysis and paralysis of accommodation are much less frequent (see Chapter 39, Volume 6).

Post-mortem studies do not help to explain why the onset of the neuropathy is delayed, often for several weeks.[167] They do show, however, that demyelination occurs in the spinal nerve roots, particularly the dorsal roots, without any significant axonal degeneration. Very little change may be found in the peripheral nerves themselves. In keeping with the persistence of the axons, the motor cells in the anterior grey columns of the spinal cord are unaffected; however, a few neurons in dorsal root ganglia may degenerate, possibly because of swelling in this confined region consequent upon myelin degradation. No changes that can be related to the paralysis are found in the central nervous system.

Experimental Diphtherial Paralysis

A lesion analogous to that of human diphtheria occurs experimentally in allergic neuritis in rabbits; in this condition myelin degeneration is selective, and greatest in the dorsal roots.[168] On the other hand, in the guinea-pig the peripheral nerves are affected throughout their length, both in allergic neuritis and in that due to diphtheria toxin. It is possible that such species differences are attributable to differences in the permeability of the so-called blood–nerve barrier, but the evidence at present available leaves much to be discovered before a final conclusion can be drawn. It is certainly true that diphtheria toxin does not enter all tissues freely and does not ordinarily pass through the wall of the capillary bed of the central nervous system: the central nervous system is not damaged unless the toxin is injected directly into the cerebrospinal fluid. The factors that control the diffusion of the toxin in different regions are also unknown. Once inside a cell, the changes that the toxin produces are akin, in their mildest form, to the change traditionally known by the term 'cloudy swelling', and to necrosis if the intoxication becomes severer. It has been shown in the chicken that not all sizes of fibres respond in the same manner.[163] Thus, small diameter fibres are earliest affected and show complete internodal break-up. Larger diameter fibres show damage a few days later, confined to the juxtanodal regions.

Pathogenesis

No explanation has been forthcoming for the delay in the onset of symptoms—a latent period that, apart from its longer duration, is reminiscent of the delay in the development of the manifestations of poisoning by organic phosphorus compounds (see page 2323). It has been suggested that diphtheria toxin is the protein component of bacterial cytochrome and may act as a chemical analogue, thus interfering with the normal function of the cytochrome of the intoxicated cell.[169] An important action of diphtheria toxin may be upon protein synthesis, by preventing incorporation of amino acids into the protein-building system.[170, 171]

So far as nerves are concerned, it is of particular interest that Schwann cells and not nerve fibres seem most susceptible to this metabolic disturbance.

It has been customary to think that it is the nerve cells and their fibres that are most vulnerable to interference with metabolic mechanisms: perhaps this view is wrong—Schwann cells may be the more vulnerable element in the peripheral nerves. The tendency for these cells to be damaged first wnen there is local ischaemia or a pressure lesion is support for this view (see page 2310).

Lead Neuropathy

Very little is known about the structural lesions in lead poisoning in man (see page 2246). Clinical descriptions suggest that the neuropathy is purely motor, and that occupational use of certain muscles is a factor in determining the localization of the paralysis: for instance, wrist-drop in the working arm was often the presenting manifestation in painters, who were, formerly, specially exposed to the risk of poisoning by lead compounds in paint. Early experiments showed that segmental or inter-nodal degeneration of myelin is conspicuous and that there is relatively little loss of axons. However, de Villaverde, working in the Ramón y Cajal Institute, in Madrid, found that axons did degener-ate, especially in the distal part of a limb.[172] It is possible, therefore, that lead lesions are not pure in the sense that only the system of Schwann cells is affected: there may also be a dying-back of axons, although it would seem that this is of secondary importance. The occurrence of both segmental myelin degeneration and Wallerian degeneration in guinea-pigs with lead poisoning confirms the complex nature of the changes.[173]

Neuropathy of Metachromatic Leucodystrophy and Other Disorders of Lipid Metabolism

In recent years it has come to be realized that peripheral nerves are as much affected by primary demyelination as are fibres in the central nervous system.[174] Metachromatic leucodystrophy (see page 2233) is essentially a dyscrasia of myelin formation, affecting particularly the metabolism of cerebro-sides, for the brain in such cases contains abnor-mally large amounts of sulphatides and sulphated cerebrosides. In this disease, the peripheral nerves, including the spinal nerve roots, show degeneration of myelin into granular masses that exhibit marked metachromasia when stained with basic stains.[175] The axons are relatively spared and appear to be little affected by the disorder of the Schwann cells; however, the rate of conduction of nervous im-pulses in such fibres is notably slowed.

Segmental myelin degeneration is also found in globoid cell leucodystrophy (Krabbe's disease—see page 2233)[176, 177] and in the infantile (Tay–Sachs) and juvenile (Batten–Mayou) forms of familial amaurotic idiocy (see page 2235 and, in Volume 6, Chapter 40).[178] This indicates the generalized nature of the disturbance of lipid metabolism in these diseases. The findings are of importance, too, in indicating that biopsy examination of a nerve is a means of confirming the diagnosis—a procedure safer and simpler than brain biopsy. The histochemical features of the demyelinated nerves are the same as those in the central nervous system (see pages 2233 and 2234).

'Hypertrophic' Neuropathy

Hypertrophic neuropathy, a condition originally described by Déjerine and Sottas,[179] occurs both sporadically and as a recessive heritable disease. It affects infants or older children. Its occurrence in adults has been reported, but there is doubt whether such cases should be regarded as instances of the same condition. The illness presents as a slowly progressive distal neuropathy, with 'glove and stocking' anaesthesia, and weakness and wasting of muscles. Scoliosis often develops and ataxia is a common feature. The most characteristic change is the diffuse swelling of nerve trunks, which makes those in the skin readily palpable.

Refsum's Disease[180] (Heredopathia Atactica Poly-neuritiformis; Thiébault–Refsum Disease[180a]).— The presentation of this condition is similar to that of hypertrophic neuropathy, as described above, but there are additional features, including ichthyosis, retinitis pigmentosa (see Chapter 40, Volume 6) and changes in bones. An unusual fatty acid, phytanic acid (3,7,11,15-tetramethylhexadecanoic acid) is present in the tissues and urine and further distinguishes this disease from the Déjerine–Sottas form.[181] Phytanic acid is an intermediate product in the catabolism of phytol, which is a constituent of chlorophyll. Phytol is ingested not only in green vegetables but also in butter and other animal fats, particularly the fat of herbivores.

Histology

Two features characterize the microscopical changes of hypertrophic neuropathy, including Refsum's disease: however, their presence is of diagnostic significance only in relation to a clinical history consistent with those diseases. First, the individual nerve fibres may be markedly separated from one another by oedema fluid that extends throughout the whole length of the nerve trunk. Even the structural components of the sensory endings are oedematous. Second, there is much thickening of the sheath of Schwann, due to hyperplasia of its cells, so that, instead of forming a single covering layer, the Schwann cells may be clustered three or four deep round each surviving axon (Fig. 35.27). These fibres have lost their myelin, but the axons persist; when, eventually, axons degenerate, those that survive commonly show evidence of regenerative growth, with development of sprouts. In transverse sections, the Schwann cell hyperplasia gives rise to a lamellated, 'onion-bulb' appearance.[182] All nerve trunks are affected to some degree, including the spinal roots and ganglia and the trunks of the autonomic nervous system. Some of the nerve cells in the spinal root ganglia may show degenerative changes. Because of this loss of cells and because of the changes in the dorsal roots, degeneration of fibres in the posterior funiculi is common.

Nature

Although the cerebrospinal fluid may contain an increased amount of protein, the lesion does not seem to be primarily inflammatory, and indeed the cellular proliferation has all the features of a reactionary rather than a degenerative process. What stimulates the proliferation of the Schwann cells is unknown. It is notable that the 'onion-bulb' hyperplasia of Schwann cells is not peculiar to the conditions described by Déjerine and Sottas and by Refsum. The same appearance has been observed in diabetic neuropathy[183] and in some cases of peroneal muscular atrophy (see page 2315).[184] Its significance is uncertain: probably it is the Schwann cell's response to repeated stimulation, from whatever cause; and probably it has no specific pathological connotation.

INFLAMMATORY DISEASES OF NERVES (TRUE NEURITIS)

Infection by Bacteria

The number of true infective diseases of peripheral nerves is small. Peripheral polyneuropathy commonly occurs following exanthematous fevers and as a complication of various acute bacterial infections, but it is highly doubtful whether the neurological disturbances in such cases are ever the result of direct invasion of the nerves by microorganisms. Such invasion is likely to occur only during the course of a septicaemia.

Among the granulomas, *leprosy* is the only one that has a special predilection for nerves (see Chapter 39, Volume 6). The maculoanaesthetic (tuberculoid) form of the disease, in which peripheral nerves are invaded, may or may not be associated with the nodular (lepromatous) form, which is essentially the cutaneous manifestation of the disease. How the lepra bacilli come to enter the distal nerve terminals is by no means clear; it may be by direct invasion of the endings in the skin. It is possible that in the breakdown products of neural tissue or in the reacting Schwann cell they find an environment conducive to their growth. The bacilli are present in large numbers, both within the cells of the infected tissues and free-lying: however, it has been suggested that many of them are dead.[185] The infected cells include Schwann cells and others that are essentially part of the normal composition of the nerves; there are also many macrophages, some of them 'foamy' cells containing the products of nerve-fibre and myelin-sheath degeneration as well as bacilli. The nerve trunks are thickened and nodular, particularly where they are situated superficially and in relation to joints, and the destruction of many of their fibres leads to patchy anaesthesia and muscle degeneration in the denervated areas. The dorsal root ganglia may eventually be invaded and their nerve cells destroyed. Although the infection spreads centripetally in nerve trunks, the spinal cord is said never to be invaded.

As in other granulomatous infections, the progress and character of the disease are dependent upon the immune state of the patient. Khanolkar[186]

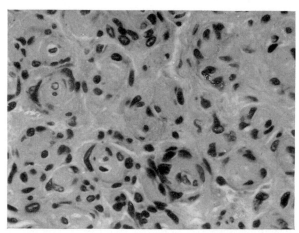

Fig. 35.27. Hypertrophic neuropathy. Transverse section of nerve showing the lamellated multiplication of the Schwann sheath. *Haematoxylin; Van Gieson's stain.* × 500.

noted that when immunity is high the incidence of neural invasion is greatest, and that the neural lesions are not readily influenced by specific therapy.

Infection by Viruses

It has been recognized for many years that nerves can be infected by neurotropic viruses: the belief that such viruses may invade the central nervous system along neural pathways has long occupied the attention of experimental pathologists. Poliomyelitis, rabies and herpes simplex virus in particular have been studied extensively from this standpoint. There seems to be little question about the ability of the virus of *herpes simplex* to ascend nerve trunks in experimental herpes infection. Whether the herpes virus is carried in the endoneurial spaces[187] or within the axons themselves[188] is a question that has not yet been convincingly answered. On balance, the evidence seems to point to the former route, for the spaces within the endoneurium, between the nerve fibres, continue directly into the cerebrospinal axis.[189, 190]

In *rabies*, which is among the gravest of the neurotropic viral diseases (see page 2149), the segmental location of the early lesions in the cerebrospinal axis seems to indicate that the virus passes along nerve trunks from the site of the bite to reach the central nervous system. Its passage, apparently, is not accompanied by any functional or structural changes in the nerve fibres in the conducting trunk: however, once it reaches the dorsal root ganglia and the spinal cord the virus causes degeneration and necrosis of the nerve cells (Figs 35.28A and 35.28B), first in the ganglia and later in the cord itself.

In contrast, the lesions of *herpes zoster* are essentially inflammatory (see page 2157): they occur mainly in the dorsal root ganglia, where destruction of nerve cells results.[191] Post-mortem studies have shown that the inflammatory reaction may extend locally into the meninges and the adjacent part of the spinal cord, with the result that motor as well as sensory nerve fibres may be damaged. The relation between the characteristic, localized skin eruption of herpes zoster and the inflammatory changes in the dorsal root ganglia is by no means clear (see Chapter 39, Volume 6).

Guillain–Barré Syndrome (Landry–Guillain–Barré Syndrome; Landry's Paralysis)

The term 'idiopathic polyneuritis' may be preferred for this acute disease, but the eponyms are too

9*

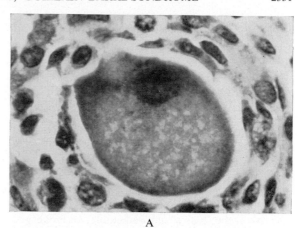

A

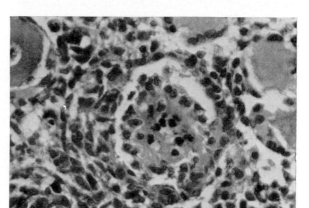

B

Fig. 35.28.§ Experimental rabies infection of the dorsal root ganglion of a spinal nerve of a rabbit. *Haematoxylin–eosin.*
A. Early swelling of a nerve cell and commencing pyknosis of its nucleus. × 930.
B. Neuronal disintegration, phagocytosis, and surrounding cellular increase. × 360.

generally familiar to be readily replaced.[192, 192a] In those areas where acute poliomyelitis has become infrequent its place as the most feared of acute neurological illnesses has largely been taken by this condition. Although its exact cause is unknown, there is strong evidence that an infective agent may be implicated. All ages are prone to attack, although children tend to be less at risk; most of the patients are young adults or are in late middle age. Recent studies have re-emphasized the association with a preceding attack of acute illness clinically suggesting a viral infection, or with a surgical procedure of some sort a few days to a few weeks before the onset of the neurological symptoms.[192b] In some cases there has been an apparent association with a known viral infection, including

influenza, mumps and herpes simplex.[192c] The
possibility of an association with inoculation with
a killed influenza vaccine (A/New Jersey/1976) has
recently been under discussion.[192c]

The onset is rapid and within three to seven days
paralysis may advance to impairment of respiratory
function. Motor weakness, usually beginning in the
lower limbs, tends to overshadow any sensory
disturbances, but dysaesthesia is common and
signs of sensory alterations may be found in most
cases.[193, 194] A characteristic feature is the finding
of high protein levels in the cerebrospinal fluid
(0·4 to 2·0 g/l), without a rise in the cell count such
as might occur in meningitis. The course is variable
and to some extent unpredictable. Recovery is
usually slow and occasionally there are relapses:
the cases fall into two main groups—those with
recovery within a few weeks or so and those in
which recovery takes many months.

The disease is rarely fatal in the acute phase,
and therefore there has been much uncertainty over
its pathological basis. Earlier investigators considered that oedema, principally of nerve roots, was
the earliest change, followed by inflammatory
infiltration and by demyelination with reactive
Schwann cell changes.[195] Recent studies, however,
have shown inflammatory infiltration in peripheral
nerves from the beginning of the illness.[196] This
infiltration is multifocal and affects most nerves
(Fig. 35.29), the cellular exudate being related to
small veins and consisting principally of small and
medium-sized lymphocytes. Macrophages are present but not numerous; plasma cells are rare.
Changes in myelin and in Schwann cells are closely
related to these cellular infiltrates. All degrees
of myelin breakdown may be seen, from
nodal widening and juxtanodal degeneration to
demyelination of whole internodal segments. Such
changes are better seen in dissociated preparations
of nerve than in histological sections. The Schwann
cell response is proliferation, so that the gaps in the
chain of cells are made good and remyelination
begins soon after damage has occurred. Axons are
usually spared, but in the severer cases axon
degeneration occurs in addition to the segmental
demyelination. It is this additional change that may
account for the slower recovery in certain cases of
the disease.

There may be very little change in the muscles.
Foci of inflammatory infiltration in relation to
nerve twigs are seen. Bundle atrophy is found if
there has been extensive axon degeneration. It may
be significant that focal inflammatory infiltration
may be found in the heart, spleen and adrenal

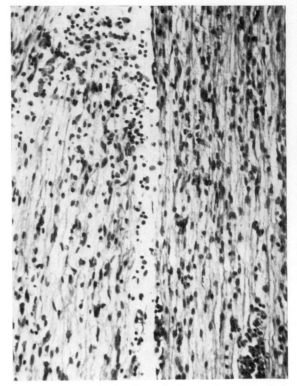

Fig. 35.29. Root of a lumbar spinal nerve in a case of the
Landry–Guillain–Barré syndrome. There is infiltration by
mononuclear cells, with an increase in the cellularity of the
nerve due to macrophage infiltration and Schwann cell
proliferation consequent upon demyelination. *Haematoxylin*;
Van Gieson's stain. ×170.

glands. Small foci of inflammation may also be
seen in the spinal cord and brain, but the chief
change in the central nervous system is chromatolysis in large motor neurons in the spinal cord and
in cranial nerve nuclei. In severer cases neuronal
degeneration and neuronophagia may be found.
When the disease is severe there may be marked
degeneration of the posterior funiculi.

The view is gaining ground that the Landry–
Guillain–Barré syndrome is a disease mediated in
some way by autoimmune mechanisms, and that
there are close similarities between it and experimental allergic neuritis.[196, 197] There is also growing
evidence that circulating lymphocytes undergo
transformation into 'blast' cells before and during
the course of the neurological illness.[198] Indeed,
there is some suggestion that the severity of the
disease may be to some extent gauged by the
extent of the 'blast' cell transformation. Studies
on experimental allergic neuritis and other immunological conditions suggest that transformed and

'sensitized' lymphocytes are in some way responsible for initiating the myelin degeneration. But whether this is a direct action upon the myelin membrane or mediated by the secretion of a cytocidal substance is unknown. The immunological attack seems, however, to be specifically upon the myelin membrane, since the Schwann cell itself and the axon membrane are not primarily affected. It is not known how lymphocytes are primed to attack myelin.

It is of interest, in view of the common association with an initial illness suggesting viral infection, or with a surgical operation, that a very similar disease occurs in 'coon-hounds'—dogs used in hunting racoons in America.[199] This develops after the dog has been bitten by a racoon. The peripheral nerves show the same changes as in the human disease. No infective agent has been discovered. The canine disease shows considerable promise of throwing further light on the pathological process in man.

A similar polyneuritis occasionally follows infectious mononucleosis (glandular fever),[195] prophylactic injections of foreign sera[200] and active immunization against rabies.[200a] However, there is considerable doubt whether the agent responsible in such cases will turn out to be the same as that in 'idiopathic polyneuritis'.

TABES DORSALIS

It is difficult to fit the pathological changes characteristic of tabes dorsalis into any recognized category. As Greenfield[201] pointed out, 'Various theories of the pathogenesis of tabes dorsalis have been put forward but none has gained general acceptance'. Tabes dorsalis is a late manifestation of infection by *Treponema pallidum* (see page 2120). It is usually of slow onset, and its symptomatology[202] is predominantly sensory. Other fibre systems may be attacked: for example, Argyll Robertson pupils, ptosis, optic atrophy and atrophy of muscles in the limbs are manifestations of involvement of other parts of the nervous system. Nevertheless, the characteristic lesion is a multifocal sensory root lesion that usually affects the thoracic roots most. Because of the multifocal distribution of the root involvement, the sensory signs and symptoms are characteristically widespread and patchy in extent. Analgesia and the occurrence of abnormal spontaneous pain ('lightning pains') are very common early manifestations. Moreover, the more discriminative aspects of sensation, such as light touch and joint-position sense, are also affected early. Thermal sensation may remain undisturbed after the other types of sensation have been lost. The conclusion to be drawn from these clinical observations is that there is interference with all forms of sensation without particular regard to fibre diameter or a marked predilection for the long fibres.

The changes in the spinal cord in tabes dorsalis become more understandable if the fate of fibres entering from the dorsal roots is considered. The fine myelinated fibres that subserve pain and thermal sensation run in the lateral part of each dorsal root into the dorsolateral tract (Lissauer's tract); they probably ascend through one or two segments of the spinal cord to end round the neurons of the substantia gelatinosa of the posterior grey column of the same side; the fibres of their second-order sensory neurons promptly cross the midline in the anterior commissure. Fibres from proprioceptive centres run in the medial part of each dorsal root and pass upward in the fasciculus gracilis and fasciculus cuneatus of the same side, and downward for a short distance in Schultze's comma tract in the cervical segments of the cord and in the septomarginal tract (Flechsig's oval tract) in the lumbar segments. A third group of fibres passes into the middle root-zone of Flechsig to end mostly upon cells of the ipsilateral posterior grey column or in the nuclei dorsales (Clarke's column). In tabes dorsalis it would appear to be this middle root-zone that is most subject to damage. Curious pictures of demyelination, probably peculiar to this disease, are thus produced (Figs 35.30A and 35.30B), so that, for instance, a relatively normal fasciculus gracilis may pass a region with complete denervation of the middle root-zone. Such findings can only result from a relatively focal, unsystematized degenerative process, and they are evidence against a diffuse affection of either the dorsal root ganglia or the roots themselves. Indeed, neither the ganglia nor the roots are affected early in tabes dorsalis unless there is concomitant syphilitic meningovascular disease. This peculiar pattern of degeneration is also against the lesion of tabes dorsalis being a manifestation of a 'dying-back' process. The direct or indirect attack by the treponeme must be regarded as its cause, and this view is supported by the serological findings and by the response to treatment. The Wassermann reaction is negative in the cerebrospinal fluid in about 30 per cent of cases, and it is negative in the blood in about the same proportion; the reaction is negative in both cerebrospinal fluid and blood in from 5 to 15 per cent of cases.

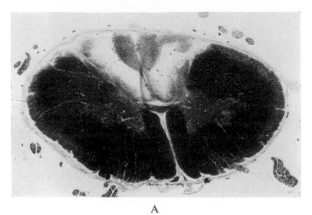

A

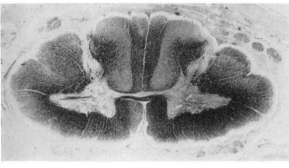

B

Fig. 35.30. Spinal cord in tabes dorsalis. *Myelin stain.* × 5.
A. Lower cervical part of cord, showing profound damage to the middle root zone and very much less fibre loss in the fasciculi graciles.
B. Cervical part of cord (above the level of major involvement) showing the curious restriction of damage to parts of the fasciculi cuneati.

See also Figs 34.38A and 34.38B, page 2120.

Specific anti-syphilis therapy arrests the progress of the disease except when there is a considerable concomitant meningovascular element. Unless, as a consequence of the present day recrudescence of syphilis, tabes dorsalis again becomes the frequent and important problem that it was formerly, it is doubtful whether the nature and pathogenesis of this condition, which seems to have no neuropathological parallel, will ever be clarified.

TUMOURS OF PERIPHERAL NERVES[203, 203a]*

Neurolemmoma

(Schwann Cell Tumour; Schwannoma)

The commonest and most important neoplasm arising in peripheral nerves is the neurolemmoma.

* *By the editor*

This tumour has had many synonyms: those in most frequent use nowadays are *neurolemmoma* (first used in the form 'neurilemoma'[204]—see footnote on page 2221) and *Schwann cell tumour*, or *Schwannoma*.[205] Other terms that still have some currency include *perineurial fibroblastoma*,[206, 207] which indicates a classic but now usually discounted view of the identity of the cell of origin of the tumour, and *neurinoma*,[208] a name now recognized to be inappropriate because it seems to imply a tumour of nerve fibres. The commonly used name neurolemmoma is criticized on the grounds that the term 'neurolemma', or 'neurilemma', is no longer valid, electron microscopy having shown that the sheath to which it referred consists of the plasma membrane of Schwann cells, together with basement membrane and possibly some connective tissue ground sustance and fibrils of collagen.[209] The name Schwannoma, or schwannoma, is said to be preferable because it indicates that the tumour is a tumour of Schwann cells.*

Neurolemmomas arise in peripheral nerves and in cranial nerves (see page 2222). The most frequent intracranial neurolemmoma is a cerebellopontine angle tumour, arising from a vestibulocochlear nerve; it must be distinguished from neurofibroma and meningioma arising in the same situation (see Fig. 34.128, page 2219). The tumours of peripheral nerves arise particularly frequently from spinal nerve roots: these tumours, unless in the cauda equina, compress the spinal cord. Some intrathecal neurolemmomas grow outward through the related intervertebral foramen, forming the so-called dumb-bell or hour-glass tumour. Less often, neurolemmomas arise from other peripheral nerves, the usual situations including the mediastinum and the major nerves of the limbs.[210] Most neurolemmomas are solitary; multiple neurolemmomas may be a feature of neurofibromatosis (see page 2339).

The tumour is a rounded or lobulate mass. When small it is firm, circumscribed, translucent, and white or of pearly appearance. When large it is often yellowish, partly opaque and partly translucent, and partly soft or pseudocystic as a result of degenerative changes.

Histology

Two patterns of tissue have long been recognized in neurolemmomas—Antoni's types A and B.[211] Many neurolemmomas combine both patterns, but

* The possible Schwann cell derivation of the so-called 'granular cell myoblastoma' is noted in Chapter 39, Volume 6.

type A predominates in most instances; those tumours that are of pure type consist of type A tissue. The distinction between the types rests primarily on the histological picture in conventional preparations: tissue culture and electron microscopy have confirmed that distinct but related cells characterize the two patterns (see next page).

Type A Tissue.—Antoni's type A pattern of neurolemmoma consists of compact fascicles of tumour cells that form an intricately interwoven pattern throughout the growth. There is often a characteristic palisade-like arrangement of the nuclei in the cellular bundles (Figs 35.31A and 35.31B). The explanation of this nuclear 'palisading', or 'regimentation', is unknown. It is important to appreciate that its presence is not pathognomonic: an identical arrangement of nuclei is commonly seen in formalin-fixed surgical specimens of smooth muscle (Fig. 35.32), such as leiomyomas and the

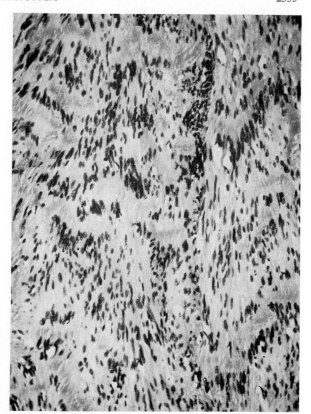

Fig. 35.31B.§ Higher magnification of part of the field illustrated in Fig. 35.31A. The partly fibrillar, partly hyaline appearance of the eosinophile cytoplasmic material between the rows of nuclei can be seen. Compare the nuclear 'palisading' in this neurolemmoma with the essentially identical appearance in the leiomyoma illustrated in Fig. 35.32. *Haematoxylin–eosin.* × 135.

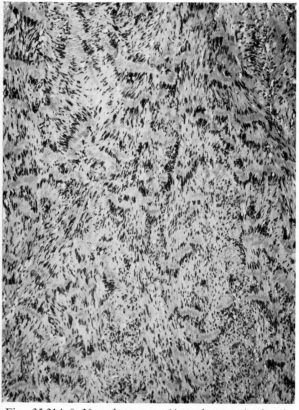

Fig. 35.31A.§ Neurolemmoma (Antoni type A tissue). 'Palisading' ('regimentation') of the nuclei of the tumour cells is conspicuous throughout the field. The tumour formed an encapsulate mass, 4 cm in diameter, arising from the right obturator nerve within the pelvis. It was an incidental finding during a gynaecological operation. See also Fig. 35.31B. *Haematoxylin–eosin.* × 55.

normal or hypertrophic muscle coat of hollow organs, particularly of the gastrointestinal tract.[212] 'Palisading' of the nuclei of smooth muscle is probably an artefact, related to effects on the contractile component of the cytoplasm that are produced by hypoxia during the process of cell death.[213] Failure to recognize that this curious disposition of tumour cell nuclei may be found in leiomyomas can lead to these tumours being mistaken for neurolemmomas. If the diagnosis is in doubt, the usually greater eosinophilia of the cytoplasm of cells of smooth muscle tumours may be a useful indication of their real nature, and confirmation should be sought by staining sections with phosphotungstic acid haematoxylin, for which the cytoplasmic myofibrils have a strong affinity.

Reticulin fibres are abundant in the type A tissue, forming a closely set series of very fine filaments that are so closely apposed to the tumour

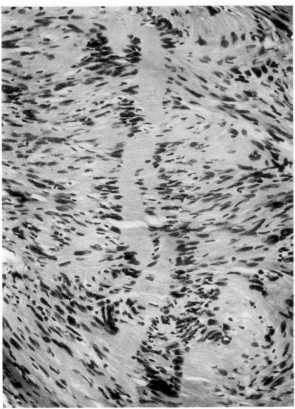

Fig. 35.32.§ Nuclear 'palisading' in a leiomyoma. Compare with Figs 35.31A and 35.31B. The cells of the leiomyoma contained myofibrils, the cytoplasm staining intensely in phosphotungstic acid haematoxylin preparations. The tumour was in the muscular coat of the stomach. It was an incidental finding in a partial gastrectomy specimen. *Haematoxylin–eosin.* × 135.

cells, in the line of their axis, that the cytoplasm is longitudinally indented and so has a ribbed or fibrous appearance in haematoxylin-eosin preparations. Collagen is usually scanty.

The eosinophile zones that are interposed between the lines of 'palisaded' nuclei may appear homogeneous and hyaline or show a more or less evident striation or lamellation that represents the cytoplasm of the cells involved in the local regimentation. When these striae are particularly fine and regularly spaced an 'organoid' appearance results that has been likened to the lamellar structure of Wagner–Meissner tactile corpuscles, particularly when the effect is confined to a small area of 'palisading' that is curved upon itself in the plane of the section. The significance of these structures, which are sometimes referred to as Verocay bodies,[208] is quite obscure; their resemblance to sensory end organs is possibly illusory.

In areas devoid of nuclear 'palisading' the bundles of tumour cells may form whorls, varying in extent and usually of rather loose texture. The whorls are reminiscent of the similar formations that may be seen in many meningiomas. Some of them appear to have developed round a small blood vessel.

Nerve fibres are found in neurolemmomas only exceptionally rarely.[214] It is generally said that they are related to the nerve from which the tumour has arisen, being either its original fibres incorporated in the growing tumour or the product of regenerative activity by injured fibres.

Type B Tissue.—Type B tissue (Fig. 35.33) is characterized by the looseness of its texture and by a tendency to degenerate. Its constituent cells are plumper and show a degree of pleomorphism that is in notable contrast to the regularity of the size, shape and chromatin content of the cells of type A tissue (see above). Large cells, of irregular outline and with a large, irregular, hyperchromatic nucleus, may be numerous at the margin of foci of type B tissue (Fig. 35.34) and may lead to a mistaken diagnosis of malignancy. Some variable features of type B tissue include 'foamy' macrophages laden with Sudanophile and birefringent lipids, some formation of granulation tissue, an infiltrate—usually sparse—of neutrophils, and some accumulation of lymphocytes and plasma cells. Thrombosis of the small blood vessels in the tumour is sometimes conspicuous and accounts for part of the accompanying degenerative changes. There may be small haemorrhages, and haemosiderin is commonly present, either free in the tissue or within macrophages.

Pseudocystic degeneration is common in type B tissue. At first it is of microscopical extent and associated with accumulation of mucinous material in the intercellular space. Later, cyst-like locules form and may range up to several centimetres in diameter.

Electron Microscopy and Tissue Culture.—Ultrastructural studies have shown distinct differences between the cells of the two Antoni types of neurolemmoma. Cells of the type A tissue have many fine, wavy cytoplasmic processes that are covered by electron-dense basement membrane material; cells of the type B tissue contain very numerous organelles and vacuoles, indicative of much greater metabolic and storage activity.[215] Tissue culture has confirmed that there are two varieties of neurolemmoma cell, corresponding to

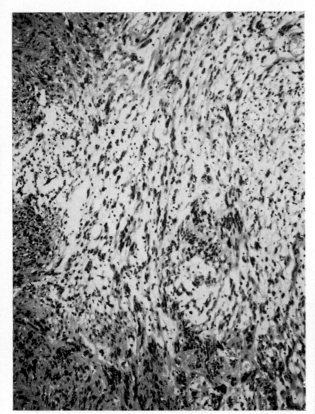

Fig. 35.33.§ Neurolemmoma. The greater part of the field is occupied by tumour tissue of Antoni's type B. This is of loose texture and contains relatively few tumour cells in comparison with the adjoining areas, which are of the Antoni type A pattern. The cells of the type B tissue are larger and plumper than those of the type A tissue, and their nucleus is generally larger. A few inflammatory cells are scattered through the field; most of them are lymphocytes. The tumour arose from the sheath of an ulnar nerve in the upper part of the forearm and measured 3 cm in its longest dimension. The patient had sensory disturbance and some atrophy of the muscles in the parts innervated by the affected nerve. The tumour was solitary. See also Fig. 35.34. *Haematoxylin-eosin.* × 85.

the cells of the two Antoni types of tissue.[216, 217] The results of electron microscopy and tissue culture support the view that neurolemmomas are tumours of Schwann cells, not of fibroblasts: this conclusion may be regarded as resolving the long debate between those who followed Verocay,[208] to whom the Schwann cell interpretation is due, and those who favoured Penfield's[206] fibroblastic derivation of the tumours.

Variants.—Epithelioid, myxomatoid and melanotic variants of neurolemmoma are referred to on page 2340.

Malignant Neurolemmoma

Some pathologists believe that all neurolemmomas should be regarded as locally malignant and, in support of this view, cite the frequency of local recurrence after surgical excision of the tumour. In fact, many neurolemmomas do not recur after local exision; further, there is some evidence that recurrence is associated with incomplete removal of the tumour at the initial operation or with possible 'seeding' of the operation site with tumour tissue in the course of piecemeal excision. The friable nature of the pseudocystic parts of tumours with a considerable component of tissue of Antoni's type B increases the risk of inadvertent contamination of the adjacent tissues during surgical manipulation; however, it may be noted that even extensive

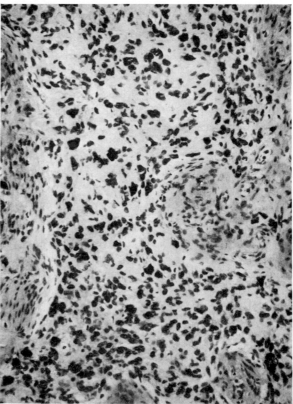

Fig. 35.34.§ Neurolemmoma. Large, pleomorphic, hyperchromatic cells at the periphery of a region of Antoni type B tissue. The adjoining tissue is of type A pattern. The tumour, an encapsulate mass, 6 cm in its greatest dimension, arose in relation to the posterior cord of a brachial plexus in a boy, aged 10 years. It was originally thought to be sarcomatous, because of the pleomorphic areas. Review of the sections and the subsequent clinical course confirmed the alternative interpretation that the tumour was benign. Compare with Fig. 35.35. *Haematoxylin-eosin.* × 135.

disruption of a tumour during the operation is by no means always followed by recurrence of the growth.[213] Locally recurrent tumours are often treated successfully by further local excision, particularly when the affected region is meticulously explored so that outlying foci of growth may be found and removed.[213]

A small proportion of neurolemmomas must be regarded as frankly malignant. Malignant change is likelier to develop in cases of neurofibromatosis.[218] Incomplete encapsulation and unequivocally invasive growth into the substance of adjoining structures, particularly when the microscopical appearances are markedly pleomorphic and tumour giant cells and mitotic figures are frequent, must be regarded as evidence of the sarcomatous nature of the tumour. Metastasis is a relatively uncommon development; the lungs are involved predominantly.[210] From the practical point of view, it has to be recognized that histological appearances are not alone sufficient indication that a given neurolemmoma is benign or malignant (Fig. 35.35). Neurolemmomas that appear to be fully differentiated have been known to metastasize through the blood stream, the secondary deposits reproducing the differentiated appearance of the primary growth. In contrast, very pleomorphic tumours, with numerous mitotic figures and looking highly malignant under the microscope, may be fully confined by their capsule and may be without recurrence or metastasis during periods of observation that in some instances have covered up to three decades.[213]

Metaplasia.—Cartilaginous, osteoid, osseous and adipose tissue may be found, sometimes in combination, in malignant neurolemmomas.[219, 220] Transformation from neurolemmoma to rhabdomyosarcoma has been observed in a number of instances, usually in tumours associated with neurofibromatosis.[221]

Neurofibroma

The tumours that properly may be called neurofibromas are much less frequent than neurolemmomas (see above). They are seen particularly in cases of von Recklinghausen's neurofibromatosis, accounting for a variable proportion of the multiple tumours that are characteristic of this disease, the rest being neurolemmomas. Solitary neurofibromas are so rare that this diagnosis may not be maintained until the possibility of neurofibromatosis has been ruled out. It must be re-

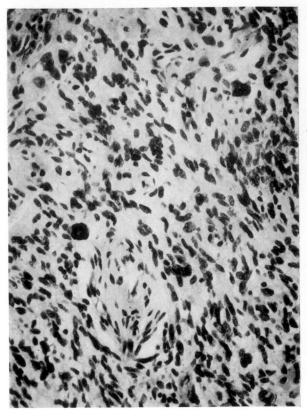

Fig. 35.35.§ Malignant neurolemmoma. This tumour, although well differentiated, and largely consisting of characteristic Antoni type A tissue with some relatively small foci of type B tissue, invaded the inferior cava. There were many secondary deposits in the lungs and throughout the body. These deposits reproduced the differentiated structure of the primary growth, which was in the retroperitoneal tissues. The field illustrated is from the primary tumour. There is nothing in it that would justify a diagnosis of malignancy. The hyperchromatic cells with bizarre nucleus may be seen in benign neurolemmomas also (compare with Fig. 35.34). *Haematoxylin–eosin.* × 215.

membered that the presence of multiple superficial tumours, immediately evident on clinical examination, is by no means invariably a feature of neurofibromatosis (see below).

Neurofibromatosis (Von Recklinghausen's Disease of Nerves[222])*

Neurofibromatosis is a familial disease with autosomal dominant inheritance. Its main features are

* The clinical picture of peripheral neurofibromatosis, with multiple tumours of the skin, a condition formerly known as *molluscum fibrosum multiplex*, had been described long before von Recklinghausen's classic account in 1882 (reference 222 on page 2347). It was well illustrated by W. G.

multiple tumours arising in nerves and the presence in the skin of so-called *café au lait* spots. The latter, which are more or less clearly defined melanotic macules, may appear in childhood, before tumours are evident; it is said that the presence of six or more of these spots, of more than 1·5 cm in diameter, is indicative of the disease.[223] The tumours may arise from any cranial or spinal nerve, including nerve roots and ganglia. The major peripheral nerves and their branches may be affected in any part of the body. Sympathetic nerves and ganglia and visceral autonomic plexuses[224] are involved in some cases. Involvement of nerves may take the form of diffuse thickening of a variable part of their length; when several nerves in a particular region are affected in this manner the thickenings are described as *plexiform neurofibromas*. Other lesions are rounded or irregular masses protruding from the surface of the nerves. Discrete sessile or, more commonly, pedunculate tumours of the skin are characteristic of the classic presentation of neurofibromatosis. This involvement of the skin may be sparse or widespread, and generalized or confined to particular regions, especially the trunk but sometimes the neck, scalp, face or limbs. The distribution of the lesions may be constant in particular families. On the trunk they commonly follow the distribution of the cutaneous nerves; the largest tumours form great pendulous masses that may weigh many hundreds of grams. The skin of the affected parts may be excessively hairy and deeply pigmented with melanin.

Gliomas of the brain,[225] optic nerves[226] or spinal cord,[227] meningiomas,[228] vascular hamartomas of the brain[229] and phaeochromocytomas[230] may be associated with neurofibromatosis. 'Central neurofibromatosis' (Wishart's disease[230a]) is a rare condition in which tumours of both vestibulocochlear nerves and of spinal nerve roots are associated with multiple meningiomas and, in some cases, neurofibromatosis of peripheral nerves (see page 2203).

Other conditions that may accompany the disease include mental retardation, delayed puberty or persistent sexual immaturity, skeletal deformity (which may be related to intraosseous neurofibromas) and syringomyelia (which is usually, but not always, secondary to an intramedullary glioma). Hypertension accompanying fibromuscular renal arterial hyperplasia (see page 178, Volume 1) has been observed.[231] Other effects on the kidneys are mentioned on page 1424, in Volume 4. Hypoglycaemia has been associated with the presence of exceptionally large intra-abdominal tumours (see page 1366, Volume 3).[213, 232]

Histology

Most of the large protuberant tumours of neurofibromatosis, including most of the 'dumb-bell' tumours that develop where affected nerves pass through cranial or intervertebral foramina, prove histologically to be neurolemmomas (see above). The small tumours of the skin often consist of fibrous tissue without specific features. The fusiform tumours, including those described as plexiform, are of the type often referred to as 'true neurofibromas': it is these that will be discussed here.

Neurofibromas consist of elongated cells that are distributed comparatively sparsely between abundant collagen fibres. Reticulin fibres are scarce and without the intimate relation to the tumour cells that is seen in neurolemmomas (see page 2336). The nucleus of the neurofibroma cell is characteristically long and slender, and of sinuous outline (Fig. 35.36). The collagen fibres tend also to have a notably sinuous disposition; they are collected loosely into bundles that traverse the tumour in any direction, but with a general orientation parallel to the length of the affected nerve. The fibres are separated by mucinous ground substance, which may be abundant. A scattering of lymphocytes and macrophages is often present; the latter commonly have foamy cytoplasm that contains neutral fat and birefringent crystalline lipids. Nerve fibres, which are part of the affected nerve, follow their course through the tumour, although often widely separated by the tissue of the latter.

Tilesius in his *Historia pathologica singularis cutis turpitudinis*, published in Leipzig in 1793, and by Robert William Smith, a surgeon in Dublin, in *A Treatise on the Pathology, Diagnosis, and Treatment of Neuroma*, published in Dublin in 1849. Robert William Smith, in 1838, was co-founder (with William Stokes) and joint Secretary of the Pathological Society of Dublin, the first pathological Society in Great Britain and Ireland (in 1883 the Society became the Section of Pathology of the Royal Academy of Medicine in Ireland, which was founded in that year). One of Tilesius's illustrations of a patient with the 'singular turpitude of the skin' is reproduced in: Beattie, J. M., Dickson, W. E. Carnegie, Drennan, A. M., *A Textbook of Pathology—General and Special—for the Use of Students and Practitioners*, 5th edn, edited by W. E. Carnegie Dickson, vol. 2, Fig. 722, page 1304; London, 1948.

Malignant Change

It is common, if casual, teaching that malignancy develops in 10 to 15 per cent of cases of neuro-

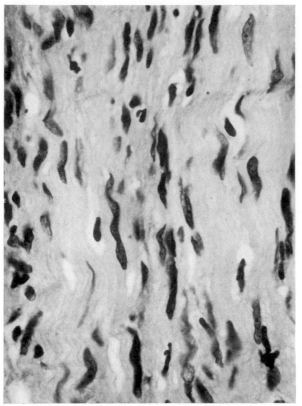

Fig. 35.36.§ Neurofibroma. This field from a plexiform neurofibroma in the thigh of a patient with classic neurofibromatosis shows the characteristically long, sinuous nuclei and the sinuous disposition of the fibrous component. *Haematoxylin–eosin.* × 550.

fibromatosis. Sarcomatous change may occur with this order of frequency among patients severely affected with the classic, florid clinical manifestations of generalized disease. If cases of less severity are taken into account, including the far from rare cases of the so-called *formes frustes*, in which overt manifestations of the disease are very limited, the overall incidence of malignant change is probably much smaller.[233, 233a] In most instances the histological picture is either that of a fibrosarcoma (when the lesion that has undergone malignant change was a neurofibroma) or that of a malignant neurolemmoma, which is perhaps more usual. Occasionally, the tumour and its metastatic deposits, which may be widespread, have the histological structure of an angiosarcoma.[233a]

Nature of Neurofibromatosis

The widespread involvement of nerves and the diffuse nature of the fibrocellular proliferation

within affected nerves suggest that neurofibromatosis may be a specific dysplasia of the fibroblastic element of nerve sheaths rather than essentially a neoplastic condition. The occurrence in florid cases of proliferation of the connective tissue of the dermis and subcutaneous tissue might support this view, as evidence of involvement of fibroblasts elsewhere than in nerves and so of a systemic alteration of connective tissue. The association with pigmentary anomalies, such as the *café au lait* spots in the skin, has been regarded as evidence of a system disorder affecting neural tissue and melanogenesis. According to this view, the development of unequivocal neoplasms—neurolemmomas and neurofibrosarcomas—is sequential and not a basic feature of the essentially dysplastic disease. However, true tumours are so regularly a feature of the disease that it is difficult to regard it as other than fundamentally neoplastic. The frequency of sarcomatous change, with metastasis, in classic cases of neurofibromatosis, the much rarer but still unequivocal liability to such change in cases of the '*formes frustes*', and the association with other types of tumours, particularly of the brain, spinal cord, eyes and sympathetic nervous system, underline the fact that the manifestations of neoplasia are of paramount clinical significance, whether the disease is to be regarded as dysplastic or as neoplastic.

Variants

Epithelioid, myxomatoid and melanotic varieties of 'neurofibroma' have been described. Some of these have been neurolemmomas with more or less extensive local variations in structure that have been thought to merit the variant designation. Others have been tumours that basically have had the structure of a true neurofibroma, as described above, but with the inclusion of foci of the variant appearance.

Epithelioid Tumours.—Some malignant neurolemmomas include areas, often quite sharply delimited, in which the tumour cells form solid aggregates that may closely simulate the appearance of undifferentiated carcinoma. Similar appearances are seen more rarely in some plexiform neurofibromas. In both situations it is possible to identify the true nature of the tumour by finding parts that retain the characteristic structure.

Myxomatoid Tumours.—Myxomatoid tissue, which may be extensive, is sometimes found in neurolemmomas, particularly in foci of Antoni type B tissue. The cells in the myxomatoid regions, although fibroblast-like or stellate, as in myxomatoid tissue in other situations, are intermixed with sparse cells of the form that is characteristic of the type B tissue (see page 2336). Mucinous material is abundant in the interstices. It is likely that these myxomatoid foci are due to degenerative changes in the tumour tissue. Similar foci are not uncommon in plexiform neurofibromas and in the larger cutaneous tumours of neurofibromatosis.

Rarely, a solitary small tumour of myxomatoid structure is found in the dermis or subcutaneous tissue, evidently having formed within the substance of a small nerve. Its probable origin is a degenerative change in the endoneurium. Some authorities regard it as a benign neoplasm and have named it *myxoma of nerve sheath*.[234]

Melanin-Containing Tumours.—Melanotic neurolemmomas and neurofibromas are the best known of the variants.[235, 236] The amount of melanin that they contain varies widely. The pigment may be readily visible in sections stained with haematoxylin and eosin, and exceptional examples are in parts black to the naked eye; at the other extreme the pigment may be so scanty that special staining is necessary for its demonstration. These pigmented growths pose interesting questions of their possible relationship to such conditions as meningeal melanosis and blue naevi of spinal nerve roots,[237] and to the problem whether, as now seems likely, Schwann cells can elaborate melanin.[238, 239]

Mucosal Neuromas with Endocrine Tumours
(Williams–Pollock Syndrome)[240, 241]

Several cases, some of them familial, have been reported in which multiple, small, pedunculate or sessile 'neuromas' at mucocutaneous junctions and on certain mucous membranes are associated with endocrine tumours and other abnormalities. The neuromas occur particularly on the margin of the eyelids and on the lips and tongue; they have been found also on the nasal, laryngeal, bronchial and vaginal mucosa.[213] The endocrine tumours have usually been phaeochromocytomas and amyloid-producing medullary thyroid carcinomas. Diffuse thickening of the lips, circumoral pigmentation, diverticular disease of the colon, megacolon, and Marfan's syndrome have been among other features in various cases.[241]

The 'neuromas' consist of well-formed bundles of myelinated nerve fibres enclosed in a perineurial sheath. The bundles course randomly through the extent of the nodule and are separated by relatively abundant, loose-textured areolar tissue. There is no fibrosis unless the lesion has been injured—for instance, through being inadvertently crushed between the teeth—or infected. The histological picture is not that of a neurofibroma; rather, it is reminiscent of the so-called 'amputation neuroma'. In the cases with intestinal symptoms there have been changes in the myenteric plexuses, including a marked increase in their content of nerve fibres and a proliferation of ganglion cells that has been described as ganglioneuromatosis.[240, 242]

'Amputation Neuroma'
(Post-Traumatic Pseudoneuroma)

The so-called amputation neuroma is not a neoplasm but a nodule formed by the proliferation of nerve fibres, including myelinated axons, Schwann cells and collagenous tissue, at a site of major injury to a nerve. Usually the injury is in the form of complete transection, as during amputation, but occasionally severe crushing has the same sequel. The lesion is a regenerative phenomenon. It is most familiar in the limbs, but comparable nodules have been found on the vagus nerves following vagotomy[213] and gastrectomy,[243] in the stump of the ureter after nephrectomy,[244] in the stump of the cystic duct after cholecystectomy,[245] in the stump of the bronchus after pneumonectomy[213] and in the spinal cord after injury.[246] The visceral nodules are generally symptomless, although persistent symptoms following cholecystectomy have been attributed to this sequel. Amputation 'neuromas' in the limbs are commonly painful and tender but may cause no symptoms. When associated with pain, this may be felt by the patient at the site of the 'neuroma' itself or it may be referred to that area that normally would have been innervated by the severed nerve. The phenomenon of the 'phantom limb', the patient experiencing sensations that seem to relate to the part that has been amputated, including painful sensations, is rarely attributable to the presence of an amputation 'neuroma'.[247]

Histology

The fully developed amputation 'neuroma' consists of a tangle of well-formed nerve fibres, enclosed in perineurium and embedded in a more or less dense mass of fibrous scar tissue. Appropriate histological methods show that some of the cords of Schwann cells lack axons.

Plantar Digital 'Neuroma'[248, 249]
(Traumatic Digital Neuropathy in Metatarsalgia)

The painful condition that is known as Morton's metatarsalgia, 'Morton's toe', or Durlacher–Morton disease,[250, 251] is due to chronic repeated injury to a plantar digital nerve in the vicinity of the heads of the related metatarsal bones. This results in expansion of the affected part of the nerve to form a nodule up to about a centimetre long and less than half that in its other dimensions. Microscopical examination shows a variable loss of nerve tissue, thickening of the perineurium, and a general increase in fibrous tissue, often with rounded, hyaline or concentrically layered scar-like foci. Earlier lesions, or lesions that are still active, include small collections of mucinous material, sometimes within the perineurial sheath and sometimes in the epineurium. Inflammatory cells, mainly lymphocytes and macrophages, may be present but are seldom very numerous.

The condition is not neoplastic. It is probably due to intermittent compression of the nerve as a consequence of local changes in anatomical relations, such as may result from lessening or loss of the concavity of the transverse arch of the foot in the region of the metatarsal heads.

Neuronal Tumours

The tumours of the precursors of the ganglion cells of the peripheral nervous system and those formed of the mature derivatives of these cells are respectively the neuroblastomas (sympathicoblastomas) and the ganglioneuromas and phaeochromocytomas (chromaffinomas).

Neuroblastoma

Neuroblastomas arise most frequently in the medulla of the adrenal glands, particularly in the first three years of life. Origin apart from the adrenals, and especially in the retroperitoneal tissues, is also frequent, particularly in older children and predominantly so in adults.[252] The extra-adrenal tumours are believed to originate in sympathetic ganglia. The neuroblastomas are considered on page 1962 in Volume 4. The olfactory neuroblastoma, which is a nasal tumour distinct from the neuroblastomas that arise elsewhere, is considered on page 226 in Volume 1.

Ganglioneuroblastoma and Ganglioneuroma

Ganglioneuroblastomas (malignant ganglioneuromas) are seen most frequently in children under six years of age. They usually arise in the retroperitoneal tissues or in the posterior part of the mediastinum;[252] others are adrenal tumours. They are considered on page 1965 in Volume 4.

Phaeochromocytoma (Chromaffinoma)

The phaeochromocytomas may be classed among the neuronal tumours as they are tumours of chromaffin cells, which, like the sympathetic nerve cells, are derived from the primitive sympathogonia. They occur at all ages and most frequently in the third, fourth and fifth decades. In about four fifths of cases they arise in the adrenal glands.[253, 254] They are considered on page 1965 in Volume 4.

Non-Chromaffin Paragangliomas[255]

There is no uniformity in current application of the term paraganglion and it is not surprising that there is corresponding uncertainty about the range of tumours that may be described as paragangliomas. An authoritative anatomical definition[256] of the paraganglia is that they are spherical masses of chromaffin cells, about 2 mm in diameter, situated within a ganglion of the sympathetic trunks or in or just outside its capsule; in adults they are generally represented by microscopic remnants only. Other authorities include among the paraganglia such structures as the para-aortic bodies (organs of Zuckerkandl), which ordinarily disappear by the middle of the second decade, and chemoreceptors such as the carotid bodies and tympanic bodies (jugular glomera), and related structures in various parts of the body. Some of these contain chromaffin cells; others do not, although they, and the non-chromaffin tumours arising from them, may be shown in some instances to produce catecholamines.[257]

As it is probable, although uncertain, that the paraganglia, in the broader sense referred to above, receive a quota of neuroblasts from neural structures developing in their vicinity and so are not exclusively of mesodermal derivation, their relation to the peripheral nervous system may be accepted and their tumours noted in the present context. The tumours in general resemble the phaeochromocytomas histologically (see page 1967 in Volume 4), except that the non-chromaffin examples by definition lack demonstrable cytoplasmic chromaffinity. Most of them are encapsulate growths consisting of solid alveolar clusters or diffuse masses of large, closely packed, mononuclear cells with opaque and often finely granular cytoplasm. The nucleus of the tumour cells is often relatively small; its chromatin may be dense or arranged in a fine vesicular pattern. Delicate collagenous stroma outlines the clusters of cells or traverses the growth; small, thin-walled blood vessels may be numerous. Those tumours that arise from chemoreceptor organs are often known as *chemodectomas*.

Most non-chromaffin paragangliomas are of very slow growth. Some reach a large size, such as those of the carotid bodies, and their surgical removal may be hazardous or impossible because of their adherence to major blood vessels, which may become totally surrounded by the tumour tissue. Others, such as those of the tympanic bodies (jugular glomera), grow invasively into adjoining structures and may prove incurable by reason of their situation (see Chapter 41, Volume 6). Invasion of blood vessels is often, but not invariably, followed by metastasis to the lungs and elsewhere.

Malignant Non-Chromaffin Paragangliomas.[255]—In addition to the metastasizing tumours just mentioned there are paragangliomas of pleomorphic structure that grow more rapidly and aggressively than the typical examples. These malignant growths are seen most frequently in the limbs (usually within or between the muscles) and in the retroperitoneal tissues. In spite of a greater variation in size and appearance of the cells, the general appearance of the malignant paragangliomas is sufficiently similar to that of the classic carotid body tumour and other slowly growing tumours of this type for the diagnosis to be evident.

Tumours of Primitive Neural Structure

There are very rare reports of malignant tumours arising in peripheral nerves and presenting a histological appearance comparable to that of the most primitive tumours of the central nervous system. Their interpretation has been controversial and some authorities reject the likelihood of neuroepithelial origin[258] that others have maintained.[259] The possibility that such tumours are metastatic carcinomas and not of neural origin is evident in a considerable proportion of the few published accounts;[258] other cases support the neural view.[260] The features of the less equivocal growths that have suggested their derivation from primitive tissue of the nervous system include rosette-like structures and tubules lined by columnar cells reminiscent of embryonic neuroepithelium.

Vascular Hamartomas and Blood Vessel Neoplasms

Capillary haemangiomatous hamartomas in the vicinity of nerves sometimes extend into the substance of the latter, without evident disability developing. The rare association of angiosarcomatous change with neurofibromatosis has been mentioned above (page 2340).

Secondary Tumours

Peripheral nerves are commonly invaded by carcinomas and other malignant tumours in their vicinity, including lymphomas. Once within the perineurium the tumour may extend for considerable distances along the nerve without necessarily causing degenerative effects, although these may develop if the tumour tissue becomes expansive at any particular level.

The observation that epithelial structures may grow within nerves in the breast in association with benign proliferative conditions of the mammary parenchyma is referred to on page 1975 in Volume 4. The importance of this occurrence is twofold—its significance to the practising histopathologist, who must interpret such findings accurately, and its challenge to the hitherto accepted principle that neural invasion by epithelial structures is an absolute criterion of malignancy. A comparable, and even rarer, observation, with similar diagnostic implications, is the occasional presence of endometrium within a pelvic nerve in cases of endometriosis.[213]

Peripheral nerves are sometimes heavily, if patchily, infiltrated by leukaemic cells, particularly in chronic myeloid leukaemia.

REFERENCES

NORMAL STRUCTURE OF PERIPHERAL NERVES

1. Greenfield, J. G., in *Greenfield's Neuropathology*, 2nd edn, by W. Blackwood, W. H. McMenemey, A. Meyer, R. M. Norman and D. S. Russell, chap. 13. London, 1963.

1a. Urich, H., in *Greenfield's Neuropathology*, 3rd edn, edited by W. Blackwood and J. A. N. Corsellis, chap. 16. London, 1976.

1b. Ramón y Cajal, S., *Rev. Cienc. méd.* (*Madr.*), 1892, **18**, 457.

2. Einarsen, L., in *Modern Scientific Aspects of Neurology*, edited by J. N. Cumings, page 1. London, 1960.
3. Schmitt, F. O., *Neurosci. Res. Prog. Bull.*, 1968, **6**, 119.
4. Porter, K. R., in *Principles of Biomolecular Organization*, edited by G. W. Wolstenholme and M. O'Connor, page 308. London, 1966.
4a. Barr, M. L., Bertram, E. G., *Nature (Lond.)*, 1949, **163**, 676.
5. Robertis, E. de, *Histophysiology of Synapses and Neurosecretion*. Oxford, 1964.
6. Gray, E. G., Guillery, R. W., *Int. Rev. Cytol.*, 1966, **19**, 111.
7. Castillo, J. del, Katz, B., *Progr. Biophys. biophys. Cytol.*, 1956, **6**, 121.
8. Gray, E. G., *Comp. Biochem. Physiol.*, 1970, **36**, 419.
9. Hörstadius, S., *The Neural Crest*. Oxford, 1950.
10. Brizzee, K. R., *J. comp. Neurol.*, 1949, **19**, 129.
10a. Plenk, H., *Ergebn. Anat. Entwickl.-Gesch.*, 1927, **27**, 302.
10b. Laidlaw, G. F., *Amer. J. Path.*, 1930, **6**, 435.
10c. Remak, R., *Arch. Anat. Physiol. wiss. Med.*, 1836, 145.
10d. Remak, R., *Observationes anatomicae et microscopicae de systematis nervosi structura*. Berolini, 1838.
11. Robertson, J. D., *J. biophys. biochem. Cytol.*, 1957, **3**, 1043.
12. Weiss, P., *Neurosci. Res. Prog. Bull.*, 1967, **5**, 371.
13. Kreutzberg, G. W., *Proc. nat. Acad. Sci. (Wash.)*, 1969, **62**, 722.
14. Weiss, P., Hiscoe, H. B., *J. exp. Zool.*, 1948, **107**, 315.
14a. Ranvier, L.-A., *Leçons sur l'histologie du système nerveux*. Paris, 1878.
14b. Schmidt, H. D., *Mth. micr. J.*, 1874, **11**, 200.
14c. Lantermann, A. J., *Arch. mikr. Anat.*, 1877, **13**, 1.
15. Hall, S. M., Williams, P. L., *J. Cell Sci.*, 1970, **6**, 767.
16. Luxoro, M., *Proc. nat. Acad. Sci.*, 1958, **49**, 152.
17. Williams, P. L., Landon, D. N., *Nature (Lond.)*, 1963, **198**, 670.
18. Langley, O. K., Landon, D. N., *J. Histochem. Cytochem.*, 1968, **15**, 722.
19. Thomas, P. K., *J. Anat. (Lond.)*, 1963, **97**, 35.
20. Tasaki, I., in *Handbook of Physiology*, published by the American Physiological Society, vol. 1, chap. 3. Washington, D.C., 1959.
21. Greenfield, J. G., Carmichael, E. A., *Brain*, 1935, **58**, 483.
22. Wohlfart, G., Swank, E. L., *Arch. Neurol. Psychiat. (Chic.)*, 1941, **46**, 783.
23. Garven, H. S. D., Gairns, F. W., Smith, G., *Scot. med. J.*, 1962, **7**, 250.
24. Coërs, C., *Acta neurol. belg.*, 1955, **55**, 741.
25. Cooper, S., in *Structure and Function of Muscle*, edited by G. H. Bourne, vol. 1, page 381. New York, 1960.
26. Landon, D. N., in *Control and Innervation of Skeletal Muscle*, edited by B. L. Andrew, page 96. Edinburgh and London, 1966.
27. Cavanagh, J. B., Passingham, R. J., Vogt, J. A., *J. Path. Bact.*, 1964, **88**, 89.
28. Adams, W. E., *J. Anat. (Lond.)*, 1942, **76**, 243.
29. Brierley, J. B., *Acta psychiat. scand.*, 1955, **30**, 553.
30. Tarlov, I. M., *Arch. Neurol. Psychiat. (Chic.)*, 1937, **37**, 555.
31. Brierley, J. B., Field, E. J., *J. Neurol. Neurosurg. Psychiat.*, 1949, **12**, 86.
32. Brierley, J. B., Field, E. J., *J. Anat. (Lond.)*, 1948, **82**, 153.
33. Wright, G. Payling, in *Modern Trends in Pathology*, edited by D. H. Collins, page 212. London, 1959.
33a. Waksman, B. H., *J. Neuropath. exp. Neurol.*, 1961, **20**, 35.
34. Cavanagh, J. B., Jacobs, J. M., *Brit. J. exp. Path.*, 1964, **45**, 309.

THE REACTIONS OF NERVE TRUNKS TO TRANSECTION
35. Waller, A., *Phil. Trans. roy. Soc.*, 1850, **140**, 423.
36. Weddell, G., Glees, P., *J. Anat. (Lond.)*, 1941, **76**, 65.
37. Causey, G., Palmer, E., *J. Anat. (Lond.)*, 1953, **87**, 185.
38. Johnson, A. C., McNabb, A. R., Rossiter, R. S., *Arch. Neurol. Psychiat. (Chic.)*, 1950, **64**, 105.
39. Adams, C. W. M., *J. Neurochem.*, 1958, **2**, 178.
40. Gutmann, G., Holubar, J., *J. Neurol. Neurosurg. Psychiat.*, 1950, **13**, 89.
41. Abercrombie, M., Johnson, M., *J. Anat. (Lond.)*, 1946, **80**, 37.
42. Olsson, G., *Int. Rev. Cytol.*, 1968, **24**, 27.
43. Mellick, R. S., Cavanagh, J. B., *Brain*, 1968, **91**, 141.
44. Rexed, B., Fredriksson, T., *Acta Soc. Med. upsalien.*, 1956, **61**, 199.
45. Noback, C. R., Montagna, W., *J. comp. Neurol.*, 1952, **97**, 211.
45a. Büngner, O. von, *Beitr. path. Anat.*, 1891, **10**, 321.
46. Jacobs, J. M., Cavanagh, J. B., *J. Anat. (Lond.)*, 1969, **105**, 295.
47. Edds, M. V., Jr, *Quart. Rev. Biol.*, 1953, **28**, 260.
48. Hoffman, H., *Aust. J. exp. Biol.*, 1950, **28**, 374.
49. Young, J. Z., *Physiol. Rev.*, 1942, **22**, 318.
50. Gutmann, E., Young, J. Z., *J. Anat. (Lond.)*, 1944, **78**, 15.
51. Weddell, G., Guttmann, L., Gutmann, E., *J. Neurol. Neurosurg. Psychiat.*, 1941, **4**, 206.
52. Romanes, G., *J. Anat. (Lond.)*, 1941, **76**, 112.
53. Brattgård, S.-O., Edström, J.-E., Hydén, H., *J. Neurochem.*, 1957, **1**, 316.
54. Watson, W. E., *J. Physiol.*, 1965, **180**, 741.
55. Watson, W. E., *J. Physiol.*, 1968, **196**, 655.
56. Watson, W. E., *J. Physiol.*, 1969, **202**, 611.
57. Duchen, L. W., Strich, S. J., *Quart. J. exp. Physiol.*, 1968, **53**, 84.
58. Cragg, B. G., *Brain Res.*, 1970, **23**, 1.
59. Einarsen, L., in *Modern Scientific Aspects of Neurology*, edited by J. N. Cumings, page 1. London, 1960.
60. Liu, C.-N., *Anat. Rec.*, 1953, **115**, 342.

CIRCULATORY DISORDERS AND THE EFFECTS OF COMPRESSION TRAUMA
61. Waller, A., *Proc. roy. Soc. Lond.*, 1862, **12**, 89.
62. Lewis, T., Pickering, G. W., Rothschild, P., *Heart*, 1931, **16**, 1.
63. Denny-Brown, D., Brenner, C., *Arch. Neurol. Psychiat. (Chic.)*, 1944, **51**, 1.
64. Landon, D. N., Langley, O. K., *J. Anat. (Lond.)*, 1971, **108**, 419.
65. Miller, H. G., Daley, R., *Quart. J. Med.*, 1946, N.S. **15**, 255.
66. Lovshin, L. L., Kernohan, J. W., *Arch. intern. Med.*, 1948, **82**, 321.
67. Garven, H. S. D., Gairns, F. W., Smith, G., *Scot. med. J.*, 1962, **7**, 250.
68. Woltman, H. W., Wilder, R. W., *Arch. intern. Med.*, 1929, **44**, 576.
69. Fagerberg, S. A., *Acta med. scand.*, 1959, suppl. 345.

70. Field, R. A., Adams, L. C., *Medicine (Baltimore)*, 1964, **43**, 275.

71. Gabbay, K. H., Merola, L. O., Field, R. A., *Science*, 1966, **157**, 209.

72. Martin, M. M., *Brain*, 1953, **76**, 594.

73. Rundles, R. W., *Medicine (Baltimore)*, 1945, **24**, 111.

74. Thomas, P. K., Lascelles, R. G., *Quart. J. Med.*, 1966, N.S. **35**, 489.

75. Greenbaum, D., Richardson, P. C., Salmon, M. V., Urich, H., *Brain*, 1964, **87**, 201.

76. Gilliatt, R. W., Willison, R. G., *J. Neurol. Neurosurg. Psychiat.*, 1962, **25**, 11.

77. Garland, H., Taverner, D., *Brit. med. J.*, 1953, **1**, 1405.

78. Mulder, D. W., Lambert, E. H., Bastron, J. A., Sprague, R. G., *Neurology (Minneap.)*, 1961, **11**, 275.

79. Martin, M. M., *Lancet*, 1953, **1**, 560.

80. Appenzeller, O., Richardson, E. P., *Neurology (Minneap.)*, 1966, **16**, 1205.

81. Rukavina, J. G., Block, W. D., Jackson, C. E., Falls, H. F., Carey, J. H., Curtis, A. C., *Medicine (Baltimore)*, 1956, **35**, 239.

82. Symmers, W. St C., *J. clin. Path.*, 1956, **9**, 187.

83. Navasquez, S. de, Treble, H. A., *Brain*, 1938, **61**, 116.

84. Andrade, C., *Brain*, 1952, **75**, 408.

84a. Urich, H., in *Greenfield's Neuropathology*, 3rd edn, edited by W. Blackwood and J. A. N. Corsellis, chap. 16 [page 731]. London, 1976.

PARENCHYMATOUS NEUROPATHIES

85. Gowers, W. R., *Lancet*, 1902, **1**, 1003.

85a. Greenfield, J. G., *The Spinocerebellar Degenerations*. Oxford, 1954.

86. Spatz, H., in *Proceedings of the First International Congress of Neuropathology, Rome, 1952*, vol. 2, page 375. Amsterdam, 1952.

87. Charcot, J. M., Marie, P., *Rev. Méd. (Paris)*, 1886, **6**, 97.

87a. Tooth, H. H., *The Peroneal Type of Progressive Muscular Atrophy*. London, 1886.

87b. Friedreich, N., *Virchows Arch. path. Anat.*, 1863, **26**, 391, 433; 1863, **27**, 1; 1876, **68**, 145; 1877, **70**, 140.

87c. Roth, M., *Brain*, 1948, **71**, 416.

87d. Marie, P., *Sem. méd. (Paris)*, 1893, **13**, 444, 447.

88. Brodal, A., Refsum, S., *Acta psychiat. scand.*, 1942, **17**, 2.

89. Werdnig, G., *Arch. Psychiat. Nervenkr.*, 1891, **22**, 437.

89a. Hoffmann, J., *Dtsch. Z. Nervenheilk.*, 1891, **1**, 95; 1893, **3**, 427.

89b. Greenfield, J. G., Stern, R. O., *Brain*, 1927, **50**, 652.

90. Conel, J. L., *Arch. Path. (Chic.)*, 1940, **30**, 153.

91. Conel, J. L., *Arch. Neurol. Psychiat. (Chic.)*, 1938, **40**, 337.

92. Follis, R. H., Jr, *Deficiency Diseases*, page 202. Springfield, Illinois, 1958.

93. Swank, R. L., *J. exp. Med.*, 1940, **71**, 683.

94. Swank, R. L., Prados, M., *Arch. Neurol. Psychiat. (Chic.)*, 1942, **47**, 97.

95. Aring, C. D., Bean, W. B., Roseman, E., Rosenbaum, M., Spies, T. D., *Arch. Neurol. Psychiat. (Chic.)*, 1941, **45**, 772.

96. Greenfield, J. G., Carmichael, E. A., *Brain*, 1935, **58**, 483.

97. Loughridge, L. W., *Lancet*, 1962, **2**, 1133.

98. Robertson, D. H. H., Knight, R. H., *Acta trop. (Basel)*, 1964, **21**, 239.

99. Collings, H., *Arch. Neurol. (Chic.)*, 1960, **3**, 656.

100. Platt, B. S., *Fed. Proc.*, 1958, **71**, 8.

101. Paul, M. F., Paul, H. E., Kopko, F., Bryson, M. J., Harrington, C., *J. biol. Chem.*, 1954, **206**, 491.

102. Lhermitte, F., Fritel, D., Cambier, J., Marteau, R., Gautier, J.-C., Nocton, F., *Presse méd.*, 1963, **71**, 767.

103. Hassin, G. B., *J. nerv. ment. Dis.*, 1930, **72**, 628.

104. Paterson, D., Greenfield, J. G., *Quart. J. Med.*, 1923–1924, **17**, 6.

105. Wyllie, W. G., Stern, R. O., *Arch. Dis. Childh.*, 1931, **6**, 137.

106. Warkany, J., Hubbard, D. M., *Lancet*, 1948, **1**, 829.

107. Colver, T., *Brit. med. J.*, 1956, **1**, 897.

108. Hunter, D. H., Bomford, R. R., Russell, D. S., *Quart. J. Med.*, 1940, N.S. **9**, 193.

109. Hunter, D. H., Russell, D. S., *J. Neurol. Neurosurg. Psychiat.*, 1954, **17**, 235.

109a. Bakir, F., Damluji, S. F., Amin-Zaki, L., Murtadha, M., Khalidi, A., Al-Rawi, N. Y., Tikriti, S., Dhahir, H. I., Clarkson, T. W., Smith, J. C., Doherty, R. A., *Science*, 1973, **181**, 230.

110. McAlpine, D., Araki, S., *Lancet*, 1958, **2**, 629.

110a. Hunter, D., *The Diseases of Occupations*, 6th edn, pages 337–342. London, Sydney, Auckland and Toronto, 1978.

111. Cavanagh, J. B., Chen, F. C. K., *Acta neuropath. (Berl.)*, 1972, **19**, 208.

112. Yoshino, Y., Mozai, T., Nakao, K., *J. Neurochem.*, 1966, **13**, 397.

113. Yoshino, Y., Mozai, T., Nakao, K., *J. Neurochem.*, 1966, **13**, 1223.

114. Erbslöh, W., *Dtsch. Z. Nervenheilk.*, 1903, **23**, 197.

115. Ridley, A., *Quart. J. Med.*, 1968, N.S. **38**, 307.

116. Ridley, A., Hierons, R., Cavanagh, J. B., *Lancet*, 1968, **2**, 607.

117. Goldberg, A., *Quart. J. Med.*, 1959, N.S. **28**, 183.

118. Cavanagh, J. B., Mellick, R. S., *J. Neurol. Neurosurg. Psychiat.*, 1965, **28**, 320.

119. Hierons, R., *Brain*, 1952, **80**, 176.

120. Denny-Brown, D., Sciarra, D., *Brain*, 1945, **68**, 1.

121. Gibson, J. B., Goldberg, A., *J. Path. Bact.*, 1956, **71**, 495.

122. De Matteis, F., *Pharmacol. Rev.*, 1967, **19**, 523.

123. Price, J. M., Brown, R. R., Peters, H. A., *Neurology (Minneap.)*, 1959, **9**, 456.

124. Cavanagh, J. B., *J. Neurol. Neurosurg. Psychiat.*, 1967, **30**, 26.

125. Cavanagh, J. B., Ridley, A., *Lancet*, 1967, **2**, 1023.

126. Biehl, J. P., Skavlem, J. H., *Amer. Rev. Tuberc.*, 1953, **68**, 296.

127. Gammon, G. D., Burge, F. W., King, G., *A.M.A. Arch. Neurol. Psychiat.*, 1953, **70**, 64.

128. Zbinden, G., Studer, A., *Z. Tuberk.*, 1955, **107**, 97.

129. Hughes, H. B., Biehl, J. P., Jones, A. P., Schmidt, L. H., *Amer. Rev. Tuberc.*, 1954, **70**, 266.

130. Evans, D. A. P., Manley, K. A., McKusick, V. A., *Brit. med. J.*, 1960, **2**, 485.

131. McClean, A. E. M., in *Mechanisms of Toxicity*, edited by W. W. Aldridge, page 219. London, 1971.

132. McCormick, D. B., Snell, E. E., *Proc. nat. Acad. Sci. (Wash.)*, 1959, **45**, 1371.

133. Holtz, P., Palm, D., *Pharmacol. Rev.*, 1964, **16**, 113.

134. Raskin, A. H., Fishman, R. A., *New Engl. J. Med.*, 1965, **273**, 1182.

135. Davies, D. R., Holland, P., Rumens, M. J., *Brit. J. Pharmacol.*, 1960, **15**, 217.

136. Johnson, M. K., *Biochem. J.*, 1969, **111**, 487.

137. Smith, H., Spalding, M. J. K., *Lancet*, 1959, **2**, 1019.

138. Cavanagh, J. B., *J. Path. Bact.*, 1964, **87**, 365.

139. Cavanagh, J. B., Patangia, G. N., *Brain*, 1965, **85**, 165.
140. Charcot, J. M., Joffroy, A., *Arch. Physiol. (Paris)*, 1869, **2**, 235.
141. Brownell, B., Oppenheimer, D. R., Hughes, T., *J. Neurol. Neurosurg. Psychiat.*, 1970, **33**, 338.
142. Kurland, L. T., Mulder, D. W., *Neurology (Minneap.)*, 1955, **5**, 182, 249.
143. Mulder, D. W., Kurland, L. T., *Proc. Mayo Clin.*, 1954, **29**, 666.
144. Wohlfart, G., *Neurology (Minneap.)*, 1957, **7**, 124.
145. Greenfield, J. G., O'Flynn, E., *Lancet*, 1933, **2**, 62.
146. Russell, J. S. R., Batten, F. E., Collier, J., *Brain*, 1900, **23**, 39.
147. Coërs, C., Woolf, A. L., *The Innervation of Muscle: A Biopsy Study*. Oxford, 1959.
148. Cavanagh, J. B., *Int. Rev. exp. Path.*, 1964, **3**, 1.
148a. Gibbels, E., *Fortschr. Neurol. Psychiat.*, 1967, **35**, 393.
149. Brain, *Lancet*, 1963, **1**, 179.
150. Denny-Brown, D., *J. Neurol. Neurosurg. Psychiat.*, 1948, **11**, 73.
151. Lennox, B., Pritchard, S., *Quart. J. Med.*, 1950, N.S. **19**, 97.
152. Croft, P. B., Wilkinson, M., *Brain*, 1965, **88**, 427.
153. Croft, P. B., Urich, H., Wilkinson, M., *Brain*, 1967, **90**, 31.
153a. Nageotte, J., *Rev. neurol.*, 1907, **15**, 933.
154. Brain, R. B., Daniel, P. M., Greenfield, J. G., *J. Neurol. Neurosurg. Psychiat.*, 1951, **14**, 590.
155. Henson, R. A., Russell, D. S., Wilkinson, M., *Brain*, 1954, **77**, 82.
156. Lambert, E. H., Rooke, E. D., Eaton, L. M., Hodgson, C. H., in *Myasthenia Gravis*, edited by H. R. Viets, page 362. Springfield, Illinois, 1961.
157. Cooke, W. T., Smith, W. T., *Brain*, 1966, **89**, 683.
158. Dyke, P. J., *Minn. Med.*, 1966, **49**, 1629.
159. Wilkinson, P. C., *Lancet*, 1974, **1**, 1301.

DISORDERS OF THE SCHWANN CELLS
160. Gombault, M., *Arch. Neurol. (Paris)*, 1880, **1**, 11.
161. Meyer, P., *Virchows Arch. path. Anat.*, 1881, **85**, 181.
162. Stransky, E., *J. Psychol. Neurol. (Lpz.)*, 1903, **1**, 169.
163. Cavanagh, J. B., Jacobs, J. M., *Brit. J. exp. Path.*, 1964, **45**, 309.
164. Allt, G., *Brain*, 1969, **92**, 639.
165. Walshe, F. M. R., *Quart. J. Med.*, 1918–19, **12**, 14.
166. Gaskill, H. C., Korb, M., *Arch. Neurol. Psychiat. (Chic.)*, 1946, **55**, 559.
166a. Bezjak, V., Farsey, S. J., *Bull. Wld Hlth Org.*, 1970, **43**, 643.
167. Fisher, C. M., Adams, R. D., *J. Neuropath. exp. Neurol.*, 1956, **15**, 243.
168. Waskman, B. H., Adams, R. D., Mansmann, H. C., *J. exp. Med.*, 1957, **105**, 591.
169. Pappenheimer, A. M., Hendee, E. D., *J. biol. Chem.*, 1947, **171**, 701.
170. Strauss, N., Hendee, E. D., *J. exp. Med.*, 1959, **109**, 145.
171. Kato, I., Pappenheimer, A. M., Jr, *J. exp. Med.*, 1960, **112**, 329.
172. Villaverde, J. M. de, *Trab. Inst. Cajal Invest. biol.*, 1926, **24**, 101.
173. Fullerton, P. M., *J. Neuropath. exp. Neurol.*, 1966, **25**, 214.
174. Jacobi, M., *Virchows Arch. path. Anat.*, 1947, **314**, 460.
175. Webster, H. de F., *J. Neuropath. exp. Neurol.*, 1962, **21**, 534.

176. Sourander, P., Olsson, Y., *Acta path. microbiol. scand.*, 1967, **70**, 147.
177. Lake, B. D., *Nature (Lond.)*, 1968, **217**, 171.
178. Kristensson, K., Olsson, Y., Sourander, P., *Acta path. microbiol. scand.*, 1967, **70**, 630.
179. Déjerine, J., Sottas, I., *C.R. Soc. Biol. (Paris)*, 1893, **45**, 60.
180. Refsum, S., *Acta psychiat. scand.*, 1946, suppl. 38.
180a. Thiébault, F., Lemoyne, J., Guillaumat, L., *Rev. neurol.*, 1939, **72**, 71; 1961, **104**, 152.
181. Klenk, E., Kahlke, W., *Hoppe-Seylers Z. physiol. Chem.*, 1963, **333**, 133.
182. Weller, R. O., *J. Neurol. Neurosurg. Psychiat.*, 1967, **30**, 111.
183. Thomas, P. K., Ballin, R. H. M., *Acta neuropath. (Berl.)*, 1968, **11**, 93.
184. Dyck, P. J., Lambert, E. H., *Arch. Neurol. (Chic.)*, 1968, **18**, 603.

INFLAMMATORY DISEASES OF NERVES (TRUE NEURITIS)
185. Rees, R. J. W., *Guy's Hosp. Rep.*, 1963, **112**, 320.
186. Khanolkar, V. R., *Indian J. med. Sci.*, 1955, **9**, suppl. 1, 1.
187. Marinesco, G., Draganescu, S., *Ann. Inst. Pasteur*, 1923, **37**, 753.
188. Goodpasture, E. W., *Medicine (Baltimore)*, 1929, **8**, 223.
189. Wright, G. Payling, *Proc. roy. Soc. Med.*, 1955, **46**, 319.
190. Boyse, E. A., Morgan, R. S., Pearson, J. D., Wright, G. Payling, *Brit. J. exp. Path.*, 1956, **37**, 333.
191. Denny-Brown, D., Adams, R. D., Fitzgerald, P. J., *Arch. Neurol. Psychiat. (Chic.)*, 1944, **51**, 216.
192. Landry, O., *Gaz. hebd. Méd. Chir. (Paris)*, 1859, **6**, 472, 486.
192a. Guillain, G., Barré, J. A., Strohl, A., *Bull. Soc. méd. Hôp. Paris*, 1915–16, **40**, 1462.
192b. Astbury, A. K., Arnason, B. G., Adams, R. D., *Medicine (Baltimore)*, 1969, **48**, 173.
192c. Leading Article, *Brit. med. J.*, 1977, **2**, 1374.
193. Bradford, J. R., Bashford, E. F., Wilson, J. A., *Quart. J. Med.*, 1918–19, **12**, 88.
194. Guillain, G., *Ann. Méd.*, 1953, **54**, 81.
195. Haymaker, W., Kernohan, J. W., *Medicine (Baltimore)*, 1949, **28**, 59.
196. Astbury, A. K., Arnason, B. G., *J. Neuropath. exp. Neurol.*, 1968, **27**, 581.
197. Waksman, B. H., Adams, R. D., *J. Neuropath. exp. Neurol.*, 1956, **15**, 293.
198. Cook, S. D., Dowling, P. C., Whitaker, J. N., *Arch. Neurol. (Chic.)*, 1970, **22**, 470.
199. Commings, J. F., Haas, D. C., *J. neurol. Sci.*, 1967, **4**, 51.
200. Miller, H. G., Stanton, J. B., *Quart. J. Med.*, 1954, N.S. **23**, 1.
200a. Ditchfield, W. J. B., in *Textbook of Virology for Students and Practitioners of Medicine and the Other Health Sciences*, by A. J. Rhodes and C. E. van Rooyen, 5th edn, sect. 4, chap. 10 [page 511]. Baltimore, 1968.
201. Greenfield, J. G., in *Greenfield's Neuropathology*, 2nd edn, by W. Blackwood, W. H. McMenemey, A. Meyer, R. M. Norman and D. S. Russell, page 173. London, 1963.
202. Worster-Drought, C., *Neurosyphilis (Syphilis of the Nervous System)*, chap. 12. London, 1940.

TUMOURS

203. Harkin, J. C., Reed, R. J., *Tumors of the Peripheral Nervous System* (Atlas of Tumor Pathology, 2nd series, fasc. 3). Washington, D.C., 1969.

203a. Russell, D. S., Rubinstein, L. J., *Pathology of Tumours of the Nervous System*, 4th edn, chaps 12 and 13. London, 1977.

204. Stout, A. P., *Amer. J. Cancer*, 1935, **24**, 751.

205. Masson, P., *Amer. J. Path.*, 1932, **8**, 367, 389.

206. Penfield, W., *Surg. Gynec. Obstet.*, 1927, **45**, 178.

207. Raimondi, A. J., Beckman, F., *Acta neuropath. (Berl.)*, 1967, **8**, 1.

208. Verocay, J., *Beitr. path. Anat.*, 1910, **48**, 1.

209. Thomas, P. K., *J. Anat. (Lond.)*, 1963, **97**, 35.

210. Ingels, G. W., Campbell, D. C., Jr, Giampetro, A. M., Kozub, R. E., Bentlage, C. H., *Cancer (Philad.)*, 1971, **27**, 1190.

211. Antoni, N., *Ueber Rückenmarkstumoren und Neurofibrome*. München, 1920.

212. Golden, T., Stout, A. P., *Surg. Gynec. Obstet.*, 1941, **73**, 784.

213. Symmers, W. St C., *personal observations.*

214. Masson, P., *Rev. canad. Biol..*, 1942, **1**, 209.

215. Waggener, J. D., *Cancer (Philad.)*, 1966, **19**, 699.

216. Murray, M. R., Stout, A. P., *Amer. J. Path.*, 1940, **16**, 41.

217. Lumsden, C. E., in *Pathology of Tumours of the Nervous System*, by D. S. Russell and L. J. Rubinstein, 3rd edn, chap. 14. London, 1971.

218. Stout, A. P., *Tumors of the Peripheral Nervous System* (Atlas of Tumor Pathology, sect. 2, fasc. 6), page F6-28. Washington, D.C., 1949.

219. D'Agostino, A. N., Soule, E. H., Miller, R. II., *Cancer (Philad.)*, 1963, **16**, 1015.

220. White, H. R., Jr, *Cancer (Philad.)*, 1971, **27**, 720.

221. Woodruff, J. M., Chernik, N. L., Smith, M. C., Millett, W. B., Foote, F. W., Jr, *Cancer (Philad.)*, 1973, **32**, 426.

222. Recklinghausen, F. D. von, *Ueber die multiplen Fibrome der Haut und ihre Beziehung zu den multiplen Neuromen*. Berlin, 1882.

223. Crowe, F. W., Schull, W. J., Neel, J. V., *Multiple Neurofibromatosis*. Springfield, Illinois, 1955.

224. Hochberg, F. H., Dasilva, A. B., Galdabini, J., Richardson, E. P., Jr, *Neurology (Minneap.)*, 1974, **24**, 1144.

225. David, M., Hecaen, H., Bonis, A., *Sem. Hôp. Paris (Ann. Chir.)*, 1956, **32**, C. 335.

226. Davis, F. A., *Arch. Ophthal.*, 1940, **23**, 735, 957.

227. Worster-Drought, C., Dickson, W. E. Carnegie, McMenemey, W. H., *Brain*, 1937, **60**, 85.

228. Hosoi, K., *Amer. J. Path.*, 1930, **6**, 245.

229. Mandeville, F. B., Sahyoun, P. F., *J. Urol. (Baltimore)*, 1949, **62**, 93.

230. Glushien, A. S., Mansuy, M. M., Littman, D. S., *Amer. J. Med.*, 1953, **14**, 318.

230a. Wishart, J. H., *Edinb. med. surg. J.*, 1822, **18**, 393.

231. Diekmann, L., Huther, W., Pfeiffer, R. A., *Z. Kinderheilk.*, 1967, **101**, 191.

232. Hayes, D. M., Spurr, C. L., Felts, J. H., Miller, E. C., Jr, *Metabolism*, 1961, **10**, 183.

233. Harkin, J. C., Reed, R. J., *Tumors of the Peripheral Nervous System* (Atlas of Tumor Pathology, 2nd series, fasc. 3), page 94. Washington, D.C., 1969.

233a. Russell, D. S., Rubinstein, L. J., *Pathology of Tumours of the Nervous System*, 4th edn, page 395. London, 1977.

234. Harkin, J. C., Reed, R. J., *Tumors of the Peripheral Nervous System* (Atlas of Tumor Pathology, 2nd series, fasc. 3), page 60. Washington, D.C., 1969.

235. Mandybur, T. I., *J. Neurosurg.*, 1974, **41**, 187.

236. Bird, C. C., Willis, R. A., *J. Path.*, 1969, **97**, 631.

237. Graham, D. I., Paterson, A., McQueen, A., Milne, J. A., Urich, H., *J. Path.*, 1976, **118**, 83.

238. Masson, P., in *Pathology Annual*, edited by S. C. Sommers, vol. 2, page 351 [abbreviated translation by H. L. Ioachim of: Masson, P., *Tumeurs humaines*, 2nd edn, chap. 8; Paris, 1956].

239. Spence, A. M., Rubinstein, L. J., Conley, F. K., Herman, M. M., *Acta neuropath. (Berl.)*, 1976, **35**, 27.

240. Williams, E. D., Pollock, D. J., *J. Path. Bact.*, 1966, **91**, 71.

241. Gorlin, R. J., Mirkin, B. L., *Z. Kinderheilk.*, 1972, **113**, 313.

242. Russell, D. S., Rubinstein, L. J., *Pathology of Tumours of the Nervous System*, 4th edn, page 423. London, 1977.

243. Gillesby, W. J., Wu, K. H., *Amer. J. Surg.*, 1965, **110**, 673.

244. Tuovinen, P. I., Alfthan, O., Rusk, J., *J. Urol. (Baltimore)*, 1965, **94**, 395.

245. Joske, R. A., Finlay-Jones, L. R., *Brit. J. Surg.*, 1966, **53**, 766.

246. Wolman, L., *J. Path. Bact.*, 1967, **94**, 123.

247. Livingston, K. E., *J. Neurosurg.*, 1945, **2**, 251.

248. Bickel, W. H., Dockerty, M. B., *Surg. Gynec. Obstet.*, 1947, **84**, 111.

249. Graham, W. D., Johnston, C. R., *Lancet*, 1957, **2**, 470.

250. Durlacher, L., *A Treatise on Corns, Bunions, the Diseases of Nails, and the General Management of the Feet*, page 52. London, 1845.

251. Morton, T. G., *Amer. J. med. Sci.*, 1876, **71**, 37.

252. Stowens, D., *A. M. A. Arch. Path.*, 1957, **63**, 451.

253. Symington, T., Goodall, A. L., *Glasg. med. J.*, 1953, **34**, 75.

254. Hermann, H., Mornex, R., *Human Tumours Secreting Catecholamines—Clinical and Physiopathological Study of the Pheochromocytomas*. Oxford, 1964.

255. Glenner, G. G., Grimley, P. M., *Tumors of the Extra-Adrenal Paraganglion Systems (Including Chemoreceptors)* (Atlas of Tumor Pathology, 2nd series, fasc. 9). Washington, D.C., 1974.

256. *Gray's Anatomy*, 35th edn, edited by R. Warwick and P. L. Williams, page 1381. [London] 1973.

257. Pryse-Davies, J., Dawson, I. M. P., Westbury, G., *Cancer (Philad.)*, 1964, **17**, 185.

258. Willis, R. A., *Pathology of Tumours*, 4th edn, page 854. London, 1967.

259. Stout, A. P., *Tumors of the Peripheral Nervous System* (Atlas of Tumor Pathology, sect. 2, fasc. 6), page F6-31. Washington, D.C., 1949.

260. Nesbitt, K. A., Vidone, R. A., *Cancer (Philad.)*, 1976, **37**, 1562.

ACKNOWLEDGEMENTS FOR ILLUSTRATIONS

Fig. 35.2. Preparation provided by Dr L. S. Illis, Wessex Neurological Centre, Southampton University Hospital Group, Southampton, while working formerly in the National Hospital for Nervous Diseases, London.

Figs 35.7, 8. Electron micrographs provided by Dr D. N. Landon, Institute of Neurology, London.

Fig. 35.9. Preparation provided by Dr V. D. MacDermot, Honorary Research Fellow, University College, London, while working formerly in St Thomas's Hospital, London.

Fig. 35.14. Redrawn from: Cavanagh, J. B., Webster, G. R., *Quart. J. exp. Physiol.*, 1955, **40**, 12. Reproduced by permission of the editor of the *Journal*.

Fig. 35.18. Redrawn from: Garven, H. S. D., Gairns, F. W., Smith, G., *Scot. med. J.*, 1962, **7**, 250. Reproduced by permission of the authors and of the editor of the *Journal*.

Fig. 35.24. Redrawn from: Wohlfart, G., Swank, R. L., *Arch. Neurol. Psychiat.* (*Chic.*), 1941, **46**, 783. Reproduced by permission of the authors and of the editor of the *Archives*.

Fig. 35.26. Redrawn from: Meyer, P., *Virchows Arch. path. Anat.*, 1881, **85**, 181.

Figs 35.28A, 28B. Preparation provided by Professor G. Payling Wright, Guy's Hospital Medical School, London.

Figs 35.31A, 31B, 32–36. Photomicrographs from the Department of Histopathology, Charing Cross Hospital Medical School, London.

36: *Skeletal Muscle*

by P. M. DANIEL *and* SABINA J. STRICH
revised by D. G. F. HARRIMAN

CONTENTS

36: *Skeletal Muscle*

by P. M. Daniel *and* Sabina J. Strich

revised by D. G. F. Harriman

NORMAL STRUCTURE AND INNERVATION

Normal human muscle varies in colour from deep red-brown to light red. Each muscle consists of cross-striated fibres attached to connective tissue at each end and packed closely together so that, in fixed material, their cross-sections are polygonal (Figs 36.1A and 36.1B). Each fibre is surrounded by

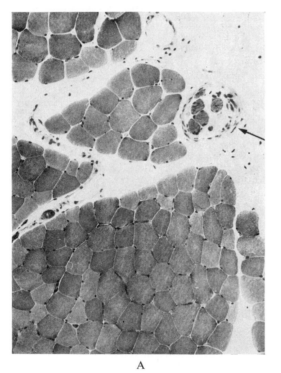

A

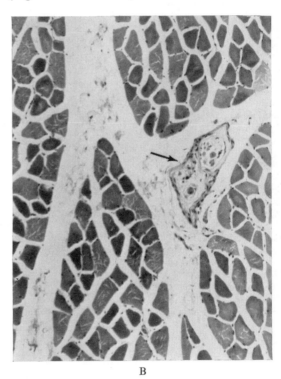

B

Fig. 36.1.§ Comparison of cryostat and paraffin wax sections of respectively fresh and fixed normal muscle, to illustrate the shrinkage artefact inseparable from the latter method of preparation.

A. Normal muscle. The muscle fibres appear polygonal in transverse section; in this cryostat section of fresh tissue they remain close to each other (compare with the shrinkage and retraction in fixed tissue, illustrated in Fig. 36.1B). A muscle spindle containing large and small intrafusal fibres is seen (arrowed): the intrafusal fibres are smaller than the extrafusal fibres (the fibres of the main mass of the muscle). The spindle is enclosed within a fibrous capsule. *Gomori trichrome stain.* × 120.

B. Normal muscle. In this paraffin-wax section of formalin-fixed material, shrinkage has led to separation of the fibres (compare with Fig. 36.1A). The uneven staining of the fibres is another common artefact and has no pathological significance. Two adjacent muscle spindles are included in the picture (arrowed). *Haematoxylin–eosin.* × 115.

§ See *Acknowledgements*, page 2381.

a delicate sheath of connective tissue, the endomysium. The cells associated with this connective tissue have large vesicular nuclei which should not be confused with subsarcolemmal or muscle nuclei. Bundles of muscle fibres are bound together by fibrous perimysium.

Each muscle fibre is one long cell and has one neuromuscular junction, the motor endplate. The muscle fibre is composed of sarcoplasm in which large numbers of transversely striated myofibrils are embedded in such a manner that the whole fibre appears cross-striated as well as being striped longitudinally. Electron microscopy, X-ray diffraction and biochemical methods have shown that a myofibril is striated because it is composed of an alternating series of interdigitating arrays of two types of protein filament, myosin and actin. When the muscle shortens the two sets of filaments slide into each other.[1]

The cell membrane of the muscle cell is called the sarcolemma. Beneath this membrane lie numerous small, dense, elongated subsarcolemmal or muscle nuclei, arranged round the periphery of the muscle fibre and indenting the sarcoplasm. Near tendinous attachments these nuclei may lie in the centre of the fibre, as they often do in the extrinsic ocular muscles. In muscle fibres elsewhere central nuclei should be regarded as abnormal.

The size of muscle fibres varies considerably, both in length and diameter, in different muscles;[2] the diameter ranges from 15 to 50 μm. These values are 25 to 30 per cent less than those for fresh muscle that has been allowed to retract after excision and then sectioned in the cryostat. Muscles with delicate actions, such as the extrinsic eye muscles or the lumbrical muscles, have the thinnest fibres (and the smallest numbers of fibres in each bundle).

A few fat cells are present between bundles of muscle fibres but such cells are not normally seen within a bundle.

Type 1 and Type 2 Fibres ('Red Muscle' and 'White Muscle')

It seems that there are two types of muscle fibre, differing in function and using different substances as their source of energy. One type contains abundant myoglobin and many mitochondria with their associated enzymes for the oxidation, in the citric acid cycle, of compounds derived from sugars, fats and amino acids. The presence of many of these oxidative enzymes can be demonstrated histochemically. These fibres are capable of sustained effort and in bulk make up the 'red muscle' of many animals. The other type of muscle fibre contains less myoglobin and few mitochondria, and so only small quantities of the oxidative enzymes, but these include all the enzymes necessary for glycolysis of glycogen and glucose to lactic acid. Such muscle fibres make up 'white muscle' and are capable of short bouts of heavy work. In man there is no clearcut division into red and white muscle, but with the appropriate histochemical techniques the two types of fibre can be seen in the same muscle, forming a mosaic pattern (Figs 36.2A and 36.2B).[3] The mitochondrion-rich 'red muscle' fibres are known as *type 1 fibres* and the mitochondrion-poor 'white muscle' fibres as *type 2 fibres*.

Ring fibres are peculiar muscle cells in which one or more peripheral myofibrils encircle the others in a spiral (Fig. 36.3). Although most familiar in some forms of myopathy (see page 2361), they are seen in normal muscle, mainly in the extrinsic muscles of the eyes and close to the tendinous insertions in other muscles. They have a tendency to increase in number in old age.

Motor and Sensory Innervation of Normal Muscle

Without a nerve supply muscle cannot function, and its fibres atrophy and many eventually disappear. The neuromuscular junction lies at the midpoint of each muscle fibre and not at the midpoint of the muscle itself. The motor endings, therefore, lie in well defined narrow bands across the muscle. The position of these bands depends on the arrangement of the muscle fibres and is different in pennate, fusiform and strap-shaped muscles.[4] Knowledge of the position of the innervation band is essential if nerve endings in a piece of muscle are to be examined. During life the motor point can be localized by electrical stimulation. Some muscle spindles (the most numerous sensory organs of striated muscle—see below) are also to be found in the region of the motor point.

The muscle fibres that are innervated by a single large neuron of the anterior grey columns (anterior horns) of the spinal cord make up a motor unit: this may comprise from 20 to many hundreds of muscle fibres. Muscles with the most delicate actions have the smallest motor units. In man, the muscle fibres in one muscle bundle are not all supplied by the same anterior column cell: there is much overlap between units, and this doubtless determines the mosaic pattern of the fibre types (Figs 36.2A and 36.2B). It is not known

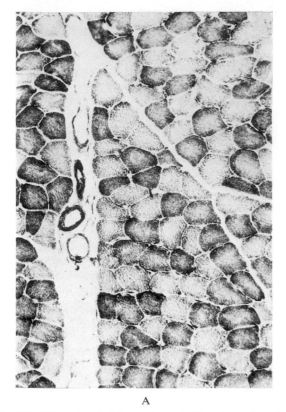
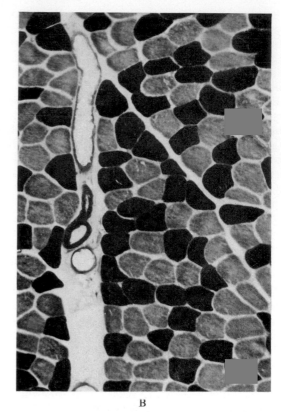

A   B

Fig. 36.2.§ Histochemical types of muscle fibre shown in serial cryostat sections. There is reciprocal staining of the two main fibre types.

A. Cryostat section of muscle, stained for the oxidative enzyme nicotinamide adenine dinucleotide tetrazolium reductase. Type 1 fibres (the 'slow' or 'red' fibres) appear dark (compare with the serial section illustrated in Fig. 36.2B). × 120.

B. Cryostat section of muscle, stained for alkali-stable myosin adenosine triphosphatase. The preparation is a serial section of that illustrated in Fig. 36.2A. With this method it is the type 2 fibres (the 'fast' or 'white' fibres) that appear dark. × 120.

how the bundles of muscle fibres supplied by an individual anterior column cell are distributed in a muscle. Branching of the axon of the anterior column cell occurs in the last few centimetres before the nerve enters the muscle[5] and also in the intramuscular plexus; branching is not seen among subterminal nerve fibres, each of which supplies one muscle fibre.

Nerve and muscle come into intimate contact, though they remain separate, at the motor endplate, or neuromuscular junction.[6] Here the fibrous endoneurium (sheath of Henle) becomes continuous with the endomysium. The nerve fibre loses its myelin sheath and divides into short terminals that come to lie in indentations of the sarcoplasm, the so-called synaptic gutters. Under the nerve ending, along the wall of the synaptic gutters, the sarcolemma shows complicated but regularly spaced folds, the subneural apparatus, which thus has a lamellate appearance. In these folds the cell membrane is very rich in acetylcholinesterase (true cholinesterase): the subneural apparatus can be stained specifically to show this enzyme (for instance, by Koelle's technique—see Fig. 35.10, page 2303).[6] In the region of the motor endplate the sarcoplasm is rich in mitochondria and there is an aggregation of muscle nuclei that are larger than those elsewhere along the muscle fibre.

Sensory fibres account for a third to half of the myelinated fibres in the nerve supplying a muscle.[7] It is for this reason that the nerves in a muscle that has a complete motor denervation still contain many normal fibres—the sensory fibres from muscle spindles and tendon organs. The commonest sensory organ in human muscles is the muscle spindle (Figs 36.1A and 36.1B). This is a long, slender, cigar-shaped, fibrous bag, often laminate, and containing from 2 to 15 thin, striated muscle

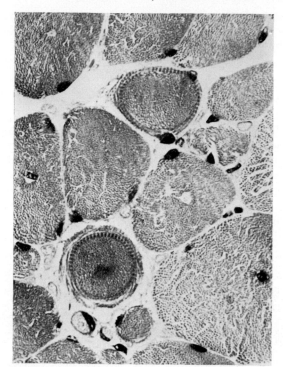

Fig. 36.3.§ Two ring fibres are included in this field. One or more of the peripheral striated myofibrils in these two fibres are out of their normal position and form a circle or spiral round the transversely sectioned, normally oriented fibrils. *Haematoxylin–eosin.* × 680.

fibres, the intrafusal fibres. Some intrafusal fibres contain a central cluster of nuclei (nuclear bag fibres); others, which are thinner, have a string of nuclei (nuclear chain fibres). Extremely complex sensory and motor endings are present in the muscle spindle.[8, 9] The cell bodies of the sensory cells lie in the dorsal root ganglia; the cell bodies of the motor nerves (gamma efferent fibres) innervating the intrafusal muscle fibres are thought to be small nerve cells situated in the anterior grey columns of the spinal cord.

At the junction of muscle fibres with tendons or aponeuroses there are sensory organs that respond to stretch, the Golgi tendon organs. Pressure receptors, the Pacinian corpuscles, may also be seen in these situations. There are simple sensory endings in the fascia overlying the muscle.

Physiological Atrophy and Hypertrophy

Prolonged bed rest, immobility due to joint disease, or general disuse leads to atrophy of muscles. The muscle fibres shrink and may look more cellular than normal. There may also be an increase in

interfascicular fat. Muscle fibres in old people may show deposition of brown lipofuscin pigments, but this is not so striking in skeletal muscle as it is in cardiac muscle (see page 43, Volume 1).

The massiveness of the muscles of many athletes, such as weight lifters, makes it clear that muscles hypertrophy when they are used more than usual. This is due to an increase in sarcoplasm and in the number of myofibrils, particularly in the smaller muscle fibres, which thus become enlarged.[10, 11] There is no evidence that the number of muscle fibres increases.

Histological Artefacts

Irregularity of staining of muscle fibres is very common and should be ignored (Figs 36.1A, 36.1B and 36.4). Severe shrinkage, leaving large spaces between muscle fibres and endomysium is also

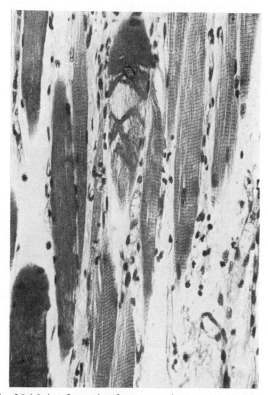

Fig. 36.4.§ Artefacts. Artefacts are quite common in biopsy preparations. Contraction bands of coagulated sarcoplasm (centre of upper half of field) are the result of exposure of still viable muscle fibres to fixative solution. Irregular staining of fibres (bottom, left) is also frequent (see also Fig. 36.1B). It may be noted that striations in muscle fibres are well seen only when the specimen has been promptly fixed. *Haematoxylin–eosin.* × 300.

often seen and depends partly on the fixative used.[12] Contraction swellings alternating with thin portions of muscle fibre are sometimes seen in longitudinal sections. They are due to the state of contraction of the muscle at the time of fixation and are not abnormal (Fig. 36.4).

PATHOLOGICAL CONDITIONS[13-15]

GENERAL CONSIDERATIONS

Diseases of muscle can be divided into the myopathies—that is, diseases in which there is intrinsic degeneration of muscle fibres (this group includes the muscular dystrophies and some types of so-called 'polymyositis')—and diseases in which muscle fibres atrophy because their nerve supply has been interrupted.

Apart from these conditions, muscle may be affected by trauma, vascular disease, infections and neoplastic changes, as are the other tissues of the body. Similarly, it may be involved in generalized diseases such as polyarteritis (Figs 36.19 and 36.20, pages 2366 and 2367) and sarcoidosis.

The responses of striated muscle to disease are limited and it is important to realize that any of the changes about to be described may be seen in any muscle disease, including myopathies, denervation, infections, and so on. This often makes the accurate interpretation of biopsy specimens very difficult. A disease may affect some muscles more than others, and even when the condition is far advanced normal and abnormal muscle may be seen side by side (Figs 36.8 and 36.11B). In many myopathies the proximal limb muscles are more severely affected than the distal ones. The muscles innervated by the cranial nerves may be particularly severely involved, or almost spared; the extrinsic eye muscles, although also innervated by the cranial nerves, behave differently again. At present no biochemical differences are known that might account for these findings.

The histological appearances of the end-stage of the various diseases of muscle tend to resemble each other closely, but early and late phases of the pathological process can often be found in different muscles (Figs 36.9 and 36.10). Biopsies should be taken therefore from slightly affected muscles as well as from those more severely involved.

Reaction of Muscle to Injury

Massive Destruction.—The results of massive destruction of a piece of muscle, as by trauma, impaired blood supply or the injection of noxious substances (Fig. 36.5), are different from those seen when individual muscle fibres are destroyed. In the former case necrosis involving all tissue components results. The necrotic area is invaded by neutrophile leucocytes, plasma cells, macrophages and fibroblasts in succession: eventually it is converted into a fibrous scar that may impede reconstitution of the contractile tissue.

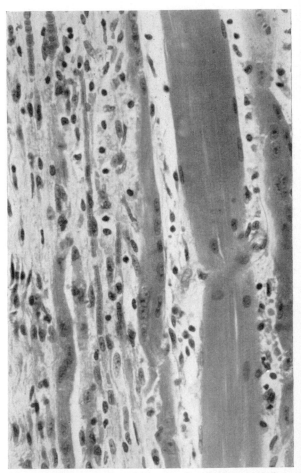

Fig. 36.5.§ Regeneration of muscle—in this instance following damage by inadvertent intramuscular injection of iophendylate ('Myodil'), an X-ray contrast medium used in myelography. Note the thin muscle fibres containing chains of large nuclei with conspicuous nucleoli. One large normal fibre is seen. Longitudinal section. *Haematoxylin–eosin.* × 380.

'*Single Fibre Necrosis*'.—At the edge of an area of destruction of muscle, or of a clean cut, or after a mild crush, and in many disease processes, single muscle fibres or parts of single muscle fibres become necrotic, the fibrous tissue framework of the muscle remaining intact. The sarcoplasm loses its striation, swells and becomes floccular (Figs 36.10B and 36.21B) or hyaline and eosinophile. The intact endomysial tube becomes filled with neutrophils and then with macrophages ('myophages'), which may appear foamy: these cells digest and clear away the debris. Into this tube the regenerating ends of the surviving muscle fibres grow to bridge the gap.[15a] Necrosis of muscle fibres and evidence of regeneration are often seen side by side in the same muscle.

Regeneration of Muscle

When a muscle fibre is damaged, it regenerates by forming either a muscle bud or sprouts of spindle-shaped cells at its surviving ends. If the damage to the endomysium has been slight, the two ends join and a normal-looking striated muscle fibre is reconstituted. Even if the connective tissue framework is destroyed the sprouting muscle fibres may bridge a considerable gap, but this process of repair can be prevented by scar formation.[16] During regeneration the sarcoplasm is basiphile and unstriated. The sarcolemmal nuclei undergo a striking change that may occur even at some distance from the lesion. They enlarge, become vesicular and show one or more prominent nucleoli (Fig. 36.5). They lie closely packed in the muscle buds; in contrast, in the thin, spindle-shaped strips of regenerating muscle fibre they lie in central rows, often separated from one another by vacuoles.

Electron microscopy has provided good evidence that regeneration of muscle is effected by cells known as satellite cells. These are mononuclear cells embedded in the surface of muscle fibres, internal to the basement membrane but external to the sarcolemma. They cannot be distinguished with the light microscope. When regeneration is required, the satellite cells undergo mitotic division and form spindle-shaped myoblasts, which fuse to become 'myotubes' and eventually muscle fibres. The muscle buds that form at the ends of damaged muscle cells are thought to consist of accumulated muscle nuclei that have no part in regeneration, but this view is controversial.[17]

It has been found that denervated or dystrophic muscle is capable of regeneration after injury unless its atrophy is very far advanced.[18]

Biochemical Abnormalities

Enzymes

Two enzymes that are normally present in muscle may be found also in the blood serum under abnormal conditions. They are of special importance: *aldolase* splits fructose 1,6-diphosphate, and *creatine kinase* reversibly catalyses the reaction creatine + adenosine triphosphate $\rightleftharpoons$ creatine phosphate + adenosine diphosphate.[19, 20] The level of both these enzymes in the serum is raised in conditions in which there is damage to or destruction of muscle fibres, such as 'polymyositis', trauma and some stages of muscular dystrophy.[19] The level is not raised when there is only muscle atrophy, as after denervation. Creatine kinase is the more sensitive index of muscle damage.

Myoglobinuria

In any case in which there is muscle necrosis, from whatever cause, myoglobin is released into the circulation and passed in the urine, sometimes in large quantities. If much myoglobin is liberated, acute renal tubular necrosis may develop (see page 1445, Volume 4).

Creatine and Creatinine Excretion[21]

The amount of *creatine* that is excreted in the urine is increased and that of *creatinine* is decreased when the total mass of muscle tissue is reduced: such findings are not an indication that the metabolism of the remaining muscle fibres is abnormal. Muscle takes up creatine from the blood and converts it into creatinine, which is excreted in the urine. Patients with reduced muscle bulk therefore excrete less creatinine. The creatine is derived from the liver, which apparently secretes it into the blood at a fairly constant rate, even when the demands of the body are low. The blood concentration of creatine may exceed the renal threshold when, owing to a reduction in the mass of muscle, its utilization is decreased. Creatinuria occurs thus in patients who have had severe poliomyelitis (even years after the acute attack). It is also found in cases of muscular dystrophy and even as a consequence of amputation of a limb.[21a]

Miscellaneous Changes in Muscle
Myositis Ossificans

Traumatic Myositis Ossificans.—Ossification may occur in traumatized muscle, especially after repeated minor stretching injuries—traditionally, although a curiosity today, in those parts of the adductor muscles of the thighs that take origin from the inferior ramus of the pubic bone ('horseman's bone' and 'rider's bone' are terms that indicate the former frequency in cavalrymen of ossification in this situation). The condition is seen oftener today in the brachialis muscle, typically after dislocation of the elbow (particularly when there has been injudicious physiotherapy in the recovery period, entailing passive stretching and deep massage of the muscle). It is also seen in the quadriceps muscle of the thigh and in the muscles of the calf following severe contusions or even—rarely—severe cramp: in such cases the formation of bone in the muscles is probably a manifestation of metaplasia in the developing scar tissue in the vicinity of an intramuscular haematoma. 'Myositis' is, strictly, a misnomer in the context of traumatic ossifying myositis: the condition is degenerative rather than primarily inflammatory.

Traumatic ossifying myositis must be distinguished from primary ossifying myositis, particularly the solitary form (see below and page 2516).

Generalized Primary Myositis Ossificans.[22]—This rare disease, first described by Münchmeyer,[23] has many synonyms. It is an inherited condition, at least in some cases, and is characterized by the progressive formation of bone, particularly in skeletal muscles but also in tendons, ligaments and aponeuroses, the capsule of joints, and sometimes visceral muscle, particularly myocardium. The skeletal muscles first to be affected are commonly the flat muscles of the back, followed by the spinal and thoracic musculature: the patient eventually becomes virtually immobilized ('poker man'). Death is generally due to respiratory complications. Symptoms of the disease start in childhood or early adult life and its course may be run in from 5 to 20 years. The pathogenesis of the lesions is scarcely understood: the ossification is believed to be the final stage in a condition of patchy intramuscular fibrosis of unknown causation.

In an occasional variant of the classic disease the lesions are less widespread and even may be solitary. Such cases may occur sporadically or among members of a family affected with the generalized form.

Injury Due to Irradiation

Muscle is one of the tissues that are most resistant to irradiation,[24] though changes ranging from simple atrophy of single fibres with fat replacement to total necrosis of muscle tissue can be produced, depending on the dose and type of radiation. Fibrosis may be very severe in the healed stage.

Effects of Impairment of Circulation

Any sustained interruption of the arterial blood supply to a muscle leads to infarction as it does in other tissues of the body. During healing, quite large areas of necrosis may be effectively bridged by muscle tissue that has grown from surviving muscle fibres at the edge of the infarct.[25]

Infarction may also result from venous occlusion: in these cases regeneration of muscle seems to be less adequate, the necrotic area being eventually replaced almost entirely by fibrous tissue. Impaired venous drainage has been invoked as a cause of *Volkmann's ischaemic contracture*[25a] and of *congenital torticollis*, but clinical evidence favours arterial obstruction followed by infarction and fibrosis of the affected muscle.[26]

Infarcts of muscle in limbs amputated for ischaemic disease are often found to be of very varied extent and distribution.

CONGENITAL MALFORMATIONS

Congenital absence of muscles or parts of muscles occurs, particularly in the shoulder girdle.[27, 28]

Many cases of malformation, or even absence, of limbs were recorded in infants of mothers who were given thalidomide during the early stages of pregnancy (see page 2197).

THE PRIMARY MYOPATHIES[29]

A myopathy is a disease in which the primary lesion appears to be in the muscle tissue itself and not in the interstitial or nervous tissue. The term is applicable to the hereditary disorders known as the muscular dystrophies, to metabolic disorders, to some infections, and to polymyositis, which is an immunological disorder in which necrosis of muscle fibres and an inflammatory reaction are features. Microscopically, the myopathies may resemble one another so closely that classification on histological grounds is difficult. A detailed clinical and family history is therefore of particular diagnostic value.

Pathological Findings Common to the Myopathies

Macroscopical Appearances

Whereas normal muscle is dark red, abnormal muscle may be pale, or wholly or partially replaced by yellow fat (Fig. 36.8A), or grey and translucent, resembling fish flesh.

Histological Findings

Microscopically, rounding of the normally polygonal cross-section of the muscle fibres and the presence of internally placed muscle nuclei (Fig. 36.6), often in chains (Fig. 36.12A), are early features of abnormality. Small foci of necrotic and regenerating (Fig. 36.7) muscle fibres, scattered throughout the muscle bundles, are frequently found on histological examination in any case of active myopathy (including the slowly progressive muscular dystrophies).

Extensive replacement of muscle by fat and sometimes by fibrous tissue accompanies all types of myopathy (Figs 36.6A and 36.10A). Severely atrophied muscle consists usually of a mass of adipose tissue in which a few recognizable muscle fibres may survive. Often the muscle tissue is represented by clumps and short rows of closely set, small, darkly staining nuclei. The amount of fibrosis varies and is particularly well marked round the nerves, which may be hardly recognizable. The muscle spindles are relatively exempt from degenerative changes and may stand out in an otherwise featureless field of fat (Fig. 36.11A).

The Muscular Dystrophies

These myopathies are hereditary muscle disorders characterized clinically by progressive weakness and wasting of muscles. It is of great importance to distinguish between the different varieties of dystrophy in view of the significant differences in their natural history and in their mode of inheritance.[30] Although a diagnosis of 'muscular dystrophy' can usually be made on biopsy, the division into the different types has to be made on clinical grounds because the pathological findings are confusingly similar. The latter include all the varieties of degenerative change that may affect muscle: as well as atrophy and replacement by fat there may be muscle fibre necrosis and an inflammatory reaction. The histological appearance depends on the stage that the

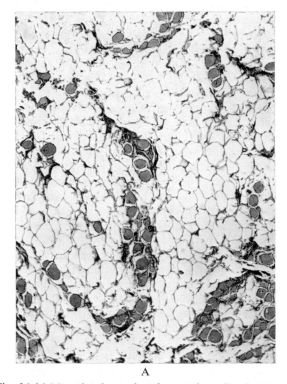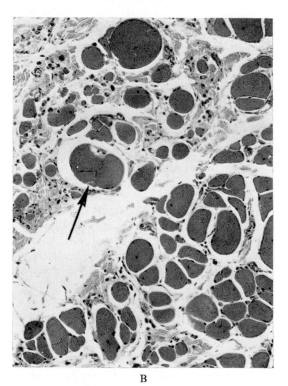

A   B

Fig. 36.6.§ Muscular dystrophy of young boys (Duchenne type of dystrophy). See also Figs 36.7 to 36.9.

A. Transverse section showing extensive replacement of muscle by adipose tissue. The few remaining fibres are rounded. *Haematoxylin–eosin.* × 65.

B. Transverse section showing rounded muscle fibres of varying diameter embedded in fat and fibrous tissue. Note splitting of muscle fibres (a split fibre is arrowed) and centrally placed nuclei. *Haematoxylin–eosin.* × 180.

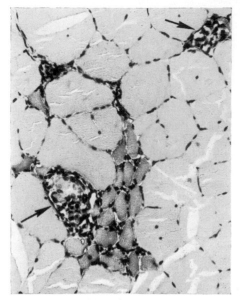

Fig. 36.7.§ Muscular dystrophy of young boys (Duchenne type). Transverse section showing a group of small, darkly staining (basiphile) muscle fibres. The presence of such fibres is regarded as evidence of regeneration. Two endomysial tubes (arrowed) are filled with phagocytes and debris of muscle fibres—evidence of recent necrosis. Centrally placed nuclei and splitting are seen in other muscle fibres. *Haematoxylin–eosin.* × 130.

condition has reached in the particular muscle examined and not on the rate of progress of the disease as a whole. Muscles in all stages of degeneration will be found in the same patient at any one time: samples of many muscles must be examined if the whole process is to be studied (Figs 36.9, 36.10 and 36.11B). Abnormalities may be seen at the myoneural junction.[31] The heart is commonly involved in dystrophies, both clinically and pathologically, the muscle showing patches of fibrosis and fatty infiltration. Smooth muscle, on the other hand, is not obviously affected. In cases of muscular dystrophy of acute onset and rapid course, myoglobinuria may occur. In many forms of muscular dystrophy the level of creatine kinase and aldolase in the serum may be raised, sometimes even before the patients become noticeably weak (see page 2355).

In *tissue cultures* of muscle from dystrophic patients the muscle fibres may become much wider and more cellular than normal, show no spontaneous contraction and soon degenerate, the culture dying out after the first subculture.[32] In other instances there may be no evident abnormalities in their growth, or only minor disorders of maturation.[33, 34]

Pseudohypertrophic Muscular Dystrophy of Young Boys (Duchenne Type) (Griesinger–Duchenne Disease*[34a, 34b])

This disease is inherited as a sex-linked recessive characteristic. The boys fail to walk properly, become 'chair-bound' by the age of 11 or 12 and usually die in their late teens, when the muscles of respiration become affected. In the final stages the patients often show deformities of the spine and limbs due to muscular imbalance. The proximal muscles are affected before the distal ones and in the early stages there may be enlargement or pseudohypertrophy of muscles (this also occurs in other forms of dystrophy). Muscles innervated by the cranial nerves are the last to be affected.

It is clearly of importance to detect the female carriers of the abnormal gene of muscular dystrophy. In a high proportion of cases this can now be done since it has been found that carriers may show very slight evidence of the disease in the form of raised serum creatine kinase or aldolase levels. There may also be mild abnormalities in muscle biopsy specimens from carriers.[35]

At necropsy, the proximal limb muscles look as though they were sculpted in fat. More distal muscles have a 'thrush breast' appearance, and the most distal of all, such as the lumbricals, may look almost normal, but often are unusually pale (Fig. 36.8).

Histologically, the classic features are groups of rounded muscle fibres of greatly varying diameter scattered in a mass of fat (Fig. 36.6A). The large fibres may be as much as twice the diameter of normal ones; they may also show longitudinal splitting. In contrast, many fibres are very small.

In the least affected muscles, rounding of some muscle fibres, internally placed nuclei and a little fat within the muscle bundles are seen (Fig. 36.9B). At another stage, there are foci of necrotic muscle fibres with evidence of regeneration (Fig. 36.7) and an inflammatory reaction; sometimes these are seen in otherwise normal muscle bundles (this is similar to the appearance in polymyositis, see page 2366). The endstage of these processes is a mass of fatty or fibrous tissue containing an occasional muscle fibre (Figs 36.6A and 36.9A), an occasional muscle

* The name of Guillaume Benjamin Amand Duchenne de Boulogne is sometimes given to tabes dorsalis, in recognition of his account of this disease in 1858–59, when he presented a comprehensive synthesis of what was known at that time (Duchenne, G. B., *Arch. gén. Méd.*, 1858, 5 sér., **12**, 641; 1859, 5 sér., **13**, 36, 158, 417). In texts in English the eponym Duchenne is ordinarily reserved for pseudohypertrophic muscular dystrophy.

an autosomal (that is, not sex-linked) dominant gene. The muscles of the face and shoulders are first and mainly affected, although after many years the whole musculature becomes involved.

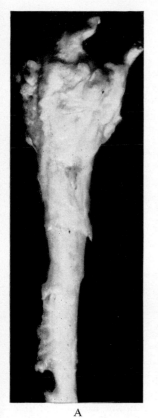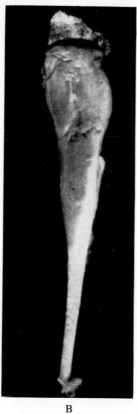

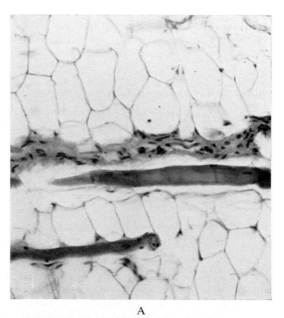

A

Fig. 36.8.§ Muscular dystrophy of young boys (Duchenne type). Two adjacent muscles of the same forearm: the flexor carpi ulnaris (Fig. 36.8A) appears white, being replaced by adipose tissue, whereas the palmaris longus (Fig. 36.8B) appears almost normal. See Figs 36.9A and 36.9B.

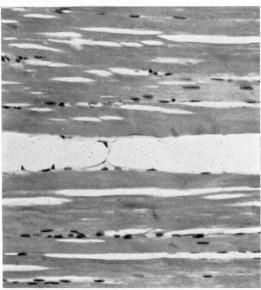

B

spindle (the muscle spindles are very resistant to such degenerative processes—Fig. 36.11A) and an occasional nerve. Nerve fibres that have lost the muscle fibre that they originally supplied are seen, either ending blindly or forming additional end-plates on surviving muscle fibres.

Progressive muscular dystrophy may begin *in utero*. Such babies are born with atrophied muscles and stiff joints, and this myopathy is one of the causes of *arthrogryposis multiplex congenita*.[36] Intrauterine denervation and cerebral defects have been implicated in the pathogenesis of the condition in some cases.[37]

Facio-Scapulo-Humeral Muscular Dystrophy (Landouzy–Déjerine Type[37a])

This is a very slowly progressive disease, starting in childhood or adolescence: the patients often survive to middle age. The disease is transmitted by

Fig. 36.9.§ Muscular dystrophy of young boys (Duchenne type). *Haematoxylin–eosin.* × 180.

A. Two surviving muscle fibres surrounded by adipose tissue. The section is from the muscle in Fig. 36.8A.

B. Relatively normal-looking muscle with only a slight increase in the amount of adipose tissue. The section is from the muscle in Fig. 36.8B.

Mildly affected individuals are frequently found in these families.

Histologically, the changes are not fundamentally different from those seen in the Duchenne type of dystrophy, though fibrosis may be more prominent (Figs 36.10A and 36.11). Acute changes, such as necrosis of muscle fibres, may be present even 30 or 40 years after the onset of the disease (Fig. 36.10B), but they are not commonly observed.

Limb-Girdle Type of Muscular Dystrophy[37b]

This condition is transmitted as an autosomal recessive characteristic. Weakness and wasting begin in muscles of the shoulder or pelvic girdle in young adults, who usually become severely disabled by middle life. The histological changes are the same as in the other dystrophies.

Ocular Muscle Dystrophy

The eye muscles are usually spared in the dystrophies, but there is one rare variety in which these muscles are affected first and most.[38] This ocular myopathy is usually a very slowly progressive condition, with onset in early or middle life, and manifested first by ptosis and then by limitation of

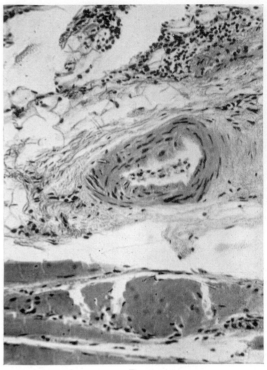

B

Fig. 36.10.§ Facio-scapulo-humeral muscular dystrophy (Landouzy–Déjerine type) in a man who had suffered from progressive weakness for 20 years.

A. Pectoralis major. The muscle tissue has been completely replaced by fibrous tissue (dark) and fat. *Haematoxylin; Van Gieson's stain.* × 45.

B. Psoas (longitudinal section). Collections of inflammatory cells are seen and there is a muscle fibre (below the blood vessel) in the acute stage of necrosis. Much of the muscle appeared normal microscopically. *Haematoxylin–eosin.* × 190.

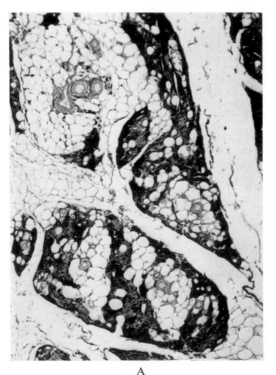

A

Fig. 36.10A.§ *Caption in adjoining column.*

ocular movements. The patient may be unaware of a disability, compensating for the effects of the disease by moving his head when altering the direction of his gaze. Diplopia is rare. The range of possible clinical manifestations is wide, from ptosis alone to involvement of the pharyngeal musculature (*oculopharyngeal dystrophy*) and of the limbs ('*oculogeneralized' myopathy*). The histological picture is the same as that in other muscular dystrophies.

The disease is usually hereditary; ordinarily the mode of inheritance is dominant. There are also many isolated cases. Ocular muscle dystrophy must be distinguished from other conditions causing ophthalmoplegia, especially myasthenia gravis.[38] If it is thought advisable to have a biopsy examination, it is noteworthy that minor but diagnostically

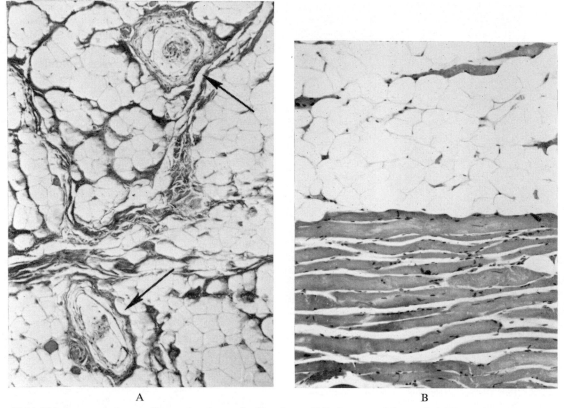

A   B

Fig. 36.11.§ Facio-scapulo-humeral muscular dystrophy (Landouzy–Déjerine type of dystrophy). The patient was a man who had suffered from progressive weakness for very many years.

A. Transverse section of a sternocleidomastoid muscle showing adipose and fibrous tissue, and two muscle spindles (arrowed) with intact intrafusal muscle fibres. *Haematoxylin; Van Gieson's stain.* × 80.

B. Longitudinal section of an infraspinatus muscle of the same patient. Part of the muscle has been almost completely replaced by adipose tissue; the adjacent part is almost normal. *Haematoxylin–eosin.* × 130.

important changes are often to be found in the deltoid muscles even when the clinical signs are wholly confined to the eyes.

Dystrophia Myotonica (Myotonia Atrophica; Steinert–Batten–Curschmann Disease[39, 39a, 39b])

Myotonic dystrophy is inherited as an autosomal dominant characteristic. Clinically, there is inability of the muscles to relax; later, weakness and atrophy develop. The muscular abnormality is part of a more widespread pathological state of which premature baldness, cataracts and testicular atrophy are other manifestations.

Histologically,[39c] the most striking feature is the presence of multiple long rows of close-set, internal nuclei in many muscle fibres (Fig. 36.12A). All the other changes characteristic of dystrophic muscle are also seen. Abnormalities of innervation have

been described in the form of diffuse branching of terminal nerve fibres, with the presence of multiple and abnormally long motor endplates on many muscle fibres (Fig. 36.12B). Two further histological changes are quite common—the presence of ring fibres (Fig. 36.3) and the formation of sarcoplasmic masses. The latter result from the retraction of the myofibrils from the periphery of muscle cells, leaving an amorphous substance: they must be distinguished from artefact.

There is a remarkable change in the muscle spindles of all the affected muscles, and this is usually severest in the lumbrical muscles of the hands and feet. The number of intrafusal fibres in normal muscle spindles is never more than 15: in this disease up to 60 intrafusal fibres may be found (Fig. 36.13). The innervation of such a spindle is grossly abnormal. Clumping of nuclei in the intrafusal muscle fibres and infiltration by inflammatory

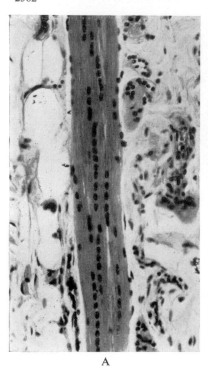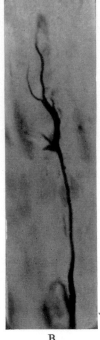

A   B

Fig. 36.12.§ Dystrophia myotonica (longitudinal sections).

A. Multiple chains of centrally placed nuclei in a single muscle fibre that is embedded in fibrous and adipose tissue. *Haematoxylin–eosin.* × 220.

B. Abnormally long motor nerve ending. *Silver impregnation.* × 800.

cells may be seen, indicating that in this type of dystrophy the spindles are affected by the disease process.[40]

Myotonia Congenita (Thomsen's Disease)

In this condition, first described by Thomsen (who, with his sons, suffered from the disease),[41] the abnormality lies in faulty relaxation. No dystrophic picture is seen, clinically or pathologically, but the fibres are hypertrophic.

Central Core Disease

This very rare familial disease was described by Shy and Magee.[42] Affected members show weakness from birth, mainly affecting the legs. The condition is compatible with a normal life span.

Histologically, the essential feature is the presence within the muscle fibre of one or more areas where mitochondria are absent (Fig. 36.14A). These 'cores' may be difficult to detect in paraffin sections stained with haematoxylin and eosin, although

trichrome stains are effective for showing them in some specimens. The clearest demonstration is in sections cut in the cryostat and stained for mitochondrial enzymes: the cores are seen in type 1 fibres only, or—in apparently undifferentiated muscle—in fibres that show uniform type 1 and type 2 enzyme activity (see page 2351).[43] Longitudinal sections of core fibres show that the striation of the myofibrils within them is preserved and that the core extends throughout the length of the muscle fibre (Fig. 36.14B): in this they differ from target fibres (see page 2372), in which there is myofibrillar disruption and involvement usually of only a short length of the muscle cell.

Benign Congenital Hypotonia ('Floppy Baby' Syndrome)

This condition manifests itself by evident weakness and 'floppiness' in babies. There is non-progressive

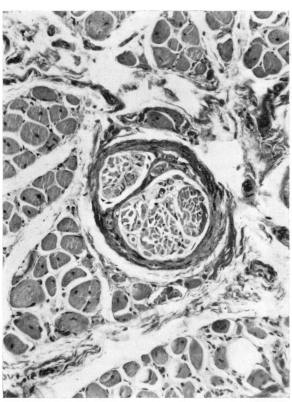

Fig. 36.13.§ Dystrophia myotonica. Transverse section of a lumbrical muscle, showing an abnormal muscle spindle. The number of intrafusal muscle fibres is about 10 times greater than in a normal spindle, and the capsule is thickened. Note that the extrafusal muscle fibres are rounded and that many of them have internally placed nuclei. *Haematoxylin–eosin.* × 200.

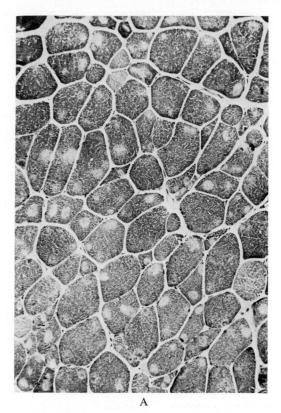
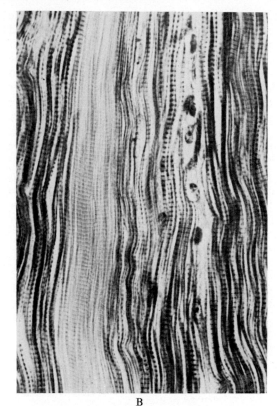

A   B

Fig. 36.14.§ Central core disease.

A. Transverse section. Almost every muscle fibre contains one or more areas of altered staining. Mitochondria are absent from the cores, which stain lightly (as here) or darkly, according to the packing of the myofibrils. *Phosphotungstic-acid–haematoxylin.* × 120.

B. Longitudinal section. The core is seen to contain striated myofibrils. It extended throughout the whole length of the fibre within the plane of this preparation. *Phosphotungstic-acid–haematoxylin.* × 680.

weakness of the muscles at birth: in about half the cases strength improves, so that the children are normal by the time they reach their teens, although they may be left with deformities. Other patients remain weak and have small muscles. There are no obvious pathological changes in the muscles,[44] but the muscle fibres may be small.

The cause of the condition and the explanation of the weakness are not known.

'Amyotonia Congenita'

This term should be avoided since it is merely a clinical 'diagnosis' for many conditions in infancy that are characterized by hypotonia and paralysis. These may be due to anything from damage to the spinal cord at birth to dystrophy or disease affecting the neurons of the anterior grey columns of the spinal cord.

10*

Rarer Congenital Myopathies

In recent years, particularly with the help of histochemical studies and electron microscopy, various congenital myopathies have been defined that previously would probably have been categorized simply as 'muscular dystrophy'. Although rare, they are important, for most are compatible with long survival, in contrast to some dystrophies, which they may resemble clinically at an early stage and from which they must be distinguished by muscle biopsy.

Mitochondrial Myopathies[45]

The mitochondrial myopathies are conditions characterized by abnormalities of the mitochondria in muscle cells. The mitochondria in scattered type 1 fibres are excessively numerous or are structurally abnormal and then often very large. Oxidative enzyme reactions produce intense staining of the mitochondria in cryostat sections: the affected fibres are then very conspicuous (Fig. 36.15). If the mitochondria are large enough they may be recognized as granules in paraffin sections stained with haematoxylin and eosin. The affected fibres contain excess lipid. The histological findings are not pathognomonic: fibres of similar appearance are occasionally found incidentally in various neuromuscular disorders, but in general their number is small in such cases.

The clinical course of the mitochondrial myopathies is variable.[46] It is clear that there is a series of different conditions within the group. Further study and classification are needed for their definition.

'Rod Body' Myopathy[47]

'Rod body' myopathy is a condition in which granules or short rod-like structures are found

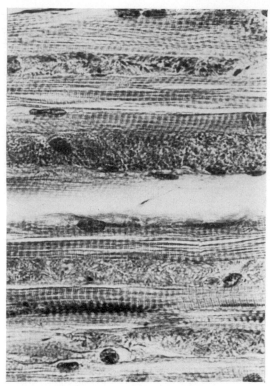

Fig. 36.16.§ 'Rod body' myopathy. Granules and short rods are present beneath the sarcolemma in several of the fibres in this field. These structures can be shown by electron microscopy to be composed of Z line material. Myofibrils, which are reduced in number, occupy the rest of the affected cells. *Phosphotungstic-acid–haematoxylin.* × 680.

beneath the sarcolemma of type 1 or type 2 muscle fibres (see page 2351) (Fig. 36.16). The granules and 'rods' are derived from the Z lines of myofibrils, and they are well demonstrated by phase contrast microscopy. The course of this myopathy is generally benign. In some cases the presentation is that of the 'floppy baby' syndrome (see above). In most cases the disease has been sporadic; it has also been reported, in one family, with autosomal dominant inheritance. It has been recognized once[48] in association with Adie's syndrome (pupillotonia and absence of tendon reflexes[48a]).

Rod bodies are occasionally found in other myopathies, including polymyositis (see below).

Centronuclear Myopathy[49]

Centronuclear myopathy is a distinct variety of myopathy in which maturation of the muscle fibres is impaired, resulting in a structural appearance that has some resemblance to the muscle tube stage of muscle fibre development. The fibres may

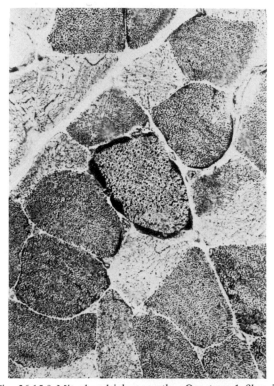

Fig. 36.15.§ Mitochondrial myopathy. One type 1 fibre in this field stands out from the others because of the densely stained crescents at its periphery and the prominent mitochondria in its sarcoplasm. The crescents consist of agglomerated mitochondria. This change, which occurs in scattered fibres in all fasciculi, may not be recognizable in paraffin wax sections. *Cryostat section. Stained for nicotinamide adenine dinucleotide tetrazolium reductase.* × 450.

be of uniform size or there may be large and small fibres. Most of the nuclei are at the centre of the cell, the rest being in the normal subsarcolemmal position (Fig. 36.17). Most cases have a benign course, but the disease is occasionally severe, leading to death during childhood. There is usually oculofacial involvement as well as involvement of the limbs.

Myopathy with Tubular Aggregates.[50]—When muscle affected by this condition is examined in paraffin wax sections, stained with haematoxylin and eosin, peripheral crescentic spaces are seen: these spaces contain a small quantity of material that looks finely granular. In sections cut in the cryostat the affected fibres can be shown by histochemical means to be of type 2 (see page 2351); the peripheral material presents increased enzyme activity

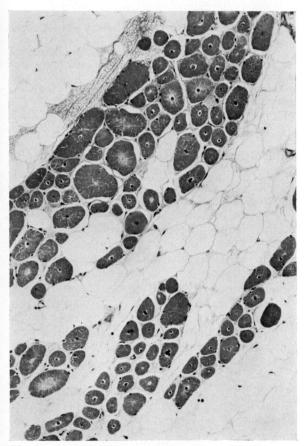

Fig. 36.17.§ Centronuclear myopathy. Most of the fibres are seen to have either a central nucleus or, according to the plane of the section, a central juxtanuclear space. Both large and small muscle fibres are present: some, of both sizes, have normally placed (subsarcolemmal) nuclei as well as the central one. *Haematoxylin–eosin.* × 160.

and reacts with stains for lipid. Ultrastructurally, the material is found to consist of arrays of tubules.

The nature of this myopathy is obscure. The histological findings are not diagnostic, for similar appearances may be seen in some other conditions.

Polymyositis

Polymyositis is an inflammatory condition of muscle due to autoimmunization. Lymphocytes from patients with the disease have been shown to be sensitized to muscle.[50a] The disease is seen about twice as often in women as in men. Most of the patients are in their 4th to 7th decade. The patient complains of weakness of the affected muscles, which may be painful and tender. The distribution of the lesions is random throughout the musculature, not restricted to particular muscle groups, as in muscular dystrophy, although the cervical and lumbar muscles are often affected. The muscles may be swollen and uncommonly firm, or they may be atrophic.

The course of the disease varies. It may end in death within a few months, or remain mild or moderately severe for years, or—especially in children—tend to recovery.

Polymyositis may be symptomatic of such generalized diseases of the connective tissues and vasculature as systemic lupus erythematosus, systemic sclerosis, polyarteritis and rheumatoid arthritis. It may be simple or difficult to distinguish the cause of the myositis in such cases: sometimes it is clearly secondary to interference with the local blood supply—for instance, in the course of polyarteritis; in other cases the extent of the muscle involvement is out of proportion to the effects ordinarily attributable to the associated disease and muscle may then be regarded as directly involved in the autoimmune disturbance.

Dermatomyositis.—When the skin is also involved (see Chapter 39, Volume 6) there may be a punctate rash of patchy or widespread distribution, and there is often congestion of the nail folds. A violaceous malar flush is an inconstant characteristic.

Dermatomyositis in childhood is mentioned on page 2367.

Histological Findings

There are two characteristic features of the histological picture of polymyositis: inflammation, which may be diffuse or focal, and necrosis of muscle, with its sequelae. Most of the inflammatory cells are lymphocytes and plasma cells. Occasional eosinophils are present also: if they are numerous ('*eosinophil myositis*'), a vain search for metazoal parasites is likely to be instituted. The infiltrate may extend diffusely between the muscle fascicles and between the muscle cells themselves; or it may be localized, forming nodules in the interstitial tissue (Fig. 36.18). The nodular foci may be large; lymphoid follicles with conspicuous germinal centres may develop in them. The blood vessels in the muscle may be cuffed with lymphocytes; in rare instances a true arteritis is found, with or without fibrinoid necrosis of the vessel wall. The rarity of arteritis helps to distinguish polymyositis from secondary myositis of polyarteritis (Figs 36.19 and 36.20). It is because of the graver outlook of polyarteritis that the rare coexistence of polyarteritis and polymyositis must be remembered and care taken not to overlook the presence of the former.

The necrosis that occurs in the muscles in polymyositis is similar to that in other myopathies. If it continues for long, variation in the diameter of

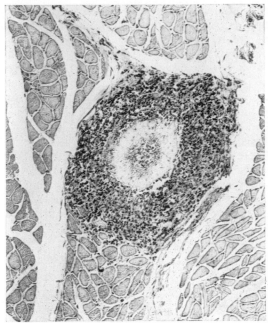

Fig. 36.19.§ Polyarteritis affecting a small artery in skeletal muscle. The wall of the vessel is necrotic and represented by the pale zone round the thrombus in the lumen. A wide cuff of inflammatory cells, most of them neutrophils but with occasional eosinophils, surrounds the artery and extends between the muscle fibres. See also Fig. 36.20. *Haematoxylin; Van Gieson's stain.* × 140.

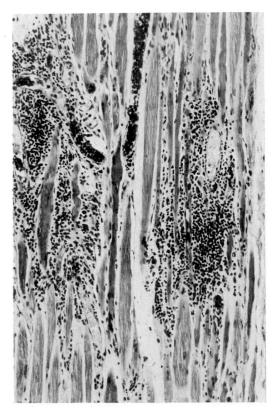

Fig. 36.18.§ Polymyositis. Accumulations of lymphocytes and plasma cells are present, particularly in the vicinity of the blood vessels. *Haematoxylin–eosin.* × 120.

the muscle fibres becomes a feature, with inward migration of the muscle nuclei, eventual loss of muscle cells, fibrosis and replacement of muscle by adipose tissue.

In some cases there is excessive formation of fibrous tissue, leading to an almost 'wooden' rigidity of the affected muscles (*myositis fibrosa*, or *myosclerosis*). In other rare instances, foci of calcification appear in the affected muscles. Calcification is less rare in the subcutaneous fat, but only in those cases in which there is an accompanying dermatitis. When calcification is present in the muscles it is a valuable diagnostic feature as it does not occur in muscular dystrophy.

Necrotizing Myopathy[51]

It has been found that in some cases in which a diagnosis of polymyositis seems to be straightforward on clinical grounds, and is supported by positive immunological findings, histological examination shows no recognizable inflammatory changes in the muscles but only necrosis, phagocytosis and regeneration (Figs 36.21A and 36.21B). Such findings are likelier in those cases in which

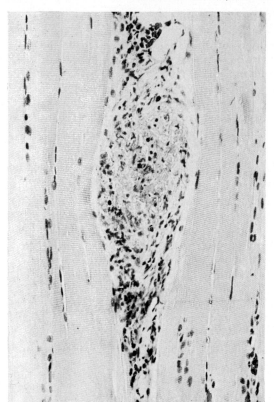

Fig. 36.20.§ Polyarteritis affecting an arteriole in muscle. Necrosis of the wall of the vessel has led to obliteration of its lumen. There is comparatively little cellular infiltrate in the vicinity of this early lesion (compare with Fig. 36.19). *Haematoxylin–eosin.* × 180.

there has been treatment with corticosteroids prior to biopsy. In these instances a diagnosis of myositis cannot be justified: a term such as necrotizing myopathy[51] or reactive myopathy may be more appropriate.

The occurrence of necrotizing myopathy in cases that present the clinical picture of polymyositis has led to much confusion in the literature, for it occurs in other diseases also. Endocrine disorders, acute and chronic infections and many metabolic disturbances may precipitate such a reaction. Terms such as menopausal myopathy and 'late-onset myopathy' have been used to designate these cases; often, too, they have simply been labelled 'polymyositis'. Opportunities for misunderstanding of the nomenclature are commonplace.

'Carcinomatous Myopathy'[52]

Both the necrotizing type of myopathy that is described in the preceding section and the classic form of polymyositis may occur, rarely, as a com-

plication of carcinomas of various types and in various sites. The explanation of this association is unknown. It may be comparable to the occurrence of various forms of degenerative changes in the central nervous system (see pages 2263, 2264, 2266 and 2267) and in peripheral nerves (see page 2326) in patients with cancer.

Diagnosis of Polymyositis and Necrotizing Myopathy from Muscular Dystrophy

It is of the greatest practical importance to distinguish polymyositis and necrotizing myopathy from the muscular dystrophies. The first two, which are not inherited, may respond to treatment with corticosteroids or recover spontaneously; the latter are often hereditary and most of them are progressive and eventually fatal. The distinction cannot always be made by biopsy because focal degeneration of muscle fibres, mild inflammatory reactions and some degree of replacement of muscle by adipose tissue occur at some stage in cases in both groups (Figs 36.7, 36.10B and 36.21A).

Dermatomyositis in Children

Particularly severe involvement of muscle is characteristic of a variety of dermatomyositis that is peculiar to childhood. The primary changes in this condition are inflammation and intimal hyperplasia of arteries and veins, leading to occlusion. The muscles show multiple small infarcts; in addition, infarcts in nerves lead to denervation.[53]

The 'adult' form of dermatomyositis and polymyositis may also be seen in children. It is characterized by atrophy of muscle cells at the periphery of the fascicles in addition to cellular infiltration of the perimysium, with fibrosis.

Myopathies in Metabolic and Endocrine Diseases

Cachectic Muscular Atrophy[54]

In the cachexia that develops in wasting diseases generally, whether due to chronic infection, endocrine disorder, malabsorption or cancer, all tissues in the body are affected to some extent. Owing to increased catabolism, skeletal muscle loses structural protein: cachexia may therefore affect muscle to a particularly marked degree, even before there is evident loss of subcutaneous fat. Taking into account the prevalence of malnutrition, cachectic muscular atrophy must be regarded as the commonest of all forms of myopathy. The muscle fibres in general show a loss of bulk, but the effect

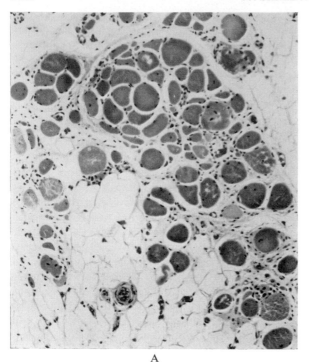

A

Fig. 36.21A.§ *Caption in adjoining column.*

effect that the units of the subneural apparatus (see page 2352) are increased in number, are small, and are spread along the muscle fibre.[56] The muscles involved, which frequently include the eye muscles, contain collections of lymphocytes, known as *lymphorrhages*;[56a] plasma cells are present among the lymphocytes. There may also be the necrosis, inflammatory response and atrophy that are to be seen in any myopathy.[57]

Muscle Changes Accompanying Hyperthyroidism

Hyperthyroidism is frequently associated with reversible muscular weakness, but the histological changes in the affected muscles are not striking. Inflammation or lymphocytic infiltration of the extrinsic eye muscles occurs in exophthalmic opthalmoplegia (see Chapter 40, Volume 6):[58] the

is variable and type 2 fibres are more susceptible than type 1 fibres (see page 2351) (Fig. 36.22). Some fibres become angular in outline; the muscle nuclei, although remaining subsarcolemmal, come to lie closer to one another. Necrosis of muscle is rare in this condition.

A similar change occurs in old age. It is then characterized by an accumulation of lipofuscin near the nuclear poles, as in myocardial cells in cases of 'brown atrophy' of the heart (see page 43, Volume 1).

Myasthenia Gravis

Myasthenia gravis is characterized by a peculiar defect in the production of acetylcholine at the motor endplates. The power of the affected muscles improves after the administration of an anti-cholinesterase such as neostigmine. A thymoma is present in about 10 per cent of cases (see page 920, Volume 2). There is reasonably conclusive evidence that autoimmune responses play a part in the causation of myasthenia gravis.[55] In some cases there is an association with hyperthyroidism (see page 1990, Volume 4).

Histology.—The motor endplates have not been examined very frequently in cases of myasthenia gravis. The terminal arborization of the nerve fibres is increased (Figs 36.23A and 23B), with the

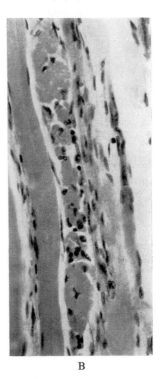

B

Fig. 36.21.§ Necrotizing myopathy. This is a non-specific myopathic reaction that may develop in the course of carcinoma, chronic infection and metabolic and endocrine disorders. It may also occur as an incomplete form of polymyositis.

A. Necrotizing myopathy. Transverse section, showing vacuolate and necrotic muscle fibres, replacement of muscle by adipose tissue, and slight lymphocytic infiltration. *Haematoxylin–eosin.* × 160.

B. Longitudinal section of the same muscle, showing a necrotic muscle fibre invaded by neutrophils. *Haematoxylin–eosin.* × 260.

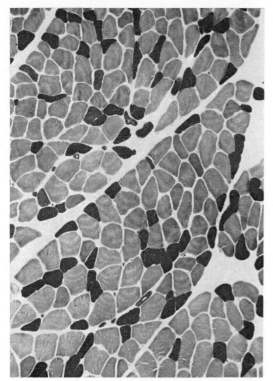

Fig. 36.22.§ Cachectic muscular atrophy. Type 2 fibres (dark) are affected more than type 1 fibres. The patient was a woman, aged 62, who had had rheumatoid arthritis for seven years. The same histological pattern may be found in many wasting diseases. *Cryostat section. Stained for myosin adenosine triphosphatase at pH 9·4.* × 120.

relation of this condition to thyroid disease is not a simple one, since the myositis may occur with or without, or following, hyperthyroidism. It may be due to the activity of the long-acting thyroid stimulator;[59] this and other possibilities are referred to on page 1994 (Volume 4).

Corticosteroid Myopathy

Therapeutic use of cortisone and its derivatives and analogues, and of corticotrophin, has shown that a myopathy may develop in susceptible people, usually affecting the proximal parts of the limbs. In the earlier stages the muscle fibres are not altered in size but there is an increase in the quantity of intracellular lipid droplets, which are demonstrable only in cryostat or conventional frozen sections. In later stages there is atrophy of the muscle fibres, especially type 2 fibres (see page 2351).[60]

Glycogen Storage Disease

In glycogenoses that affect skeletal and cardiac muscle there is an excess of glycogen within the muscle fibres, which take on a foamy or vacuolate appearance (see page 44, Volume 1).[61] Clinically, these conditions have to be distinguished from other childhood diseases characterized by hypotonia and paralysis.

McArdle's Disease.[61a]—This is a rare myopathy with abnormal glycogen metabolism, in which a deficiency of the enzyme phosphorylase has been demonstrated in the muscle fibres. The disease is a glycogenosis (glycogen storage disease Cori type V—see page 1276, Volume 3). It is characterized by painful cramps following moderate or severe exercise. Weakness and wasting may develop, with accompanying muscle fibre necrosis and atrophy. More glycogen than normal is seen in the muscle fibres, often in the form of granules that may completely fill parts of a fibre.[62]

Vitamin Deficiencies

It is noted below that lack of vitamins E (tocopherol) and A frequently gives rise to muscular disorders in animals.

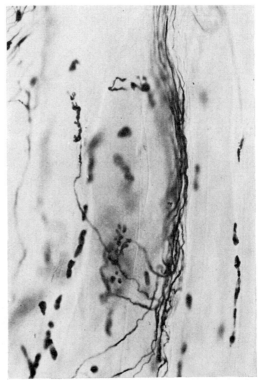

Fig. 36.23A.§ Myasthenia gravis. Motor endplate showing linear elongation and small, deformed expansions. *Methylene blue.* × 300.

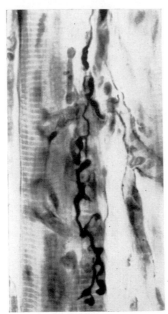

Fig. 36.23B.§ Myasthenia gravis. Motor nerve ending, showing elongation and club-like terminations. *Silver impregnation.* × 580.

In man, myopathy due to vitamin E deficiency has been said to occur in patients with congenital biliary atresia or with fibrocystic disease (cystic fibrosis of the pancreas).[63]

Periodic Paralysis

The condition known as periodic paralysis may be familial or sporadic. It is due to an abnormality of potassium metabolism. The exact nature of the abnormality is unknown; it seems not to be the same in all affected families. The attacks of paralysis may be associated with hypokalaemia or with hyperkalaemia; in some cases the serum potassium level remains unchanged. In the past a possible role of excessive secretion of aldosterone in the causation of the symptoms was overstressed.[64] The weakness, which may be severe, may last from a few hours to one or even two days. Biopsy during attacks characteristically shows vacuolation of muscle cells; a similar appearance is sometimes also seen in specimens obtained in the interval between attacks. In longstanding cases myopathic changes develop—necrosis, variation in fibre calibre, and fibrosis (Fig. 36.24).

Myoglobinuria

Idiopathic Paroxysmal Myoglobinuria.—This condition, which is sometimes familial, is associated with acute degeneration of muscle fibres. It is followed by regeneration.[65]

Myoglobinuria.—This may occur when large quantities of muscle are destroyed, whatever the cause of the destruction. Thus it may appear in any myopathy (including—occasionally—muscular dystrophy), after infarction of muscle, and apparently after the ingestion of poisoned fish (*Haff* disease*).[66, 67] Severe myoglobinuria, such as follows extensive injury to muscle, may lead to renal failure (crush syndrome—see page 1445, Volume 4).

Primary Amyloidosis

Skeletal muscle amd cardiac muscle (Fig. 1.36, page 43 in Volume 1) are characteristically, and sometimes heavily, affected in primary amyloidosis.[67a] The fibres become coated and then replaced by amyloid.

Myopathies in Animals[68]

Muscular dystrophy comparable with that seen in man is rare in animals. Sporadic cases have been reported in dogs and ducks,[69] but it is in mice that the condition has been most fully studied.[70] It has been shown that the disease in mice is carried by a recessive autosomal gene.[71] The animals are small at birth and show progressive weakness of the muscles. The histological picture

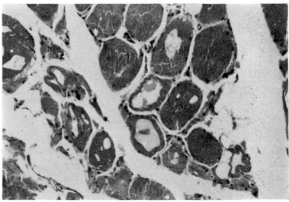

Fig. 36.24.§ Periodic paralysis. There is vacuolation of many of the fibres. The condition was of long standing in this case and there is an accompanying myopathic variation in fibre calibre. It should be noted that similar vacuoles are to be seen in occasional fibres in a proportion of cases of many other varieties of myopathy. *Haematoxylin–eosin.* × 230.

* The name 'Haff' disease' indicates the source of the poisoned fish—the German word *Haff* describes a sea bay partly enclosed by a spit of land, particularly on the Baltic coast.

is somewhat similar to that seen in human cases. Goats suffering from a hereditary condition closely resembling dystrophia myotonica have also been studied extensively.[72]

Most of the diseases of animals that are commonly described in the literature as 'muscular dystrophies' are in fact non-hereditary myopathies in which the major features are necrosis of muscle fibres and regenerative phenomena (the changes shown in Figs 36.7 and 36.21B are indistinguishable from the picture seen in these animal myopathies). The myopathies of animals are most frequently due to vitamin deficiency, especially deficiency of vitamin E. Similar histological changes of unknown aetiology are seen in sheep[73] and in hamsters.[74] Virus infections, such as those due to the Coxsackie viruses, also produce necrosis, followed by regeneration of muscle fibres.

An acute disorder of uncertain aetiology, paralytic myoglobinuria (equine nutritional myopathy),[74a] is one of several forms of myopathy that are seen in horses. The condition comes on after forced exercise in animals that have been rested and well fed for some days (hence the name, 'Monday morning disease', by which it is sometimes known). The affected animals may die of renal tubular necrosis associated with the presence of myoglobin casts, a condition comparable to the lesions accompanying the crush syndrome in man (see page 1445, Volume 4). Acute necrosis of muscle fibres is seen histologically. There is little or no inflammatory reaction.

'POLYMYALGIA RHEUMATICA'[75]

The condition that is known to clinicians as polymyalgia rheumatica is not an entity but a syndrome of variable causation. It is a fairly common cause of disability, accounting for 1·3 per cent of 2222 patients attending certain arthritis clinics in England during a period of about two years.[75a] Usually there is no obvious pathological basis for the patient's symptoms, which are mainly pain and stiffness, particularly affecting the shoulder girdle, neck and back, and particularly in the mornings. In most cases there is recovery within one to three years. Biopsy shows no evident abnormality of the muscles in such cases.

In some cases the condition is symptomatic of the presence of visceral neoplastic disease. In another important group of cases there is an association with giant cell arteritis (temporal arteritis—see page 140, Volume 1): in such cases the condition is sometimes described as 'polymyalgia arteritica'.[75b] In some patients the myalgia is the presenting manifestation. In others, blindness has developed as a complication of the arteritis,[75c] even after relief from the myalgic symptoms, which usually respond to notably small doses of a corticosteroid such as prednisone. The low dosage that relieves the myalgia is quite insufficient to arrest the progress of any associated arteritis.

REACTION OF MUSCLE TO DENERVATION[76]

When a muscle is deprived of its nerve supply, either through interruption of the peripheral nerve that supplies it or by destruction of neurons of the anterior grey columns of the spinal cord, it loses bulk and becomes pale and later somewhat translucent. The subsarcolemmal nuclei tend to enlarge and migrate into the centre of the muscle fibres, which slowly shrink in diameter, without losing their striations (Fig. 36.25A). Rounding of the muscle fibre in cross-section is usually seen. The

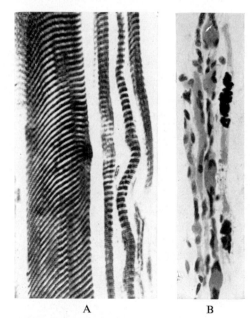

A   B

Fig. 36.25.§ Denervation of muscle (longitudinal sections). See also Figs 36.26 to 36.28.

A. Preservation of cross striation in three muscle fibres (right of picture) that have atrophied as a consequence of denervation. One normal muscle fibre is seen. *Phosphotungstic-acid–haematoxylin.* × 600.

B. Denervation of long standing (due to motor neuron disease). The muscle fibres are thin and irregular in outline, and there is clumping of sarcolemmal nuclei. Much of the muscle has been replaced by fat. *Haematoxylin–eosin.* × 350.

subsarcolemmal nuclei appear to increase in number and the interstitial fibrous tissue becomes more prominent. Necrosis of single muscle fibres may be seen (this is particularly common in some experimental animals, for instance the rabbit). Cholinesterase remains histochemically demonstrable at the motor endplate for about six weeks.[76a] For a long time after denervation, clumps of muscle nuclei, sometimes spaced at regular intervals, are seen in remnants of still cross-striated sarcoplasm (Fig. 36.25B). Eventually, after years, disappearance of the muscle fibres is complete and the muscle is represented by fat and fibrous tissue, although occasional minute cross-striated fibres may be seen 20 or more years after denervation. The time taken for these degenerative changes to develop varies greatly, even within a single muscle, and also from species to species.

When a nerve fibre degenerates all the muscle fibres supplied by it atrophy. This leads to shrinking of whole bundles of muscle fibres, which are then seen lying adjacent to normal (innervated) bundles (Fig. 36.26). The change is best seen in transverse sections.

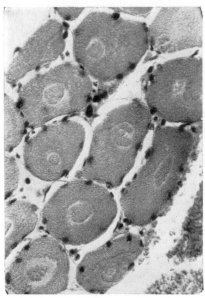

Fig. 36.27.§ Longstanding denervation due to poliomyelitis. Transverse section, showing 'target' appearance of muscle fibres that have not undergone denervation atrophy. See also Figs 36.28A and 36.28B. *Haematoxylin–eosin.* × 325.

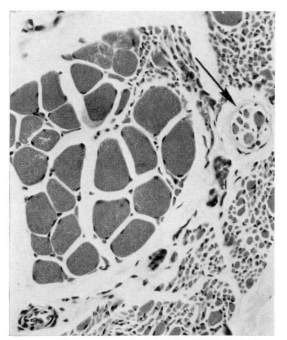

Fig. 36.26.§ Denervation of muscle in Werdnig–Hoffmann disease. Transverse section showing a bundle of normal muscle fibres adjacent to denervated bundles that consist of small muscle fibres with an occasional fibre of normal size. Note the normal-looking muscle spindle (arrowed). This picture is typical of denervated muscle and is seen, for instance, in cases of motor neuron disease and of poliomyelitis. *Haematoxylin–eosin.* × 220.

The muscle spindles probably atrophy and become fibrotic only if both their sensory supply and their motor supply is cut.[77] In partially denervated muscle the fibres that retain their innervation may or may not hypertrophy. A curious change has been described in incompletely denervated muscle: fibres that have not atrophied show a core and two concentric layers of abnormal muscle substance and, in cross section, look like targets (Figs 36.27, 36.28A and 36.28B).[78] The appearance must not be confused with that of central core disease (see page 2362).

Reinnervation of Muscle.—After section of a peripheral nerve the regenerating axons grow down the neurolemmal tubes and reinnervate the original motor endplates; new endplates may also form.[79] If reinnervated, the muscle fibres eventually regain their normal girth. The neuromuscular junction cannot be re-established if denervation atrophy of the muscle fibre has gone too far. It is believed that if more than three years have elapsed between injury and suture of a severed nerve, no useful reinnervation may be expected.[80]

In muscle that has lost only part of its motor nerve supply another process is seen. A denervated muscle fibre provides a strong stimulus to adjacent nerve fibres to sprout, and it attracts these sprouts, which in turn form new motor endplates. The re-

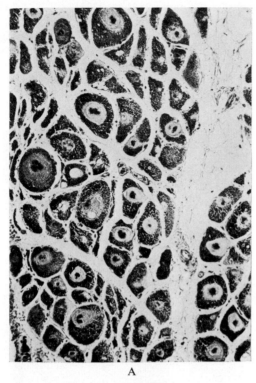
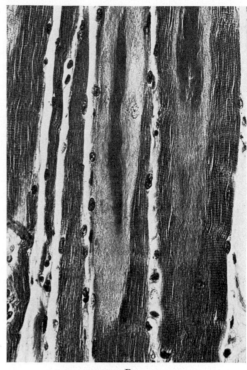

A   B

Fig. 36.28.§ 'Target' fibres in motor neuron disease.

A. This cross section of muscle in a case of motor neuron disease shows the characteristic target-like appearance that may develop in muscle fibres that have not undergone denervation atrophy. *Phosphotungstic-acid–haematoxylin.* × 180.

B. A longitudinal section shows that the 'target' change extends for only a short distance within the fibres. Contrast with the extent of the lesion that characterizes central core disease (Fig. 36.14B). *Phosphotungstic-acid–haematoxylin.* × 300.

sult of this is that a terminal nerve fibre may come to supply many muscle fibres (Figs 36.29A, 36.29B and 36.30), although normally it supplies only one, and a single muscle fibre may come to possess several motor endplates. Branching of terminal nerve fibres may be the only histological evidence of past denervation or of lesions in the more distal branches of the motor nerves. The innervation pattern can, of course, only be seen if the specimen of muscle is taken from the region of the motor point, and only if the nerve fibres are stained either with silver or intravitally with methylene blue.[81] It has been pointed out that, by sprouting from surviving axons, one motor cell may come to supply three times the number of muscle fibres that it normally innervates.[82] It is said that good function can be obtained from a muscle as long as 10 per cent of its motor nerve cells survive.[83]

Conditions Leading to Denervation

Denervation is due to trauma or to disease of the lower motor neuron. The lesions may be in the peripheral nerve, the ventral root or the motor cell body in the spinal cord or brainstem.

The most frequent diseases affecting the cell body of the lower motor neuron are: *acute poliomyelitis* (see page 2141), in which the virus affects a varying number of nerve cells in the anterior grey columns of the spinal cord; *motor neuron disease*, including amyotrophic lateral sclerosis (progressive muscular atrophy), which is a chronic progressive disease of unknown aetiology in which motor nerve cells disappear (see page 2262); and Werdnig–Hoffmann disease, a familial condition of childhood with a non-sex-linked, recessive mode of inheritance, characterized by progressive loss of motor cells in the brainstem and spinal cord (see page 2263).[84, 85] In cases of *congenital abnormalities of the spinal cord*, such as meningomyeloceles, denervation of the muscles may also be found. In all these conditions there is irregular loss of nerve cells in the anterior columns, which produces patchy atrophy of groups of muscle fibres, bundles of atrophic fibres being scattered among normal bundles (Fig.

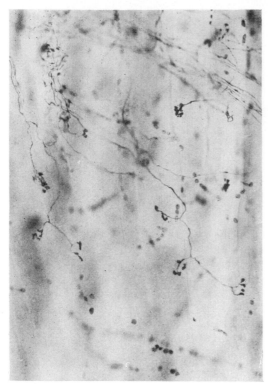

Fig. 36.29A.§ Denervation and reinnervation of muscle following peripheral neuropathy. Collateral branches from surviving subterminal nerve fibres have grown and reinnervated some previously denervated muscle fibres, the subterminal fibres thus coming to supply endplates to three or more muscle fibres instead of one. Compare with Fig. 36.29B. See also Fig. 36.30. *Methylene blue.* × 180.

36.26). This clear-cut pattern may be obscured by reinnervation of muscle fibres by sprouts from surviving nerve fibres.

The reinnervation that occurs early in denervating diseases is responsible for an interesting (and diagnostically useful) change in the histochemical pattern of type 1 and type 2 fibres. This is known as 'type grouping' (Fig. 36.31) and reflects the development in human muscle of large areas consisting of the same muscle fibre type. It occurs before group atrophy, and it is thought to be due to the reinnervation of muscle fibres of one type by branches of axons that properly supply fibres of the other type. The reinnervating axon has the capacity to transform the muscle cells into the type that it normally supplies.[86]

Denervation occurs in any of the diseases that cause peripheral neuropathy, such as polyarteritis (see page 2310), compression by carcinomatous deposits, and the Guillain–Barré syndrome (Landry––Guillain–Barré syndrome, or 'idiopathic poly-

neuritis'—see pages 2331 to 2333).

If a lesion affects the more distal branches of a motor nerve fibre, only small groups of muscle fibres or even individual fibres atrophy. Under such conditions abnormal branching of the terminal nerve fibres may be the only demonstrable abnormality (Fig. 36.30).

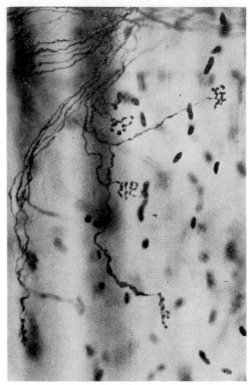

Fig. 36.29B.§ Normal innervation of muscle, for comparison with Fig. 36.29A. *Methylene blue.* × 300.

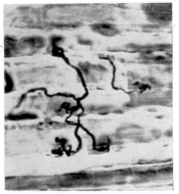

Fig. 36.30.§ Denervation and reinnervation of muscle following poliomyelitis. Sprouts from one surviving nerve fibre supply motor endplates to three muscle fibres. *Silver impregnation.* × 200.

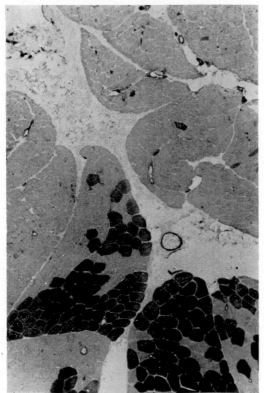

Fig. 36.31.§ 'Type grouping' of muscle fibres in neurogenic disease. When muscle is undergoing denervation, and unaffected axons react by reinnervating the denervated muscle fibres, it may happen that a neuron that normally supplies one main type of muscle fibre reinnervates fibres of the other main type. The reinnervating neuron has the capability of transforming muscle fibres into the fibre type that it ordinarily supplies: in consequence, large groups of muscle fibres of the same histochemical type develop. Compare the type grouping in this illustration with the mosaic pattern of normal muscle in Figs 36.2A and 36.2B. *Cryostat section. Stained for myosin adenosine triphosphatase at pH 9.4. × 50.*

Peroneal Muscular Atrophy (Charcot–Marie–Tooth Disease[86a, 86b]).—This is a hereditary, slowly progressive disease of the spinal cord and peripheral nerves (see page 2315). The muscles show the appearances seen in denervation, but there is also an unusual degree of fibrosis of their substance, which fixes the joints. This disease may accompany other degenerative disorders of the nervous system, such as Friedreich's ataxia (see pages 2266 and 2316).

Hereditary Denervation in Animals

Two forms of hereditary denervation in mice have been described. In one, *dystonia musculorum*, there is sensory denervation of muscle and other struc-

tures.[87] The other resembles human motor neuron disease in that there is progressive disappearance of motor neurons, with accompanying motor denervation (see page 2262).[88]

INFECTIONS AND INFESTATIONS

Bacterial Infections

Any systemic bacterial infection, either acute (such as staphylococcal septicaemia) or chronic (such as tuberculosis) may cause myositis. Caseating tuberculosis of a psoas muscle was formerly a familiar instance of the so-called 'cold abscess' that occurred as a complication of tuberculous infection of the bodies of the vertebrae (see page 2412).

Some infections affect muscles particularly: the most important are clostridial infections causing gas gangrene. *Clostridium welchii* and other clostridia grow only under such anaerobic conditions as exist in necrotic muscle tissue. Their toxins (mainly the alpha-toxin, a lecithinase) cause a spreading necrosis, and the necrotic tissue provides a medium in which the bacteria can multiply further. Histologically, the necrosis is accompanied by an acute inflammatory reaction with much exudate in which the Gram-positive bacilli can be seen.

Zenker's Hyaline Degeneration

In lobar pneumonia, typhoid fever and some other generalized bacterial infections, muscles may show foci of hyaline necrosis, and some regeneration, as first described by Zenker in 1863.[89, 89a] This necrosis is apparently not due to bacterial invasion: it is believed to be of the same nature as the necrosis that occurs in the primary myopathies (see page 2357).

Suppurative Myositis

With the exception of rare cases of diffuse streptococcal myositis, affecting a single muscle or group of muscles (and usually the result of direct inoculation of infected material), suppuration in the skeletal musculature is characterized by abscess formation. Multiple small abscesses, commonly of little more than microscopical size, are found in cases of pyaemia.

Large abscesses, single or multiple, may occur in any muscle. Such lesions may result from injection of drugs: antibiotics, chemotherapeutic agents (particularly preparations intended for intravenous administration and given intramuscularly in error), hormonal preparations, antisera and vaccines (including bacillus Calmette–Guérin inadvertently administered by intramuscular injection) were among the causes in a series of 40 cases collected in a recent study in western Europe.[90] In some of these cases of iatrogenic abscess there was a serious accompanying neuritis, often permanently crippling, from involvement of nerves in the suppurative lesion, particularly the sciatic nerve. Similar abscesses, usually in the thigh, are sometimes seen in drug addicts, but are comparatively rare among them, perhaps because of the infrequent use of the intramuscular route when drugs are self-administered.

Tropical Pyomyositis

The condition known as tropical pyomyositis is characterized by large, solitary or multiple, intramuscular abscesses in the limbs or trunk.[91] In many cases it has been shown to be caused by *Staphylococcus aureus*; in others no micro-organisms have been isolated and the cause is unknown. Debility is commonly a predisposing factor, but some patients are apparently in good health and free from malnutrition when the disease develops.

Histological examination may show the commonplace features of a localized abscess. In some cases the contents of the abscess have the characteristics of caseous material rather than of pus, and the wall of the cavity may then consist of organizing granulation tissue in which macrophages, including epithelioid cells and multinucleate giant cells, greatly outnumber neutrophils. Similar histological appearances may be found in tuberculous myositis or when chromomycotic 'cold abscesses'[92] extend from the subcutaneous tissue into the musculature; the causative organisms may be overlooked in these cases if not carefully sought. Chronic abscesses due to therapeutic agents (see above) may also present this granulomatous type of histological picture.

Abscesses between muscles, not within their substance, may be associated with local infestation by nematodes, particularly the Guinea worm (*Dracunculus medinensis*).[93]

Viral Infections

The only viruses known to grow in human muscle are the Coxsackie viruses, which produce acute necrosis of muscle fibres:[94] this is followed by invasion by macrophages and then regeneration. In adults, they cause epidemic myalgia (Bornholm disease*).[95] They may infect the fetus, giving rise to congenital myopathy; the virus may be recoverable from the tissues for many months after birth.[96]

Protozoal Infections

Toxoplasmosis

The protozoal parasite, *Toxoplasma gondii* (see Fig. 1.39, page 46 in Volume 1), may infect skeletal muscle fibres and cause severe myositis,[97] with necrosis of infected fibres.

American Trypanosomiasis (Chagas's Disease)

Skeletal muscle fibres are less often found to be infected by *Trypanosoma cruzi*, the cause of American trypanosomiasis, than myocardial fibres (see page 46, Volume 1).[98]

Infestation by Sarcocystis Species[99]

The protozoal parasite *Sarcocystis* is occasionally found encysted in skeletal and cardiac muscle fibres of various domestic and wild animals in any part of the world. It was formerly a very frequent finding in laboratory rodents, but has become exceptionally rare since the introduction of modern methods of breeding, feeding and housing. The parasite is sometimes referred to as a sarcosporidium and the infestation as sarcosporidiosis.

The cysts have been found incidentally in human muscle, both skeletal[100] and cardiac.[101] In rare instances fever and localized swelling of infected muscles have been observed.[102, 103] The organism in cases of human infection is sometimes specified as *Sarcocystis lindemanni*, but it is probably identical with the species that are parasitic in mice and rats (*Sarcocystis muris*) or in rabbits (*Sarcocystis cuniculi*).[104]

Histological examination in symptomatic cases in man (Fig. 36.32) shows an inflammatory reaction, often with numerous eosinophils, round ruptured parasitic cysts (Fig. 36.32C). Intact cysts evoke no reaction (Figs 36.32A and 36.32B). They measure from 50 to 300 μm in length and from 20 to 15 μm in width, being disposed lengthwise in the infected muscle fibre. The size of the trophozoites may vary from case to case, but usually they are from 10 to 14 μm long (shorter trophozoites are

---

* Bornholm disease (Sylvest's disease) is named after the Danish island of Bornholm, in the Baltic Sea, where it was described in 1930 by Sylvest (Sylvest, E., *Ugeskr. Læg.*, 1930, **92**, 798).

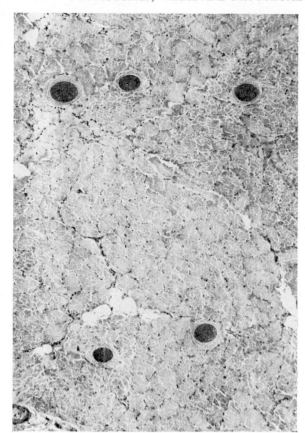

Fig. 36.32.§ Sarcocystis infection. The patient was a man who had been working for some years as a cleaner in the animal house of a biological institute. He developed several painful swellings in muscles of his trunk and limbs, accompanied by slight fever and an eosinophilia of $1.2 \times 10^9/l$ (1200/μl) in the blood. The condition subsided without treatment. There were no electrocardiographic abnormalities. The three photographs are of tissue excised from the site of a swelling in a soleus muscle. Requests for information about the possible occurrence of sarcocystis infection among the laboratory animals in the institute were refused.

Fig. 36.32A.§ Five cysts of *Sarcocystis* species are seen in this cross-section of the muscle. Each infected fibre is considerably distended by the presence of the cyst. See also Fig. 36.32B. *Haematoxylin–eosin.* × 65.

Occasionally, man may become the intermediate host by ingesting the free ova. Larvae hatch from these ova and are distributed to skeletal and heart muscle, and occasionally to other organs of the host, giving rise to the condition known as cysticercosis.[106] Ordinarily, this occurs only in cases of infestation by *Taenia solium* (see page 677, Volume 2). The larvae encyst between the muscle fibres, part of the cyst wall being formed by the host's tissue. The fully developed larval cyst is an ovoid or spheroidal structure that measures from 0.5 to 1.0 cm across. The cyst may attract many eosinophils. Eventually the lesions become calcified and radiologically opaque. They may be palpable in the tongue and sometimes in other situations.

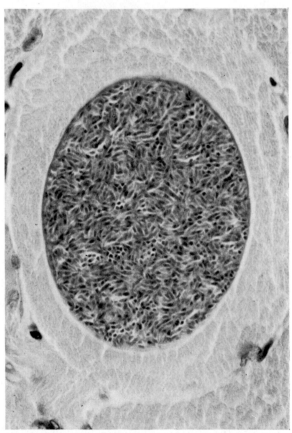

Fig. 36.32B.§ The upper left-hand cyst in Fig. 36.32A. The elongated trophozoites, somewhat tapered at one end, each contain an elongated nucleus near the blunter end. They are enclosed by the smooth, delicate wall of the cyst. Trophozoites that are cut across appear as clusters of rounded bodies. The clustering of the trophozoites results from their formation by multiple binary fission. There is no evident reaction of the parasitized tissue to the presence of the intact cyst. *Haematoxylin–eosin.* × 630.

liable to be mistaken for the trophozoites of *Toxoplasma gondii*).

Metazoal Infestations[105]

Cysticercosis

Some parasitic worms spend part of their life cycle in larval form in muscle. The adult forms of *Taenia solium* (pig tape worm) and *Taenia saginata* (beef tape worm) live in the intestine of the definitive hosts, which include man (see page 1081, Volume 3).

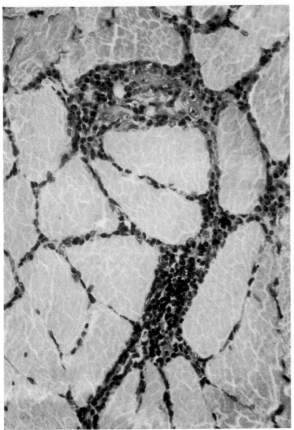

Fig. 36.32C.§ Focal myositis (same specimen as Figs 36.32A and 36.32B). Eosinophils predominate in the exudate; there are a few conspicuous macrophages. Although there is no trace of a ruptured cyst and no trophozoites could be recognized with certainty in this field, the picture is typical of the reaction that develops in muscle in the vicinity of a sarcocystis cyst that has disintegrated. The reaction is believed to be a manifestation of hypersensitivity. The trophozoites are destroyed rapidly once liberated from the cysts. *Haematoxylin–eosin.* × 250.

Trichinosis (Trichinellosis; Trichiniasis)

The adult *Trichinella spiralis* (*Trichina spiralis*) can live in the intestine of many animals, including pigs and man. The main source of human infestation is uncooked pork. The trichina embryos pass through the intestinal mucosa and thence in the blood stream to the muscles. This dissemination may be accompanied by a systemic reaction. In the muscles the larvae can be seen curled up in oval cysts that are about 0·5 mm long: the cysts lie within the muscle fibres, the cyst wall being formed by the host's tissues. Once the parasites have encysted they do no further harm to the host, unless they have settled in the heart or in the brain.

'Myospherulosis' (Sperulocystic Disease)

This condition, which is of uncertain nature, affects subcutaneous tissue much oftener than muscle. It is considered in Chapter 39, Volume 6.

SARCOIDOSIS

Random biopsy of skeletal muscle (usually of a gastrocnemius) in 42 cases of proven sarcoidosis showed sarcoid granulomas in 23 (55 per cent).[107] Clinical manifestations of involvement of the muscles occur in a much smaller proportion of cases. They are said to develop particularly in older women and they take the form mainly of weakness and wasting.[108]

TUMOURS AND TUMOUR-LIKE LESIONS

Benign Tumours and Tumour-Like Lesions

Benign rhabdomyomas are very rare in voluntary muscle.[109] They have been described more frequently as lesions of the myocardium: however, in this situation it seems that they are not true tumours but the manifestation either of a localized form of glycogen storage (nodular glycogenic infiltration) or of hamartomas associated with tuberose sclerosis (see pages 66 and 81, Volume 1).

Primary Malignant Tumours

Rhabdomyosarcoma.—Malignant neoplasms of striated muscle are rare (see also page 2514). They occur more frequently in organs that contain *smooth* muscle, such as the male and female genitalia, and the urinary bladder, and in the nasopharynx.

Rhabdomyosarcomas of skeletal muscles[110] are most commonly found in the legs. They usually grow rapidly and they may metastasize by way of the blood stream and, occasionally, by lymphatics. Histologically, the cells are frequently large and may contain two or more nuclei. Here and there the cytoplasm shows cross-striation, but this may be difficult to find. Cells with large, peripherally placed vacuoles—'spider cells'—may be seen: the vacuoles are full of glycogen. Similar 'spider cells' are seen in examples of nodular glycogenic infiltration of the myocardium (Fig. 2.4A, page 82 in Volume 1).

Fibrosarcoma.—Fibrosarcomas are rarer in skeletal muscles than myosarcomas. They probably arise from the fibrous connective tissue.

Neoplastic Muscle Tissue in Teratomas

Neoplastic muscle tissue is often a constituent of malignant teratomas of the ovaries and testes or arising elsewhere (Fig. 36.33).

Secondary Tumours and Leukaemic Infiltration

Metastatic deposits of carcinomas may be found in skeletal muscles, but only very rarely, even when searched for. Leukaemic infiltration, in contrast, is frequent; occasionally, the leukaemic cells form tumour-like aggregates.

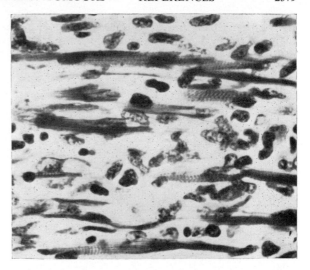

Fig. 36.33.§ Longitudinal section of cross-striated muscle fibres in a malignant teratoma in the region of the falx cerebri. *Haematoxylin–eosin.* × 350.

REFERENCES

NORMAL ANATOMY AND HISTOLOGY

1. Huxley, H. E., in *Muscle*, edited by W. M. Paul, E. E. Daniel, C. M. Kay and G. Monckton, page 3. Oxford, 1965.
2. Sissons, H. A., in *Disorders of Voluntary Muscle*, edited by J. N. Walton, 3rd edn, page 7. Edinburgh and London, 1974.
3. Dubowitz, V., in *Disorders of Voluntary Muscle*, 3rd edn, edited by J. N. Walton, page 325. Edinburgh and London, 1974.
4. Coërs, C., Woolf, A. L., *The Innervation of Muscle*, page 14. Oxford, 1959.
5. Eccles, J. C., Sherrington, C. S., *Proc. Roy. Soc. B*, 1930, **106**, 326.
6. Coërs, C., *Int. Rev. Cytol.*, 1967, **22**, 239.
7. Sherrington, C. S., *J. Physiol.*, 1894, **17**, 211.
8. Cooper, S., Daniel, P. M., *Brain*, 1964, **86**, 563.
9. Barker, D., in *Myotatic, Kinesthetic and Vestibular Mechanisms*, edited by A. V. S. de Reuck and J. Knight, page 3. London, 1967.
10. Denny-Brown, D., *Res. Publ. Ass. nerv. ment. Dis.*, 1960, **38**, 147.
11. Schiaffino, S., Hanzlickova, V., *Experientia (Basel)*, 1970, **26**, 152.
12. Goldspink, G., *Nature (Lond.)*, 1961, **192**, 1305.

PATHOLOGICAL CONDITIONS: GENERAL CONSIDERATIONS

13. Adams, R. D., Denny-Brown, D., Pearson, C. M., *Diseases of Muscle*, 2nd edn. London, 1962.
14. Bethlem, J., *Muscle Pathology—Introduction and Atlas*. Amsterdam and London, 1970.
15. Harriman, D. G. F., in *Greenfield's Neuropathology*, 3rd edn, edited by W. Blackwood and J. A. N. Corsellis, chap. 19. London, 1976.
15a. Forbus, W. D., *Arch. Path. Lab. Med.*, 1926, **2**, 486.
16. Clark, W. E. Le Gros, *J. Anat. (Lond.)*, 1946, **80**, 24.
17. Shafiq, S. A., in *Regeneration of Striated Muscle, and Myogenesis*, edited by A. Mauro, S. A. Shafiq and A. T. Milhorat, page 122. Amsterdam, 1970.

18. Baloh, R., Cancilla, P. A., Kalyanaramau, K., Munsat, T., Pearson, C. M., Rich, R., *Lab. Invest.*, 1972, **26**, 319.
19. Pearce, J. M. S., Pennington, R. J., Walton, J. N., *J. Neurol. Neurosurg. Psychiat.*, 1964, **27**, 1, 96, 181.
20. Ebashi, S., Toyokura, Y., Momoi, H., Sugita, H., *J. Biochem. (Tokyo)*, 1959, **46**, 103.
21. Pennington, R. J. T., in *Disorders of Voluntary Muscle*, 3rd edn, edited by J. N. Walton, page 489. Edinburgh and London, 1974.
21a. Zierler, K. L., Folk, B. P., Magladery, J. W., Lilienthal, J. L., Jr, *Bull. Johns Hopk. Hosp.*, 1949, **85**, 370.
22. McKusick, V., *Heritable Disorders of Connective Tissue*, 3rd edn, page 400. St Louis, 1966.
23. Münchmeyer, E., *Z. rat. Med.*, 1869, **34**, 1.
24. Warren, S., *Arch. Path. (Chic.)*, 1943, **35**, 347.
25. Clark, W. E. Le Gros, Blomfield, L. B., *J. Anat. (Lond.)*, 1945, **79**, 15.
25a. Volkmann, R. von, *Zbl. Chir.*, 1881, **8**, 801.
26. Griffiths, D. Ll., *Brit. J. Surg.*, 1940–41, **28**, 239.

CONGENITAL MALFORMATIONS

27. Bing, R., *Virchows Arch. path. Anat.*, 1902, **170**, 175.
28. Le Double, A.-F., *Traité des variations du système musculaire de l'homme*. Paris, 1897.

THE MYOPATHIES

29. Bosanquet, F. D., Daniel, P. M., Parry, H. B., in *The Structure and Function of Muscle*, edited by G. H. Bourne, vol. 3, page 321. New York and London, 1960.
30. Walton, J. N., in *Muscle*, edited by W. M. Paul, E. E. Daniel, C. M. Kay and G. Monckton, page 501. Oxford, 1965.
31. Coërs, C., in *Muscle*, edited by W. M. Paul, E. E. Daniel, C. M. Kay and G. Monckton, page 453. Oxford, 1965.
32. Geiger, R. S., Garvin, J. S., *J. Neuropath. exp. Neurol.*, 1957, **16**, 532.

33. Dubowitz, V., *Develop. Med. Child Neurol.*, 1971, **13**, 238.
34. Kakulas, B. A., Papadimitriou, J. M., Knight, J. O., Mastaglia, F. L., *Proceedings of the Second Pan-Oceanian Congress of Neurology, Melbourne, 1967*, page 79. Melbourne, 1967.
34a. Griesinger, W., *Arch. Heilk.*, 1865, **6**, 1.
34b. Duchenne, G. B., *Arch. gén. Méd.*, 1868, 6 sér., **11**, 5, 179, 305, 421, 552.
35. Roy, S., Dubowitz, V., *J. neurol. Sci.*, 1970, **11**, 65.
36. Banker, B. Q., Victor, M., Adams, R. D., *Brain*, 1957, **80**, 319.
37. Fowler, M., *Arch. Dis. Childh.*, 1959, **34**, 505.
37a. Landouzy, L., Déjerine, J., *C.R. Acad. Sci. (Paris)*, 1884, **98**, 53.
37b. Walton, J. N., Gardner-Medwin, D., in *Disorders of Voluntary Muscle*, edited by J. N. Walton, 3rd edn, chap. 15 [page 575]. Edinburgh and London, 1974.
38. Kiloh, L. G., Nevin, S., *Brain*, 1951, **74**, 115.
39. Steinert, H., *Dtsch. Z. Nervenheilk.*, 1909, **37**, 58.
39a. Batten, F. E., Gibbs, H. P., *Brain*, 1909, **32**, 187.
39b. Curschmann, H., *Dtsch. Z. Nervenheilk.*, 1912, **45**, 161.
39c. Adie, W. J., Greenfield, J. G., *Brain*, 1923, **46**, 73.
40. Daniel, P. M., Strich, S. J., *Neurology*, 1964, **14**, 310.
41. Thomsen, J., *Arch. Psychiat. Nervenkr.*, 1876, **6**, 702.
42. Shy, G. M., Magee, K. R., *Brain*, 1956, **79**, 610.
43. Bethlem, J., Wyngaarden, G. K. van, Meijer, A. E. F. H., Fleury, P., *J. neurol. Sci.*, 1971, **14**, 293.
44. Walton, J. N., *J. Neurol. Neurosurg. Psychiat.*, 1957, **20**, 144.
45. Hulsmann, W. C., Bethlem, J., Meijer, A. E. F. H., Fleury, P., Schellens, J. P. M., *J. Neurol. Neurosurg. Psychiat.*, 1967, **30**, 519.
46. Abu Haydar, N., Conn, H. L., Afifi, A., Wakid, N., Ballas, S., Fawaz, K., *Ann. intern. Med.*, 1971, **74**, 548.
47. Engel, A. G., *Mayo Clin. Proc.*, 1966, **41**, 713.
48. Harriman, D. G. F., *Advanc. Ophthal.*, 1970, **23**, 55.
48a. Adie, W. J., *Brit. med. J.*, 1931, **1**, 928.
49. Harriman, D. G. F., Haleem, M. A., *J. Path.*, 1972, **108**, 237.
50. Morgan-Hughes, J. A., Mair, W. G. P., Lascelles, P. T., *Brain*, 1970, **93**, 873.
50a. Currie, S., Saunders, M., Knowles, M., Brown, A. E., *Quart. J. Med.*, 1971, N.S. **40**, 63.
51. Denny-Brown, D., *Trans. Coll. Phycns Philad.*, 1960–61, **28**, 14.
52. Currie, S., Saunders, M., Knowles, M., Brown, A. E., *Quart. J. Med.*, 1971, N.S. **40**, 63.
53. Banker, B. Q., Victor, M., *Medicine (Baltimore)*, 1966, **45**, 261.
54. Haslock, D. I., Wright, V., Harriman, D. G. F., *Quart. J. Med.*, 1970, N.S. **34**, 335.
55. Kalden, J. R., Williamson, W. G., Johnson, R. J., Irvine, W. J., *Clin. exp. Immunol.*, 1969, **5**, 319.
56. Coërs, C., Desmedt, J. E., *Acta neurol. belg.*, 1959, **59**, 539.
56a. Buzzard, E. Farquhar, *Brain*, 1905, **28**, 438.
57. Russell, D. S., *J. Path. Bact.*, 1953, **65**, 279.
58. Kroll, A. J., Kuwabara, T., *Arch. Ophthal.*, 1966, **76**, 244.
59. Kriss, J. P., Pleshakov, V., Rosenblum, A. L., Holderness, M., Sharp, G., Utiger, R., *J. clin. Endocr.*, 1967, **27**, 582.
60. Harriman, D. G. F., Reed, R., *J. Path.*, 1972, **106**, 1.

61. Bethlem, J., *Muscle Pathology—Introduction and Atlas*, page 45. Amsterdam and London, 1970.
61a. McArdle, B., *Clin. Sci.*, 1951, **10**, 13.
62. Pearson, C. M., Rimer, D. G., Mommaerts, W. F. H. M., *Amer. J. Med.*, 1961, **30**, 502.
63. Weinberg, T., Gordon, H. H., Oppenheimer, E. H., Nitowsky, H. M., *Amer. J. Path.*, 1958, **34**, 565.
64. McArdle, B., in *Disorders of Voluntary Muscle*, 3rd edn, edited by J. N. Walton, page 726. Edinburgh and London, 1974.
65. Korein, J., Coddon, D. R., Mowrey, F. H., *Neurology (Minneap.)*, 1959, **9**, 767.
66. Günther, H., *Ergebn. inn. Med. Kinderheilk.*, 1940, **58**, 331.
67. Berlin, R., *Acta med. scand.*, 1948, **129**, 560.
67a. Martin, J. J., Bogaert, L. van, Damme, J. van, Peremans, J., *J. neurol. Sci.*, 1970, **11**, 147.
68. Hadlow, W. J., in *Comparative Neuropathology*, edited by J. R. M. Innes and L. Z. Saunders, page 147. New York and London, 1962.
69. Rigdon, R. H., *Amer. J. Path.*, 1961, **39**, 27.
70. West, W. T., Murphy, E. D., *Anat. Rec.*, 1960, **137**, 279.
71. Michelson, A. M., Russell, E. S., Harman, P. J., *Proc. nat. Acad. Sci. (Wash.)*, 1955, **41**, 1079.
72. Brown, G. L., Harvey, A. M., *Brain*, 1939, **62**, 341.
73. Bosanquet, F. D., Daniel, P. M., Parry, H. B., *Lancet*, 1956, **2**, 737.
74. Homburger, F., Baker, J. R., Nixon, C. W., Wilgram, G., *Arch. intern. Med.*, 1962, **110**, 660.
74a. Carlström, B., *Skand. Arch. Physiol.*, 1931, **61**, 161; 1931, **62**, 1; 1932, **63**, 164.

'POLYMYALGIA RHEUMATICA'
75. Hunder, G. G., Disney, T. F., Ward, L. E., *Proc. Mayo Clin.*, 1969, **44**, 849.
75a. Dixon, A. S., Beardwell, C., Kay, A., Wanka, J., Wong, Y. T., *Ann. rheum. Dis.*, 1966, **25**, 203.
75b. Hamrin, B., *Acta med. scand.*, 1972, suppl. 533.
75c. Fessel, W. J., Pearson, C. M., *New Engl. J. Med.*, 1967, **276**, 1403.

REACTION OF MUSCLE TO DENERVATION
76. *The Denervated Muscle*, edited by E. Gutmann. Prague, 1962.
76a. Snell, R. S., McIntyre, N., *Brit. J. exp. Path.*, 1956, **37**, 44.
77. Tower, S. S., *Brain*, 1932, **55**, 77.
78. Tomonaga, M., Sluga, E., *Virchows Arch. Abt. A*, 1969, **348**, 89.
79. Gutmann, E., Young, J. Z., *J. Anat. (Lond.)*, 1944, **78**, 15.
80. Bowden, R. E. M., Gutmann, E., *Brain*, 1944, **67**, 273.
81. Coërs, C., Woolf, A. L., *The Innervation of Muscle*, page 7. Oxford, 1959.
82. Wohlfart, G., *Neurology*, 1957, **7**, 124.
83. Sharrard, W. J. W., *J. Bone Jt Surg.*, 1955, **37B**, 540.
84. Conel, J. L., *Arch. Neurol. Psychiat. (Chic.)*, 1938, **40**, 337.
85. Conel, J. L., *Arch. Path. (Chic.)*, 1940, **30**, 153.
86. Dubowitz, V., *J. Neurol. Neurosurg. Psychiat.*, 1967, **30**, 99.
86a. Charcot, J. M., Marie, P., *Rev. Méd.*, 1886, **6**, 97.
86b. Tooth, H. H., *The Peroneal Type of Progressive Muscular Atrophy*. London, 1886.
87. Duchen, L. W., Strich, S. J., *Brain*, 1964, **87**, 367.

88. Duchen, L. W., Falconer, D. S., Strich, S. J., *J. Physiol.*, 1965, **183**, 53 P.

INFECTIONS AND INFESTATIONS

89. Zenker, F. A., *Ueber die Veränderungen der willkührlichen Muskeln im Typhus abdominalis*, part 1, *Casuistik*. Erlangen, 1863.
89a. Forbus, W. D., *Arch. Path. Lab. Med.*, 1926, **2**, 318.
90. Symmers, W. St C., *unpublished observations*, 1969–74.
91. Horn, C. V., Master, S., *E. Afr. med. J.*, 1968, **45**, 463.
92. Symmers, W. St C., *Brit. med. J.*, 1971, **2**, 337.
93. Anand, S. V., Evans, K. T., *Brit. J. Surg.*, 1964, **51**, 917.
94. Dalldorf, G., *Ann. Rev. Microbiol.*, 1955, **9**, 277.
95. Lépine, P., Desse, G., Sautter, V., *Bull. Acad. nat. Méd. (Paris)*, 1952, **136**, 66.
96. Freudenberg, E., Roulet, F., Nicole, R., *Ann. paediat. (Basel)*, 1952, **178**, 150.
97. Chandar, K., Mair, H. J., Mair, N. S., *Brit. med. J.*, 1968, **1**, 158.
98. Andrade, Z. A., Andrade, S. G., *personal communication to W. St C. Symmers*, 1972.
99. Frenkel, J. K., in *Pathology of Protozoal and Helminthic Diseases with Clinical Correlation*, edited by R. A. Marcial-Rojas and E. Moreno, chap. 15 [pages 358–361]. Baltimore, 1971.

100. Liu, C. T., Roberts, L. M., *Amer. J. clin. Path.*, 1965, **44**, 639.
101. Hewitt, J. A., *J. Path. Bact.*, 1933, **36**, 133.
102. Pugh, A. M., *Trans. roy. Soc. trop. Med. Hyg.*, 1950, **44**, 1.
103. Mandour, A. M., *Trans. roy. Soc. trop. Med. Hyg.*, 1965, **59**, 432.
104. Levine, N. D., *Protozoan Parasites of Domestic Animals and of Man*. Minneapolis, 1961.
105. Garnham, P. P. C., in *The Structure and Function of Muscle*, edited by G. H. Bourne, vol. 3, page 109. New York and London, 1960.
106. Jolly, S. S., Pallis, C., *J. neurol. Sci.*, 1971, **12**, 155.

SARCOIDOSIS

107. Wallace, S. L., Lattes, R., Malia, J. P., Ragan, C., *Ann. intern. Med.*, 1958, **48**, 497.
108. Gardner-Thorpe, C., *Neurology (Minneapolis)*, 1972, **22**, 971.

TUMOURS AND TUMOUR-LIKE LESIONS

109. Goldman, R. L., *Cancer (Philad.)*, 1963, **16**, 1609.
110. Soule, E. H., Geity, M., Henderson, E. D., *Cancer (Philad.)*, 1969, **23**, 1336.

ACKNOWLEDGEMENTS FOR ILLUSTRATIONS

Figs 36.1A, 2A, 2B, 3, 4, 14A, 14B, 15–18, 20, 22, 23A, 24, 28A, 28B, 29A, 29B, 31. These illustrations were prepared with the support of grants to D. G. F. Harriman from the Medical Research Council [United Kingdom], the Board of Governors of the United Leeds Hospitals and the West Riding of Yorkshire Medical Research Trust.

Figs 36.1B, 5, 6A, 6B, 7, 8A, 8B, 9A, 9B, 10A, 10B, 11A, 11B, 12A, 12B, 13, 19, 21A, 21B, 23B, 25A, 25B, 26, 27, 30, 33.

These illustrations were prepared by P. M. Daniel and Sabina J. Strich from material studied while in receipt of a grant from the Muscular Dystrophy Associations of America, Incorporated.

Fig. 36.17. Reproduced by permission of the editor from: Harriman, D. G. F., Haleem, M. A., *J. Path.*, 1972, **108**, 237.

Figs 36.32A, 32B, 32C. Photomicrographs provided by W. St C. Symmers.

37: *Bones*

by H. A. SISSONS

CONTENTS

37: *Bones*

by H. A. SISSONS

Technical Note

The histological preparations illustrated in this chapter are paraffin wax sections. When bone is present the tissue has been decalcified, unless the contrary is stated in the caption.

BONE STRUCTURE AND PHYSIOLOGY[1-4]

As a preliminary to an account of diseases of bone, it is necessary to consider the normal structure of bone, its mode of growth, and something of its physiology.

Bone Structure

Bone is a specialized form of connective tissue. Its intercellular matrix is loaded with hydroxyapatite, a mineral that may be represented approximately by the formula $3Ca_3(PO_4)_2.5Ca(OH)_2$. The presence of this material gives bone its rigidity, and also makes it the body's storehouse for calcium and therefore an important part of the homoeostatic mechanism for controlling the level of calcium in the blood and tissue fluids. In addition to the mineral, or 'bone salt', the intercellular material of bone consists of collagen fibres bound together by amorphous, polysaccharide ground substance. The bone cells, or osteocytes, are situated in lacunae in the calcified matrix: these are connected with each other and with the vascular spaces of the tissue by a system of fine canaliculi that contain cytoplasmic extensions of the osteocytes. It is through the canaliculi that the nutritional and respiratory exchanges of these cells takes place.

Histology.[5, 6]—The skeleton is made up of compact and cancellous bone. In the adult, both of these types of bone have an almost entirely lamellar structure. The collagen fibres of *lamellar bone* are arranged in sheets (lamellae): in any lamella the fibres are parallel to each other, but their orientation differs from that of fibres in adjacent lamellae.

The lamellar structure is barely visible in sections stained with haematoxylin and eosin (Figs 37.1 and 37.2), but it is obvious in specially stained preparations or in sections examined with a polarizing microscope. In the embryo or the young child, and under a variety of pathological conditions in adult life, another type of bone tissue is encountered. This is termed *non-lamellar bone* ('coarsely-fibred', or 'woven', bone), and it fails to show the oriented arrangement of collagen fibres characteristic of lamellar bone (Fig. 37.3). Cortical bone contains numerous *Haversian systems,** or *osteons*. These are roughly cylindrical structures, running more or less longitudinally in the bone,[7] and thus appearing circular or ovoid in transverse sections (Figs 37.1 and 37.2; Fig. 37.44B, page 2426). Their lamellae are arranged concentrically round a central canal containing one or more blood vessels—usually capillaries. Each osteon is separated from the surrounding tissue by a *cement line* that stains darkly with haematoxylin (Fig. 37.1). Some cortical bone, however, particularly toward the endosteal and periosteal surfaces, consists of non-Haversian bone, the lamellae—*circumferential lamellae*—being arranged parallel to these surfaces. Haversian systems are not present in cancellous bone, the trabeculae consisting of lamellar bone divided by occasional cement lines.

Bone Formation and Bone Destruction

During growth, and also in adult life, bone is deposited and resorbed as a result of the activities

* The Haversian systems are named after Clopton Havers (*circa* 1657-1702), a physician in London, who described the canals in cortical bone and the bony lamellae surrounding them (long known respectively as Haversian canals and Haversian lamellae). His name is also carried by the intra-articular pads and fringes of adipose tissue that he regarded as contributing to the lubrication of joints (Haversian 'glands', or folds). His book, *Osteologia nova, or Some New Observations of the Bones and the Parts Belonging to Them, with the Manner of Their Accretion and Nutrition*, was published in London in 1691.

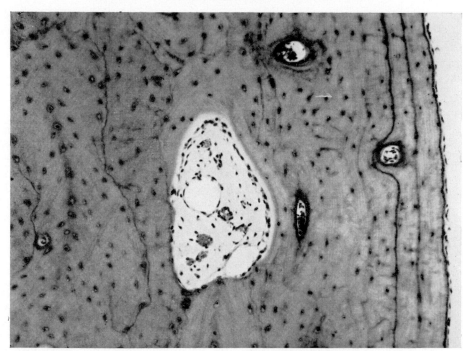

Fig. 37.1. Normal bone. Cortex of shaft of a child's femur, showing a developing Haversian system with its lining of palely staining osteoid tissue covered by osteoblasts. The lamellar structure of the bone is just visible. The tissue is divided by a number of crenated cement lines. Two smoothly contoured 'arrest lines' are present beneath the periosteal surface at the right: these indicate periods of temporary cessation of bone formation. *Haematoxylin–eosin,* × 150.

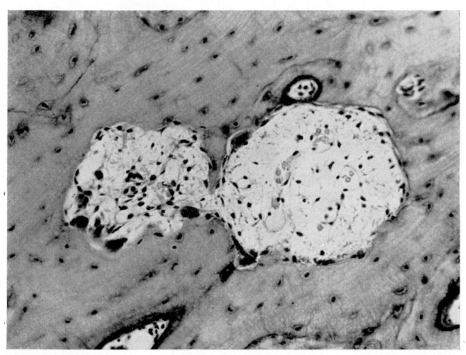

Fig. 37.2. Normal bone. Cortex of shaft of a child's femur, showing an area of active osteoclastic resorption. The eroded bone surface is irregular and crenated, and presents a number of Howship's lacunae, in which multinucleate giant cells (osteoclasts) are situated. The basophile staining of the bone surface in the nearby vascular channels indicates that this part of the surface is in an inactive phase. *Haematoxylin–eosin.* × 220.

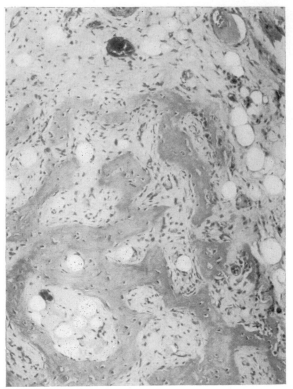

Fig. 37.3. Non-lamellar bone—fracture callus. The irregular bone trabeculae show no lamellar arrangement of their collagen fibres. *Haematoxylin–eosin.* × 120.

of connective tissue cells that form a continuous layer covering its surface. It should be noted that the 'surface' of bone includes not only the periosteum and endosteum, but the surface of the vascular canals penetrating cortical bone and also that of the trabeculae of cancellous bone.

While bone deposition and bone resorption are the results of the activities of morphologically distinct types of cell known respectively as osteoblasts and osteoclasts, these cells should not be regarded as immutable. The various types of cell making up skeletal connective tissue—osteocytes, cartilage cells, osteoblasts, reticulum cells and undifferentiated connective tissue cells—are closely related. Under normal conditions, *osteoblasts* may become embedded in bone matrix to form *osteocytes.* Recent evidence suggests that *osteoclasts* are derived from precursors in the bone marrow that reach bone as blood-borne mononuclear cells.[7a] Under pathological conditions additional types of cell conversion are encountered, as, for example, in the development of fracture callus, when periosteal cells—which normally form bone—

are found to produce cartilage (see page 2402). Bone tumours, too, provide evidence of the close relationship and interconvertibility of a wide range of cell types.

Bone Deposition

When they are actively depositing lamellar bone, osteoblasts appear as a layer of plump cells covering the involved part of the bone surface. The cells show conspicuous cytoplasmic basiphilia, due to the presence of ribonucleic acid, and they contain numerous mitochondria. Differentiating osteoblasts contain glycogen, but this is absent from the cells that are actively forming bone. The osteoblasts and the tissues immediately adjacent to them contain alkaline phosphatase; the amount of the enzyme appears to decrease with the onset of calcification, and it is thought to be concerned in some way with the formation of the protein matrix of bone. Surfaces of active bone deposition show a narrow zone of osteoid tissue between the osteoblasts and the underlying bone (Fig. 37.1). Osteoid tissue is bone matrix without its mineral material: it represents the initial stage in the formation of bone tissue, and subsequently undergoes calcification. The interface between calcified bone and osteoid tissue is sometimes referred to as the *calcification front*:[8] it is coloured intensely by stains for lipids[9] and by certain other dyes.[10] In rickets and osteomalacia (see page 2418), in which there is interference with calcification, excessive amounts of osteoid tissue accumulate. The histological identification of osteoid tissue is discussed on page 2421; its histochemical features have been the subject of a review.[11]

It is possible, by the use of certain vital markers, to measure the rate at which bone is deposited on microscopical surfaces. Certain bone-seeking isotopes,[12] lead,[13] and tetracycline antibiotics,[14–16] which are taken up on surfaces of bone deposition, have been used for this purpose, and the appositional growth rate has been found to be up to 10 to 15 μm weekly in man and in the dog. When the rate of appositional growth is low, osteoblasts are less conspicuous and the surface layer of osteoid tissue is thinner than when growth is more active. Studies with tritiated thymidine[17–19] show that the osteoblasts do not undergo mitosis but are formed by the proliferation and maturation of *osteoprogenitor cells.* New cells are continuously being formed on a growing surface and subsequently are left in the bone tissue as mature osteocytes.

Bone Resorption[6]

Areas of active bone resorption can be identified by the presence of multinucleate giant cells (osteoclasts) in eroded bays—the so-called *Howship's lacunae*[20]—on the bone surface (Fig. 37.2). In contrast to surfaces of bone deposition, resorption surfaces are irregular and crenated, and bear no relation to the direction of the adjacent bone lamellae: they are devoid of anything resembling an osteoid border, and this suggests that the various constituents of bone—mineral, collagen and polysaccharide—are removed simultaneously. The osteoclasts are often grouped in clusters: they usually occupy only a small part of the eroded surface, the remainder of which is covered by nondescript cells. This is responsible for the often-expressed view that resorption of bone can occur in the absence of osteoclasts. However, it seems reasonable to assume that the osteoclast has a short functional life, and that, having produced erosion of bone, it disappears quickly, leaving an irregular —but inactive—area of bone surface.[6, 20a] That osteoclasts bring about resorption of bone was first suggested by Koelliker,[21] in 1873, and this view is still held by most authorities: the enzymatic or chemical mechanism by which the cells bring about the removal of bone is not yet known. Osteoclasts themselves vary greatly in size and in the number of their nuclei; their cytoplasm does not show the intense basiphilia characteristic of osteoblasts. Where an osteoclast is in contact with the bone surface, a striated border is present: the question whether this is part of the cell or part of the bone[6] appears to have been resolved by electron microscopy in favour of the former interpretation (see below, *Ultrastructure*).

Calcification of bone matrix appears to be a necessary precursor of resorption. In rickets, it has been noted[22, 23] that uncalcified osteoid tissue fails to be resorbed: in normal bone, resorption does not involve surfaces that are covered by osteoid tissue.

In the normal adult a considerable part of the available bone surface is inactive, neither deposition nor resorption of bone taking place. Such inert surfaces have a smooth outline, but they fail to show osteoid borders: in sections stained with haematoxylin and eosin there is a superficial linear zone of haematoxyphilia (Fig. 37.2).

Ultrastructure

Electron microscopy has provided important information about the cells of bone.[24–27] The osteoblast, in common with other cells that synthetize collagen, has much endoplasmic reticulum (Figs 37.4 and 37.5). It is this material that gives the cells their characteristic cytoplasmic basiphilia on light microscopy.

Osteoclasts have strikingly different ultrastructural features (Figs 37.6 and 37.7). Their cytoplasm contains many mitochondria but there is little endoplasmic reticulum. The striated border, where the osteoclast is in contact with the bone surface, has a complex appearance due to folding of the cell membrane and the presence of numerous small vacuoles and vesicles, some of which may contain crystals of bone mineral. These features, of course, are consistent with the role of the osteoclast as the active agent of bone resorption.

Osteocytes show less evidence of metabolic activity than osteoblasts and osteoclasts (Fig. 37.8). They are generally regarded as inactive cells, although variation in their size and appearance have led to suggestions that they may be concerned in a process of *osteocytic resorption*.[28, 29] The importance of this process, and even its occurrence, is not unchallenged.

Scanning electron microscopy is being applied to the study of bone surfaces, with interesting results that are still in an early stage of assessment.[30]

'Turnover' of Bone Tissue

It is not only during growth of the skeleton that the processes of bone deposition and bone resorption are active: they continue throughout adult life and are responsible for a continuous remodelling—or *turnover*—of bone tissue. Normally, the two opposed processes are balanced in any part of the skeleton. As long ago as 1853, Tomes and de Morgan[31] were aware, from histological study of normal bone, of the continuous remodelling of adult bone tissue. They observed resorption cavities and developing Haversian systems in cortical bone, and they were the first to realize that the Haversian architecture of this tissue resulted from alternating periods of resorption and deposition at any given point. In fact, each Haversian system, or osteon, has been preceded by a resorption cavity, and has been formed by the deposition of concentric lamellae of bone on the inner wall of this cavity. The position of osteons changes slightly with each cycle of resorption, and as age increases a good deal of cortical bone comes to consist of incomplete residues of earlier osteons. In transverse sections, the cement lines bounding Haversian systems indicate the outlines of the antecedent resorption cavities: they are *reversal lines*, indicating a change

11

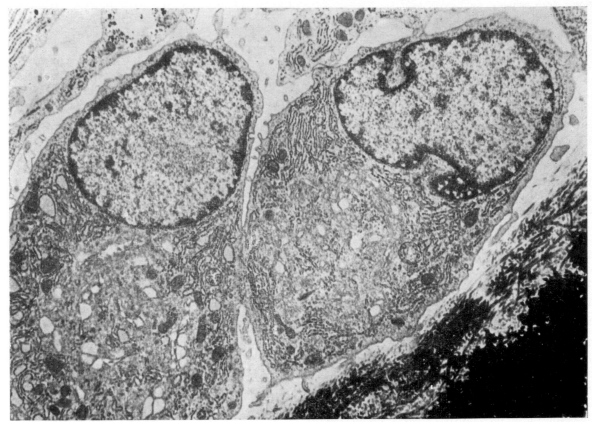

Fig. 37.4. Electron micrograph of normal osteoblasts on partly calcified surface of developing cancellous bone of metaphysis (rat). × 5000.

from resorption to deposition, and this explains their irregular and crenated contour (Fig. 37.1).

The concept of continuous remodelling of bone tissue has come to be of great interest, not only in normal bone, but also in connexion with the study of metabolic bone diseases (see page 2424). Quantitative histological evaluation of the local rates of bone turnover for different parts of the skeleton is now possible,[32] particularly when use is made of vital bone markers.[14, 33, 34]

A technique that is finding increasing application in this connexion is the use of radioactive 'bone-seeking' isotopes for the determination of the over-all rate of calcium accretion.[35–37] The subject is a complex one, and the following account is only a very brief outline. There is a dynamic equilibrium, with a rapid exchange rate, between the calcium of the blood and part of the calcium in bone tissue: following its injection into the blood, an isotope such as ^{45}Ca quickly becomes diluted in the 'exchangeable pool', from which it is removed partly by excretion in the urine and faeces and partly by incorporation into the less readily exchangeable parts of the skeleton. If the amount of urinary and faecal excretion is known, the rate of dilution of the isotope in the blood gives a measure of the rate of incorporation of calcium into the skeleton. Much of this incorporation of calcium appears to result from the deposition of new tissue, although slow exchange processes are also at work:[38] the calcium accretion rates that have been obtained are thought to give a good indication of the overall rate of bone accretion. Values of approximately 10 mg of calcium per kilogram of body weight per day have been obtained in normal adults. Abnormally high rates occur in patients with Paget's disease of bone and in those with hyperparathyroidism, conditions in which histological observations also indicate very active bone formation (see pages 2436, 2438 and 2431; in osteoporosis the calcium accretion rate has not been found to depart from normal (see page 2427).

Neglecting any slow exchange processes, and assuming that accretion in the normal skeleton is

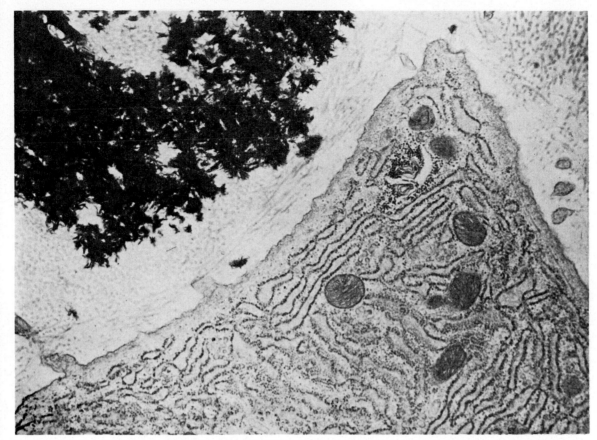

Fig. 37.5. Electron micrograph of part of a normal osteoblast in contact with bone surface (rat). The cytoplasm contains conspicuous endoplasmic reticulum. A thin layer of uncalcified bone (osteoid tissue) separates the cell from the bone mineral, which appears black. × 15 000.

balanced by an equal amount of resorption, a value of 10 mg of calcium per kilogram of body weight per day represents, for a person weighing 70 kg, whose skeleton contains approximately 1000 g of calcium, a turnover of 0·07 per cent of the skeleton each day, or a mean life of approximately seven years for bone tissue. Despite the assumptions involved, this at least indicates the order of magnitude of the rate of turnover of bone tissue under normal conditions.

There is evidence to suggest that different parts of the skeleton have different rates of turnover, and that the rate for cancellous bone is greater than that for cortical bone: this may explain the severer involvement of cancellous bone in generalized osteoporosis (see page 2426).

Control of Bone Deposition and Bone Resorption

The factors controlling bone deposition and bone resorption are numerous, and the ways in which they influence cellular activity are not always clearly understood. Bone responds to changes in mechanical stress by changes in structure. Vascular factors have been much discussed in connexion with the control of osteoblastic and osteoclastic activity, but apart from the occasional demonstration of hyperaemic changes in areas of active bone destruction, little is known of their exact role. Bone formation, in common with other processes of tissue synthesis, is impaired under conditions of poor nutrition and also by various toxic and metabolic substances: little is known of the factors controlling it, even under physiological conditions.

Parathyroid Activity

Bone resorption appears to be under the general control of the parathyroid glands, increased secretion of parathyroid hormone resulting in increased bone resorption, apparently as a result of increased osteoclastic activity. This results in

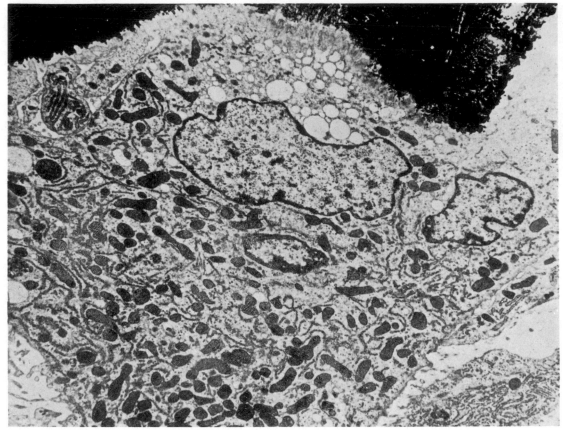

Fig. 37.6. Electron micrograph of a normal osteoclast in contact with resorbing surface of cancellous bone of metaphysis (rat). There are numerous mitochondria in the cytoplasm. × 6000.

the mobilization of bone salt, an effect that tends to elevate the serum calcium. As a low serum calcium is a stimulus to parathyroid activity, it can be seen that the parathyroid glands and the skeleton constitute a homoeostatic mechanism for the control of the serum calcium.[39] In hypoparathyroidism the serum calcium is not maintained at its normal level, but remains low; in hyperparathyroidism the serum calcium is increased, and there may be evidence of greatly increased osteoclastic bone resorption (see page 2431).

Calcitonin

The physiological role of the plasma-calcium-lowering hormone, calcitonin, is still the subject of intensive study. Calcitonin was initially thought to be secreted by the parathyroids,[40] but later work shows that it is of thyroid origin (see pages 1980 and 2041 in Volume 4).[41–44] The mechanism by which it lowers the serum calcium has been the subject of much investigation: evidence from tissue culture,[45, 46] as well as from studies on animals,[47, 48] indicates that the primary action of the hormone is to inhibit bone resorption. Increased density of trabecular bone and a reduction in the number of osteoclasts have been observed to follow administration of calcitonin to parathyroidectomized rats.[49]

The role of calcitonin in bone pathology is not yet known in any detail.

Maturation of Osteons

We have seen that Haversian systems, or osteons, result from the concentric deposition of lamellar bone in cylindrical resorption cavities. At an early stage of its development an osteon appears in cross-section as a thin layer of bone adjacent to the cement line bounding the system: ultimately it consists of a cylinder of bone with a narrow central canal. Examination of undecalcified bone sections by radiomicrography has established that osteons vary in the degree of their mineralization (Figs

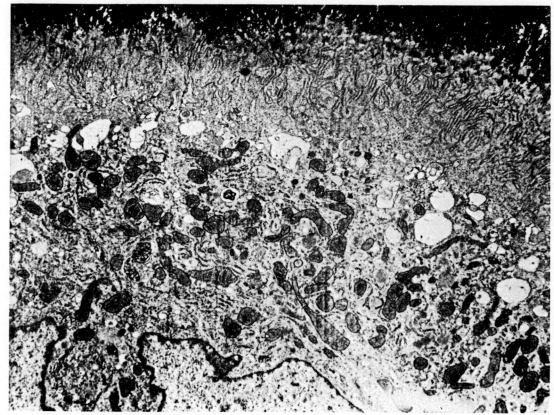

Fig. 37.7. Electron micrograph of part of a normal osteoclast to show the striated border of the cell. Calcified bone is seen at the upper margin of the field. × 12 000.

37.10 and 37.44).[50, 51] There is, in fact, a progressive increase in the mineralization of lamellar bone following its formation; this process may not be complete for many months.[52] The amount of matrix does not appear to change during the maturation of the bone, the mineral content increasing as a result of the replacement of water.[53] There is some evidence that the arrangement of the collagen fibres can change as the age of the osteon increases.[54]

Recently formed and still incompletely mineralized osteons are the site of maximum uptake of bone-seeking radioactive isotopes,[55-57] such as ^{45}Ca. Some, at least, of the calcium in these structures is evidently in rapid equilibrium with the serum calcium, and thus is part of the 'exchangeable pool'. As the tissue becomes more completely mineralized its calcium becomes less readily available for such exchange reactions.

Age Changes in Bone

Throughout life, bone tissue shows progressive ageing changes: these become important after middle age, and must not be mistaken for changes due to disease. In old age the amount of bone tissue in most situations becomes reduced, the change particularly affecting cancellous bone and the inner parts of the cortex of the long bones. Histological study shows that bone trabeculae become more slender and cortical bone more porous.[58-62] Information on the amount of bone tissue normally present in different parts of the skeleton can be obtained by a variety of other methods, including weighing individual bones,[63] measurement of the cortical thickness[64, 65] or area,[66, 67] determination of radiographic density[68, 69] and calcium content,[70, 71] and measurement of the apparent density of macerated bone specimens.[72] All these methods show an appreciable decrease of skeletal mass in normal individuals after about 50 years of age: it is consequently difficult to draw a dividing line between age changes of this type and minor degrees of osteoporosis (see page 2426).

Certain additional microscopical changes are encountered in ageing bone.[73] Death of osteocytes

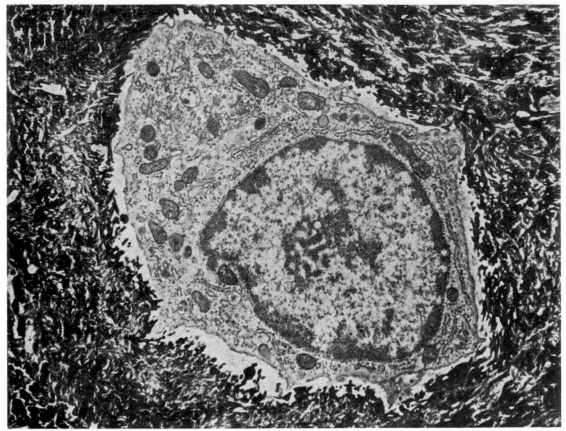

Fig. 37.8. Electron micrograph of a normal osteocyte in a metaphysis (rat). The cell is completely surrounded by calcified bone matrix. × 6000.

occurs, and an increasing number of empty osteo-cyte lacunae can be identified in sections: in cortical bone (Fig. 37.9) many of these are situated in areas of interstitial bone. In radiomicrographs of undecalcified bone sections (Fig. 37.10) some of the lacunae are seen to have become filled with bone salt. Although some Haversian canals are occupied by amorphous calcified material (Figs 37.9 and 37.10), with obliteration of blood vessels, it has not been established that the loss of osteocytes is due to impairment of blood supply: in fact, the diminution in their number may precede the development of evident abnormalities of the vessels.

Bone Growth

During development, bone is formed either by *intramembranous ossification* or by *endochondral ossification*. The bone itself has the same ultimate histological structure, but in endochondral ossifica-tion it is laid down on a scaffolding of calcified cartilage. Most bones are composite structures, being formed partly by intramembranous and partly by endochondral ossification: there is no evidence that their behaviour under pathological circumstances in the child or adult is in any way related to the manner of their embryological formation.

Endochondral Ossification

Endochondral ossification is the process by which most bones grow in length. It is best seen in the region of the epiphysial cartilage plate of a developing long bone (Fig. 37.11). It comprises a coordinated sequence of cellular processes.[5] These are: the multiplication, growth and degeneration of the cartilage cells in the epiphysial plate (the appearances of the degenerating cartilage are sometimes described as 'hypertrophic'); the vas-cularization of the empty cell spaces of the de-generated ('hypertrophic') cartilage by blood vessels, accompanied by connective tissue cells from the

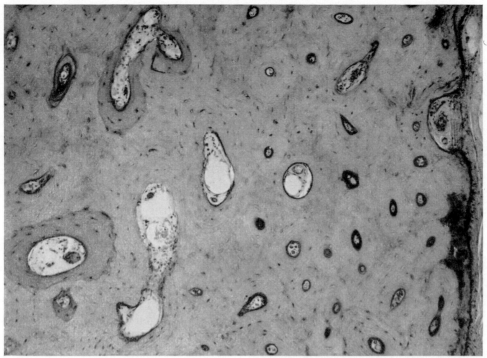

Fig. 37.9. Cortical bone: age changes. Cortex of femoral shaft of a man aged 84. Many of the osteo-cyte lacunae are empty, and some of the Haversian canals are occupied by amorphous basiphile material. Same specimen as in Fig. 37.10. *Haematoxylin–eosin.* × 80.

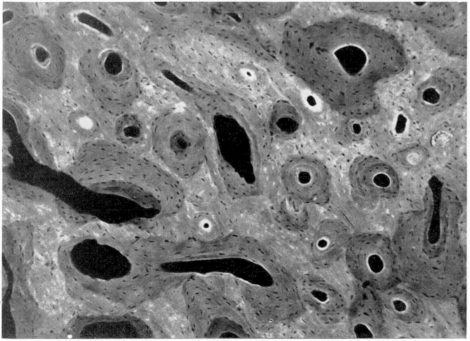

Fig. 37.10. Cortical bone: age changes. Radiomicrograph of an undecalcified section from the bone illustrated in Fig. 37.9. Some of the osteocyte lacunae are calcified; one Haversian canal is plugged with heavily calcified material, which appears white in the illustration. × 80.

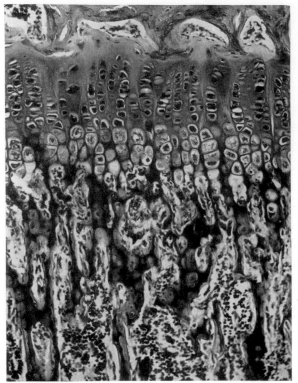

Fig. 37.11. Endochondral ossification: epiphysial cartilage plate of a tibia of a rat. The cartilage cells are arranged in columns: those on the lower aspect of the plate are degenerate ('hypertrophic'). The metaphysial trabeculae contain cores of unresorbed cartilage covered by bone, which stains more palely. *Haematoxylin–eosin.* × 130.

metaphysical surface of the palte; the formation, by the ingrowing connective tissue cells (osteoblasts), of a network of bone trabeculae on the framework of the unresorbed cartilage; and, finally, the remodelling of this bony tissue. Under normal circumstances, these processes proceed in equilibrium, with the result that the metaphysial bone trabeculae extend continuously into a receding zone of 'hypertrophic' cartilage, so extending the length of the bony shaft. The proliferating and maturing cartilage cells are arranged in columns in the plate, and their degeneration and the vascularization at the metaphysial surface appear to be a consequence of the calcification of the cartilage matrix in this region. When calcification fails to occur, as in rickets (see page 2418), the cells fail to degenerate, the plate becomes thicker, and its cell columns become irregular. Endochondral ossification is not seen in the normal adult skeleton, but can be reactivated under pathological conditions, particularly in fracture callus (page 2402).

Factors Influencing Bone Growth

The general control of bone growth and the effects of dietary, hormonal and other factors on it have been reviewed elsewhere.[74]

Endocrine Influences.—A very great volume of clinical and experimental evidence has established the importance of hormonal factors in the control of skeletal growth and maturation.[75] Normal skeletal growth is dependent on the presence of the growth hormone of the pituitary, which appears to have a direct effect on the proliferation of many types of cell, including those of the growing epiphysial cartilage plate. During adolescence, thyroid hormone, gonadal hormones, and adrenal androgens are important both in influencing bone growth and in bringing about skeletal maturation, with cessation of growth and epiphysial fusion. Excess or deficiency of each type of hormone is found to have a characteristic effect on growth and development of bone (see pages 2427 to 2430).

Other Factors.—Epiphysial growth can be retarded by local factors, including externally applied pressure, the application of heat or cold, and ionizing radiation. The restricted dietary intake and other metabolic disturbances associated with general illness leave their mark on epiphysial growth, resulting in Harris's 'transverse lines of growth arrest', due to temporary interference with cartilage proliferation.[76, 77] Accelerated growth of the epiphysial plate is sometimes encountered in osteomyelitis or following a fracture of a long bone: it has been suggested that this is an effect of increased vascularity on the growing region.[78] Local interference with the blood supply of the metaphysial surface of the growing plate results in failure of calcification and vascularization of the cartilage, with consequent local thickening.[79]

Calcification of Bone and Cartilage

Much attention has been paid to the chemical mechanisms concerned in the deposition of bone salt. Early work was concerned with the availability of calcium and phosphate ions in the body fluids, and with mechanisms that might increase the concentrations of these ions in the neighbourhood of areas of calcification. In 1923, Howland and Kramer[80, 81] observed that the presence or absence of rickets in children could be correlated with the simple product of calcium and phosphorus concentrations in the plasma: this emphasized that certain minimum ionic concentrations are necessary for calcification to occur. In the same year,

Robison[82] announced the presence, in ossifying cartilage, of an enzyme—phosphatase—that hydrolyses hexose 1-phosphoric acid, yielding free phosphate ions: he suggested that this might be a factor in calcification. Certain difficulties are encountered, however, in envisaging the role of this enzyme in calcification: (1) the pH at which it operates (pH 9·4) is far removed from that of body fluids; (2) phosphoric esters suitable for hydrolysis by the enzyme are lacking; (3) similar enzymes are present in tissues that do not calcify. Current opinion is that alkaline phosphatase is likelier to be concerned in the synthesis of the protein material of the bone matrix than in the actual process of calcification. The level of alkaline phosphatase in the blood, however, is an important indication of the metabolic activity of the skeleton, being raised in conditions—both generalized and local—in which osteoblastic activity is increased. Other enzymes, which belong to the glycolytic cycle that is so important in muscle, have been discovered in calcifying cartilage, but their role in calcification is still not established.

Adequate concentrations of calcium, phosphate, and hydrogen ions are not by themselves sufficient to explain calcification, and recent interest has centred on local mechanisms that might be responsible for initiating this process. A number of chemical constituents of bone matrix, including the polysaccharide known as chondroitin sulphate, have been suggested for such a role, but so far without any definite conclusions being reached. Certain types of collagen, precipitated from solution, have the ability to initiate calcification from solutions containing appropriate mineral constituents,[83] and the suggestion has been made that the collagen macromolecule itself may be concerned in this initiating or 'nucleating' mechanism. This suggestion is supported by studies of calcifying bone tissue with the electron microscope:[84, 85] these have shown a close relation between the smallest bone crystals and collagen fibres. In cartilage, the earliest crystals of mineral material have been shown to form within 'matrix vesicles': these are regarded as initiating calcification.[85a] As well as these nucleating factors, which initiate calcification, there must also be important factors that inhibit the occurrence of calcification in tissues other than bone collagen.[86]

DEVELOPMENTAL ABNORMALITIES

The skeleton is liable to a number of types of developmental abnormality. Some of these are

11*

local, involving a single bone or a group of bones, which may be absent, present in diminutive form, fused with neighbouring bones, or duplicated. The related soft tissues may also be affected. The morbid anatomy of such abnormalities of the limbs has been comprehensively documented.[87] They were frequent among the children affected by thalidomide (see page 2197).[87a] Spina bifida, the failure of development of the neural arches of certain vertebrae, is an example of a local abnormality involving the axial skeleton; in cleft palate, the facial skeleton is involved. The aetiology of many types of local developmental abnormality is obscure, but some, at least, are genetical.[88] It has been found that a single gene abnormality, particularly if it is dominant, can result in a variety of skeletal abnormalities: in one example,[89] different members of a family showed cleft hand, gross malformation of the legs with absence of the tibiae, and deformities of the arms, all apparently the results of the variability of expression of a single gene.

In contrast to such localized abnormalities of development, there are conditions in which either the whole skeleton is abnormal or there are numerous and widespread lesions.[90] Some of the more important of these generalized anomalies are considered in the following paragraphs.

Osteogenesis Imperfecta[91-94]

This is a generalized abnormality of the skeleton that results from a specific gene abnormality, inherited as an autosomal dominant. In some cases the bony abnormality is evident at birth (*osteogenesis imperfecta congenita*): the condition is then invariably fatal. In others it becomes apparent during childhood or adolescence (*osteogenesis imperfecta tarda*). The bony abnormality is frequently associated with blueness of the sclerae and with deafness, and occasionally with excessive mobility of joints. The sclerae appear blue because they are abnormally thin, thus allowing the pigment of the choroid to be seen; the deafness results from otosclerosis. There may be an associated abnormality of dentine formation (*dentinogenesis imperfecta*—see page 974, Volume 3).

In the congenital form there are multiple fractures and deformities of the bones (Fig. 37.12). The cortical bone is greatly reduced in amount: histologically, instead of being lamellar in structure, it consists of a spongy network of non-lamellar bone, with areas of cartilaginous and bony callus in the region of fractures. The changes are usually

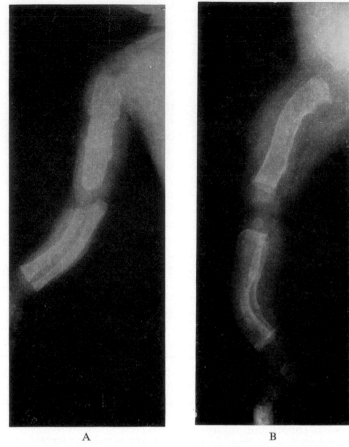

A　　　　　　　　　　　B

Figs 37.12A and 37.12B. Osteogenesis imperfecta. Radiographs of an upper and a lower limb of a stillborn infant, showing fractures and deformities of long bones. The normal cortical outline is absent.

regarded as the result of a functional abnormality of osteoblasts; the proliferating cartilage of the growth plates at the ends of the long bones is relatively normal.

In older individuals, the changes are less striking. The bones are abnormally slender, and the thickness of cortical bone is greatly reduced. The tibiae and femora are often bowed, and the pelvis is often narrowed: these deformities result from the thinning of the bones, and not from any failure of mineralization. As well as being slender, the bones appear to be abnormally brittle, the condition sometimes being known as *fragilitas ossium*. Fractures of long bones are frequent, and are ordinarily the outstanding clinical manifestation. Fracture repair usually occurs in a normal fashion, but occasionally bulky masses of cellular, 'hyperplastic' callus develop and may even be confused with sarcoma.[95] In these older individuals, sections of

bones sometimes show absence of the normal lamellar and Haversian architecture of the tissue, but there does not appear to be any particular histological abnormality that is pathognomonic of the condition.

Achondroplasia[96, 97]

Like osteogenesis imperfecta, achondroplasia is the result of a specific gene abnormality. It is inherited as an autosomal dominant, about half the offspring of an achondroplastic parent being affected. Most cases of the disease represent the occurrence of a fresh mutation, usually associated with paternal ageing.[98] It is the commonest cause of dwarfism, occurring once in about 10 000 births. About 80 per cent of achondroplastic dwarfs are stillborn or die during the first year of life; those surviving early childhood have a normal expectation of life.

There is selective interference with the proliferation of cartilage cells, particularly in the growth plates of the long bones of the limbs and in the synchondroses of the base of the skull. As a result, the limbs are very short in relation to the more normal proportions of the trunk (Figs 37.13 and 37.14). The base of the skull is also shortened and the foramen magnum reduced in size. The width of the shaft of the long bones is not affected, although their shortening gives them an illusory appearance of excessive width at the metaphyses.

Histology

Histologically, there is evidence of diminished proliferation of cartilage cells in the growth

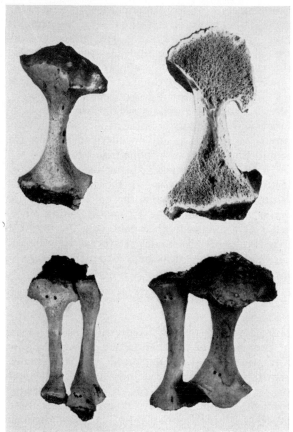

Fig. 37.14.§ Achondroplasia. Bones of upper and lower limbs of an achondroplastic fetus at term. The cartilaginous ends of the bones have been removed during preparation of the specimens.

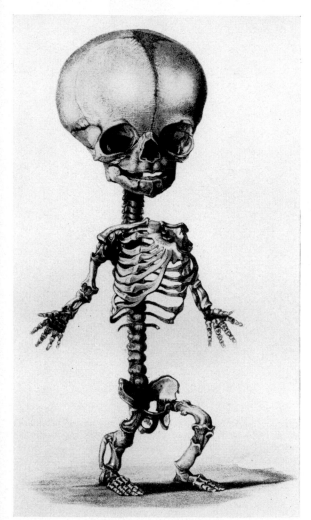

Fig. 37.13. Achondroplasia. The skeleton of an achondroplastic fetus at term (reproduced from: Liston, R., *Elements of Surgery*, 2nd edition; London, 1840). Note the disproportionate shortening of the limb bones.

cartilages at the ends of the long bones. The normal columnar arrangement of cartilage cells is absent, there being only a few normally oriented cells on the metaphysial surface of the plate. Calcification of cartilage matrix occurs normally in the neighbourhood of any hypertrophic cells that are formed: osteoblastic bone formation, whether in the metaphysis or the shaft, is unaffected.

Osteopetrosis[99, 100]

This rare disease, which was described by Albers-Schönberg[101] in 1904, is characterized by excessive radiographic density of the entire skeleton. It usually becomes evident in early childhood, but it is clear that the disorder of bone development begins during fetal life. It appears to result from a specific gene abnormality, which is inherited as an autosomal recessive.[102] Death may result

§ See *Acknowledgements*, page 2488.

from anaemia or from intercurrent infection, but some patients survive without any abnormality other than their dense bones. The pathogenesis of the condition is not completely understood, but the skeletal abnormality appears to result from failure of removal of calcified cartilage and bone trabeculae that normally takes place at the meta-physes: excessive amounts of bone are also present in areas where endochondral ossification does not occur, indicating a similar interference with the remodelling activities of bone tissue itself.

The bones are thickened and heavy, hard and brittle: the metaphyses of the long bones are frequently expanded, and the cut surface of the dense metaphysial bone frequently shows transverse and longitudinal streaks (Fig. 37.15). The marrow cavity is largely replaced by calcified cartilage or dense trabecular bone: the remaining marrow is usually fibrotic.

Histology

Histologically, interest centres in the processes of endochondral ossification and membrane bone formation. In the epiphysial cartilage plates, growth appears to proceed fairly normally, although the overall length of the bones is somewhat reduced. On the metaphysial surface of the plate, however, large amounts of calcified cartilage matrix persist, and become incorporated in a dense medullary plug of cartilage and bone: there is little or none of the normal osteoclastic removal and remodelling of cartilage and bone. In areas where membrane bone formation occurs, immature non-lamellar bone persists without much evidence of normal remodelling activities.

Anaemia is a frequent complication, and is usually attributed to obliteration of the bone marrow: its severity, however, is not always related to the degree of bony change. The abnormal bone is liable to fracture; osteomyelitis has also been reported, particularly in relation to abnormally erupting teeth. Changes in the bones of the skull may result in compression of cranial nerves, with such manifestations as optic atrophy and deafness.

Enchondromatosis

In this rare condition, multiple cartilaginous nodules are present within bones. The lesions, which usually become apparent during the period of growth, may range from microscopical nodules to bulky cartilaginous tumours. Enchondromatosis

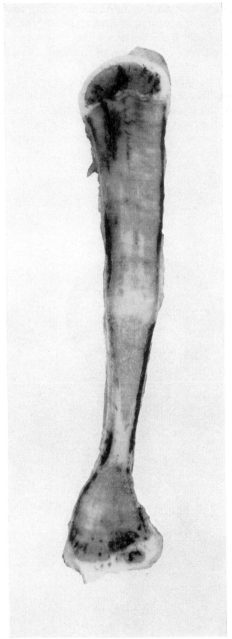

Fig. 37.15.§ Osteopetrosis. Longitudinally divided humerus of a child with growing epiphyses. Note the complete replacement of the marrow cavity by calcified tissue: histological examination showed this to consist partly of cartilage and partly of bone.

is sometimes known as *Ollier's disease*,[103] a name that has been given also to the condition of multiple exostoses (see page 2400). As Ollier's cases of enchondromatosis showed a predominantly unilateral distribution of bone lesions, some authorities apply the eponym only to such cases. Other synonyms are multiple enchondromas and dys-chondroplasia. The aetiology of enchondromatosis is unknown: it is not familial, and it is to be distinguished from multiple exostoses, to which it is in no way related.[104] The term *Maffucci's syndrome* has been applied to cases of enchondro-matosis associated with haemangiomas of soft tissues.[105-107]

Common sites for enchondromas include the small bones of the hands and feet (Fig. 37.16), the long bones of the limbs (Fig. 37.17)—particularly the region of the knees and the lower end of the radius and ulna—and the pelvis. As already noted, a particular case may show predominant involvement of one side of the body: sometimes the majority of lesions are confined to a single limb. Long bones that are severely affected are usually shortened and often angulated or otherwise de-formed (Fig. 37.17). In the long bones, the lesions develop in the metaphysial region in continuity

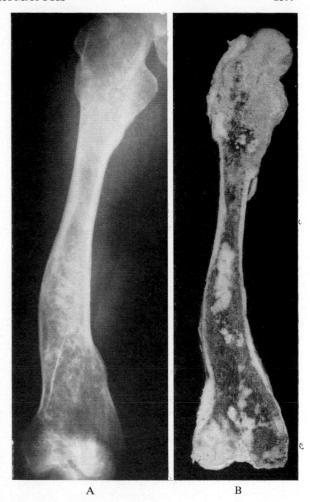

A   B

Fig. 37.17.§ Enchondromatosis.

A.§ Radiograph of a femur from the case illustrated in Fig. 37.16. The bone is shortened and bent, and shows scattered opaque foci throughout the marrow cavity. See also Fig. 37.17B.

B.§ The femur illustrated in Fig. 37.17A has been divided longitudinally. Rounded cartilaginous nodules can be seen on the cut surface.

with the epiphysial cartilage plate: later they become separated from the plate and remain as cartilaginous nodules in the metaphysial spongiosa or marrow cavity. It has been suggested that enchondromas can also develop from periosteal rests of cartilage that grow inward to reach the marrow cavity.[108]

Histology

Histologically, the lesions consist of rounded nodules of cartilage (Fig. 37.18), which may or

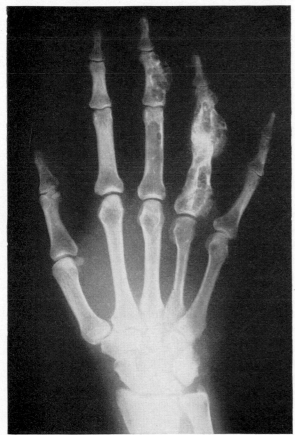

Fig. 37.16. Enchondromatosis. Radiograph of a hand, showing multiple cartilaginous tumours in the phalanges. Same case as in Figs 37.17A and 37.17B.

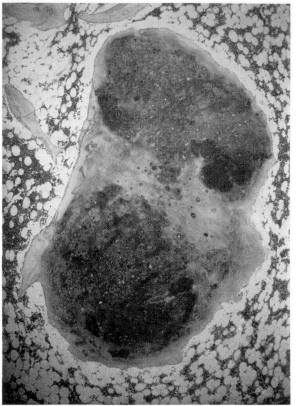

Fig. 37.18. Enchondromatosis. Typical appearance of a cartilaginous nodule from the marrow cavity of an affected bone. *Haematoxylin–eosin.* × 35.

may not be calcified. Even in the absence of malignant change they tend to be more cellular than the usual solitary enchondroma.

Outcome

Growth of the cartilaginous nodules may stop with skeletal maturation; in other cases it continues and may result in bulky tumours, particularly of the bones of the hands and feet. Chondrosarcoma sometimes develops in a lesion of enchondromatosis,[109, 110] but there is insufficient published information to give an accurate idea of its incidence.

Hereditary Multiple Exostoses

This abnormality of skeletal development is characterized by the presence of multiple cartilage-capped exostoses and by abnormality of the contour of the terminal parts of the shaft of long bones. The term *diaphysial aclasis* was applied to it by Keith[111] to describe the characteristic failure of normal remodelling of bone. The condition results

from a specific gene abnormality that is inherited as an autosomal dominant, about half the offspring of an affected person showing bony lesions.[112] Although rare, this is probably the commonest of the generalized developmental abnormalities of the skeleton. Like enchondromatosis (see above), it is sometimes referred to as Ollier's disease (Ollier described multiple exostoses in 1889,[112a] 10 years before his account of enchondromatosis[103]).

The lesions develop during the growing period, usually in late childhood: occasionally the abnormality is not noticed until later in life. The exostoses are externally projecting masses of cancellous bone, each covered by a cap of cartilage (Fig. 37.19). They commonly occur in the long bones of the limbs, developing in the metaphysis near the periphery of the epiphysial cartilage plate, from which they become separated as growth of the bone continues. They appear to arise as areas of cartilaginous metaplasia in the periosteum.[113] Common sites are the femur and tibia in the region of the knee joint, the upper end of the humerus, both ends of the fibula, and the lower end of the radius and ulna. The contour of the metaphysial part of an involved bone is often irregular (Fig. 37.19) and it may be impossible to distinguish between the remodelling abnormality and the actual exostosis. Involved bones show a variable degree of shortening, due to reduced growth at the epiphysial cartilage plate.

The microscopical structure of the exostoses is identical with that of a solitary exostosis (see page 2450).

Outcome

The growth of exostoses usually ceases at the time of skeletal maturation. Chondrosarcoma sometimes develops in the cartilage cap. The incidence of malignant change varies greatly in reported series: in one study it was present in 10 per cent of the cases.[114]

Other Generalized Developmental Abnormalities

There is a considerable number of other generalized abnormalities of bone development.[90] They are rare conditions of obscure aetiology and pathogenesis: it is consequently not easy to define them or to discuss their relation to one another in other than clinical terms. In *metaphysial dysostosis, dysplasia epiphysialis multiplex* and *dysplasia epiphysialis punctata* the abnormality chiefly affects developing epiphysial cartilage. In *Hunter–Hurler disease* (see page 2237) and in the *Morquio–*

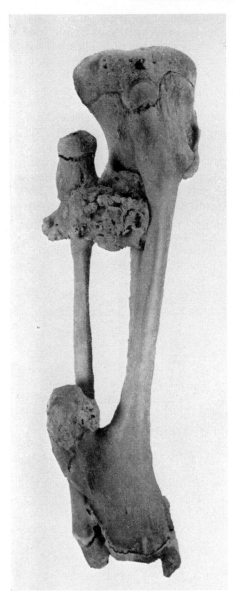

Fig. 37.19.§ Multiple exostoses in a tibia and fibula. A bulky exostosis of the upper end of the fibula has indented the adjacent tibia; a similar exostosis of the lower end of the tibia projects in front of the fibula. The surface of the upper part of the metaphysis of the tibia is irregular.

Brailsford type of osteochondrodystrophy,[115, 116] both of which are familial, the whole skeleton is affected by dwarfing and by a variety of bone deformities that appear to result from metabolic defects characterized by widespread deposition in the tissues of particular mucopolysaccharides, which are also found in the patient's urine.[88]

Camurati–Engelmann disease[117, 118] and *infantile cortical hyperostosis* are characterized by abnormal and excessive periosteal bone formation involving the shaft of the long bones and occasionally other parts of the skeleton. In *melorrhoeostosis* and *osteopoikilosis* local areas of abnormally dense bone are present.

Fibrous dysplasia of bone, another condition of obscure aetiology, is probably best regarded as an abnormality of bone development involving the later rather than the earlier stages of the process. Because of its special features and general importance it is discussed separately (see page 2439).

REACTION TO TRAUMA

Repair of Fractures[119]

Fracture of a bone initiates a series of tissue changes, the ultimate result of which is the restoration of structure and function to normal. Knowledge of the repair of fractures is based largely on the study of animal material;[120–123] comparatively few papers describe the histological findings in man.[124, 125]

As well as disrupting bony structures, a fracture severs innumerable blood vessels in the marrow spaces and in the Haversian canals of cortical bone. The periosteum is usually separated from the surface of the bone in the region of the fracture: it may be lacerated, and the surrounding soft tissues may also be damaged. The vascular damage results in immediate haemorrhage in the region of the fracture: the resulting haematoma occupies the gap between the bone ends, and usually extends for some distance subperiosteally.

Formation and Role of Callus.—The tissue damage resulting from the fracture stimulates proliferation of the adjoining cells: this gives rise to a mass of tissue, composite in its structure and origin, termed *callus*, that ultimately establishes bony continuity between the fractured parts (see Figs 37.20 and 37.21). All the tissue components in the neighbourhood of the fracture take part in the formation of the callus. In a long bone, the periosteum forms a collar of tissue known as *external callus*; the cells covering the endosteal surface of the bone and the trabecular surfaces near the fracture give rise to *medullary*, or *internal*, *callus*. At the margin of the haematoma, capillary blood vessels and connective tissue cells invade the clot (Fig. 37.22). The osteocytes of the cortical bone contribute little or nothing to callus formation: near the fracture line many of them have undergone necrosis as a result of

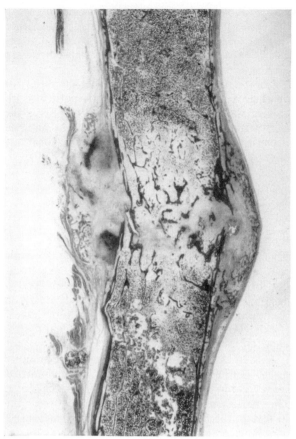

Fig. 37.20.§ Fracture repair. Rib fracture, showing periosteal displacement and early callus formation. (Human material.) See Fig. 37.21. *Haematoxylin–eosin.* × 4.

vascular damage, while those that are alive are imprisoned in their lacunae in the bone tissue.

The external callus (Fig. 37.23) results from the proliferation of the deep layer of the periosteum, either where this is in contact with the bony surface or where it has been separated from it by the fracture. Initially, it consists of trabeculae of non-lamellar bone, together with fibrous tissue and cartilage. Cartilage forms where the callus develops most rapidly and is usually located in the thickest part of the external callus at the actual line of the fracture. Cartilaginous callus is seen in man (Figs 37.21 and 37.24) as well as in experimental fractures in small laboratory animals. Movement between the bone ends is a stimulus to the formation of callus, and, in particular, to the formation of cartilaginous callus: when it is completely prevented, as in a compression arthrodesis, union is quickly effected by the development of a very small amount of bony callus, without any formation of cartilage.[126]

The cells of the cartilaginous areas of callus show the same sequence of proliferation and 'hypertrophy' as is seen in the normal epiphysial cartilage plate (see page 2392): the hypertrophic cartilage becomes calcified, and is replaced by endochondral bone. The distinction between bony and cartilaginous callus is not always a clear one, tissue frequently being present that shows some of the histological features of each (Fig. 37.25). The internal callus (Figs 37.21 and 37.26) consists of bone trabeculae and fibrous tissue developed from endosteal cells and marrow components: areas of cartilage may also be present (Fig. 37.24).

The result of the development of callus in these situations is that the bone ends become loosely united by tissue containing a fine framework of slender trabeculae of non-lamellar bone. As bone formation continues, the fracture becomes less

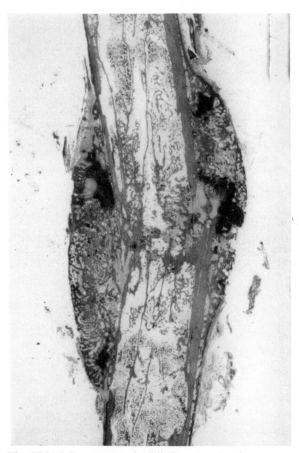

Fig. 37.21.§ Fracture repair. Rib fracture, showing a stage of repair later than that illustrated in Fig. 37.20. Abundant external callus unites the bone ends; callus is also present in the marrow cavity. The darkly staining parts of the external callus are cartilage. (Human material.) *Haematoxylin–eosin.* × 4.

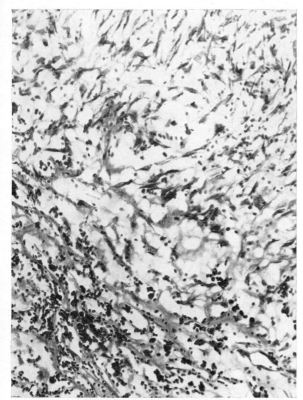

Fig. 37.22. Fracture repair. Granulation tissue replacing central haematoma. (Experimental fracture of rabbit's tibia.) *Haematoxylin–eosin.* × 175.

mobile, and ultimately reaches the stage of 'clinical union'. With the passage of time, remodelling activities convert the callus to a maturer structure consisting of lamellar bone and ultimately showing a normal cancellous and cortical architecture. The amount of bony callus and its distribution appear to be largely governed by the stresses and strains to which the fracture site is subjected: bone is deposited where these are greatest and is removed where it does not serve a useful mechanical function. This is in accord with the generalization, known as *Wolff's law*,[127] that a bone, normal or abnormal, develops the structure that is most suited to resist the forces acting on it. An angulated fracture becomes buttressed on the concave (weight-bearing) side, while over-riding bone ends (not subjected to weight-bearing stresses) are removed.

The period occupied by the process of fracture repair varies greatly. In small laboratory animals, callus formation is active within a few days of fracture and firm union has developed in two to three weeks; in most human fractures a considerably longer period is required. The application of

isotope techniques for the study of bone turnover (see page 2388) indicates that active remodelling of fracture sites in man continues for as long as 12 months.[128]

Non-Union of Fractures

The process of fracture repair occasionally fails, non-union resulting. The reasons for this are not always known, but factors such as ischaemia of the bone ends, undue mobility of the fracture, interposition of soft tissue between the bone ends, and infection are important. In cases of established non-union the bone ends are covered by dense fibrous tissue: this is a barrier to bridging of the gap by callus. If non-union is prolonged, a pseud-arthrosis results, the opposed surfaces undergoing cartilaginous metaplasia to form a false joint.

'Pathological Fracture'

A variety of osteolytic lesions may be complicated by *pathological fracture*, a term used to indicate a fracture predisposed to by a pathological change in

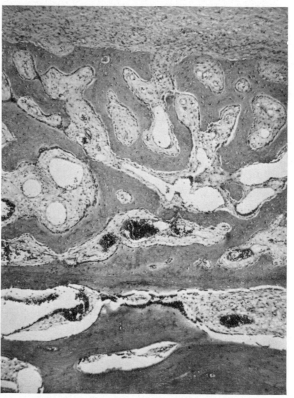

Fig. 37.23. Fracture repair. Periosteal bony callus. (Human material.) *Haematoxylin–eosin.* × 40.

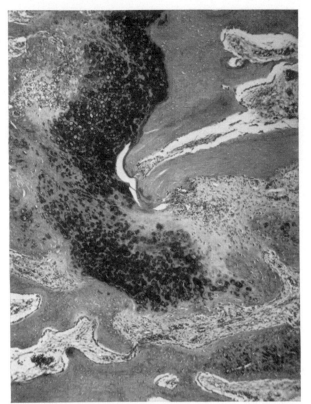

Fig. 37.24. Fracture repair. Cartilaginous callus. (Human material.) *Haematoxylin–eosin.* × 40.

the bone. Such fractures may result from the application of forces that would not have broken the bone if it had been healthy. The underlying lesion often interferes with the process of fracture repair. Osteoporosis is important among conditions predisposing to fractures in old people, and particularly fractures of the femoral neck, which occur with sharply increasing incidence as age increases, and with a great predominance among women in the older age groups.[129]

Bone Grafts

The reparative processes that follow the insertion of a bone graft[119, 130] are comparable to those concerned in fracture repair. Stored bone grafts are, of course, completely non-viable. With fresh homografts a few superficial cells may survive temporarily until the onset of a homograft reaction after about 10 days.[131] Even with a fresh autograft, however, the bulk of the grafted bone is necrotic because of its separation from an effective blood supply. In each case the graft becomes vascularized

by the ingrowth of blood vessels from the periphery: these are accompanied by osteogenic cells, which, as in callus, form a network of trabeculae of non-lamellar bone. This newly-formed bone unites the fragments of the bone graft and joins them to the surrounding bony structures: progressive remodelling ultimately produces normal cortical or cancellous bone at the site of the graft.

Bone Induction

The role of bone induction—the formation of bone by other connective tissues under some biological stimulus—is often discussed in relation to fracture repair and bone grafting. Bone induction can be produced in the connective tissue of the abdominal wall by the transplantation of urinary bladder mucosa,[132] and there is some—although conflicting—experimental evidence to suggest that extracts of bone tissue may have a similar effect.[133] There is little to suggest that this process plays any appreciable part in fracture repair or bone grafting, for in these circumstances an abundance of osteogenic connective tissue is already present.

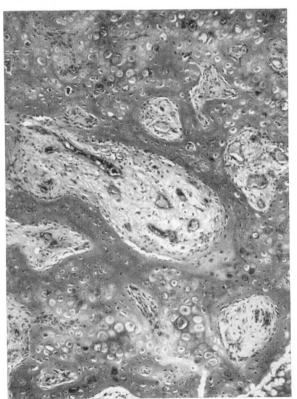

Fig. 37.25. Fracture repair. Chondro-osseous tissue in fracture callus. (Human material.) *Haematoxylin–eosin.* × 70.

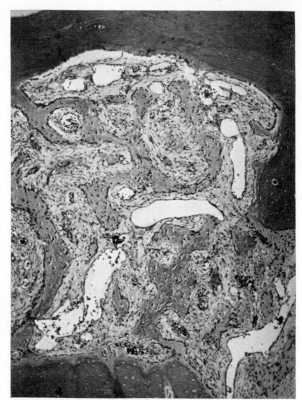

Fig. 37.26. Fracture repair. Endosteal (medullary) callus. The marrow spaces are occupied by osteogenic tissue with slender trabeculae of non-lamellar bone. (Human material.) *Haematoxylin–eosin.* × 40.

VASCULAR DISTURBANCES

The great majority of notable vascular disturbances of bone tend to result in ischaemia and consequent necrosis. Hyperaemia has been mentioned as a possible stimulus to osteoclastic resorption (see page 2389), and is an incidental feature of a variety of disorders of bone, particularly Paget's disease (see page 2437).

'*Vanishing bone disease*', or *massive osteolysis*, is a condition of obscure aetiology in which bone is progressively replaced by vascular tissue (see page 2459).[134]

Some other conditions that are related to vascular disturbances are considered in the following paragraphs.

Ischaemic Necrosis of Bone

Ischaemia of bone leads to necrosis, and this is manifested by death of osteocytes and the consequent presence in sections of empty osteocyte lacunae. It has been noted (see page 2392) that with increasing age, and in the absence of any other abnormality, an increasing number of empty lacunae can be seen, particularly in the interstitial tissue of cortical bone. Under pathological conditions, bone necrosis can take the form either of more marked, but still patchy, loss of cells, or of a circumscribed infarct. The patchy necrosis need not be accompanied by other bone changes; the marrow remains viable, and the general bone structure may be quite unaltered.

Necrosis of Bones of the Legs Due to Atherosclerosis

In cases of atherosclerosis in which gangrene of the distal part of the lower limb has resulted, examination of the more proximal bones of the leg may show widespread, patchy necrosis of bone, sometimes accompanied by frank infarction.[135]

Infarction Complicating Fracture of the Femoral Neck

The vascular damage associated with a fracture usually causes some necrosis of bone, but in most cases this is not extensive. Fracture of the femoral neck, however, often results in gross infarction of the femoral head, as a result of disruption of some or all of the blood vessels supplying it.[136–138] The infarct may involve the whole of the femoral head or only part of it. The necrotic bone and bone marrow can be recognized by the complete absence of cells (Fig. 37.27). The articular cartilage usually remains viable, as its metabolic needs are low and its nutrition and respiratory exchange take place through the synovial fluid as well as through the blood vessels of the underlying bone.

Following infarction, particularly when the fracture is immobilized by impaction or by surgical nailing, the necrotic areas of bone may become revascularized by the ingrowth of blood vessels and connective tissue from the periphery. Osteoblasts form new bone (Fig. 37.28), often on the surface of necrotic trabeculae (a process sometimes termed *creeping substitution of bone*[139]), and the structure can slowly revert to normal. The necrotic bone tissue may undergo a process of collapse,[140] usually as a late complication of a united fracture. There appears to be no change in the mineral content of the necrotic bone:[141] the appearance of increased radiological density that an area of infarcted bone often shows is the result of the occupation of marrow spaces by calcified debris, fragmented trabeculae, or new bone, the relative opacity often

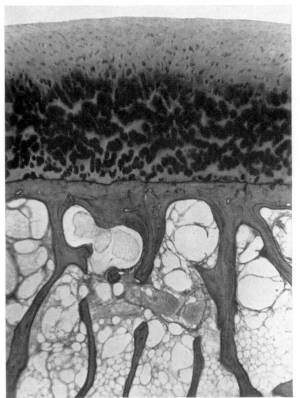

Fig. 37.27. Bone necrosis. Head of a femur, some months after fracture of the neck of the bone. The subchondral bone and bone marrow are completely necrotic. See Fig. 37.28. *Haematoxylin–eosin.* × 20.

being accentuated by the disuse osteoporosis of the surrounding bone tissue.

Infarction of the Femoral Head without Fracture

In young children, infarction of the centre of ossification of the femoral head results in flattening of the articular surface.[142, 143] This is the condition that is usually known as Legg–Perthes disease, or Calvé–Legg–Perthes disease,[144–146] although it was described first by H. Waldenström.[147] Idiopathic infarction of the femoral head is seen in adult life too,[148, 149] particularly in alcoholics, in patients receiving corticosteroid therapy and following renal transplantation. The disease in adults usually leads to collapse of the femoral head and secondary osteoarthritis.

Caisson Disease

Infarction of substantial areas of bone tissue, often subchondral in situation, is occasionally seen in caisson disease (decompression sickness—see page 281 in Volume 1),[150, 151] presumably as the result of obstruction of the smaller arteries in the bone by bubbles of nitrogen.

Other Causes of Ischaemic Necrosis of Bone

Ischaemic bone necrosis frequently accompanies inflammatory lesions. It is the basis of sequestrum formation in suppurative osteomyelitis, tuberculosis and syphilis. It also occurs in Gaucher's disease (see page 759 in Volume 2),[152] in which its pathogenesis is obscure. In cases of sickle cell anaemia and other haemoglobinopathies (see page 469 in Volume 2)[153–155] it is believed to result from obstruction of the small vessels by aggregates of abnormal erythrocytes; thrombosis, increased viscosity of the blood and anaemia may be contributory causes.

'Osteochondritis'[156]

Infarction of bone is the basis of a group of bone lesions that are often referred to by the terms idio-

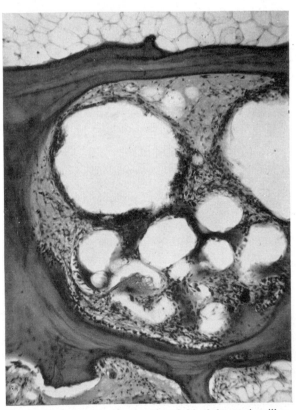

Fig. 37.28. Bone necrosis. Another field of the section illustrated in Fig. 37.27. Part of the necrotic tissue in this field has been revascularized: the marrow space in the centre of the picture contains a variety of cells, and osteoblasts are depositing bone on the surface of a necrotic bone trabecula. *Haematoxylin–eosin.* × 75.

pathic bone necrosis and 'osteochondritis'. The aetiology of these lesions is not clear, but it is thought that in many cases they result from trauma: they occur in young individuals, and usually involve areas of bone adjacent to articular cartilage. When a small area of subchondral bone abutting on the articular surface of a major joint is involved (usually a femoral condyle or the lower articular surface of the humerus), the infarction is followed by separation of an osteocartilaginous loose body into the joint, and the lesion is described by the term 'osteochondritis dissecans'. In other situations, the articular cartilage usually retains its continuity, and infarction is followed by mechanical collapse as revascularization of the affected part and removal of necrotic bone proceed. Common sites for the lesions are the upper femoral epiphysis (*Calvé–Legg–Perthes disease*—see above), the tibial tuberosity (*Osgood–Schlatter disease*[157, 158]), the navicular bone of the tarsus (*Köhler's disease*[159]), the head of the second metatarsal ('*Köhler's second disease*',[160] *Freiberg's infraction*[161]) and the carpal lunate bone (*Kienböck's disease*[162]).

Hypertrophic Pulmonary Osteoarthropathy[163, 164]

Certain pulmonary lesions, including bronchial carcinoma, bronchiectasis, and metastatic tumours in the lungs may be associated with clubbing of the fingers and toes, periosteal bone formation, and painful swelling of joints (see page 405 in Volume 1). The term *hypertrophic pulmonary osteoarthropathy* was applied to the syndrome by Marie.[165] The mechanism of production of the lesions is not known, although vascular changes have been suggested as the causative factor.[166] There is oedema and lymphocytic infiltration of the soft tissues of the clubbed fingers, with oedema and a mild non-specific reaction in the synovial membrane of the joints. The bone changes consist of exaggerated periosteal bone formation, with lymphocytic accumulation in the periosteum. It is usually the shafts of the long bones that are involved, particularly the tibia and fibula and the radius and ulna; the changes are usually symmetrical.

IRRADIATION DAMAGE[167, 168]

Bone tissue can be damaged by irradiation from external sources (X-rays, gamma rays), and also by irradiation (usually alpha or beta particles) from radioactive materials that have been deposited within the skeleton.

Large doses of external irradiation produce necrosis of bone, and the necrotic tissue shows an increased susceptibility to fracture and to infection. Many cases have been reported in which fracture of the femoral neck has followed pelvic irradiation in women.[169, 170] In young patients epiphysial growth is depressed or even completely arrested by large doses of external irradiation.

Radium poisoning, following occupational ingestion or therapeutic injection, has provided information on bone damage following skeletal deposition of radioactive material.[171–173] Widespread bone changes are produced, and take the form of a combination of patchy rarefaction and apparently increased density. Sections show widespread patchy necrosis of bone, with obliteration of vascular canals by calcified material; foci of bone resorption are also present. The damaged bones sometimes undergo spontaneous fracture. Infection, particularly of jaw bones, also occurs.

The production of bone tumours by ionizing radiation,[174] both from external sources and from internally deposited radioactive materials has been confirmed by a considerable amount of experimental work, as well as by experience following therapeutic irradiation and radium poisoning in man. The tumours are usually osteosarcomas, and may develop after a latent period of many years. The question of a 'threshold dosage' for bone damage and bone tumour formation from internally deposited radioactive materials is of considerable interest in connexion with the definition of permissible levels of strontium-90 in human bone as a result of atomic fall-out.[167, 175]

INFLAMMATORY CONDITIONS

Bone can be involved in a variety of inflammatory conditions: the sites of the lesions and their pathological features depend, to a great extent, on the type of infecting organism.

Pyogenic Infections

Haematogenous suppurative osteomyelitis occurs most commonly in infants and young children, and has been reported even in the neonatal period. The primary lesion responsible for the underlying bacteriaemia is not always evident. *Staphylococcus aureus* is the organism most commonly responsible, but streptococci, pneumococci, meningococci, brucellae and salmonellae are also encountered. The metaphyses of the long bones, particularly the femur, tibia and humerus, are the usual sites of involvement, and it has been suggested that the peculiar pattern of vascularity associated with endochondral ossification (see page 2392) favours the lodgement of bacteria carried in the blood stream.[176] Infection of bone is not always haematogenous: osteomyelitis can follow the direct introduction of bacteria into bone, as may occur with a compound fracture or in the jaws in association with dental sepsis.

In the classic staphylococcal case, the initial lesion is an area of acute exudative inflammation involving the marrow spaces of the metaphysis. The inflammatory change quickly spreads through the cancellous bone to reach the periosteum, which becomes stripped from the underlying cortex as a subperiosteal abscess forms. One effect of these changes is to produce immediate and sometimes widespread necrosis of the bone. The bacterial toxins themselves contribute to this, but the obliteration of blood vessels by the inflammatory process is also an important factor. A long bone receives the major part of its blood supply from within the marrow cavity, through the main nutrient arteries and their endosteal and metaphysial branches, and these vessels, and their accompanying veins, are inevitably involved by an extending inflammatory lesion inside the bone. An abscess originating at one end of a long bone may extend along the marrow cavity to reach the other end: this usually results in necrosis of the entire shaft. It is rare for an inflammatory lesion of this type to extend through the epiphysial plate of cartilage to involve the epiphysis; the protection afforded to the latter by the plate indirectly prevents spread of the infection into the adjacent joint. Osteomyelitis of the upper part of the femur, however, not infrequently extends to involve the hip joint: this is explained by the intracapsular location of the metaphysis.

In the absence of treatment, suppurative inflammatory lesions of bone usually become chronic. The central part of a bone is a favourable site for the continued growth of infecting organisms, and a process of chronic infection, usually punctuated by episodes of acute inflammation, is the rule. Pyaemia is common, and in the absence of treatment leads to death.

In cases in which the patient survives the acute stage of the infection, certain reparative processes ensue. The necrotic areas of bone become separated from the adjacent viable tissue by a process of *sequestration* (Figs 37.29 to 37.31). Removal of bone is restricted to the margin of the sequestrum, where this is in contact with viable tissue: it is brought about by the same process of osteoclastic resorption that is seen in normal bone and in other pathological conditions (see page 2387). While some, or all, of the original shaft is undergoing separation as a sequestrum, the periosteum forms a shell of new bone, termed an *involucrum*, round the old shaft (Figs 37.30 and 37.31). The involucrum is fixed to the viable part of the bone where the periosteum retains its attachment, but is separated from the underlying sequestrum by pus or granulation tissue. Sinuses, termed *cloacae*, often communicate between the central abscess and the overlying soft tissues, or even the skin surface. At first, the sinuses are lined by inflamed granulation tissue, but if they persist for long periods they may acquire an epithelial lining through ingrowth of epidermis. Cases have been recorded in which, after many years, a squamous carcinoma has originated in such a sinus.[177] Sequestra are not at first evident radiologically, but they become visible as their separation from the surrounding tissue proceeds. They appear denser than the surrounding bone, but this is ascribed to the rarefaction of the surrounding tissue rather than to any increase in the mineral content of the necrotic bone itself (see page 2424).

Chemotherapy, particularly in association with adequate surgical drainage, has entirely altered the course of staphylococcal osteomyelitis. Treated lesions subside rapidly, often without appreciable sequestration or involucrum formation, and the advanced forms of the disease are seen less often than in the days before antibiotics.

Quite apart from treatment, in certain instances the infection is localized from the start, and a circumscribed abscess, often known as *Brodie's abscess*,[178] results. It consists of pus surrounded by a wall of dense fibrous tissue: the surrounding bone is often sclerotic.

Brucella Infection

Bone and joint lesions have been reported in cases of brucella infection, particularly infection by *Brucella melitensis*[179] and *Brucella suis*,[179a] although *Brucella abortus* also may occasionally cause synovitis and periosteitis or osteomyelitis.[180]

The vertebral column is the most frequent site of *brucella osteomyelitis*:[181] the usual lesion is a chronic abscess involving one or two vertebrae and associated with destruction of bone and patchy sclerosis. Clinical distinction between such lesions and tuberculosis is sometimes difficult.

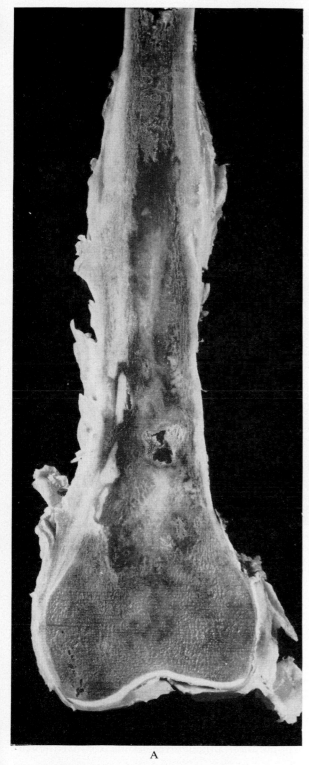

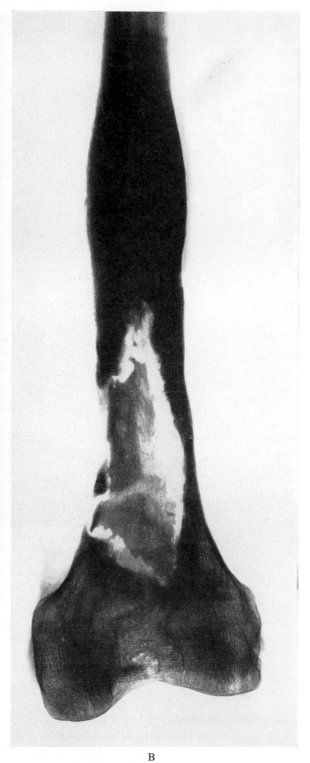

A

B

Fig. 37.29.§ Chronic suppurative osteomyelitis.

A.§ Femur divided longitudinally.

B.§ Radiograph of a slab of bone from the same specimen. Note the eroded cortical sequestrum, replacement of marrow by fibrotic granulation tissue, and diffuse periosteal bone formation.

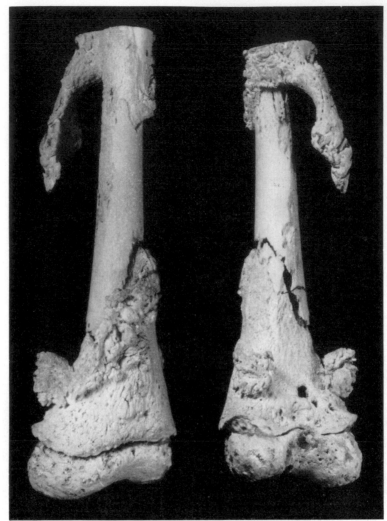

Fig. 37.30.§ Chronic suppurative osteomyelitis. Macerated femur (lower end: anterior aspect at left of picture, posterior at right). A massive sequestrum of the shaft is present: the sequestrum was covered by a large subperiosteal abscess. The bony excrescences were formed as part of the periosteal reaction on the surface of the bone and in the abscess wall: they constitute the involucrum.

Salmonella Infection with Suppuration

Some forms of salmonella infection of bone are suppurative; others are not. Both are considered below.

Salmonella Infections

Infection by Salmonella typhi.—Focal osteitis and osteomyelitis are occasional complications of typhoid fever (see page 1068 in Volume 3).[182] The long bones of the limbs and the vertebral bodies are the usual sites. In some cases involvement of bone develops during the course of the acute illness; rather oftener it becomes manifest only during convalescence. Sometimes a skeletal lesion is not recognized until years later. The histological picture is usually characterized by predominance of large mononuclear cells in the inflammatory reaction ('typhoid cells'—see page 575 in Volume 2); in some instances neutrophils are present, but in small numbers—the picture is not that of true suppuration although the lesion is conventionally referred to as a 'typhoid abscess'.

Typhoid infection of bone tends to become chronic. It may persist for months or years.[182a]

poisoning. Infection of bone by these organisms is most frequent in children, particularly in association with sickle cell anaemia and other haemoglobinopathies:[183, 183a] the lesions usually involve long bones, and are often multiple.

Tuberculosis

Tuberculosis of bone is almost invariably the result of haematogenous spread from a tuberculous lesion elsewhere in the body. Children are more frequently involved than adults. In general, the incidence of bone and joint tuberculosis has fallen greatly in recent years. The ends of the long bones are most commonly involved (Fig. 37.32); in contrast to pyogenic infections the lesion not infrequently involves the epiphysis, and it may extend into the joint. Another common site is the spine (*Pott's disease*,[184] or *David's disease*[185]—see below). The tuberculous lesion typically appears as a focus of bone destruction, with replacement of the affected

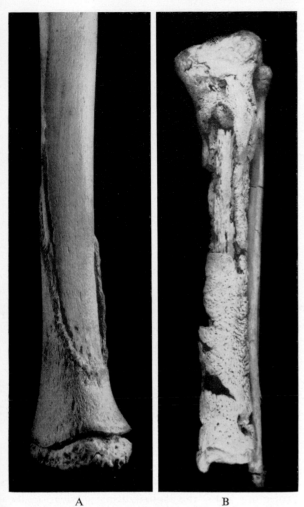

A   B

Fig. 37.31.§ Chronic suppurative osteomyelitis.

A.§ Macerated tibia (lower end). Most of the shaft is necrotic and is in process of sequestration. This part of the bone was covered by a subperiosteal abscess: the site of attachment of the periosteum is marked by reactive bone formation.

B.§ Macerated tibia and fibula (another specimen). The sequestrated shaft of the tibia is surrounded by a bulky involucrum in which there are many cloacae.

Infection by Other Salmonellae.—Enteric fever caused by paratyphoid salmonellae may be complicated by infection of bone, as occurs in typhoid fever (see above). True abscesses may develop in some of these infections, particularly in the cases caused by *Salmonella paratyphi C* in Asia and eastern Europe.

Many other species of salmonella are occasional causes of osteitis and osteomyelitis. They include *Salmonella typhimurium*, *Salmonella enteritidis* and other salmonellae that are associated with food-

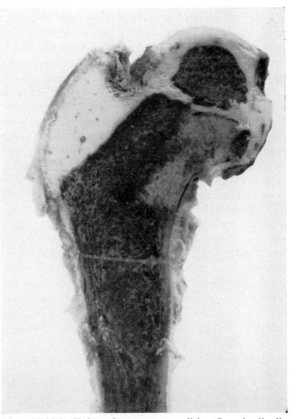

Fig. 37.32.§ Tuberculous osteomyelitis. Longitudinally divided femur: the pale area adjacent to the lower aspect of the epiphysial cartilage plate consists of tuberculous granulation tissue and caseous material.

tissue by whitish, solid or semisolid, caseous material: extension into the adjacent soft tissues is not uncommon, the resulting lesion being traditionally referred to as a *cold abscess* (see page 2376).

The bone lesions of tuberculosis have the same general histological features as tuberculosis in other situations, and consist of a central caseous mass surrounded by tuberculous granulation tissue. There is usually localized necrosis of bone, with the formation of small sequestra; the tuberculous process is predominantly osteolytic, and little or no new bone formation is seen. The lesions extend slowly and they may remain quiescent for long periods, appearing as pockets of caseous material encapsulated by fibrous tissue.

Tuberculosis of the Spine

In the spine, tuberculous lesions almost invariably commence in a vertebral body: they usually extend to involve the intervertebral discs and the bodies of the immediately adjacent vertebrae (Fig. 37.33). Bone destruction often results in anterior angulation of the spine (*kyphosis*), and this may be extreme. Displacement of the periosteum and adjacent soft tissues by tuberculous material results in a *paravertebral abscess*: this may be a conspicuous radiological feature of tuberculous disease of the spine. A paravertebral abscess may erupt through the displaced and thickened periosteum that confines it: the infection may then extend widely in the soft tissues. In the cervical or thoracic spine it may compress or even rupture into the pharynx or oesophagus, or it may extend into the mediastinum or pleural cavity. A characteristic complication is spread within the sheath of one of the muscles attached to the spine, usually a psoas muscle: such a *psoas abscess* (more correctly, a pseudoabscess, since its contents are caseous) may track downward to present as a fluctuant, subcutaneous swelling below the inguinal ligament. Although bone destruction may continue for months or years, it is usual for a tuberculous lesion of the spine ultimately to heal, or at least to become inactive: the involved vertebrae become fused into a bony block, with or without pockets of residual caseous material.

Involvement of the Spinal Cord.—Sometimes the spinal cord is compressed, with consequent paraplegia—the so-called *Pott's paraplegia*.[186] Cord involvement may occur at any time, even in cases that had seemed to be healed. The usual cause of damage to the cord is compression by a caseating

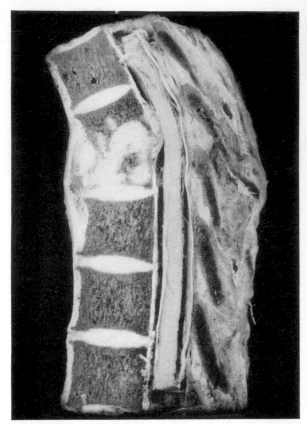

Fig. 37.33.§ Tuberculous osteomyelitis. Longitudinally divided spine: two vertebral bodies and the intervertebral disc between them are largely replaced by tuberculous granulation tissue.

granulomatous mass or tuberculous 'abscess' projecting into the spinal canal; occasionally dislocation of a vertebral body or the backward displacement of a large sequestrum is responsible. The dura is an effective barrier against the spread of the infection to the leptomeninges and the cord. In some instances of paraplegia of late onset, in the absence of reactivation of the tuberculous lesion, the symptoms appear to be the result of gradual shortening of the spinal cord itself. Angulation of the spine, even when extreme, is not alone likely to produce paraplegia.

Syphilis

Bone lesions may occur in both congenital and acquired syphilis. Improvements in the diagnosis and treatment of the early stages of the disease have led to a great reduction in their frequency.

Congenital Syphilis

In the newborn, the changes of congenital syphilis take the form of involvement of the ends of the long bones by granulomatous lesions (the so-called *syphilitic osteochondritis*), together with a diffuse periosteal reaction along the shaft (*syphilitic periosteitis*).[187] The growing surface of the epiphysial cartilage plate is marked by an irregular, whitish-yellow line that consists of unresorbed calcified cartilage: the marrow spaces of the adjacent metaphysial spongiosa are occupied by fibrotic granulation tissue. In some instances, separation of epiphyses may occur as a result of fracture through the weakened metaphysis. The periosteal changes take the form of the deposition of successive layers of bone in the mildly inflamed tissues. The histological abnormalities of bone in congenital syphilis were formerly regarded as specific inflammatory changes induced by the treponemes.[188] It is clear, however, that in addition to such specific changes, non-specific interference with bone growth and various nutritional disturbances contribute to the process in many cases.

Tertiary Syphilis

The bone changes of congenital syphilis in older children and in adults resemble those of the tertiary stage of the acquired disease. In the latter, the characteristic changes take the form of diffuse periosteal bone formation, with or without the development of localized gummatous lesions. The involved bones, which typically are the tibiae, clavicles, and skull, are thickened and dense. The gummas form circumscribed areas of granulomatous replacement of bone, with necrosis. The most characteristic of these lesions is the condition that Virchow named *caries sicca*:[189] this involves the vault of the skull (Fig. 37.34) and begins as a series of superficial excavations that extend into the diploë but rarely perforate the inner table. Later in their evolution the lesions come to form a series of more or less contiguous nodules on the surface of the bone, with intervening stellate depressions.

Yaws

Bone lesions similar to those of tertiary syphilis are seen in the late stage of yaws.[190]

Infections by Actinomycetes and Fungi[191, 191a]

With the exception of the mycetomas (see below), infections of bone that are caused by actinomycetes or by fungi are comparatively infrequent. In rare instances the organism responsible is implanted directly into the bone at the time of a penetrating injury; usually, infection results through extension of an adjacent lesion or in the course of haematogenous dissemination from cutaneous or visceral foci. Once established, the infection in bone is usually slowly progressive. In some instances it may spread from bone into the related joints. Spinal infection[192] is particularly to be feared, because of the risk of neurological complications.

In almost all cases the organisms can be seen in tissue sections stained with haematoxylin and eosin. Demonstration of the true fungi is facilitated by use of the Grocott–Gomori hexamine (methenamine) silver nitrate stain; actinomycetes are often seen best when stained by a Gram method. Cultures may be necessary for specific identification of the organisms; in most cases their value is greatest as a guide to the sensitivity of the infecting strain to drugs that may be used in the attempt to control the disease by conservative measures. In some instances, serological studies provide useful confirmatory evidence of the nature of the infection and of its continuing activity once treatment has been begun.

Actinomycosis.—In many parts of the world, but in temperate climates particularly, infection by *Actinomyces israelii* is the commonest cause of skeletal mycosis. Nevertheless, bone is not frequently involved in cases of visceral actinomycosis. In contrast, the bone of the jaw is often infected in cases of cervicofacial actinomycosis, in which the portal of entry of the organism into the tissues is usually through tooth sockets. An unusual, but by no means rare, manifestation of actinomycosis is dactylitis, the result of direct implantation of the organism into the soft tissues or periosteum of a finger by the teeth of a person in whose mouth the actinomyces is present as a commensal. Actinomycotic dactylitis has been seen in dentists, accidentally bitten by their patients, and in young men who strike others in the mouth.[193]

Actinomycotic infection of the spine,[193a] particularly of the vertebral bodies, may develop as a result of direct extension of intrathoracic actinomycosis and, more rarely, of cervicofacial actinomycosis. It may be confined to one vertebra; more usually there is involvement of several successive vertebrae.

Mycetoma.[194, 195]—A score or so of distinct species of true fungi and actinomycetes may be recognized as causes of the distinctive clinical and pathological

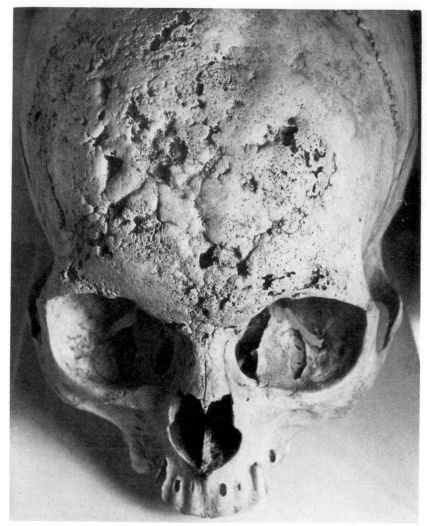

Fig. 37.34. Syphilis. Characteristic appearance of caries sicca involving frontal bone.

condition that is variously known as mycetoma, 'Madura foot' and maduramycosis. It may be stressed at the outset that such mycetomas have nothing in common with aspergilloma and other mycotic diseases of the lungs that are characterized by the presence of an intracavitary fungal ball colony and that sometimes are referred to misleadingly as pulmonary mycetomas (see pages 347 and 350 in Volume 1). The disease that is properly named mycetoma is of worldwide distribution. However, it is specially prevalent—and a cause of much suffering and incapacity—in some parts of the world, particularly in the Sudan and in West Africa and certain areas of Latin America.

In tropical and subtropical lands the organisms that most commonly cause mycetoma are *Madurella*

mycetomatis (see Fig. 39.182 in Volume 6) and *Madurella grisea*, *Actinomadura madurae* (Fig. 9.89, page 618 in Volume 2), *Streptomyces somaliensis* (Fig. 9.90, page 619) and *Actinomadura pelletieri* (Fig. 9.91, page 619), and *Nocardia brasiliensis* (Fig. 9.88, page 618). There are quite well-defined geographical differences in the prevalence of the different species. In temperate climates, indigenous cases of mycetoma are rare: the usual cause is *Petriellidium boydii* (formerly known as *Monosporium apiospermum* and, more commonly, as *Allescheria boydii*), which has been identified as the organism responsible for cases of mycetoma in the British Isles (see Fig. 39.183 in Volume 6)[193] and elsewhere in north-western Europe. The organisms that cause mycetoma are present in soil as saprophytes; they are carried into the tissues when the skin is pierced by the thorns or spines of plants. The initial lesion is in the superficial tissues—usually of a foot—and the infection spreads slowly to involve muscles, tendons, bones and joints (Figs 37.35A–E). A ramifying system of abscesses and sinuses lined by fibrotic granulation tissue develops. The involved bones become excavated as the fungal colonies grow within them: these lesions, which are often referred to by the mineralogical term geode,* may range in diameter from a few millimetres to 3 or 4 cm, according to the species of organism responsible.[195] Mycetomas usually progress only slowly, and they seldom extend beyond the anatomical region in which they originate. Involvement of lymph nodes (see page 617 in Volume 2) and spread by the blood stream are rare.

Blastomycosis.—The disease caused by *Blastomyces dermatitidis* has traditionally been known as North American blastomycosis. This designation is no longer appropriate, now that it is known that the disease occurs throughout the African continent. Cases originating in Africa seem to have a greater tendency than those occurring in America to present with skeletal lesions. Involvement of the spine,[196, 197] leading to collapse of vertebral bodies

* A geode, in mineralogy, is a cavity in rock, lined by crystals.

and neurological complications, and involvement of the long bones of the limbs, resulting in pathological fracture, are the most frequent manifestations. The histological reaction is a sclerosing tuberculoid granuloma, often with a suppurative element (the so-called suppurating pseudotubercle). The rounded, double-contoured fungal cells, commonly about 8 μm in diameter, are easily identified in active lesions (see Fig. 39.188 in Chapter 39, Volume 6) but may escape notice in older, fibrotic foci (Figs 37.35F and 37.35G).

Histoplasmosis.—Skeletal involvement is less characteristic of infection by *Histoplasma capsulatum* than of African histoplasmosis, which is caused by the larger *Histoplasma duboisii*.[198] In contrast to infection by *Histoplasma capsulatum*, in which the parasitized cells are mononucleate macrophages, infection by *Histoplasma duboisii* is characterized by parasitization of typical foreign body multinucleate giant cells (see Figs 39.187A and 39.187B in Chapter 39, Volume 6). The skeletal lesions of African histoplasmosis are usually few in number and may be solitary. They are osteolytic but generally well circumscribed.

Other Fungal Infections.—Any mycosis may involve bone. Of those that have not been mentioned above, two should be noted because skeletal lesions

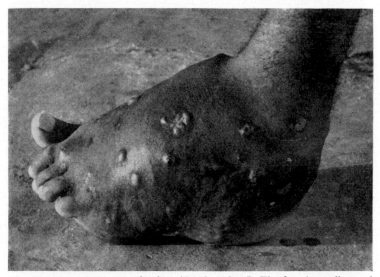

Fig. 37.35A.§ Mycetoma of a foot ('Madura foot'). The foot is swollen and deformed as a result of the chronic infection. Multiple sinuses have developed; some are seen to be discharging and others have become dry and appear as small elevations of the skin, covered by the epidermis that has sealed their opening. See also Figs 37.35B to 37.35E.

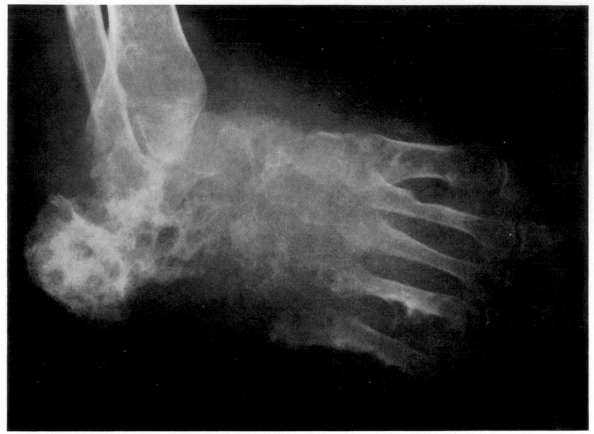

Fig. 37.35B.§ Radiograph of the foot illustrated in Fig. 37.35A. There is widespread destruction of bone. The rounded cavities that contain the colonies of the causative organism are particularly evident in the calcaneus and in the cuboid and navicular bones. There is extensive periosteitis of the metatarsal bones, with some erosion of the cortex and development of foci of infection in the medulla; protuberant spicules of new bone formation are seen in places. See also Figs 37.35C to 37.35E.

may be the presenting manifestation as well as a major clinical feature. These are cryptococcosis,[199] in which bones are involved in 5 to 10 per cent of cases, and coccidioidomycosis.[200] In both conditions the lesions in general resemble those of blastomycosis (see above), differing mainly in the appearance of the fungal elements themselves (see Figs 7.48 and 7.50, pages 354 and 358 in Volume 1, and Figs 39.185 and 39.190 in Chapter 39, Volume 6). In contrast to most other mycoses, coccidioidomycosis of bone tends to extend to involve joints.

METABOLIC AND ENDOCRINE DISORDERS

Bone structure is affected in a large number of metabolic and endocrine conditions: [201, 202, 202a] the more important of these are considered in the present section.

Scurvy[203]

This condition results from a deficient intake of vitamin C (ascorbic acid): it is characterized by anaemia, swelling and ulceration of the gums, loosening of the teeth, and haemorrhage in a variety of tissues, including skin, mucous membranes, periosteum and joints. Wolbach's histological studies of experimental scurvy in the guinea-pig[204–206] led to the conclusion that, in the absence of the vitamin, certain connective tissue cells are unable to elaborate or maintain the normal intercellular materials—specifically collagen, osteoid tissue and dentine. The associated capillary weakness has been ascribed to deficiency of the intercellular cement substance or of the supporting connective tissue framework.

Scorbutic lesions are rarely encountered now: when they are seen it is usually in young children.

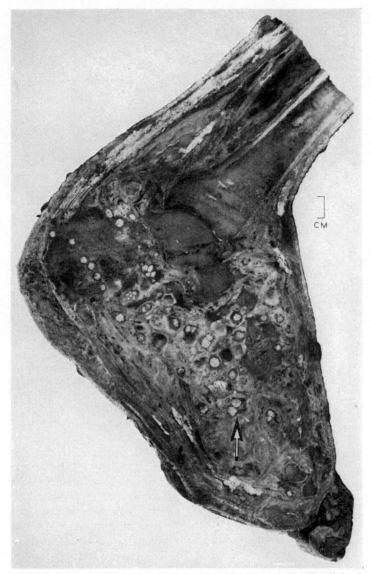

Fig. 37.35C.§ The foot illustrated in Figs 37.35A and 37.35B, divided longitudinally in the plane of the first intermetatarsal space after amputation. The destruction of the distal group of tarsal bones is evident. There are many pale, rounded colonies of the causative organism (*Actinomadura madurae* in this case). The colonies occupy spaces excavated in the infected bones and in the soft tissues. The pair of colonies indicated by the arrow is shown in Fig. 37.35E. See also Fig. 37.35D.

Bone lesions take the form of subperiosteal haemorrhages, which are sometimes massive (Fig. 37.36). In addition, the bones are usually porotic, and characteristic changes in the epiphysial cartilage plate and adjacent metaphysis have been described.[207, 208] Growth and calcification of cartilage continue, although at a reduced rate. Osteoblastic activity is arrested and there is no formation of bone on the cartilage lattice: this consequently becomes fragmented as an outcome of normal mechanical stresses. The weakened metaphysial bone may fracture and the epiphysis separate (Fig. 37.36).

The repair of wounds, including fractures, is arrested or retarded in scurvy. In teeth the formation of dentine is impaired.[209]

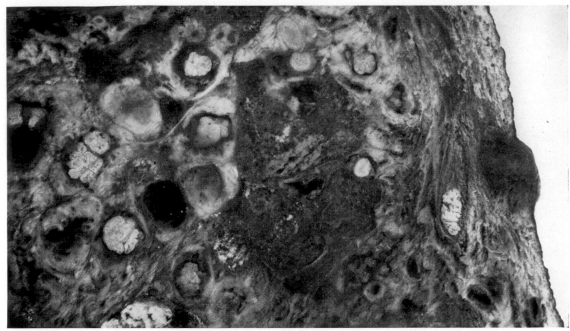

Fig. 37.35D.§ Enlargement of part of the cut surface of the specimen illustrated in Figs 37.35A to 37.35C, to show details of the pathological changes and of the appearances of the colonies of the streptomycete. The pale tissue round the colonies is for the most part composed of fibrosing granulation tissue, notably ill-provided with blood vessels. The narrow space between the colonies and the granulation tissue ordinarily contains pus, but much of this has drained away following division of the specimen. Colonies are present both in bone and in the soft tissues. The dark protrusion at the cutaneous surface consists of hyperaemic granulation tissue round the terminal part of the track of a sinus. See also Fig. 37.35E.

Rickets* and Osteomalacia[210]

These conditions are characterized by failure of calcification of bone tissue. This is evident morphologically in the accumulation of large amounts of uncalcified bone matrix—*osteoid tissue*—and un-

* Rickets was known formerly as rachitis (properly, rhachitis), a term now seldom used except in its adjectival form. The Greek origin of this name indicated no more than a disease of the spine, the suffix -itis originally lacking the specific connotation of inflammation that it now ordinarily carries. Francis Glisson (1597–1677), Regius Professor of Physic at Cambridge, introduced the name rachitis in the belief that rickets had its seat in the spine. His book, *De rachitide sive morbo puerili, qui vulgo The Rickets dicitur* (London, 1650) is commonly cited as the first account of rickets. In fact, it was preceded by the shorter, but important, description by Daniel Whistler (1619–1684)—physician, professor of geometry and Registrar (reputedly malfeasant) of the Royal College of Physicians of London, who made it the subject of his inaugural disputation for the doctorate in medicine in Leyden in 1645 (*De morbo puerili Anglorum, quem patrio idiomate indigenae vocant The Rickets*; Lugduni Batavorum [Leyden], 1645). Rickets soon came to be widely known as the English disease. Arnold Boate, or Bootius (*circa* 1600–*circa* 1653), included a detailed account of rickets under the name 'pectoreal tabes' in his *Observationes*, which included the experience of many years of practice in

calcified cartilage. In the past, rickets and osteomalacia usually resulted from a deficient intake of vitamin D, but dietary rickets and osteomalacia are now rare in prosperous countries. The basic similarity between the two conditions was observed in 1885 by Pommer,[211] in Germany, who gave the first accurate account of their pathology.

The main effect of vitamin D is to improve the absorption of calcium in the intestine. The change in bone that results from deficient intake of vitamin D is failure of calcification of hypertrophic cartilage and osteoid tissue: this appears to be due to reduction in the concentration of calcium and phosphate ions in the blood.[212] It is important to note that large doses of vitamin D affect bone directly, stimulating resorption, and even interfering with the calcification of osteoid tissue.[213–215]

In the growing child, deficiency of vitamin D causes rickets. The growing epiphysial cartilage

Ireland and also preceded Glisson's account (*Observationes medicae de affectibus omissis*, chap. 12; London, 1649).

The name rickets is said to be of Middle English origin (*wricke*, sprain) and only by association related to the Greek *rhachitis*.

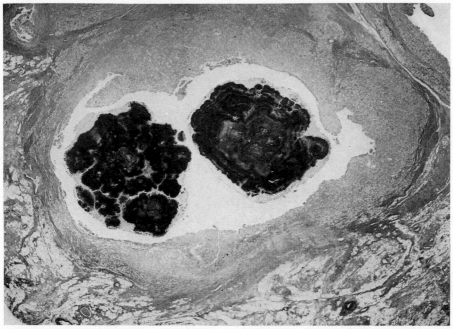

Fig. 37.35E.§ A rectangular block of tissue containing the two colonies marked with the arrow in Fig. 37.35C was dissected from the specimen and sectioned histologically. The photomicrograph shows the concentric pattern of the colonies that results from alternation of phases of active growth and phases of consolidation over periods of many months or years. The colonies have shrunken during histological processing and some of the purulent exudate that surrounded them has disappeared following dissection of the tissue, with the result that they seem to lie in an empty space. The tissue immediately surrounding the cavity is densely fibrotic; there is almost no penetration into it of branches of the blood vessels in the vicinity. It is probable that the interposition of this poorly vascularized fibrous tissue between the colonies and the nearby interstitial tissue prevents adequate diffusion of drugs from the blood to the site of infection; this may be one reason why chemotherapy and treatment with antibiotics is so often ineffective even in those cases in which the actinomycete or fungus responsible for the infection is sensitive to drugs *in vitro*. It is notable that in cases of mycetoma caused by *Nocardia brasiliensis*, which are much likelier to respond to chemotherapy than are infections by the streptomycetes and true fungi, the granulation tissue round the abscesses and sinuses is much better provided with capillary blood vessels and much less frequently converted into dense scar tissue. *Grocott–Gomori hexamine (methenamine) silver.* × 12.

plates of the long bones become thickened and irregular, and the ends of the bones may be enlarged. There are similar changes at the costochondral junctions (Fig. 37.37), which are expanded to form the *rickety rosary*, and in the frontal bones of the skull, which become bossed. The bones are abnormally soft, and deformities such as bowing of the tibia and femur usually develop.

Histology

Histologically, the rachitic epiphysial cartilage plate is thickened and irregular (Fig. 37.38). In human material, the changes are usually complicated both by the effects of intermittent healing and by the presence of other nutritional deficiencies.

The subject has been studied extensively in the rat, in which rickets can be produced by imbalance of calcium and phosphorus intake as well as by vitamin D deficiency. In experimental rickets, deposition of bone salt in the cartilage matrix fails to occur normally in the region of the hypertrophic cells (see page 2394):[216] as a result, the uncalcified cartilage is not vascularized and its hypertrophic cells persist for an abnormally long time. New cartilage cells continue to be formed, and the plate consequently increases in thickness (Fig. 37.39); the cells fail to maintain their normal columnar arrangement. The increase in thickness of the plate depends on the continued formation of cartilage cells: if this ceases, as it sometimes does in severe malnutrition, the epiphysial changes

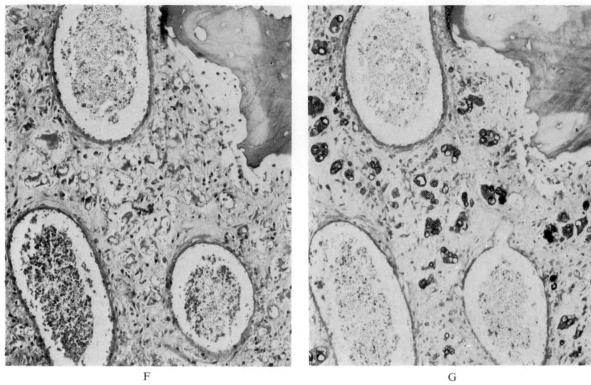

F   G

Figs 37.35F and 37.35G.§ Blastomycosis. The patient was a white South African visitor to London, on her first journey outside southern Africa. She stumbled in a theatre, sustaining a fracture of the neck of the humerus as she lightly struck one arm against a pillar. Radiological examination showed an extensive osteolytic lesion through which the fracture had occurred. There was no history of earlier symptoms associated with the lesion. It was regarded as probably a metastatic carcinoma. As no sign of a primary tumour was found the fracture was explored surgically. The photographs illustrate the findings in the biopsy specimen, which consisted of densely fibrotic tissue that in places enclosed conspicuous vascular channels, such as those in the field photographed. There was no neoplastic tissue. The fungal cells could readily be overlooked in the haematoxylin–eosin preparation (F); they are easily seen in the hexamine–silver preparation (G). Most of them are within mononucleate or multinucleate macrophages. No mycotic lesions were found elsewhere. It was initially decided that the infection should not be treated but kept under observation. The fracture healed with simple immobilization. Subsequently, although the patient had no symptoms, and there was no evident disease, other doctors prescribed an intensive course of amphotericin. She has remained well during a follow-up period of eight years. F: *Haematoxylin–eosin.* × 135. G: *Grocott–Gomori hexamine (methenamine) silver.* × 135.

of rickets cannot develop. It is usually possible to demonstrate belated calcification of isolated areas of hypertrophic cartilage, even in severe rickets: this is accompanied by local vascularization and is responsible for the irregular contour of the metaphysial surface of the plate (Figs 37.37 and 37.39). Resumption of calcification follows correction of the biochemical abnormality, deposition of bone salt occurring in the region of the cartilage cells that have most recently become hypertrophic.

In addition to the interference with calcification of the growing epiphysial cartilage plates, the rachitic skeleton shows excessive amounts of osteoid tissue on the surface of trabeculae and other bony structures. Increased amounts of osteoid tissue are also seen in osteomalacia, the adult counterpart of rickets. The osteoid tissue results from a failure of calcification of bone matrix at the time of its formation: there is no evidence to support the view that there is any appreciable selective withdrawal of bone salt from already calcified tissue—the so-called *halisteresis phenomenon.* Osteoblastic activity is usually increased in osteomalacia, and this is responsible for the elevation of the serum alkaline phosphatase that is a frequent accompaniment of vitamin D deficiency. As more and more of the skeleton comes to consist of osteoid tissue, the bones become soft: bowing of long bones, deformities of the pelvis,

result of parathyroid hyperplasia induced by a low concentration of calcium in the plasma (see also page 2052 in Volume 4).[202]

Diagnosis

The histological diagnosis of rickets and osteomalacia depends on the identification of osteoid tissue.[219, 220] In decalcified preparations, provided that treatment with strong acids has been avoided, osteoid tissue stains less intensely with haematoxylin than calcified bone (Fig. 37.40): it therefore appears pink in haematoxylin–eosin preparations. This differential staining reaction does not depend on the presence of bone salt but on some other constituent of the matrix of calcified bone tissue, probably mucopolysaccharide in nature. While this method is reliable in experienced hands, the accuracy of recognition of osteoid tissue is greatly influenced by variations in the procedures of

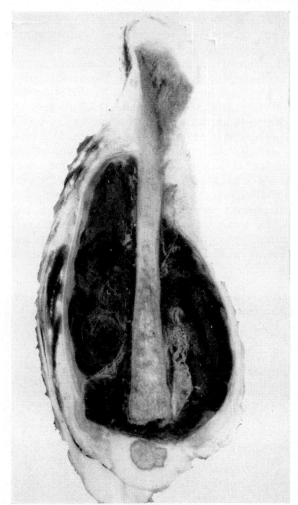

Fig. 37.36.§ Scurvy. Extensive subperiosteal haemorrhage, with separation of the lower epiphysis of the femur.

and even scoliosis may develop and may become extreme.

'*Pseudofractures*' *in Osteomalacia.*—The transverse bands or fissures known as *incomplete fractures*, *pseudofractures*, or *Looser's zones*, are characteristic of osteomalacia.[217, 218] These take the form of bands of rarefaction in cortical bone, occupied by uncalcified or incompletely calcified callus-like tissue: their most frequent sites are the humeral and femoral necks, the pubic rami, the ribs, and the lateral border of the scapulae. They occur also in Paget's disease (see page 2436).

Osteoclastic Resorption in Osteomalacia.—Active osteoclastic resorption of bone is sometimes seen in osteomalacia. It has been suggested that this is the

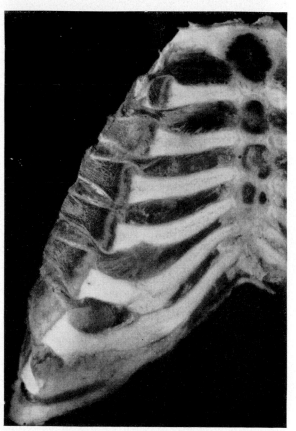

Fig. 37.37.§ Rickets. Costochondral junctions of an infant with dietary rickets. The ends of the ribs are expanded and contain a wide zone of abnormal tissue (osteoid tissue and uncalcified cartilage).

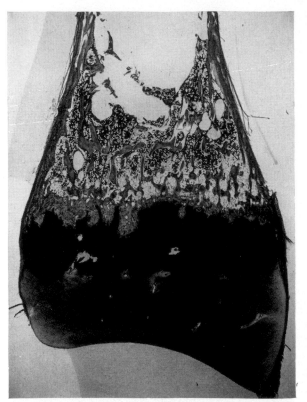

Fig. 37.38. Rickets. Lower end of radius: the growth cartilage is thickened and its metaphysial surface is broken by projecting tongues of paler material that consists largely of osteoid tissue. *Haematoxylin–eosin.* × 5.

Other Causes of Rickets and Osteomalacia

With improving standards of nutrition, the incidence of dietary rickets and osteomalacia has fallen greatly in many communities, and interest has turned to cases in which the same type of bony change has resulted from factors other than a dietary deficiency of vitamin D.[223] Rickets and osteomalacia not infrequently occur in coeliac disease and in idiopathic steatorrhoea, as a result of interference with alimentary absorption of both vitamin D and calcium. Osteomalacia may occur as a complication of gastrectomy and some other operations on the stomach.[224] It is also one of the components of renal osteodystrophy (see page 2432). Vitamin-D-resistant rickets also occurs in certain renal tubular disorders, including renal tubular acidosis, phosphaturic rickets and the

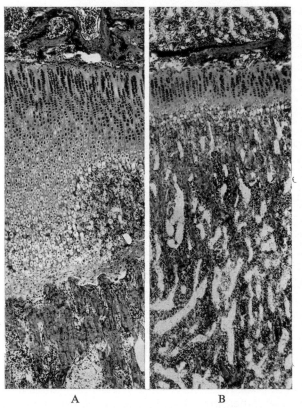

A   B

Fig. 37.39. Rickets (and normal appearances for comparison). *Haematoxylin–eosin.* × 40.

A. Greatly thickened epiphysial cartilage plate in experimental rickets in a rat. On each side of the field the metaphysial surface of the plate shows an area of calcification and vascularization.

B. Epiphysial cartilage plate of a normal rat for comparison with Fig. 37.39A.

decalcification and staining: the method is, therefore, unsuitable for everyday use. A better diagnostic procedure depends on the recognition of osteoid tissue in sections of undecalcified bone by its failure to give the von Kossa reaction for calcium (Fig. 37.41): this reaction depends on the fact that, when the tissue is calcified, the bone salt reacts with silver nitrate to form silver phosphate, which is subsequently converted to metallic silver and appears black in the section. Sections of undecalcified cancellous bone can be prepared with an ordinary sledge microtome after embedding either in paraffin wax[221] or in plastics:[222] the method is therefore applicable to a range of diagnostic material, and biopsy specimens taken from the iliac crest with a trephine are particularly suitable. Cortical bone cannot be sectioned in this way: thin sections can instead be prepared by grinding and then examined stained or unstained (Fig. 37.42A); alternatively, the presence of bone salt can be determined by its absorption of X-rays (radiomicrography) (Fig. 37.42B).

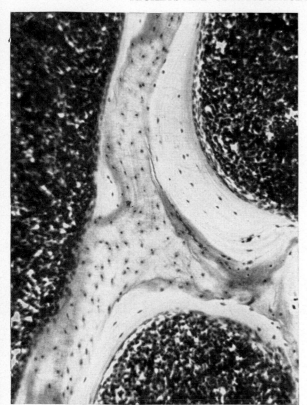

Fig. 37.40. Rickets. The superficial osteoid tissue stains less intensely with haematoxylin than the underlying bone. *Decalcified tissue; haematoxylin–eosin.* × 125.

de Toni–Fanconi syndrome (see pages 1450 and 1451 in Volume 4 and page 2434 in this chapter).

Hypophosphatasia.—It may be noted here that bone changes morphologically similar to those of rickets are present in a rare, genetically determined condition known as hypophosphatasia,[225–227] in which there is a deficiency of alkaline phosphatase. This association is of interest in view of the uncertainty regarding the exact role of alkaline phosphatase in bone formation (see page 2395).

Vitamin A Deficiency and Excess

Vitamin A Deficiency

The main result of deficient intake of vitamin A is the occurrence of changes in certain epithelial structures, including those of the respiratory tract, alimentary system and genitourinary system and the cornea and accessory glands of the eyes[228] (see Chapter 40, Volume 6). Certain neurological manifestations of deficiency of vitamin A during the growth of animals[229] have been shown to result from the effect of the deficiency on growing bone: in the rat the retarded growth of the axial skeleton results in mechanical compression of nerve roots and of parts of the central nervous system.[230] No comparable manifestations of vitamin A deficiency have been reported in man.

Experimental Vitamin A Excess

Large doses of vitamin A can produce exaggerated bone resorption in laboratory animals.[231] Studies on tissue cultures have shown that vitamin A has a selective lytic effect on cartilage matrix.[232]

Osteoporosis

The term osteoporosis is applied to any condition in which there is a reduction in the amount of bone tissue. The total amount of calcium in the skeleton may be greatly reduced, but the degree of calcification of such bone tissue as is present is normal, unless osteomalacia is also present. Osteoporosis may be local or general, and may result from a

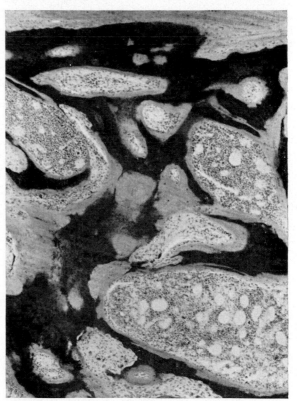

Fig. 37.41. Osteomalacia. Undecalcified section stained for calcium by the von Kossa technique: the osteoid tissue does not react whereas the calcified bone is blackened. × 90.

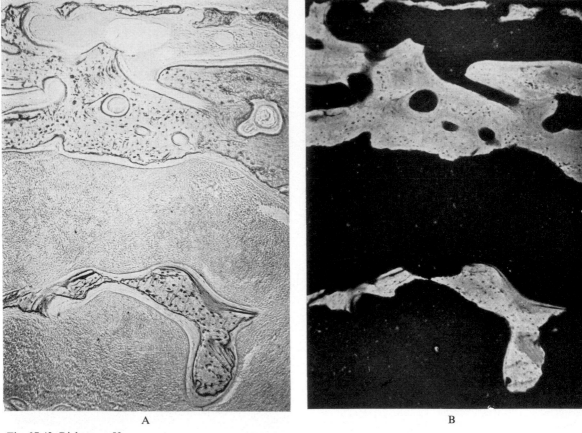

A   B

Fig. 37.42. Rickets. × 50.

A. In this unstained, undecalcified section the superficial osteoid tissue appears clear, in contrast to the more highly refractile bone.

B. Radiomicrograph of the area illustrated in Fig. 37.42A. The calcified bone is seen because it obstructs passage of X-rays, whereas the uncalcified osteoid tissue allows them to pass and therefore appears black in the radiograph.

variety of causes. From the histological point of view, interest centres on the mechanism of production of the bone changes. The maintenance of normal skeletal structure depends on a balance between the continuously active processes of bone deposition and bone resorption (see page 2387). Reduction in the amount of bone tissue present must inevitably follow any continued departure from this balance in favour of resorption. It appears that sometimes an increase in resorption is responsible and sometimes a decrease in deposition. Bony rarefaction can develop even in the presence of increased deposition, if resorption is disproportionately increased: such a situation is frequently seen at the margin of an osteolytic tumour or other local lesion of bone. It is also possible for formation and resorption to be balanced when a reduced amount of bone tissue

is present: this is the situation when osteoporosis is at a non-progressive stage.

Disuse Osteoporosis

Immobilization of a limb results in local osteoporosis, which can be regarded as a skeletal form of disuse atrophy.[233, 234] Bony rarefaction can be recognized radiologically within a few weeks of the commencement of immobilization: at this early stage the bone changes consist of focal osteoporosis of cancellous bone, particularly adjacent to the subchondral bony plate of articular surfaces (Fig. 37.43) and in the metaphyses of long bones. With more prolonged immobilization or disuse, such as is seen in limbs paralysed by poliomyelitis, bone changes involve cortical as well as cancellous bone (Fig. 37.44). At this later stage, the trabeculae

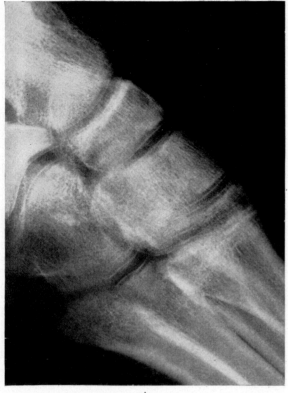
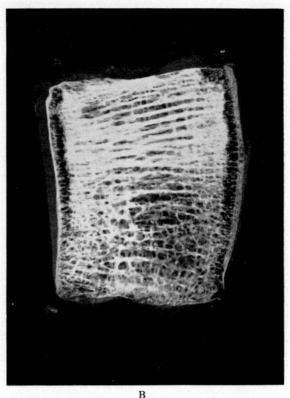

A   B

Fig. 37.43.§ Disuse osteoporosis, the result of three months' immobilization.

A.§ Radiograph of the bones of the foot.

B.§ Radiograph of a slab of tissue from the same foot after amputation, showing extreme thinning of bone trabeculae deep to the subchondral plate.

most concerned in the transmission of weight-bearing stresses are the ones that are least affected in the atrophy.[235] This is evident in Fig. 37.45: in the osteoporotic talus the systems of bone trabeculae passing anteriorly toward the metacarpals and posteriorly toward the calcaneus, and representing pathways of mechanical stress under normal conditions, are less affected than other parts of the bone.

Little information has been available on the histological mechanism of disuse osteoporosis until recent years. An experimental study of osteoporosis of the bones of the tarsus following division of the calcanean tendon showed evidence of exaggerated osteoclastic activity during the period of development of the bone changes:[236] a similar observation has been made in a case of disuse osteoporosis in man.[201] In an experimental study, using tetracycline labelling, it was found that the relation between bone formation and bone resorption changed during a period of five months follow-ing division of tendons:[237] resorption increased and bone formation decreased.

Local osteoporosis also occurs in the neighbour-hood of diseased joints, particularly in rheumatoid arthritis and tuberculous arthritis. A rapidly developing local osteoporosis, known as *Sudeck's atrophy*,[238] sometimes follows fractures or other injuries. It is painful, and is accompanied by reflex vascular changes in the skin of the involved part: neurovascular factors are thought to be responsible for the bone changes, which are probably mediated by an increased rate of circulation in the areas involved.

General immobilization results in more wide-spread osteoporosis. Balance studies have shown losses of up to 9 per cent of the total body calcium over a period of months;[239] the loss of calcium is occasionally accompanied by hypercalcaemia.[240, 241] The condition of weightlessness associated with space flight is accompanied by a similar loss of calcium.[242]

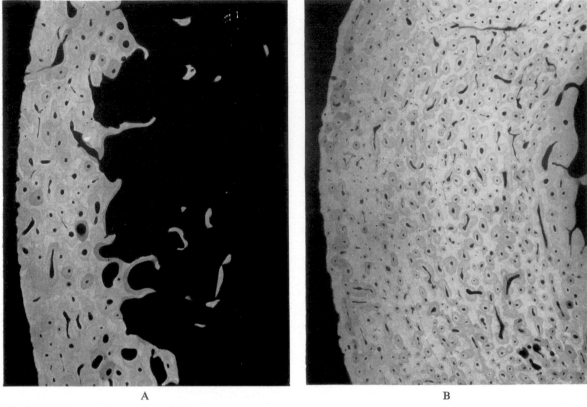

A   B

Fig. 37.44. Disuse osteoporosis. × 15.

A. Radiomicrograph of part of the cortical bone of the femoral shaft in a case of immobilization atrophy of many years'
   duration, resulting from poliomyelitis.

B. Similar preparation from a normal femur for comparison.

Idiopathic Osteoporosis[243–245]

In the majority of examples of generalized osteoporosis the cause of the bone changes is not
definitely established, and the term *idiopathic
osteoporosis* is consequently employed. The discovery that oestrogens and androgens relieved the
symptoms in some cases of this type[246] suggested
that the condition is due to an imbalance between
the anabolic and antianabolic hormones of the
adrenal cortex and gonads:[247, 248] however, direct
evidence of this is not available in osteoporotic
individuals, nor has it been definitely established
that corticosteroid therapy leads to retention of
calcium. In experimental animals, restriction of
calcium intake in the presence of vitamin D leads
to osteoporosis, and it has been suggested that
calcium deficiency might be the cause of idiopathic
osteoporosis in man:[249, 250] again, conclusive evidence of reduced calcium intake in osteoporosis,
or of retention of calcium under conditions of
increased dietary intake, is lacking.

Idiopathic osteoporosis is most commonly seen
after middle age and occurs in women oftener
than in men. It is not easy to distinguish minor
degrees of osteoporosis from normal conditions,
as the normal ageing changes in healthy individuals
take the form of a less pronounced loss of bone
from the same parts of the skeleton.[251–253] Indeed,
idiopathic osteoporosis can be regarded as an
exaggeration of the ageing process. The bone
changes are not accompanied by any abnormalities
of blood biochemistry: in particular, the values for
calcium, phosphorus and alkaline phosphatase are
normal.

The loss of bone tissue mainly affects the spine
and the pelvis; the bones of the limbs are less
severely involved. The trabeculae of the cancellous
bone of the vertebral bodies become thin, and
pressure on the weakened bone by the intervening
intervertebral discs leads to concavity of the upper
and lower surfaces. The vertebral bodies become
reduced in height, anteriorly more than posteriorly,

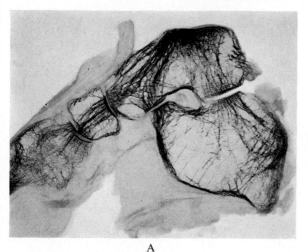
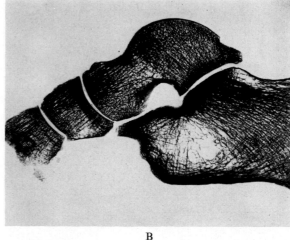

A B

Fig. 37.45. Disuse osteoporosis.

A. Radiograph of a slab of tissue from the ankle of a limb that had been completely paralysed for twenty years as a result of poliomyelitis.

B. Similar preparation from a normal ankle for comparison.

with the result that the affected individual becomes shorter and develops kyphosis. The cortex of the shafts of the long bones shows less change, but here, too, there is reduction in the amount of bone through the enlargement of the vascular canals: as in the local osteoporosis of immobilization this change is most marked in the inner part of the cortex. Osteoporosis is an important predisposing cause of fractures in elderly people, particularly fracture of the femoral neck.[254]

Little histological information is available on the dynamic cellular aspects of idiopathic osteoporosis, and it is not clear whether reduced bone formation or exaggerated resorption is responsible for the development of the bone lesions. Isotope techniques for the determination of calcium accretion rates (see page 2388) have been applied to cases of idiopathic osteoporosis by several workers, without any departure from normal values being found.[249, 255] Unless the change in the rate of accretion necessary to produce osteoporosis is too small to be detected by available techniques, or unless the cases have been studied at a stabilized stage, this negative finding suggests that exaggerated resorption must be the cause of the bony rarefaction. Morphological observations on the increasing rarefaction of 'normal' bones in old age indicate that increased resorption is responsible for the reduction in the amount of bone present:[256] it would not be surprising to find the same factor operating in cases of idiopathic osteoporosis.

12*

Endocrine Osteoporosis

Osteoporosis as a feature of Cushing's syndrome and of hyperthyroidism is referred to respectively in the next paragraph and on page 2430.

Cushing's Syndrome

Generalized osteoporosis is a feature both of Cushing's syndrome,[257] which results from the over-production of the antianabolic adrenocortical hormones, and from the therapeutic use of large doses of cortisone and related compounds.[258-260] The bone changes are clearly the result of the excess of adrenocortical hormones: they are similar to but often severer than those seen in idiopathic osteoporosis.[261]

The spine is the part of the skeleton most severely involved, and the changes can be extreme (Fig. 37.46). The bone trabeculae in the osteoporotic vertebrae are abnormally thin (Fig. 37.47). Some authors have commented on the scarcity of osteoblasts and of areas of recently formed bone on the surface of the bone trabeculae,[261] and it is clear that these changes indicate a decrease in osteoblastic bone formation: this is usually regarded as an adequate explanation for the progressive reduction in the amount of skeletal tissue, as increased osteoclasis has not been observed. The collapse of the vertebral bodies is due to fracture of the thin and weakened trabeculae. Sometimes angulation or discontinuity of individual trabeculae is all that

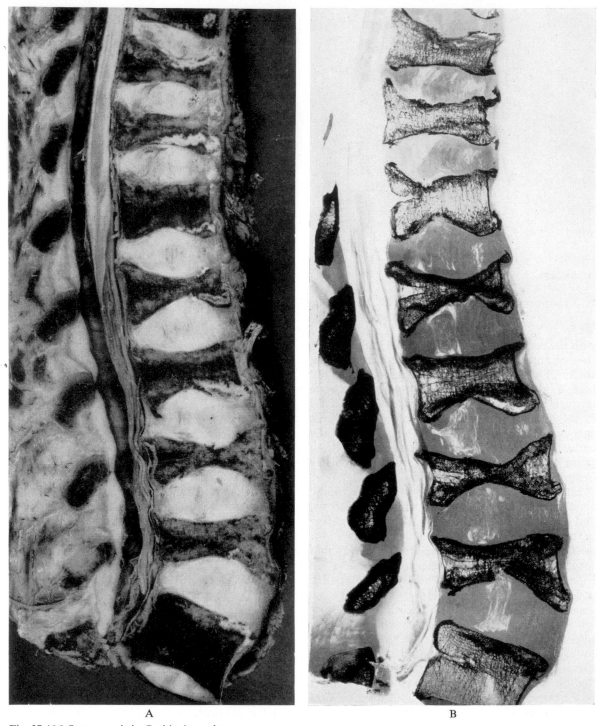

A

B

Fig. 37.46.§ Osteoporosis in Cushing's syndrome.

A.§ Longitudinally divided spine (lower dorsal and lumbar regions), showing collapsed vertebral bodies and expanded
intervertebral discs.

B.§ Radiograph of a slab of tissue from the cut surface of the same specimen.

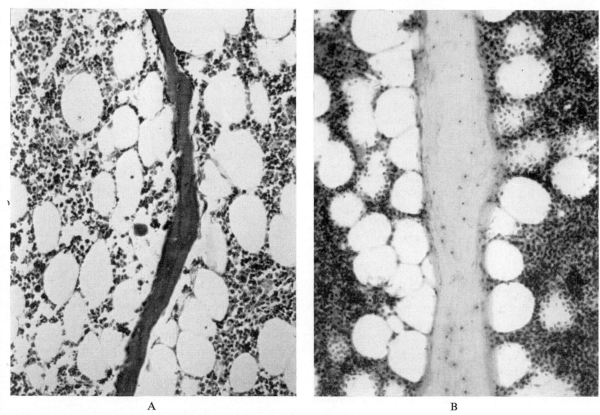

A B

Fig. 37.47.§ Osteoporosis in Cushing's syndrome. *Haematoxylin–eosin.* × 85.

A.§ A bone trabecula from the central part of a severely osteoporotic vertebra.

B.§ A comparable trabecula from a normal vertebra for comparison.

can be seen to indicate a previous 'microfracture', but on other occasions there is more massive collapse of part of a vertebral body. Compression fractures of vertebral bodies usually involve the tissue near the upper or lower surface: in some cases the impacted trabeculae produce a relatively radio-opaque band (Fig. 37.46), which can be seen in clinical radiographs.

Not only is osteoblastic activity diminished, but fracture callus fails to develop in a normal manner: despite this, many of the numerous fractures of ribs that occur in Cushing's syndrome unite. In experimental animals bone growth can be inhibited[262, 263] and the repair of fractures retarded[264, 265] by the administration of cortisone. It is possible that large doses of cortisone may induce bone resorption as well as inhibiting osteoblastic bone formation.[266]

Pituitary Dysfunction

Overproduction of growth hormone, which is usually associated with an acidophil adenoma of the pituitary gland, causes gigantism if it occurs before the time of skeletal maturation and acromegaly if it occurs later (see pages 1886 and 1894 in Volume 4).

Gigantism

In gigantism, there is a proportionate overgrowth of all parts of the skeleton. The excessive growth is usually most marked at adolescence and may continue into young adult life because of delay in the closure of the epiphysial cartilage plates of the long bones. This retardation of skeletal maturation is due to interference with the production of pituitary gonadotrophins and to the lack of gonadal and other hormones. Height is greatly increased, sometimes to over 250 cm (over 8 feet).[266a] In cases which the hormonal abnormality continues into adult life, acromegalic characteristics become superimposed on the picture of gigantism.

Acromegaly

In acromegaly,[267] there is some overgrowth of the entire skeleton, but it is particularly the skull and mandible, the spine and the thoracic cage, and the bones of the hands and feet that are affected. The lower jaw is greatly enlarged and projects forward, and the hands and feet are increased in all their dimensions. In most situations, the coarsening of bony structure is the result of reactivated periosteal bone formation: in the condyle of the mandible, at the costochondral junctions, and in the bone abutting on the articular cartilage of the phalanges, the process of endochondral ossification can become re-established with consequent increase in the overall length of the bones.[268, 269] Deformation of articular surfaces commonly leads to osteoarthritis.

Pituitary Dwarfism

Deficiency in production of pituitary growth hormone during childhood, usually the result of destruction of the anterior lobe of the pituitary by a tumour or cyst, results in cessation of growth, including that of the skeleton, with consequent dwarfism.[270] The bones are slender, and normal skeletal proportions are maintained. The growth of the epiphysial cartilage plates ceases, but they remain unclosed because of the deficiency in the production of pituitary gonadotrophins and the lack of gonadal and other hormones concerned in normal skeletal maturation.

Thyroid Dysfunction

Hyperthyroidism

Hyperthyroidism is not infrequently associated with osteoporosis, and it is believed that the bone changes are the result of exaggerated resorption (see page 1992 in Volume 4).[271–273]

Hypothyroidism

In the child, hypothyroidism (cretinism) produces retardation of skeletal growth, and there is delay in the appearance and development of epiphysial centres of ossification. The skeleton retains infantile proportions. Radiologically, the epiphysial centres that are present show a stippled and fragmented appearance, known as *epiphysial dysgenesis*;[274] histological studies have shown an interference with endochondral ossification.[275] Similar bone changes can be produced experimentally by surgical resection of the thyroid and by destruction of thyroid tissue with radioactive iodine.[276–278] Both in cretins and in experimental hypothyroidism the epiphysial cartilage plates are thickened: proliferation of cartilage cells is somewhat reduced, their 'maturation' does not occur and calcification and vascularization is retarded and irregular.[275, 279, 280]

Parathyroid Dysfunction

Hyperparathyroidism[202, 281–283]

Oversecretion of parathyroid hormone can be primary or secondary. *Primary hyperparathyroidism* is the result of a tumour (usually an adenoma) of one or more glands, or of primary parathyroid hyperplasia (see page 2049 in Volume 4). *Secondary hyperparathyroidism* is associated with secondary parathyroid hyperplasia and is seen in rickets and osteomalacia[284–287] and in renal failure (see pages 2052 to 2054 in Volume 4): a low level of serum calcium is thought to be the initial stimulus to parathyroid overactivity.

An excess of parathyroid hormone appears to influence calcium and phosphorus metabolism by its effects on the kidneys and on bone.[202] It causes increased renal excretion of phosphate, and also stimulates osteoclastic resorption by a direct effect on bone, as shown both by studies of the local effects of explanted parathyroid tissue[287a, 287b] and by tissue culture.[287c, 287d] In primary hyperparathyroidism the amount of calcium in the serum is increased and that of phosphorus is diminished, and the urinary excretion of calcium is abnormally large. When bone lesions are present, the amount of alkaline phosphatase in the serum is usually raised.

The essential skeletal changes of primary hyperparathyroidism take the form of diffuse fibrous replacement of bone, or 'osteitis fibrosa cystica'. This condition was described in 1891 by von Recklinghausen,[288] and the bone lesions of primary hyperparathyroidism are sometimes known as *von Recklinghausen's disease of bone* (or Engel–Recklinghausen disease, in recognition of a description of the lesions by Engel that antedated von Recklinghausen's account by 27 years[288a]). Von Recklinghausen distinguished 'fibrous osteitis' from other types of rarefying bone disease, including osteomalacia, Paget's disease and osteolytic carcinomatous deposits, but he was unaware of its relation to hyperparathyroidism, and he did not distinguish between the truly diffuse and the focal fibrosing lesions of bone—that is, between hyperparathyroidism and polyostotic fibrous dysplasia (see page 2439). Later, Erdheim[289] noted the association between von Recklinghausen's disease and parathyroid hyperplasia, but concluded that the parathyroid changes were secondary to the bone disease, as occurs in osteomalacia. It was not until 1926 that Mandl,[290] by the curative extirpation of a parathyroid tumour in a case of generalized osteitis fibrosa, demonstrated that parathyroid overactivity was the cause of the bone disease.

The bone lesions of primary hyperparathyroidism range from minor degrees of generalized bone rarefaction to conspicuous areas of bone destruction associated with cysts (Fig. 37.48) or 'brown tumours' (see below). Gross changes appear in only a minority of cases: when they do occur the involved bones may be greatly expanded, and in advanced cases—rarely seen today—extreme deformity of the weakened bones can occur. Small focal erosions of cortical bone, particularly in the phalanges, are characteristic of hyperparathyroidism,[291] whether primary or secondary (see Figs 37.50 and 37.54); similarly, the lamina dura (the fine layer of dense bone surrounding the roots of

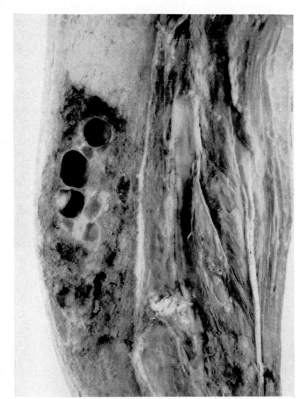

Fig. 37.48.§ Hyperparathyroidism. Expanding lesion of the shaft of a tibia—the lesion consists of haemorrhagic fibrous tissue and includes several large cysts.

the teeth) disappears,[292] although it is unchanged in most other forms of bony rarefaction.

Histology.—The lesions are characterized by exaggerated osteoclasis, and by the replacement of bone and bone marrow by spindle-celled fibrous tissue (Fig. 37.49). Bone trabeculae may be hollowed by local resorption, with fibrous replacement: the term *dissecting resorption* is applied to this process, which occurs also in cases of renal osteodystrophy (see page 2433). New bone formation is usually conspicuous (Fig. 37.49), and cortical and cancellous bone ultimately become replaced by a network of slender trabeculae of non-lamellar bone. Although the lesions are diffuse, some parts of the skeleton may be more severely involved than others. Iliac crest biopsy in cases of hyperparathyroidism[293] shows increased osteoclastic and osteoblastic activity, even in the absence of radiological changes. It is not clear why resorption of bone in hyperparathyroidism is followed by fibrous replacement, as this is not seen in most other types of bone resorption: perhaps the greater rate of removal of bone in hyperparathyroidism is responsible.

The 'brown tumours' are areas of fibrous scarring, with collections of osteoclasts, haemorrhages, and pseudocyst formation.* In the past, they were regarded as giant cell tumours (osteoclastomas), but the two types of lesion are now usually recognized to be quite distinct.[283] The brown tumours regress, as do the other bone changes, after surgical removal of the hyperplastic or adenomatous parathyroid tissue.

Bone lesions comparable with those of clinical hyperparathyroidism have been produced in experimental animals by continued administration of parathyroid hormone.[294, 294a]

Metastatic calcification, predominantly involving the kidneys, occurs in primary hyperparathyroidism, and may result in impairment of renal function.

Hypoparathyroidism[295]

Hypoparathyroidism may occur as an unexplained primary deficiency, or as the result of surgical removal of parathyroid tissue in operations on the thyroid gland (see page 2047 in Volume 4). The serum phosphorus is raised as a result of diminished renal excretion of phosphate, and the serum calcium is lowered, these changes being the reverse of those

* The name 'brown tumour' is given also to the tumour-like lesions of pigmented villonodular synovitis (see page 2509), including localized nodular synovitis (the so-called giant cell tumour of tendon sheaths).

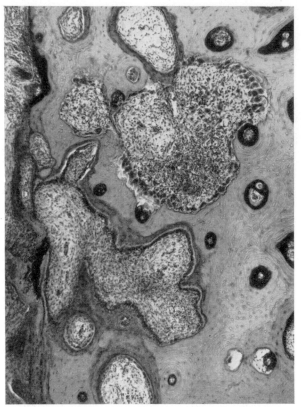

Fig. 37.49. Hyperparathyroidism. Active osteoclastic resorption and osteoblastic new bone formation in cortical bone. *Haematoxylin–eosin.* × 60.

encountered in hyperparathyroidism The signs and symptoms are the consequence of hypocalcaemia and include tetany and convulsions. Ectopic calcification, particularly of the basal ganglia of the brain, is common. Some increase in bone density has been reported in cases of hypoparathyroidism,[296] but bone changes in this condition are not conspicuous.

Bone Changes in Renal Diseases

There are two types of renal disease in which structural alterations in bone tissue occur. In straightforward renal failure, loss of glomerular and tubular function leads to uraemia, and a complex set of bone changes, collectively known as *azotaemic renal osteodystrophy*, may result. In contrast to this there are certain disorders of the renal tubules, associated with loss of phosphate and sometimes of other substances, that lead to bone changes of a rachitic or osteomalacic type. These conditions may be considered here.

Bone Changes of Renal Failure (*Azotaemic Renal Osteodystrophy*)

Prolonged renal failure is almost invariably accompanied by changes in bone tissue, and renal osteodystrophy is consequently one of the commonest metabolic diseases of bone. The bone changes consist of fibrous replacement of bone—the so-called 'osteitis fibrosa'—and this may be associated with rickets or osteomalacia, or with osteosclerosis. In children the picture is usually further complicated by interference with growth. There are several valuable reviews of the pathological changes in the bones,[297–300] and of the chemical aspects[202, 301] of renal osteodystrophy.

In renal osteodystrophy, the serum calcium is usually normal or low and the serum phosphorus is often greatly increased: uraemia and acidosis are also present. A number of factors have been invoked to explain the bone changes. Both the histology of the bone lesions, which closely resemble those of primary hyperparathyroidism, and the frequent occurrence of parathyroid enlargement,[299, 302–304] indicate the importance of secondary hyperparathyroidism in renal osteodystrophy. The fall in serum calcium, particularly in its ionized component, is the likeliest stimulus to parathyroid hyperplasia, and may also play a part in the failure of mineralization. Other factors that have been suggested in relation to the pathogenesis of the bone lesions are acidosis, increased serum phosphorus, and an acquired resistance to the effects of vitamin D. No single explanation appears applicable to all cases.

Bone Changes Accompanying Renal Failure in Children.

—In children, the bones may be bowed and otherwise deformed, and the epiphysial cartilage plates are thickened and irregular, somewhat as in dietary rickets (Figs 37.50 and 37.51). The bones, particularly the phalanges, show the periosteal erosions characteristic of hyperparathyroidism (Fig. 37.50). There is usually abundant osteoid tissue at bone surfaces, and fibrous replacement of bone indicates the presence of parathyroid overactivity As in primary hyperparathyroidism, osteoclastic resorption and osteoblastic bone formation are both active in affected parts of the skeleton. The architecture of both cancellous and cortical bone becomes very irregular, and in some longstanding cases parts of the skeleton present a characteristic radiographic appearance of 'woolly density'.

Bone Changes Accompanying Renal Failure in Adults.

—In adult patients, deformities are rare.

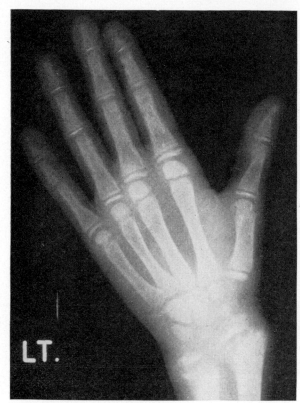

Fig. 37.50. Renal osteodystrophy in a child. Radiograph of a hand, showing the 'rachitic' appearance of the epiphysial cartilage plates of the radius and ulna, and also cortical erosions characteristic of hyperparathyroidism. See also Fig. 37.51.

Radiologically, their bones usually show a general loss of density, with widespread erosion of the cortex. In longstanding cases in adults, as in children, the bone architecture may be greatly altered, and the bones come to show a patchy appearance of increased density. This is sometimes particularly obvious in the skull (Fig. 37.52) and the spine, and in the latter situation it gives a banded appearance to vertebral bodies (Fig. 37.53). Histologically, both cortical and cancellous bone show exaggerated osteoclastic resorption, with replacement of bone by fibrous tissue (Fig. 37.54): this is responsible for the characteristic cortical erosion (Fig. 37.50). Bone trabeculae are sometimes hollowed by areas of local resorption and fibrous replacement (Fig. 37.55): this process—also seen in primary hyperparathyroidism—is termed *dissecting resorption*. As in primary hyperparathyroidism, new bone formation is abundant (Fig. 37.56), and it is evident that active structural reorganization of the involved areas is in progress. The appearance of increased radiological density is produced by the accumula-

tion, in certain areas, of large numbers of slender and irregularly outlined trabeculae, mostly made up of non-lamellar bone (Figs 37.57 and 37.58). This histological appearance is usually referred to as 'osteosclerosis',[297, 300, 305, 306] but it must be remembered that the tissue in question is very different from that in other forms of osteosclerosis, and in fact is usually quite soft. This compacted type of bone tissue may show a superficial histological resemblance to bone in Paget's disease (see page 2436), but it lacks the mosaic of cement lines that is characteristic of the latter.

'Osteosclerosis', as described above, is rarely a prominent feature in primary hyperparathyroidism. Other features of renal osteodystrophy that help to distinguish it from primary hyperparathyroidism are the rarity of cysts and 'brown tumours', and the presence, in some cases, of an osteomalacic component.

Metastatic calcification is a frequent accompaniment of renal osteodystrophy. It involves arteries, subcutaneous tissue, heart, lungs and kidneys.[307]

Rickets and Osteomalacia Due to Disorders of the Renal Tubules[308, 309]

Quite apart from frank renal failure with uraemia, certain abnormalities of renal tubular function can

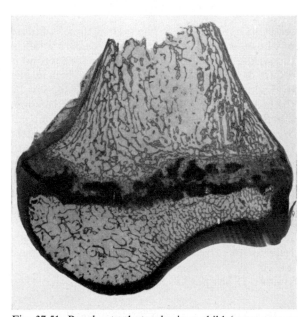

Fig. 37.51. Renal osteodystrophy in a child (same case as Fig. 37.50). Section of the lower end of a femur: the epiphysial cartilage plate is thickened and irregular, and even at this magnification the abnormal pattern of bone trabeculae in the metaphysis is evident. These structures showed extensive fibrous replacement. *Haematoxylin–eosin.* × 2.

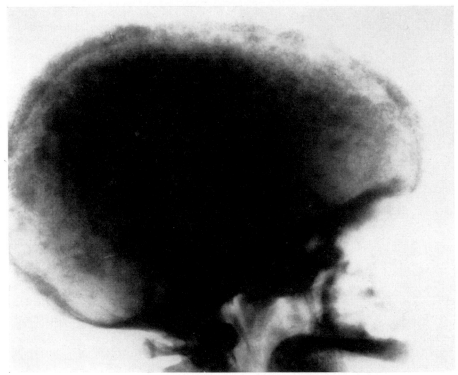

Fig. 37.52. Renal osteodystrophy. Radiograph of skull, showing mottled appearance produced by diffuse rarefaction and patchy increase in density.

result in bone changes. The first of these is failure of phosphate reabsorption, which leads to a fall in the serum phosphorus concentration. The second is failure of reabsorption of bicarbonate, which results in acidosis: reduction in ammonia production by the kidneys causes increased excretion of calcium, together with other abnormalities of mineral excretion. These defects may be present separately or together, and they are sometimes associated with renal glycosuria and aminoaciduria. Each type of abnormality leads to rickets and osteomalacia, presumably through the alterations in the level of calcium and phosphorus in the serum. The resulting rickets or osteomalacia is described as vitamin-D-resistant, enormous doses of vitamin D being required to correct the bony abnormality (see page 2422). The mechanism of the therapeutic effect of vitamin D has not yet been explained.

Phosphaturic Rickets.—A simple inability to re-absorb phosphate occurs as a familial disorder that is apparently inherited as a dominant characteristic.[309, 310] Typical rachitic changes result from the functional deficiency.

De Toni–Fanconi Syndrome (De Toni–Debré–Fanconi Syndrome)[311, 311a, 311b*]—The de Toni–Fanconi syndrome is characterized by inability to reabsorb phosphate, renal glycosuria and amino-aciduria. A distinctive deformity of the proximal part of the renal tubule has been demonstrated in caes of this condition (see page 1452, Volume 4).[312] Deposition of cystine in tissues such as the lymph nodes, bone marrow and spleen sometimes occurs in this condition, which appears to be inherited as a recessive characteristic.[310] In a number of cases, the renal lesion ultimately progresses to more wide-spread tubular and glomerular damage, with uraemia.[313]

Hypophosphataemic Osteomalacia Associated with Tumours.—There is a rare form of vitamin-D-resistant osteomalacia (or late onset rickets) that is characterized by impaired reabsorption of phos-phate by the renal tubules.[313a] In addition to phosphaturia and hypophosphataemia there may be glycosuria and aminoaciduria. In a significant proportion of cases this condition has been asso-ciated with a connective tissue tumour of bone or

* See footnote on nomenclature on page 1451 in Volume 4.

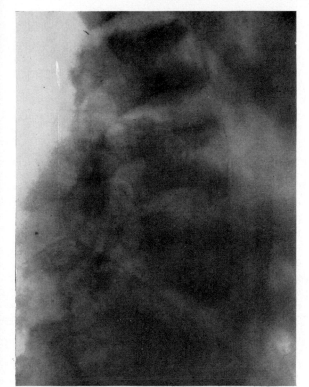

Fig. 37.53. Renal osteodystrophy. Radiograph of lumbar spine (lateral view), showing banded appearance of vertebral bodies. See also Figs 37.57A, 37.57B and 37.58.

PAGET'S DISEASE OF BONE[314]

In 1877, James Paget described a series of patients, all over 40 years of age, with enlargement and deformity of various bones.[314a] The aetiology of the condition was—and still is—obscure, and Paget used the term *osteitis deformans* to describe it. In its fully developed form it is quite rare, but it is now recognized that lesser degrees of skeletal involvement, often without clinical manifestations, are not uncommon. The classic studies of Schmorl,[315] published in 1932, provide dependable information on the incidence of Paget's disease and the distribution of the lesions: the collection of such information was made possible by Schmorl's recognition of the histological features that have come to be accepted as pathognomonic of the condition. [315–317]

Paget's disease is rarely seen in patients under 40 years of age, and usually develops after the age of 50. Juvenile cases with somewhat similar clinical and pathological features have occasionally been reported:[318–321] they are sometimes referred to by the term *hyperphosphatasia*; they are probably quite

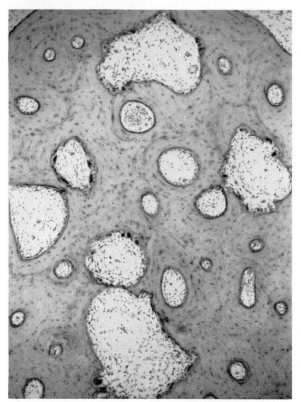

Fig. 37.54. Renal osteodystrophy. Cortical bone of femoral shaft, showing exaggerated osteoclastic resorption. *Haematoxylin–eosin.* × 60.

soft tissue.[313b] The tumours may be pleomorphic, including a range of distinct tissues of mesodermal derivation. In some of these cases the biochemical disorder has been improved or cured by excision of the tumour; in cases in which the tumour was malignant, excision has usually been without effect, probably because the growth was not removed entirely. It seems probable that the tumour secretes a factor that interferes with renal tubular function.[313b] The association of hypophosphataemic osteomalacia with widespread metastasis of prostatic carcinoma to bone has been observed[313c] and indicates a further aspect of the relation between neoplasia and osteomalacia that will need to be taken into account in diagnosis of the cause of this syndrome.[313b] It may be noted that the tumours that have been associated with this syndrome are not of endocrine type; further, hypophosphataemic osteomalacia is not a sign of oversecretion of any known hormone: these facts indicate that it is premature to regard the syndrome as a manifestation of ectopic hormone secretion.

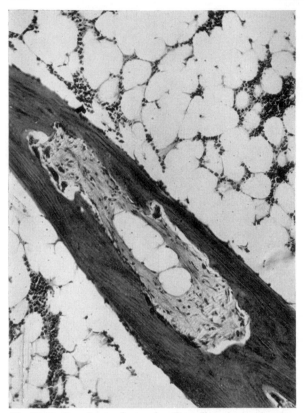

Fig. 37.55. Renal osteodystrophy. Cancellous bone, showing hollowing of a bone trabecula by 'dissecting resorption'. *Haematoxylin–eosin.* × 120.

unrelated to true Paget's disease. The incidence of Paget's disease appears to vary considerably in different parts of the world, relatively few cases having been reported in African or Asian populations: accurate comparative figures, however, are lacking. Schmorl's studies showed that, in Dresden, Paget's disease was present in about 3 per cent of unselected hospital necropsies on individuals over 40 years of age.[315] A similar figure was obtained in a survey of its incidence at necropsy in Yorkshire.[317] There is a moderate preponderance of men in most reported series. A study of about 1000 abdominal radiographs in each of 14 towns in England and Wales, as filed in the records of general hospitals, showed radiological evidence of the disease in 5·4 per cent of people aged 55 years and over (7 per cent of men and 3·8 per cent of women), with a rather greater prevalence in Lancashire than elsewhere.[321a] In some cases only a single bone is affected: in others many bones are involved. The vertebral column, including the sacrum, is most commonly affected: other common sites include the skull, pelvis and femora. The

tibiae are less frequently involved, although tibial bowing is one of the characteristic features of the fully developed form of the disease. Whether solitary or multiple, the bone lesions in Paget's disease are focal, being clearly demarcated from the adjacent uninvolved bone tissue.

The disease is said to be associated with Hashimoto's thyroiditis oftener than chance would explain (see page 2010, Volume 4).[321b]

Gross Appearances

The gross appearance of the lesions varies (Figs 37.59 to 37.61). At an early stage the involved area of bone may be porotic. Later, the cortical and cancellous bone comes to be replaced by a characteristic network of coarse trabecular structures, and this, together with an increase in the thickness of cortical bone, can result in a radiological appearance of increased density. Certain deformities are characteristic. The femoral neck, when involved, is often bent to a position of coxa vara (Fig. 37.59A). The tibia becomes greatly thickened and bowed (Fig. 37.61), and the abnormal cortical bone is often marked by numerous transverse fissures (incomplete fractures), usually referred to as *Looser's zones* (see page 2421), where a gap in the bony tissue is occupied by fibrous tissue or incompletely calcified callus. Skull involvement usually takes the form of thickening of the bones of the vault (Fig. 37.59B), with loss of the distinction between the inner and outer tables: less often, areas of focal rarefaction are encountered, a condition that is sometimes termed *osteoporosis circumscripta*.[322, 323] Involvement of the base of the skull may occur, and is occasionally accompanied by deafness or other evidence of cranial nerve compression, or by *platybasia* (flattening of the base of the skull over the supporting cervical spine).[324]

Histology

Histologically, the lesions of Paget's disease show disordered and extremely active bone remodelling. At an active stage of the development of a lesion, osteoclastic bone resorption and osteoblastic bone deposition are both evident (Figs 37.62 to 37.64); the latter may result in the presence of considerable amounts of non-lamellar bone (Fig. 37.63). In these active lesions, the marrow spaces of the bone are occupied, wholly or in part, by vascular fibrous tissue (Fig. 37.64). In more established lesions, in which lamellar bone has been formed, the bony structures show the characteristic mosaic areas (Fig. 37.62) that were recognized by Schmorl[315] as the definitive histological feature of Paget's disease.

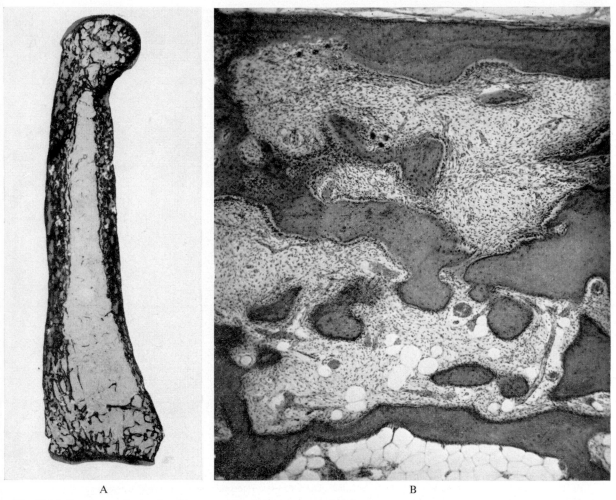

Fig. 37.56. Renal osteodystrophy. *Haematoxylin–eosin.*

A. Phalanx of a finger, showing patchy replacement of cortical bone by fibrous tissue. × 4.

B. Higher magnification of part of the cortex in Fig. 37.56A: much of the bone is replaced by fibrous tissue; two collections of osteoclasts are present, and parts of the bone surface are covered by osteoblasts and palely staining osteoid. × 50.

The mosaic areas are outlined by markedly crenated cement lines, each indicating a surface where bone resorption has been followed by bone deposition: the bizarre arrangement of the cement lines indicates the disorganization of bone remodelling that is a characteristic feature of the disease. In established lesions, the extent of the structural disorganization of cortical bone is such that no oriented vascular canals or Haversian systems remain, the bone being made up of a network of thick, irregularly outlined trabeculae. Some lesions that may be presumed to have reached a quiescent stage have plentiful mosaic areas but lack active remodelling.

Effects of Paget's Disease

Bones involved by Paget's disease are more liable to fracture than normal bones: after fracture, repair proceeds in a normal fashion.

The lesions of Paget's disease are sometimes very vascular, and there may be a great increase in blood flow through the affected bone.[325–327] In effect, these lesions are arteriovenous shunts, and in extreme cases the consequent increase in cardiac output results in cardiac failure (see page 60 in Volume 1).[328, 329] Atherosclerosis and hypertension are commonly present in patients who have Paget's disease: they also may lead to heart failure.

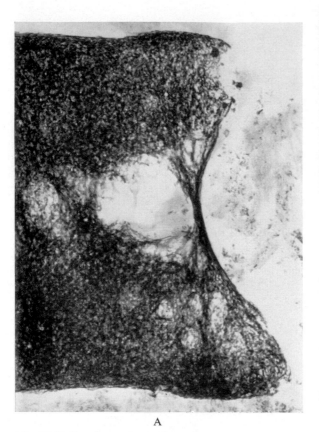
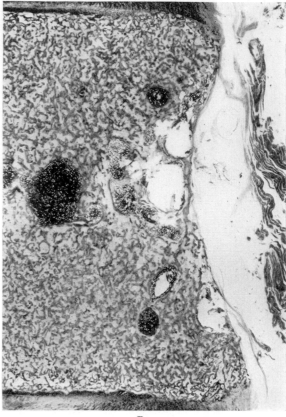

A   B

Fig. 37.57. Renal osteodystrophy. × 4.

A. Radiograph of a slab of bone from one of the vertebrae shown in Fig. 37.53.

B. Histological preparation from another vertebral body in the same case. The normal bone trabeculae have been replaced by a close meshwork of slender, irregular trabeculae: these are so numerous that the overall radiological appearance is one of increased bone density. See Fig. 37.58. *Haematoxylin–eosin.*

Biochemical Findings

The use of isotopes for the study of mineral exchange in cases of Paget's disease has shown high rates for the skeletal accretion and resorption of calcium, with an increase in the size of the exchangeable pool.[330-332] These findings are clearly related to the activity of bone remodelling. Calcium accretion of from 32 to 176 mg per kilogram of body weight per day has been reported, in contrast to normal values of about 9 mg. The serum calcium and phosphate levels are usually normal in Paget's disease, but active lesions are associated with high values for the serum alkaline phosphatase. The urinary excretion of hydroxyproline, thought to be derived from the breakdown of collagen and thus an indication of the amount of bone remodelling, is increased in Paget's disease.

Calcitonin Therapy

Calcitonin, the plasma-calcium-lowering hormone of the thyroid (see pages 1940 and 2041 in Volume 4), finds a clinical application in the treatment of Paget's disease, particularly when there is bone pain or hypercalcaemia.[333] Its administration is followed by a fall in the concentration of alkaline phosphatase in the serum and of hydroxyproline in the urine; the number of osteoclasts in biopsy specimens of bone is also reduced.

Malignant Change

It is now well established that Paget's disease is a precancerous condition.[334] It appears that about 30 per cent of primary malignant bone tumours developing after the age of 40 years occur in

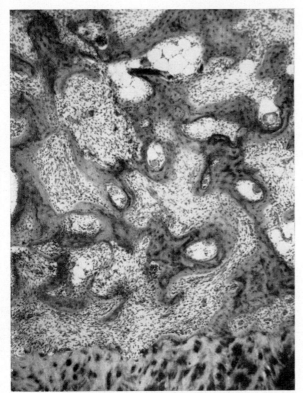

Fig. 37.58. Renal osteodystrophy. Higher magnification of part of the vertebra shown in Fig. 37.57B. The irregular trabeculae consist of non-lamellar bone; the palely staining material covering part of their surface is osteoid tissue. *Haematoxylin–eosin.* × 55.

individuals with Paget's disease, although these constitute only about 3 per cent of the population in their age group. The likelihood of malignant change in any individual with Paget's disease is quite small, although it is thought to occur in as many as 5 to 10 per cent of the cases in which the skeleton is severely involved.[335] In one series of 76 cases of bone sarcoma developing in Paget's disease, 84 per cent of the patients were men.[336] Any part of the skeleton may be involved, but tumours have been observed most frequently in the major long bones, and in the pelvis and skull.[337] The majority of the tumours are pleomorphic osteosarcomas: some of them contain conspicuously bizarre, and numerous, multinucleate tumour giant cells. Other types of malignant skeletal tumours, including chondrosarcoma and fibrosarcoma, may be found; in contrast, the typical giant cell tumour ('osteo-clastoma') is rarely encountered. The bone tumours that develop in Paget's disease are highly malignant. In a number of reported cases multiple bone sarcomas were present: in at least some of these the lesions seem to have been independent primary tumours and not metastatic.[338]

FIBROUS DYSPLASIA OF BONE[339–341]

Fibrous dysplasia of bone is characterized by the development in one or more bones of circumscribed lesions consisting of bone-forming fibrous tissue. The term *monostotic* (or *solitary*) *fibrous dysplasia* is used when the condition affects a single bone and *polyostotic fibrous dysplasia* when there are multiple lesions. The histological appearances are the same in both types of case.

Occasionally, a patient with polyostotic fibrous dysplasia presents areas of cutaneous pigmentation and evidence of endocrine disturbance, especially precocious puberty: the term *Albright's syndrome** is used to describe this association.[342, 343] The aetiology of fibrous dysplasia is unknown: although it appears to be an abnormality of skeletal development, there is no evidence that it is familial. In the past, cases of polyostotic fibrous dysplasia were often confused with hyperparathyroidism under the terms 'osteitis fibrosa' and 'fibrocystic disease of bone'. In 1931, Hunter and Turnbull[344] distinguished the two types of case, contrasting the diffuse nature of the osteitis fibrosa of hyperparathyroidism and the focal nature of the bone lesions in cases not associated with that condition. The term *fibrous dysplasia* was introduced by Lichtenstein,[339, 345] originally with reference to the polyostotic form of the disease and later to include the solitary lesions with a similar histological structure.

Fibrous dysplasia is by no means rare. Its cause is not known. The monostotic form is commoner than the polyostotic. The disease usually becomes evident during childhood or adolescence; the sexes appear to be affected with equal frequency. The bones that are commonly involved include the femora and tibiae, the facial skeleton and the ribs. In cases of the polyostotic form the lesions are often confined to one limb or one region of the body. They commence in the central part of the affected bone and often produce some expansion of the cortex. They consist of fibrous tissue that replaces the cancellous bone and the marrow (Figs 37.65 to 37.67). The fibrous tissue contains a variable amount of bone, which gives it firmness and a gritty texture. Small or large cysts are quite commonly present.

* Albright's syndrome of polyostotic fibrous dysplasia is distinct from the osteodystrophy that he also described (see pages 2047 and 2048 in Volume 4).

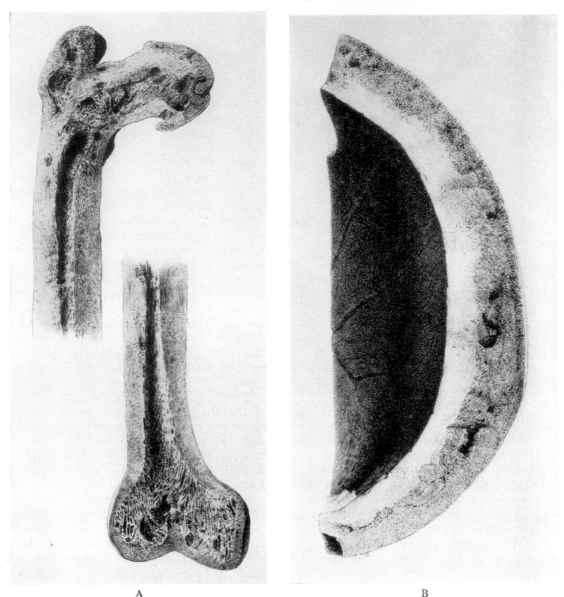

A   B

Fig. 37.59. Paget's disease, as illustrated in Sir James Paget's account (*Med.-chir. Trans.*, 1877, **60**, 37).

A. Macerated femur, showing coarse trabeculation and thickening of the cortex.

B. Macerated skull, showing thickening of the bone and loss of the demarcation between the inner and outer tables.

Histology

The histological appearance is characteristic (Figs 37.68 to 37.71). The abnormal tissue is a spindle-celled fibrous tissue in which there are trabeculae of non-lamellar bone. The bony component often forms curved sheets, appearing in sections as a distinctive network (Figs 37.68 to 37.70). Osteoclasts are often present and may be numerous (Fig. 37.71). There may be foci of cartilage.

Course and Complications

The lesions usually grow only slowly. Some become quiescent at the time of skeletal maturation: others continue to grow during adult life. Reactivation after long periods of quiescence is not uncommon, and is sometimes associated with pregnancy. A lesion of fibrous dysplasia occasionally increases rapidly in size as a result of haemorrhage or cyst formation. Recurrent fractures are

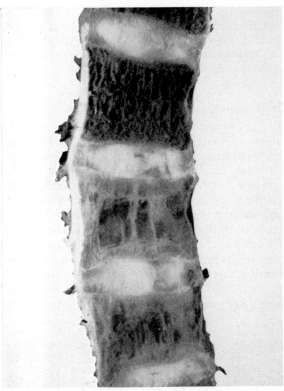

Fig. 37.60.§ Paget's disease of spine. The two lower vertebral bodies show the coarse trabeculation characteristic of the disease; the vertebral body above them is normal.

often the major disability. Even in the absence of fracture, severe deformities can occur: a common site is the upper end of the femur, which can become extremely bowed under the stresses of weight-bearing. In a few cases fibrosarcoma has developed in lesions of fibrous dysplasia,[346] but this is a most infrequent complication.

Differential Diagnosis

Certain fibro-osseous lesions of the jaws, previously described as '*fibrous osteomas*',[347] appear to be examples of fibrous dysplasia (see page 941, Volume 3). The same may possibly be true of the fibro-osseous thickening of cranial and facial bones that is referred to as '*leontiasis ossea*'.[348]

As already noted, fibrous dysplasia is to be distinguished from the changes in bone that accompany hyperparathyroidism (see page 2430). The lesions of hyperparathyroidism are more diffuse, and they lack the distinctive network of non-lamellar bone that is usually present in sections of some parts of the lesions of fibrous dysplasia. The biochemical changes of hyperparathyroidism (hypercalcaemia and hypophosphataemia) are not a feature of fibrous dysplasia, although transient hypercalcaemia may result if the patient is immobilized, particularly in cases with multiple bone

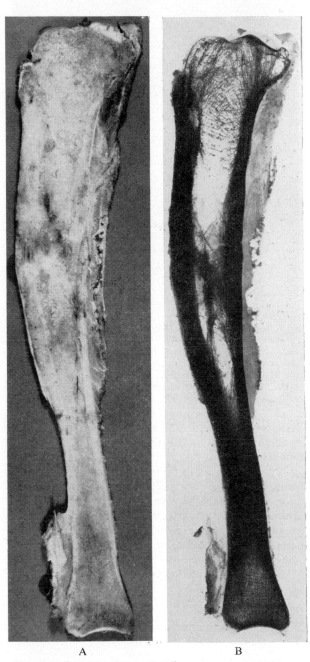

A   B

Fig. 37.61.§ Paget's disease of tibia.

A.§ Longitudinally divided tibia, showing bowing of the bone and thickening and coarse trabeculation of its cortex.

B.§ Radiograph of a slab of bone from the surface of the same specimen.

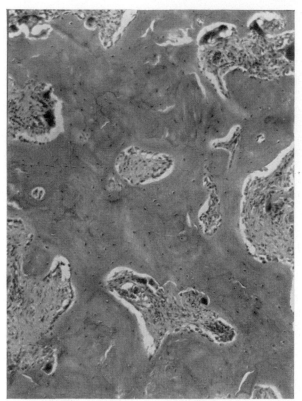

Fig. 37.62. Paget's disease. The coarse trabeculae show the characteristic mosaic of cement lines. The spaces between the trabeculae are occupied by fibrous tissue, and both osteoclastic resorption and osteoblastic bone deposition are evident. *Haematoxylin–eosin.* × 85.

lesions and fractures. In some cases there is a moderate elevation of the serum alkaline phosphatase.

A solitary lesion of fibrous dysplasia is sometimes confused with a non-ossifying fibroma of bone (see page 2455). If adequate histological material is available, the two diseases should be readily distinguishable, as the non-ossifying fibroma characteristically is devoid of any bone formation.

MISCELLANEOUS CONDITIONS

Bone Cysts

There are two types of primary cystic lesion of bone, the *simple cyst* and the *degenerative cyst.** They are considered in this section.

* Both the simple bone cyst and the degenerative bone cyst are more accurately described as pseudocysts, being without any proper cellular lining lamina and probably formed through breakdown of the cancellous bone, fluid accumulating locally in place of the original tissue. However, they are so familiar to surgeons and pathologists as 'bone cysts' that they are referred to here by this term.

Secondary cystic change—strictly, pseudocystic change—can occur in a variety of bone lesions, including fibrous dysplasia and hyperparathyroidism. The condition known as *aneurysmal bone cyst* is discussed on page 2458.

Simple Bone Cyst[349]*

This type of lesion, also known as *solitary cyst* and *unicameral cyst*, occurs in the metaphysis of long bones in children; the humerus is the bone most commonly involved. The cyst (Fig. 37.72) takes the form of a rounded cavity, lined by a thin membrane of fibrous tissue; it contains clear fluid. The overlying cortical bone may be thinned and somewhat expanded by the cyst, which grows by accumulation of fluid and progressive attenuation of the surrounding bone. Fracture is a fairly frequent complication: haemorrhage results, and the formation of granulation tissue and fracture callus may greatly increase the thickness of the lining of the

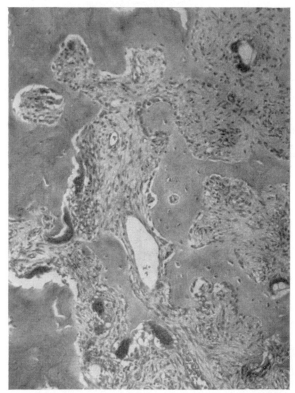

Fig. 37.63. Paget's disease. This field includes some newly formed trabeculae of non-lamellar bone: these do not show the characteristic mosaic of cement lines (compare with Fig. 37.62). *Haematoxylin–eosin.* × 95.

* See footnote in adjoining column.

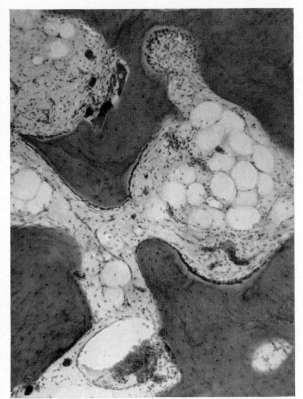

Fig. 37.64. Paget's disease. Osteoclastic resorption and osteoblastic bone deposition are evident. The marrow spaces are occupied by vascular fibrous tissue. *Haematoxylin–eosin.* ×85.

cyst. The presence of a cyst does not interfere with the growth of the nearby epiphysial cartilage plate: consequently, the lesion appears to migrate from the epiphysis as new bone is formed at the metaphysial surface of the plate.

Degenerative Bone Cyst*

Subchondral cystic lesions, consisting of degenerate fibrous tissue and a collection of fluid, occur in relation to articular lesions of osteoarthritis (see page 2502). Somewhat similar cysts occasionally occur in the absence of osteoarthritis:[350–352] they involve the subchondral bone in the neighbourhood of a joint but do not communicate with the joint cavity.

Lipidoses and Related Conditions

Bone lesions are encountered in some of the lipidoses.[353] Somewhat similar changes occur in

* See footnote in left-hand column of opposite page.

other diseases, possibly related to the lipidoses, and these may be considered here also.

Gaucher's Disease

In this condition (see page 759 in Volume 2), large amounts of the cerebroside, kerasin, accumulate in the reticuloendothelial cells of the spleen, liver, lymph nodes and bone marrow. The affected cells are large, and their cytoplasm has a characteristic ground-glass-like appearance (see Figs 9.181 and 9.182 on page 760 in Volume 1); the lipid contents do not react with the usual fat stains. The condition usually appears in childhood.

The bones may show a number of macroscopically evident abnormalities in addition to the microscopical finding of replacement of the marrow by the lipid-filled cells.[354] There is often a characteristic expansion of the lower end of each femur, giving the bone a shape that is likened to that of an Erlenmeyer flask. The cortex of the femur is thinned and there may be angulation of the neck of the bone. Foci of ischaemic necrosis sometimes develop, particularly in the femoral head.[355]

Niemann–Pick Disease[356]

Gross lesions are seldom found in the bones in cases of this rare and usually rapidly fatal lipidosis (see page 761 in Volume 2), in which the phospholipid sphingomyelin accumulates in histiocytes in the spleen, liver, lymph nodes, bone marrow and central nervous system.

Hand–Schüller–Christian Disease and Eosinophil Granuloma of Bone

Hand–Schüller–Christian Disease.[357]—In this condition the accumulation of cholesterol-laden histiocytes results in a syndrome comprising diabetes insipidus, exophthalmos and multiple osteolytic lesions, which occur particularly in the skull (see page 763 in Volume 2). The lesions in bone, which are characterized by a dense accumulation of histiocytes and eosinophils, may be indistinguishable from those of eosinophil granuloma of bone (see below).

Eosinophil Granuloma of Bone.[358, 359]—There is argument whether eosinophil granuloma of bone is related to Hand–Schüller–Christian disease, and

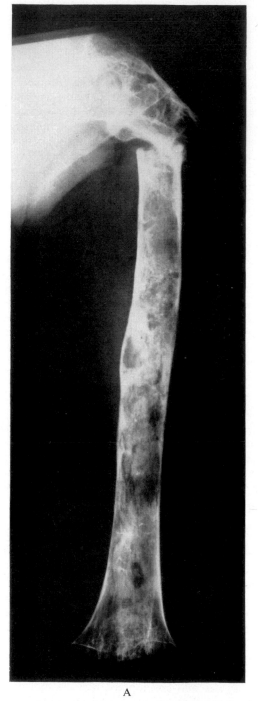 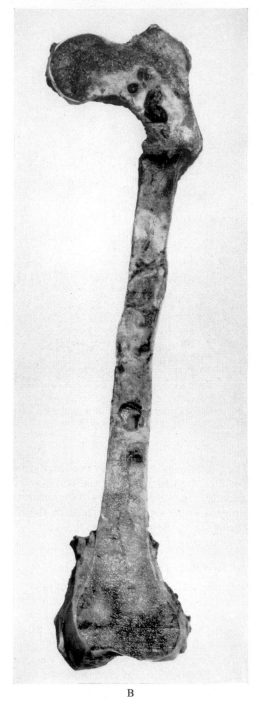

A   B

Fig. 37.65.§ Fibrous dysplasia: femur. Same case as in Figs 37.66 and 37.67.

A.§ Radiograph showing numerous areas of rarefaction and a pathological fracture.

B.§ Longitudinally divided femur: the cortex is thinned and much of the cancellous bone and marrow
cavity is replaced by fibrous tissue; several cysts are present.

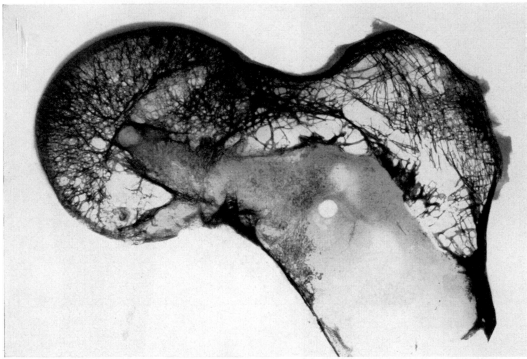

Fig. 37.66. Fibrous dysplasia: femur. Radiograph of a slab of tissue from the specimen shown in Fig. 37.65: the cancellous bone of the lower part of the neck of the femur is replaced by fibrous tissue; the fine shadows are trabeculae of non-lamellar bone in the abnormal tissue.

whether either of these is related to Letterer–Siwe disease (see below) and to the form of malignant histiocytosis that is sometimes known as 'histiocytosis X' (see page 858 in Volume 2). Eosinophil granuloma of bone occurs in children and young adults and is characterized by the development of solitary or multiple osteolytic lesions. These consist of dense accumulations of lipid-laden histiocytes and numerous eosinophils. The histiocytes appear foamy or vacuolate in paraffin wax sections; in frozen sections their cytoplasm gives the staining reactions of neutral fat and cholesterol, which can also be identified in the affected tissue by chemical analysis.

The prognosis appears to depend on the age of the patient and the multiplicity of the lesions: solitary lesions in older children usually regress spontaneously, while cases with widely disseminated lesions—particularly in very young children—may have a rapidly progressive course.

Letterer–Siwe Disease.—As indicated above, some authorities[360, 361] regard this condition as a more rapidly developing and generalized form of eosinophil granuloma of bone (see page 858 in Volume 2).

Bone Changes in the Haemoglobinopathies

Various changes have been recognized radiologically in the bones in cases of sickle cell anaemia, thalassaemia and other conditions characterized by the presence of abnormal forms of haemoglobin, particularly in children.[362–365] The view of most authorities is that the changes are the result of compression and displacement of bony structures by the proliferating erythropoietic cells of the marrow, sometimes accompanied by infarction of bone (see page 2406).[365a]

The tables of the vault of the skull are thinned; the outer table is often displaced outward, and vertical spiculation may be seen on the external aspect of the inner table. The long bones are sometimes expanded, and their cortex may be thinned. In some cases the expanded bones become sclerotic. The relatively few studies of the histological picture have established the presence of bone necrosis and non-specific reactive changes.[366–368]

Salmonella osteomyelitis (see page 2411) has been reported as a complication of the bone lesions in cases of haemoglobinopathy, particularly in younger patients.[368a]

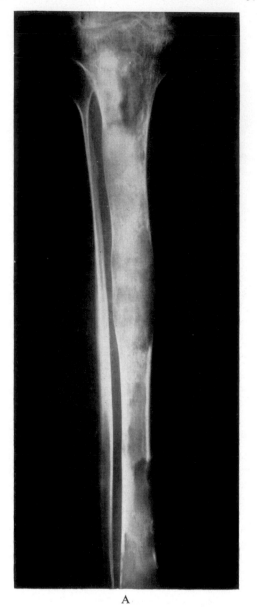

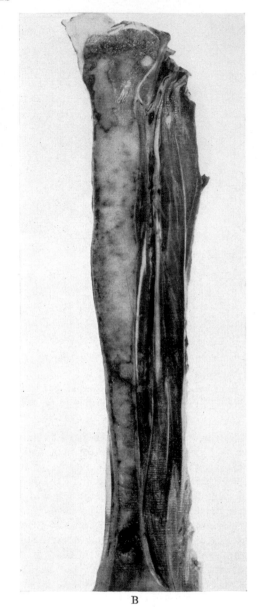

A   B

Fig. 37.67.§ Fibrous dysplasia: tibia. Same case as in Figs 37.65A and 37.66.

A.§ Radiograph showing several osteolytic areas in the lower part of the tibia; the upper part contains a larger, expanding lesion that is relatively radio-opaque.

B.§ Longitudinally divided tibia: the clearly outlined margin of the fibrous tissue is evident. See Fig. 37.67C.

TUMOURS OF BONE

Primary Tumours

There are many different types of bone tumours, and these vary widely in their clinical presentation, pathology and behaviour. Current nomenclature and classification are embodied in a World Health Organization publication.[369] The most compre-

hensive account of the pathology of tumours of bone is that by Jaffe;[370] other monographs include those by Dahlin,[371] Spjut and his associates[372] and Lichtenstein.[373]

Primary tumours of bone account for only about 0·25 to 1·0 per cent of all deaths from cancer, although bone is one of the tissues from which sarcomas most frequently arise. While the incidence

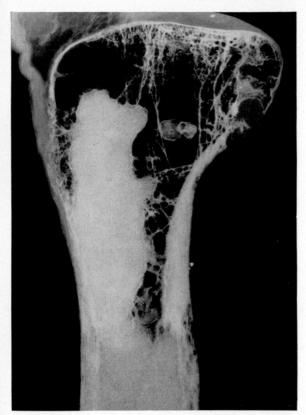

Fig. 37.67C.§ Radiograph of a slab of tissue from the upper end of the specimen shown in Fig. 37.67B: the radiographic density of the lesion results from the presence of numerous slender bone trabeculae in the abnormal tissue.

of most other types of cancer increases steadily with increasing age, there is an unexplained peak of incidence of malignant bone tumours at about 15 to 20 years: a second rise begins after the thirtieth year and continues throughout life.[374, 375]

The aetiology of tumours of bone is obscure. While malignant bone tumours can be produced experimentally by a variety of agents, including ionizing radiations, oncogenic hydrocarbons, and beryllium and other metals, there is no evidence to suggest that such factors are important in the production of 'spontaneous' bone tumours in man. Paget's disease of bone is a precancerous condition (see page 2438). Malignant change also occurs as a complication of certain benign cartilaginous lesions of bone (exostoses and enchondromas), while a few cases are on record in which there has been sarcomatous change in fibrous dysplasia of bone.

In recent years there has been considerable interest in the possibility, as yet unestablished, that

some malignant bone tumours in man may have a viral cause.[376, 377] Viruses, particularly leucoviruses, have been shown to produce bone tumours in small laboratory animals, and cell-free extracts of some human and spontaneous animal osteosarcomas have been shown to cause tumours or tumour-like lesions to develop in animals.

Classification of Primary Tumours of Bone

Table 37.1 lists the various types of primary tumours currently recognized. Most of these arise from skeletal connective tissue, which comprises all the related and more or less specifically differentiated connective tissue cells of bone. Such tumours show differentiation of bone, cartilage, fibrous tissue, giant cells, and other skeletal structures, and they are identified histologically by the type and degree of this differentiation. Other bone tumours evidently take origin from the non-osseous components of the skeleton, including the haemopoietic and lymphoreticular elements.

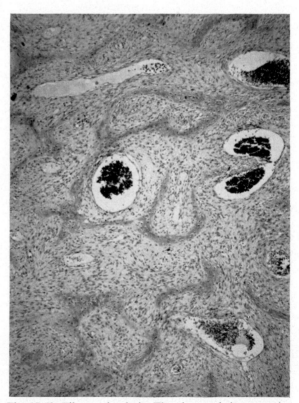

Fig. 37.68. Fibrous dysplasia. The abnormal tissue consists of fibrous tissue with spindle-shaped cells and slender trabeculae of non-lamellar bone. *Haematoxylin–eosin.* × 50.

Table 37.1. *Classification of Primary Tumours of Bone*

BENIGN TUMOURS	MALIGNANT TUMOURS
Taking origin from skeletal connective tissue	
Osteoma	Osteosarcoma:
Osteoid osteoma	Central osteosarcoma
Benign osteoblastoma	Juxtacortical osteosarcoma
Cartilage-capped exostosis	Chondrosarcoma:
(solitary or multiple)	Juxtacortical chondro-
Enchondroma	sarcoma
(solitary or multiple)	'Mesenchymal' chondro-
Chondroblastoma	sarcoma
Chondromyxoid fibroma	Fibrosarcoma
Non-ossifying fibroma	Fibrous histiocytoma
Desmoplastic fibroma	Giant cell tumour
Taking origin from other skeletal components	
Vascular tumours:	Ewing's tumour
Haemangioma	Lymphoreticular and haemo-
Lymphangioma	poietic tumours:
Lipoma	Myelomatosis
Neurolemmoma and neuro-	Hodgkin's disease
fibroma	'Lymphosarcoma'*
Other benign tumours	'Reticulum cell sarcoma'*
	Leukaemia
	Chordoma
	'Adamantinoma' of limb
	bones
	Angiosarcoma
	Liposarcoma

* The terms lymphosarcoma and reticulum cell sarcoma are still used by most specialists in the pathology of bone tumours rather than 'lymphocytic lymphoma', 'immunoblastic lymphoma', 'histiocytic lymphoma' and other terms currently favoured by those whose work is particularly concerned with the lymphomas other than Hodgkin's disease (see pages 819 to 853 in Volume 2).

Each tumour named in Table 37.1 is a reasonably well-defined clinicopathological entity. The extent of the histological subdivision is justified by the correlation between the structure of the tumours and their other characteristics—age and sex incidence, anatomical distribution, and biological behaviour.[374] Tumours are occasionally encountered that do not appear to belong to any of the listed categories: they are rare, and the majority of bone tumours can be assigned to one or other of the histological types named in the table.

An indication of the relative frequency of the different types of primary bone tumour can be obtained from a published survey of the 3987 examples that were diagnosed at the Mayo Clinic, Rochester, Minnesota, in the years 1909 to 1966.[371] The survey showed the following diagnostic distribution of the tumours—

Benign Tumours

Osteoid osteoma	102
Benign osteoblastoma	28
Cartilage-capped exostosis	464
Enchondroma	117
Chondroblastoma	24
Chondromyxoid fibroma	20
Non-ossifying fibroma	50
Desmoplastic fibroma	3
Haemangioma	47
Other benign tumours	15
Total	870

Malignant Tumours

Osteosarcoma (central type)	650
Osteosarcoma (juxtacortical type)	25
Chondrosarcoma ('primary'*)	299
Chondrosarcoma ('secondary'*)	35
'Mesenchymal' chondrosarcoma	10
Fibrosarcoma	100
Giant cell tumour	169
Ewing's sarcoma	210
'Reticulum cell sarcoma'	195
Myelomatosis	1286
Chordoma	122
Other malignant tumours	16
Total	3117

Benign Tumours

Osteoma

An osteoma is a very slowly growing tumour-like lesion that consists of well-formed mature bone of predominantly lamellar structure. It is a rare condition and usually regarded as a hamartoma. Its occurrence is all but restricted to the skull, including the mandible. An occasional site is a nasal sinus, particularly a frontal sinus (see page 231 in Volume 1): most osteomas in the sinuses are ivory-like masses of dense bone but some are of cancellous structure.

Osteoid Osteoma

This tumour was described and named by Jaffe in 1935;[378] previously, it had been regarded as an inflammatory condition. The growth of the lesion sometimes appears to be self-limited, and this has led some authorities to continue to doubt its neoplastic nature.

* See page 2463.

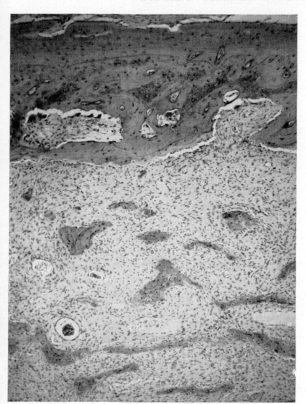

Fig. 37.69. Fibrous dysplasia. The edge of a lesion, showing the erosion of the overlying cortex by the abnormal tissue. *Haematoxylin–eosin.* × 45.

An osteoid osteoma is a rounded mass of gritty, reddish-grey tissue, usually less than a centimetre in diameter, sharply demarcated from the surrounding bone, and appearing radiologically as a localized osteolytic area, which is often enclosed by a wide zone of reactive periosteal bone formation (Fig. 37.73A). The patient is usually an adolescent or young adult, and males are more frequently affected than females. The tumour is often in the shaft of a long bone, although other parts of the skeleton may be affected. There is often severe local pain and tenderness. Histologically (Fig. 37.73B), the lesion consists of vascular osteoblastic tissue, containing much osteoid matrix and some calcified bone, the latter often being situated in the central part of the lesion.

Benign Osteoblastoma

The term benign osteoblastoma was introduced in 1956 by Lichtenstein[379] and Jaffe[380] to designate a type of benign osteoblastic tumour that is somewhat similar to the osteoid osteoma (see above)

and that is sometimes referred to as the *giant osteoid osteoma*.[381] It is evident that these two conditions, osteoid osteoma and benign osteoblastoma, are related; nonetheless, it is appropriate to retain the two terms because of differences in the size, site, radiological appearance and clinical presentation of these tumours and in the surrounding bony reaction.[382, 383]

Most of the patients are children or young adults: males and females are equally affected. Although encountered in other sites, the tumour most frequently occurs either in the vertebral column or in the short tubular bones of the hands and feet. In the spine, the lesion is usually situated in the neural arch, although in some cases the body of a vertebra is involved (Fig. 37.74). The clinical features are not distinctive: pain is frequently present, and there is sometimes evidence of compression of the spinal cord. The lesions are larger than the average osteoid osteoma: histologically, they are made up of the same components as the latter, consisting of osteoblastic tissue with osteoid matrix and calcified bone (Figs 37.74B to 37.76). A

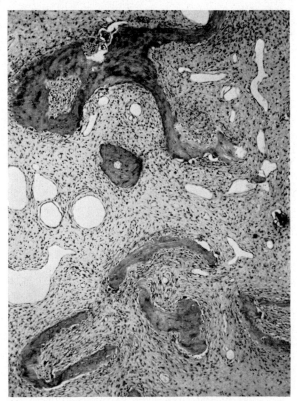

Fig. 37.70. Fibrous dysplasia. Fibrous tissue and non-lamellar bone. A few osteoclasts are present on the surface of the trabeculae. *Haematoxylin–eosin.* × 50.

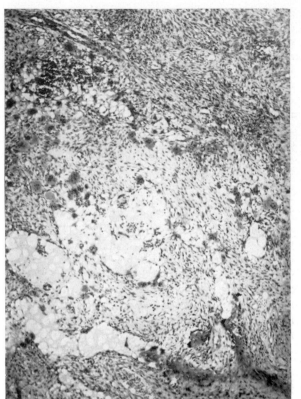

Fig. 37.71. Fibrous dysplasia. An area of fibrous tissue containing small cysts and numerous osteoclasts. *Haematoxylin–eosin.* × 50.

superficial histological examination sometimes suggests a diagnosis of osteosarcoma, but although the tissue may be quite cellular it lacks the pleomorphism and anaplasia of the malignant tumour.

A similar lesion is sometimes found in the jaws in relation to a premolar or molar tooth (*cementoblastoma*—see page 984 in Volume 3).

Cartilage-Capped Exostosis

A *cartilage-capped exostosis* may occur as a solitary lesion, or as part of the condition known as *hereditary multiple exostoses* (see page 2400).

The solitary lesion takes the form of a sessile or pedunculate bony mass attached to the metaphysial part of a long bone (Figs 37.77A to 37.77C). The lower end of the femur and the upper end of the tibia are the sites most commonly involved, but lesions may also occur at the upper end of the humerus, the lower end of the radius, and the lower end of the tibia. The exostosis appears to form in consequence of cartilaginous metaplasia in the periosteum in the neighbourhood of the epiphysial plate. The aberrant cartilage forms the growing cap of the lesion: as growth proceeds, the cartilage becomes replaced by cancellous bone as a result of endochondral ossification (Fig. 37.77D). The base of the exostosis remains attached to the cortical bone of the shaft, and appears to migrate from the epiphysis as normal endochondral ossification proceeds on the growing surface of the cartilage plate and gradually removes the latter from its original proximity to the lesion.

Exostoses develop during childhood, and the growth of the cartilage cap usually ceases at the time of skeletal maturation. During growth, the cartilage cap forms a fairly complete covering over the apex of the lesion (Figs 37.77B and 37.77C): later it becomes thin and inactive, and it may become incomplete. Sometimes the deeper tissue of the exostosis contains areas of necrotic—and often calcified—cartilage, and of fibrous tissue.

Malignant change is a particularly rare complication of a solitary exostosis: it usually takes the form of a chondrosarcoma arising in the tissues of the cartilage cap. It occurs with greater frequency

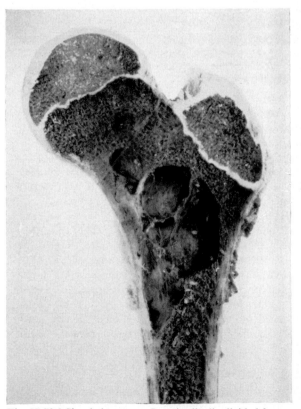

Fig. 37.72.§ Simple bone cyst. Longitudinally divided femur, showing a cyst in the region of the neck. This was an incidental finding at necropsy in a young child.

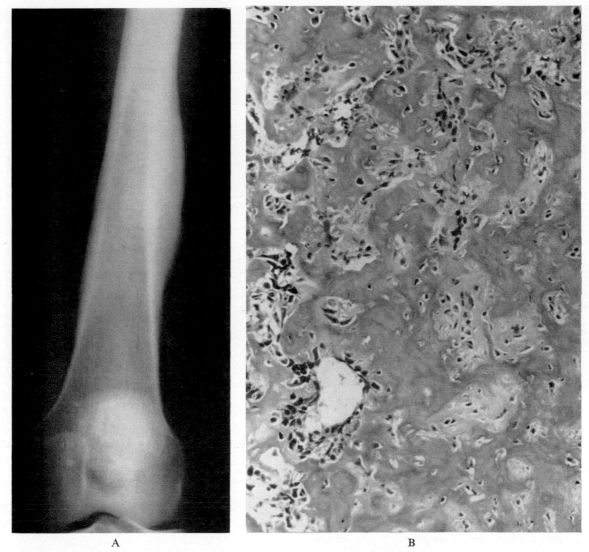

A   B

Fig. 37.73. Osteoid osteoma: femur.

A. Radiograph showing diffuse periosteal bone formation, at the centre of which there was a small focus of rarefaction (too indistinct to show in this reproduction of the original film).

B. Tissue from the area of rarefaction mentioned in the caption of Fig. 37.73A: the pale osteoid tissue and the more darkly staining calcified bone are seen. *Haematoxylin–eosin.* × 175.

in cases of hereditary multiple exostoses (see page 2400).

Enchondroma

An *enchondroma* may occur as a solitary lesion, or as part of the generalized condition of *enchondromatosis* (see page 2398).

The solitary lesion takes the form of a rounded cartilaginous tumour arising within a bone—usually a limb bone (Fig. 37.78). Males and females are

affected with equal frequency, and the condition is commonly encountered in childhood and early adult life. The phalanges of the fingers and the metacarpal bones are the commonest sites, but other bones, such as femur, humerus or tibia, may be involved. The tumour tissue has a bluish-white, characteristically cartilaginous appearance: focal areas of calcification appear as opaque, white, gritty areas. The margin of the lesion is clearly outlined, and the surrounding cortical bone may be thinned and expanded.

13

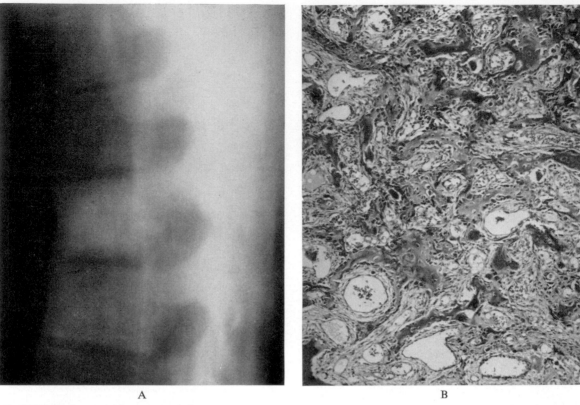

A   B

Fig. 37.74. Benign osteoblastoma: vertebra.

A. Tomograph of dorsal spine, showing an abnormally dense vertebral body.

B. This section of the lesion illustrated in Fig. 37.74A shows osteoblastic tissue with trabeculae of non-lamellar bone and occasional osteoclasts. *Haematoxylin–eosin.* × 55.

Histology

Histologically, typical cartilage matrix is abundant, and contains small spaces enclosing cartilage cells. The tumour tissue is usually avascular, and areas of degenerate and calcified matrix are found: calcification is sometimes followed by vascularization and replacement by bone, as in normal endochondral ossification. Solitary enchondromas are, on the whole, less cellular than the lesions of enchondromatosis. They differ from malignant cartilaginous tumours in that the cells of the benign lesion are small and have a compact, darkly-staining nucleus, but histological distinction between benign and malignant cartilaginous tumours is sometimes difficult (see page 2467). Indeed, cartilaginous tumours of all degrees of malignancy occur, and occasionally the history indicates that an originally benign tumour has undergone transformation into a malignant one. Malignant change is likeliest to occur in tumours of the major long bones, and is rarely encountered in those arising in the small bones of the hands.

Chondroblastoma

The lesion now known as chondroblastoma[384] (or benign chondroblastoma) was briefly noted by Ewing in 1928,[385] who referred to it as the *calcifying giant cell tumour*. The first detailed account was by Codman,[386] who described it under the name of *epiphysial chondromatous giant cell tumour*. His cases all involved the upper part of the humerus, and, like Ewing, he regarded the condition as a variant of giant cell tumour of bone. In 1942, Jaffe and Lichtenstein[387] suggested that it was a specific type of tumour, distinct from giant cell tumour, and they called it *benign chondroblastoma of bone*. They noted that it consists of rounded cells that contrast with the spindle-shaped cells of the usual giant cell tumour, and that it contains areas of

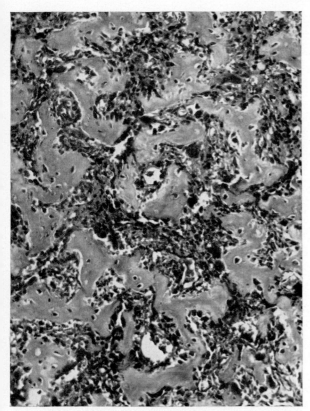

Fig. 37.75. Benign osteoblastoma. Another example of this tumour, showing cellular osteoblastic tissue and prominent trabeculae of non-lamellar bone. Overhasty examination of sections showing this type of picture may result in a mistaken diagnosis of osteosarcoma. *Haematoxylin–eosin.* × 120.

chondroid tissue and foci of calcification. Their observations led them to believe that the cells of the lesion were primitive cartilage cells—hence the name that they gave it. Although occasional giant cells are present in these lesions, Jaffe and Lichtenstein did not regard them as part of the 'primary pattern' of the tumour. They showed that the lesion almost always involves the epiphysis of a long bone (Fig. 37.79A), that it occurs mainly in patients below the age of 20 years, and that there is a preponderance of males. Radiologically, the lesions are osteolytic, although there is sometimes evidence of slight scattered calcification of the tumour tissue.

Histology

The histological appearance is distinctive (Figs 37.79B and 37.79C), the tumour consisting predominantly of cellular tissue composed mainly of round, hyperchromatic cells with a scattering of multinucleate giant cells of osteoclast type; there

are always chondroid areas, and patches of focal calcification. Recurrence is uncommon, in spite of the fact that these tumours are usually treated by local resection or curettage. Metastasis has been recorded only very rarely.[388, 389] In one case, a chondrosarcoma appeared at the site of a chondroblastoma that had been treated with X-rays;[390] this complication was interpreted as the independent development of a post-irradiation sarcoma and not attributed to malignant transformation of the chondroblastoma. The distinction between chondroblastoma and giant cell tumour (see page 2469) depends ultimately on the differences in histological structure; it is further substantiated by differences in age and sex incidence, distribution and, particularly, behaviour. The distinction from chondromyxoid fibroma (see below) is not as clear-cut: cases have been reported that showed histological features of both types of tumour.[391]

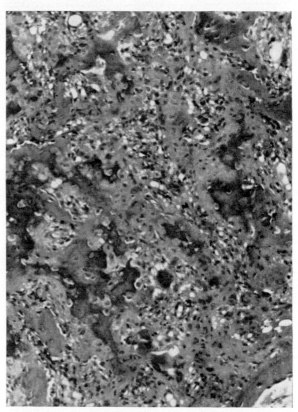

Fig. 37.76. Benign osteoblastoma. This field contains abundant osteoid tissue and occasional darkly staining areas of abnormal calcified bone. The resemblance to osteoid osteoma is close (compare with Fig. 37.73B), but the calcified tissue is scattered throughout the lesion in the osteoblastoma and not localized in a central mass as it would be in an osteoid osteoma. *Haematoxylin–eosin.* × 140.

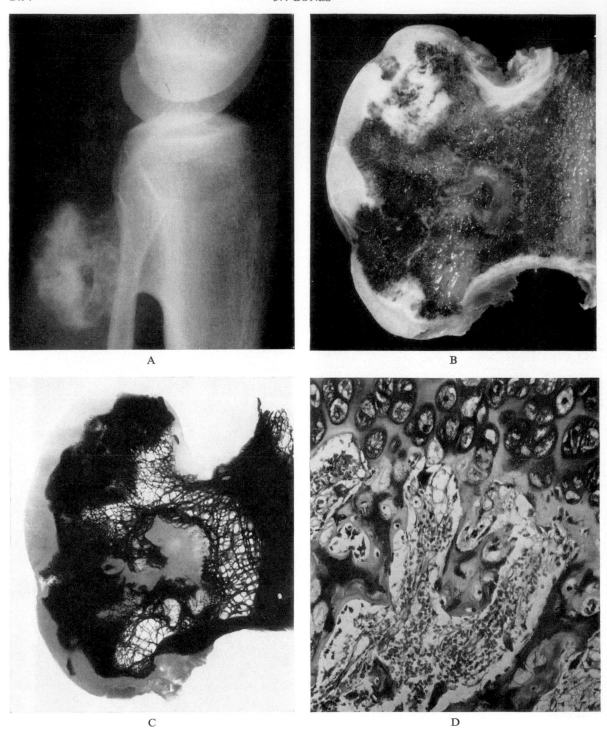

A

B

C

D

Fig. 37.77.§ Solitary exostosis: tibia.

A.§ Radiograph of knee, showing a pedunculate mass attached to the upper part of the shaft of the tibia.

B.§ Cut surface of the divided specimen, after resection, showing the cap of pale cartilaginous tissue.

C.§ Radiograph of a slab of tissue from the cut surface of the specimen shown in Fig. 37.77B, showing the amorphous shadow of the calcified cartilage and the trabecular structure of the underlying cancellous bone.

D.§ Histological appearance at the deep surface of the growing cartilaginous cap, showing irregular endochrondral ossification. *Haematoxylin–eosin.* × 90.

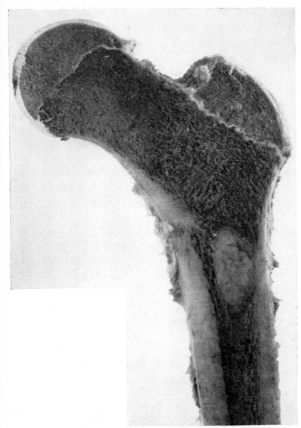

Fig. 37.78.§ Solitary enchondroma. A circumscribed cartilaginous tumour in the upper part of the shaft of a femur. An incidental necropsy finding in a boy aged 14 years.

It is important to note that the term 'chondroblastoma' was used by Geschickter and Copeland[392] to denote a quite different, and unequivocally malignant, bone tumour that most authorities would now regard as a chondrosarcoma.

Chondromyxoid Fibroma

This entity was described by Jaffe and Lichtenstein in 1948.[393] Before their account, examples of the condition had probably been regarded as chondrosarcomas: it is now recognized that the tumour is benign. The sexes are affected with equal frequency;[391, 394] most of the patients are adolescents and young adults. The tumour occurs in long bones, most frequently a tibia. It is usually situated toward the end of the shaft, and often produces an expansion that is limited to part of the circumference. In radiographs, a chondromyxoid fibroma usually appears as a clearly defined, oval or rounded, osteolytic lesion, often associated with expansion and thinning of the overlying cortical bone (Fig. 37.80A).

Histology

Histologically, the typical chondromyxoid fibroma is made up of spindle-shaped or stellate cells, separated by abundant fibrous or chondroid matrix that contains numerous vacuoles (Fig. 37.80B). The tumour often has a lobular outline, the lobules being separated by vascular connective tissue. An occasional chondromyxoid fibroma contains areas of more closely-packed, rounded cells (Fig. 37.81), that, with the presence of scattered multinucleate giant cells, may suggest a diagnosis of benign chondroblastoma: it has been noted that the distinction between these two conditions is not well defined (see above).[391]

Non-Ossifying Fibroma

This is the name currently applied[395, 396] to a group of lesions occurring in the metaphysial

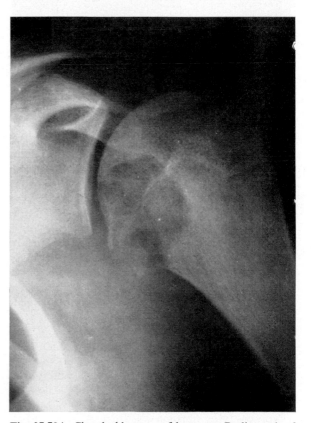

Fig. 37.79A. Chondroblastoma of humerus. Radiograph of shoulder, showing osteolytic lesion in the head of the humerus. See Figs 37.79B and 37.79C.

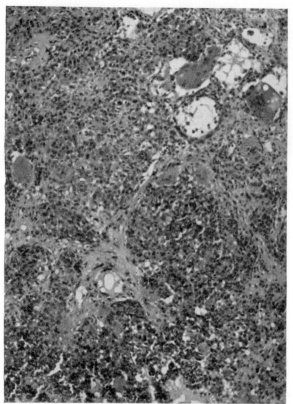

Fig. 37.79B. A histological field in the lesion shown in Fig. 37.79A, with predominance of rounded tumour cells and occasional multinucleate giant cells. *Haematoxylin–eosin.* × 115.

regions of the long bones of children and adolescents—particularly femur, tibia and fibula. Boys are somewhat more frequently affected than girls. The lesions are sharply circumscribed and osteolytic: they are often applied to the inner surface of the cortex and surrounded by a thin, encapsulating shell of bone. Histologically, they consist of a mixture of fibrous tissue (that characteristically shows a whorled pattern of interlacing bundles) and giant cells. Scattered deposits of haemosiderin and collections of lipid-containing foam cells are often present and may give the tissue a brownish colour. Some lesions of this type appear to be self-limited in their growth and are completely symptomless. Not uncommonly, they are encountered incidentally in the course of radiological examination: they are then often described by radiologists as *fibrous metaphysial defects*.[397] Multiple lesions are occasionally present.

Non-ossifying fibroma was formerly regarded as a fibrous or 'xanthic' (xanthomatoid) variant of the giant cell tumour of bone. It is occasionally con-

fused with fibrous dysplasia of bone (see page 2439), but can be distinguished from this condition by the absence of bone formation in the abnormal tissue.

Desmoplastic Fibroma

In 1958 Jaffe[398] described five cases of a tumour that he named desmoplastic fibroma. It occurs in the long bones of adolescent or young adult patients and consists of mature fibrous tissue: the name was intended to indicate a similarity to the structure of the familiar 'desmoid tumour' of the abdominal wall and other soft parts. The growth is regarded as distinct from other types of fibroma of bone, particularly non-ossifying fibroma and chondromyxoid fibroma (see above). Further series of cases have been reported,[399, 400] and the existence of the desmoplastic fibroma as an entity appears to be established.

The essential histological features are the uniformity of the tumour cells and the densely col-

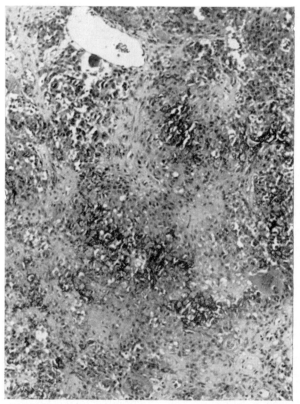

Fig. 39.79C. Same specimen as Fig. 37.79B. Field of 'chondroid' tissue with focal calcification. *Haematoxylin–eosin.* × 115.

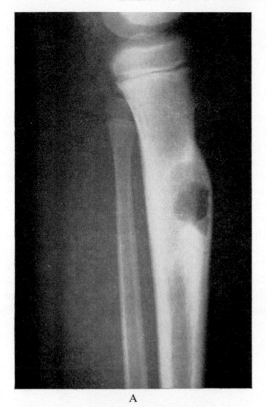
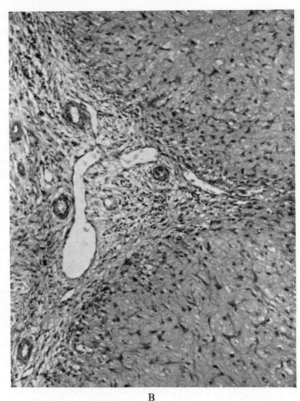

A   B

Fig. 37.80. Chondromyxoid fibroma: tibia.

A. Radiograph showing expansion of the shaft of the bone by the osteolytic tumour.

B. Histological structure of the lesion illustrated in Fig. 37.80A, showing lobulate masses of tumour tissue composed of stellate and spindle-shaped cells and a vacuolate, chondroid, intercellular matrix. *Haematoxylin–eosin.* × 110.

lagenous nature of the tissue. Distinction from slowly growing fibrosarcomas can pose difficulties.

Benign Vascular Tumours of Bone

The subject of vascular tumours of bone presents difficulties that have not yet been resolved; consequently, the terminology is not generally established. *Haemangiomas* and *aneurysmal bone cysts* are relatively common lesions (see below). *Glomus tumours* of bone have been described;[401, 402] they are very rare. The name *haemangioendothelioma* (see page 2477) is sometimes given to locally invasive and destructive tumours that appear to be intermediate between haemangiomas and angiosarcomas in structure and behaviour.

Haemangioma

Intraosseous haemangiomas occur quite commonly in vertebral bodies and occasionally in other parts of the skeleton, particularly the vault of the skull. Vertebral haemangiomas were found in about 10 per cent of a large series of necropsies in which the spine was carefully examined.[403] Like haemangiomas of other tissues, these lesions are malformations (hamartomas) rather than true tumours. They are often symptomless.

The vertebral lesions occupy part or the whole of a vertebral body, and consist of thin-walled cavernous blood vessels (Figs 37.82 and 37.83).[404, 405] Radiologically, the involved areas show sparse, coarse trabeculation.

Haemangiomas of bone are occasionally multiple, and such lesions may be accompanied by haemangiomatosis of soft tissues.[406]

Lymphangioma

Most angiomas of bone are haemangiomas. Lymphangiomas have rarely been recorded;[407–409] they

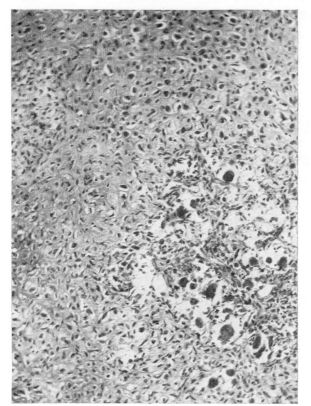

Fig. 37.81. Chondromyxoid fibroma. Another example, this one showing predominance of rounded tumour cells and occasional multinucleate giant cells. *Haematoxylin–eosin.* ×120.

are usually multiple and sometimes occur in association with similar growths in the soft tissues.

Aneurysmal Bone Cyst

An aneurysmal bone cyst is an unusual vascular lesion of bone. Its nature is somewhat obscure.[410–412] Prior to its recognition by Jaffe[413] and Lichtenstein,[414] examples of this lesion were usually regarded as haemorrhagic or cystic giant cell tumours. There is no doubt, however, that the two conditions should be distinguished, on the grounds both of structure and of behaviour. It has been suggested that aneurysmal bone cyst is a variety of haemangioma of bone,[415] but the validity of this explanation remains uncertain.

Aneurysmal bone cyst occurs in older children and young adults: there is no predominance of either sex among reported cases. The majority of lesions occur in the shaft of a long bone (Fig. 37.84) or in the spine (Fig. 37.85). Radiologically, the lesion appears as a 'ballooned' distension of

the periosteum, and it was this appearance that suggested the name aneurysmal bone cyst. On surgical exploration, the lesion appears as a blood-filled, cystic structure, eroding bone and displacing the periosteum: the central cavity is divided by ragged septa of reddish-brown tissue.

Histology.—The tenuous cyst lining and the septa consist of fibrous tissue enclosing numerous vascular channels (Fig. 37.85C). Giant cells and haemosiderin are often conspicuous, and the fibrous tissue usually contains scattered foci of bone formation. The rapid development and large size of these lesions sometimes suggest that they are malignant, but in fact they are benign.

One histological study indicated that, in a significant proportion of cases, aneurysmal bone cysts had occurred as the result of a secondary process of cystic change complicating some other lesion, such as a non-ossifying fibroma, chondroblastoma or giant cell tumour.[416] This view does not appear to be confirmed by other studies.[417]

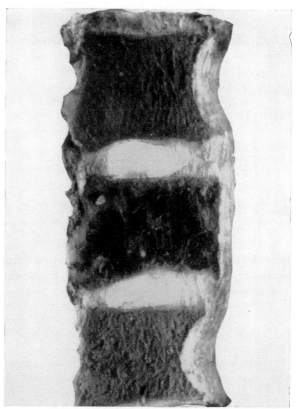

Fig. 37.82.§ Haemangioma. Three lumbar vertebrae have been divided longitudinally: the marrow of the middle one is replaced by cavernous vascular tissue. The lesion was an incidental finding at necropsy.

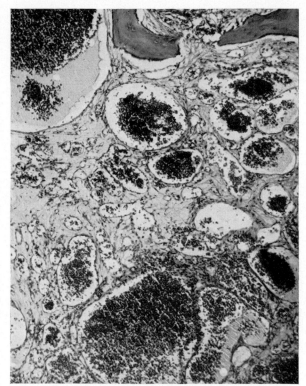

Fig. 37.83. Haemangioma of bone showing blood-filled vascular channels of various sizes. *Haematoxylin–eosin.* × 65.

'Vanishing Bone Disease'[418]

'Vanishing bone disease' has several synonyms, including disappearing bone disease, phantom bone disease and *massive osteolysis*. It is known also as Gorham's disease,[418a] although cases had been described earlier by others, including a possible example in 1838, attributed to J. B. S. Jackson, of Boston, Massachusetts (Jackson's 'boneless arm'[418b]). It occurs most frequently in childhood or early adult life and with about equal frequency in the sexes. A history of trauma, usually mild, is often obtained but may be coincidental. The disease is characterized by slowly progressive atrophy and absorption of bone. In the less severe cases one bone only, and only part of it, is affected. In classic cases practically all the osseous matter of one, two or several bones is absorbed, only a fibrous strand remaining in its place. Any bone may be affected, with some preponderance of involvement of the bones of the limb girdles, the mandible, and the bones of the hands and feet.

The condition eventually ceases to progress in most cases. Occasionally, however, there is total

13*

disablement. Some patients die of the disease or its complications.

'Vanishing bone disease' has been attributed to angiomatosis (usually haemangiomatosis but occasionally lymphangiomatosis).[418] How the angiomatous state that has been observed histologically to affect the vasculature of the bones leads to such extensive and severe osteolysis is uncertain.

Lipoma

Lipomas are rare in bone and few cases have been reported.[419, 420] Radiologically, they appear as circumscribed osteolytic lesions that may produce expansion or erosion of the surrounding bone. Histologically, they consist of mature adipose tissue.

Neural Tumours and Neurofibromatosis

Rarely, examples of neurolemmoma arising in bone have been reported,[421–424] but not all the cases are fully convincing.

Abnormalities of bones are occasionally encountered in cases of von Recklinghausen's *neurofibromatosis*:[424] rarely, these take the form of an intraosseous tumour. Sometimes, there is localized or diffuse erosion of the cortex by neurofibromatous tissue that has developed in the periosteum or adjacent soft tissues; sometimes, the bone lesion is not a tumour but an abnormality such as spina bifida, scoliosis, or accelerated or retarded growth of a bone. Congenital pseudarthrosis of the tibia may occur in neurofibromatosis; it is rare for neurofibromatous tissue to be identified in its vicinity.

Other Benign Tumours

It is rarely the case that a benign bone tumour cannot be classified in one of the recognized categories described above. However, not every tumour can be so readily identified: some show histological features that are characteristic of more than one of these forms, while others have a distinctive, but as yet undefined, structure. As more cases of tumours in the latter categories are collected, it will be possible eventually to identify their nature and make appropriate additions or modifications to the classification that represents the present consensus of understanding of benign skeletal tumours (Table 37.1, page 2448).

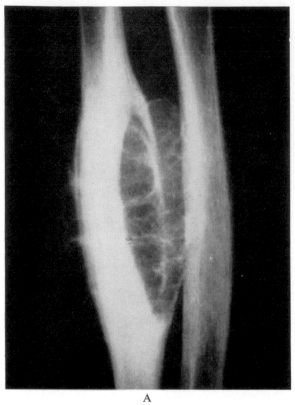

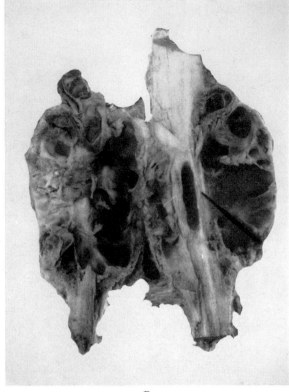

A   B

Fig. 37.84.§ Aneurysmal bone cyst: ulna.

A.§ Radiograph showing characteristic expansion of the shaft of the bone.

B.§ Macroscopical appearance of the lesion illustrated in Fig. 37.84A: the pointer indicates a gap in the cortical bone through which the cystic lesion has 'ballooned'.

Malignant Tumours

Osteosarcoma: 1. *Central or Medullary Osteo-sarcoma*[424a]

An *osteosarcoma* is a malignant bone tumour having a predominantly osteoblastic pattern of differentiation, as indicated by the formation of osteoid or bony intercellular material. The terms *osteogenic sarcoma** and *osteoblastic sarcoma* are sometimes used for these tumours, which are usually regarded as the commonest of the primary malignant tumours of bone tissue.

Most osteosarcomas occur between the ages of 10 and 30 years, and males are more frequently affected than females. Many of the tumours

* The term 'osteogenic sarcoma' has often been used to indicate that the tumour so described is a bone-forming sarcoma. However, some writers have used it in the much wider sense of a sarcoma originating in bone, a usage analogous to that of the term 'bronchogenic carcinoma', meanind a tumour arising in the bronchial tree.

developing after middle age are associated with Paget's disease. The tumours commonly develop toward the ends of the shaft of long bones, although no part of the skeleton is exempt. The lower end of a femur is the commonest site. Most tumours appear to arise centrally, and expand the bone as they grow (Fig. 37.86). Invasion of soft tissue often occurs, and pathological fracture is not infrequent. The cut surface of an osteosarcoma may show areas of tumour bone interspersed with vascular, unossified areas and patches of necrotic tissue. The amount of ossified tumour tissue can vary greatly, individual tumours sometimes being described as *sclerosing* or *osteolytic*, although usually showing areas of each type.

Radiographic Appearances

The radiographic appearance of an osteosarcoma is often diagnostic, particularly when much of the

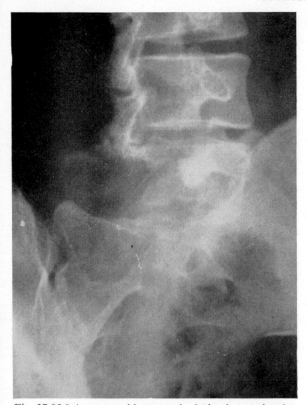

Fig. 37.85.§ Aneurysmal bone cyst in the lumbosacral region.

A. Radiograph showing an expanding osteolytic lesion of the fifth lumbar vertebra and the adjacent part of the sacrum. See also Figs 37.85B and 37.85C.

Some areas consist of relatively undifferentiated spindle-celled tissue, with little bone formation, while others include large amounts of calcified tumour bone. The cells of the relatively undifferentiated areas are usually pleomorphic, and frequently have a large, bizarre nucleus; in the more ossified areas cytological evidence of malignancy may be less conspicuous. Variable amounts of tumour cartilage are sometimes seen in predominantly osteoblastic tumours: they may occasionally cause confusion with chondrosarcoma, although the latter diagnosis is applicable only to cartilaginous tumours that show no formation of tumour bone (calcification of chondrosarcomatous tissue and its eventual replacement by non-neoplastic bone can correspondingly cause confusion with osteosarcomas — see page 2446). Tumour giant cells are sometimes conspicuous, particularly in tumours arising as a complication of Paget's disease (Fig. 37.88C). Many osteosarcomas contain areas in which conspicuous vascular structures are present (Fig. 37.88D). Pre-existing bone trabeculae are usually destroyed in areas of bone occupied by tumour tissue, but they

tumour is heavily ossified and when tumour tissue extends beyond the confines of the cortex (Fig. 37.86A). When ossification is inconspicuous or absent, however, it may be difficult or impossible to distinguish an osteosarcoma from other types of malignant bone tumour on radiographic evidence alone. New bone produced by the displaced periosteum may give the involved area an appearance of vertical spiculation, and the wedge of ossification known to radiologists as *Codman's triangle* may mark the point where the growing edge of the tumour has separated the periosteum from the underlying cortical bone: these features are not pathognomonic of osteosarcoma, for they are found in other conditions in which periosteal displacement occurs.

Histology

The histological appearances of osteosarcoma vary considerably from case to case, and even within a given tumour (Figs 37.87 and 37.88).

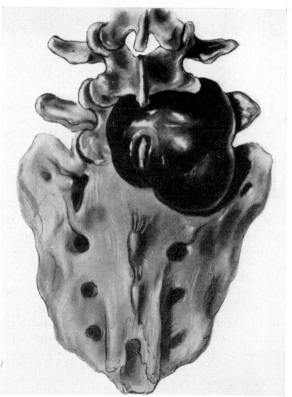

Fig. 37.85B.§ Drawing to show the extent of the lesion as found at operation.

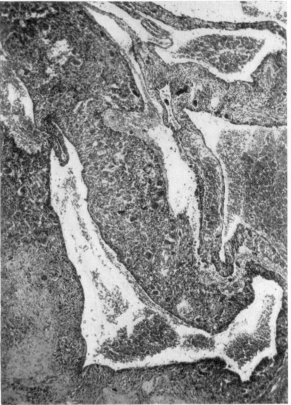

Fig. 37.85C.§ Large, blood-filled spaces separated by thin septa of vascular fibrous tissue containing numerous giant cells. Same specimen as in Figs 37.85A and 37.85B. *Haematoxylin–eosin.* × 50.

occasionally persist. Reactive bone, newly formed at the site of the tumour by non-neoplastic cells stimulated by the destructive process, may also be invaded and destroyed by the tumour tissue: its histological identification and distinction from bone formed by the tumour cells themselves can be difficult.

Biopsy Diagnosis.—Because of the variability of the histological appearance in different parts of a tumour, open biopsy—with its more adequate sample of tissue—is preferred to aspiration biopsy, although the latter method has been effectively used by some experienced workers.[425–427] Aspiration biopsy is of special value when the anatomical situation of the lesion, or the plans for its subsequent treatment, make open biopsy either hazardous or impossible.

Biochemical Findings

An increase in the amount of alkaline phosphatase in the serum is a usual, but not invariable, feature of osteosarcoma, the enzyme apparently being produced by the proliferating osteoblastic tumour cells.[428] The results of other biochemical investigations are usually normal.

Course and Prognosis

Osteosarcomas are very malignant tumours, the mortality being high, irrespective of the type of treatment adopted: most series of cases show that only a small percentage of the patients live for five years.[428a] Osteosarcomas metastasize by the blood stream: secondary tumours develop in the lungs, and occasionally in other organs, or in other bones. Metastasis to regional lymph nodes is rare, but not unknown.[428b] The secondary deposits show the same range of histological structure as the primary growth; they are often characterized by the formation of large amounts of tumour bone.

Osteosarcoma: 2. *Juxtacortical Osteosarcoma*

The juxtacortical osteosarcoma differs from the usual form of osteosarcoma in that it develops in relation to the external surface of a bone, has a more highly differentiated histological appearance, and has a distinctly better prognosis after surgical treatment. It was described by Geschickter and Copeland[428c] under the misleading name *parosteal osteoma.* They studied 16 cases, most of them in young adults. Growth was less rapid than with the usual type of osteosarcoma, and local excision or amputation was associated with a higher rate of cure, although 4 out of 13 patients eventually died with secondary deposits in the lungs. Jaffe and Selin[428d] used the term *juxtacortical osteogenic sarcoma* to describe the same condition, and to stress its malignancy.

Histology

Histologically, tumours of this group consist of mature, well-differentiated tumour bone, cartilage and fibrous tissue. Areas of more obviously sarcomatous tissue are sometimes present, particularly at a late stage when there is invasion of adjacent muscle or underlying cortical bone; in their absence, the histological distinction from benign conditions, such as localized myositis ossificans (see pages 2355 and 2516), can be difficult.

Chondrosarcoma[429, 429a]

A *chondrosarcoma* is a malignant bone tumour characterized by differentiation of cartilage cells

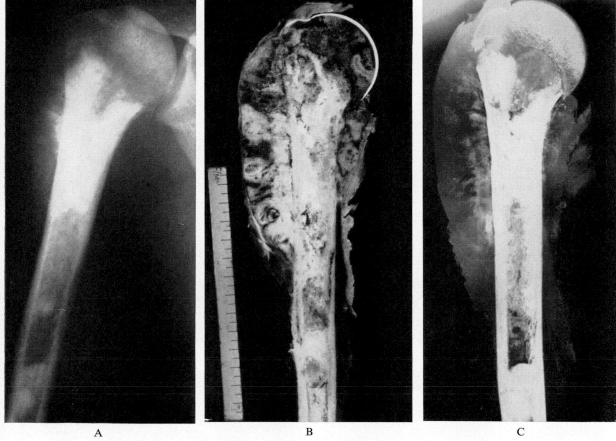

A   B   C

Fig. 37.86.§ Osteosarcoma: humerus.

A.§ Radiograph of shoulder, showing a sclerosing tumour of the upper part of the shaft of the humerus.

B.§ Longitudinally divided humerus.

C.§ Radiograph of a slab of tissue from the specimen.

and cartilaginous intercellular matrix. The term is applied only to purely cartilaginous tumours, those showing both bony and cartilaginous differentiation of tumour tissue being classified as osteosarcomas (see page 2461).

Lesions of all grades of malignancy occur, and it is not always easy to distinguish between benign and malignant cartilaginous tumours. Some chondrosarcomas arise *de novo*; others, which are sometimes ambiguously referred to as 'secondary' chondrosarcomas, have their origin in a previously benign cartilaginous lesion (a cartilage-capped exostosis or an enchondroma—see pages 2450 and 2451). Chondrosarcomas are sometimes classed as central (medullary) or peripheral (juxtacortical), according to their apparent site of origin.

Chondrosarcomas develop later than osteosarcomas, usually occurring between the ages of 30 and 50 years. Men are more frequently affected than women. In contrast to the majority of benign cartilaginous tumours, which occur toward the periphery of the limbs, chondrosarcomas usually arise in the pelvis, ribs and proximal long bones, and very few develop in the small bones of the hands and feet.

A *central chondrosarcoma* is usually a rounded lesion (Fig. 37.89); it is often accompanied by demonstrable erosion or invasion of the surrounding bone. A *peripheral chondrosarcoma* appears either as a periosteal mass of lobulate cartilaginous tissue or, when it develops from the cartilage cap of an exostosis, as a mass of tissue projecting from and sometimes surrounding the exostosis. Macroscopically, a well-differentiated chondrosarcoma closely resembles normal cartilage, being translucent and bluish-white in appearance. It often

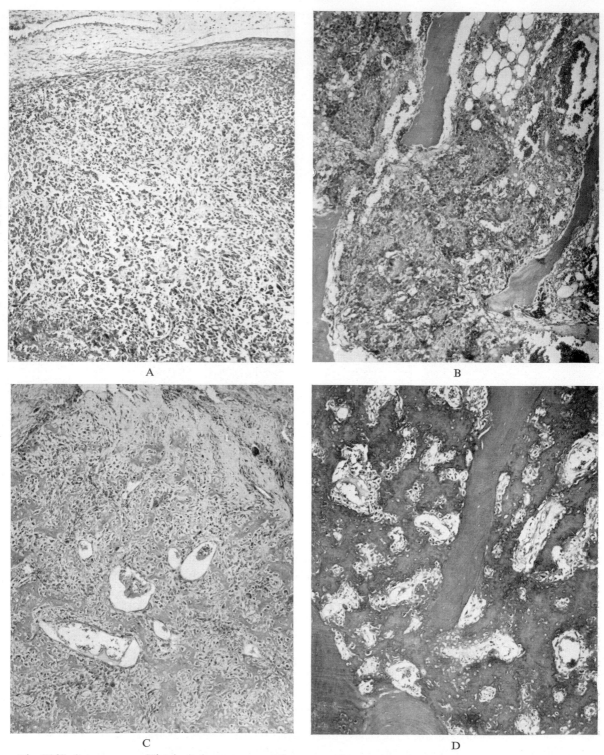

A

B

C

D

Fig. 37.87. Osteosarcoma. Histological appearance of the tumour illustrated in Fig. 37.86. *Haematoxylin–eosin.* ×65.

A. Tissue from the growing margin of the tumour, showing relatively undifferentiated, spindle-shaped cells.

B. Another part of the tumour, with clumps of the cells infiltrating marrow spaces in cancellous bone.

C. A field showing pronounced bony differentiation, as indicated by the bony matrix surrounding the tumour cells.

D. An area from the central, sclerotic part of the tumour, showing dense tumour bone occupying the marrow spaces.

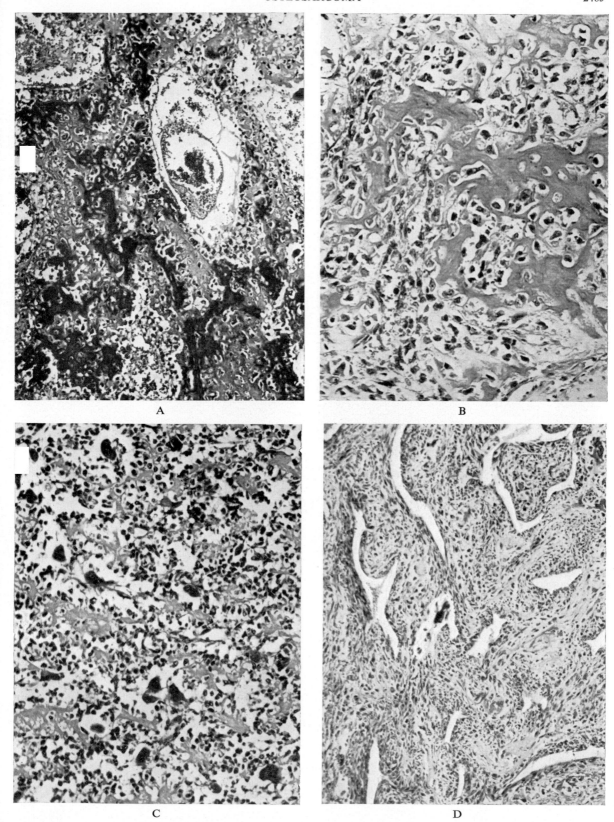

Fig. 37.88. *Captions at foot of next page.*

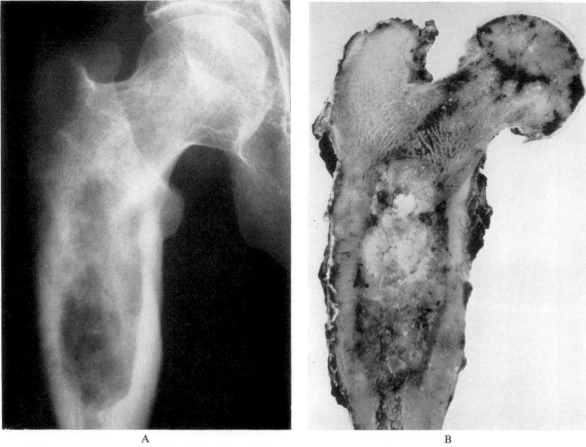

A   B

Fig. 37.89.§ Chondrosarcoma (central chondrosarcoma): femur.

A.§ Radiograph showing expanding lesion.

B.§ Longitudinally divided femur showing lobulate cartilaginous tumour expanding the cortical bone and beginning to invade it.

has a lobulate or nodular outline (Figs 37.89B and 37.90). Areas of calcification and replacement by non-neoplastic bone may be present. Degenerating areas may appear gelatinous. Poorly differentiated chondrosarcomas show less resemblance to normal cartilage; they also may have a gelatinous appearance. When scattered calcification and replacement by bone are present in a chondrosarcoma, the

irregularly mottled pattern that results may allow precise radiographic identification of the lesion.

Histology

The general histological pattern of a slowly-growing chondrosarcoma is similar to that of a benign chondroma. Areas of well-differentiated

Fig. 37.88 [page 2465]. Osteosarcoma: photomicrographs illustrating the variety of histological pictures that may be seen in different tumours. *Haematoxylin–eosin.*

A.§ Conspicuous bony differentiation in an osteosclerotic tumour: the darkly staining matrix is calcified and the rest is tumour osteoid. × 90.

B. Part of another bone-forming tumour, showing the relation of the tumour cells to the intercellular matrix. × 255.

C. An area of cellular tumour tissue in an osteosarcoma complicating Paget's disease of bone, showing some bony differentiation and scattered multinucleate giant cells. × 135.

D. An area of 'telangiectatic' tumour tissue, characterized by the presence of numerous vascular spaces. × 85.

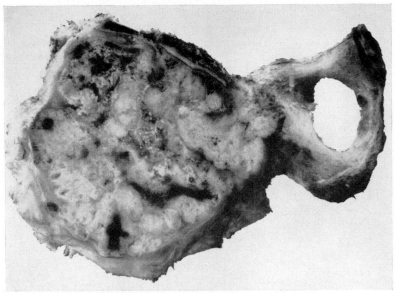

Fig. 37.90.§ Chondrosarcoma of ilium.

tumour cartilage consist of small round cells separated by abundant cartilaginous matrix (Fig. 37.91A). The tumour tissue contains very few blood vessels. Rapidly growing, frankly malignant chondrosarcomas consist of more cellular and less differentiated cartilaginous tissue: they are often more vascular than the slowly growing tumours. Chondroid intercellular matrix may be absent in some or many parts of a tumour of this type, and the cells in such areas are spindle-shaped rather than round.

Lichtenstein and Jaffe[429] emphasized the relation between histological structure and clinical behaviour among cartilage tumours, and put forward criteria for the histological recognition of malignancy. Large cells, large nuclei (Fig. 37.91B), and the presence of numerous binucleate or multinucleate cells, particularly when these cells are notably large, are all features that suggest malignancy. It should be remembered, however, that the lesions of enchondromatosis may show a disturbing degree of cellularity without necessarily behaving in a malignant fashion (see page 2398). In many chondrosarcomas, only part of the lesion is found to provide histological evidence of malignancy, and it may be necessary to examine many sections before an unequivocal diagnosis can be made. It is for this reason that a biopsy report of 'chondroma' should not be accepted without the most careful consideration if the clinical and radiological findings suggest malignancy.[430]

Course and Prognosis

Chondrosarcomas are less malignant than osteosarcomas. Growth is usually slow, and the prognosis following adequate surgical treatment is much better than that of other types of malignant bone tumour.[429, 431–433] Metastasis, which occurs by the blood stream, is a late feature, and local extension and recurrence are usually problems of greater importance. Chondrosarcomas sometimes show extensive invasion of regional veins, and large intravascular masses may extend for long distances within the lumen, in continuity with the primary growth.

'Mesenchymal' Chondrosarcoma[434, 435]

Not all cartilage tumours present the familiar histological pattern described above. The name mesenchymal chondrosarcoma was introduced to describe a group of these atypical growths. In addition to cartilage the tumours of this group are formed of very vascular, mesenchyme-like tissue that consists of spindle-shaped cells and undifferentiated round cells. They are rare and highly malignant. They occur in adults and have been identified in various sites, including ribs, vertebrae and pelvis, and tarsal and metatarsal bones. In some cases there are multiple tumours: this may indicate multicentric origin.

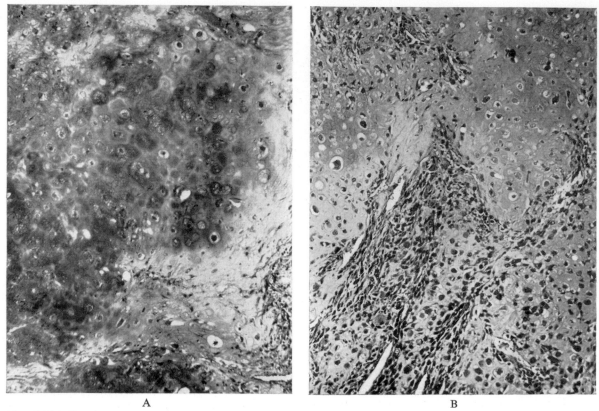

A   B

Fig. 37.91.§ Chondrosarcoma. *Haematoxylin–eosin.* × 70.

A.§ An area of well-differentiated cartilaginous tissue.

B.§ A more cellular, clearly malignant part of the tumour illustrated in Fig. 37.91A: many of the tumour cells are large and have large nuclei.

Fibrosarcoma[436, 437]

A *fibrosarcoma* is a malignant tumour showing differentiation of fibroblasts and intercellular formation of collagen: the presence of bony or cartilaginous differentiation excludes a tumour from this group. Fibrosarcomas of bone were formerly classed with osteosarcomas—the view that they should be regarded as a separate group has now gained wide acceptance. They are relatively rare and they occur at a rather later age than osteosarcomas. Their usual site is the long bones of the limbs. Some fibrosarcomas are highly malignant, but usually the outlook is less serious than in cases of osteosarcoma. The majority of fibrosarcomas develop in the absence of any pre-existing pathological condition. In a few cases the tumour represents malignant change complicating fibrous dysplasia of bone (see page 2441).

Fibrosarcomas are usually osteolytic. Their cut surface may appear whitish, with darker areas of necrosis and haemorrhage. Histologically, they consist of spindle-celled tissue with a certain amount of intercellular collagen. The more malignant members of the group are highly cellular, and contain pleomorphic areas with hyperchromatic and atypical nuclei, numerous mitotic figures, and tumour giant cells. The less malignant tumours are less cellular, and contain a larger amount of collagen. It is not possible to make a histological diagnosis of fibrosarcoma on the basis of a limited biopsy specimen: many representative sections must be examined in order to establish that the lesion is not an osteosarcoma.

As with other types of primary malignant bone tumour, metastasis occurs by the blood stream. The secondary tumours develop most commonly in the lungs.

Malignant Fibrous Histiocytoma[438]

Recently, the term malignant fibrous histiocytoma has been introduced to distinguish a group of primary bone tumours that previously were classed among the fibrosarcomas. They differ from the latter in combining a fibre-forming component of spindle-shaped cells with a conspicuous component formed of large mononuclear cells that are considered to be tumour histiocytes. These cells have a large, vesicular, hyperchromatic nucleus with one or two small, eosinophile nucleoli or a single large inclusion-like nucleolus. Some have foamy-looking cytoplasm, due to the presence of lipid; some are stippled with haemosiderin; and some show evidence of phagocytic activity in the presence of engulfed red blood cells or lymphocytes in their cytoplasm. A proportion of bizarre tumour giant cells may also be present. No osteoid is produced by the tumour cells: this observation, if confirmed on examination of a large number of samples of tissue from a given tumour, distinguishes the malignant fibrous histiocytoma from osteosarcomas. The more difficult distinction from fibrosarcomas is based on the presence of the tumour histiocytes, as described above.

These comparatively infrequent tumours are of considerable malignancy. They have some tendency to metastasize to regional lymph nodes as well as, more characteristically, by the blood stream to the lungs. Comparable tumours arise in soft tissues.

Giant Cell Tumour (Osteoclastoma)[432, 439–443]

The giant cell tumour, or osteoclastoma, is a bone tumour showing conspicuous osteoclastic differentiation within a stroma-like tissue formed of ovoid or spindle-shaped cells and devoid of bony or cartilaginous differentiation. At one time such tumours were regarded as benign, but increasing experience has shown that they are often aggressive and at least potentially malignant. This view has received increasing emphasis as certain benign lesions, previously regarded as giant cell tumours or variant giant cell tumours, have been recognized to be entities separable from this category—for example, chondroblastoma (page 2452) and non-ossifying fibroma (page 2455).[432, 439–441]

The giant cell tumour is not a common condition. It occurs oftenest between the ages of 20 and 40 years and is rarely seen in younger patients. This helps to distinguish it from the lesions that formerly were regarded as its variants, which occur in children or adolescents. Men and women are affected with about equal frequency.[442, 443]

Following adequate local treatment, about half these tumours are likely to have a favourable outcome, about one third will recur locally, and the remainder can be expected to behave as frankly malignant tumours and metastasize to the lungs. Most giant cell tumours arise at the ends of long bones, the commonest sites being the lower end of a femur, the upper end of a tibia and the lower end of a radius.

The typical giant cell tumour is an osteolytic lesion producing some expansion of the bone (Figs 37.92A and 37.92B). The tumour tissue is soft and friable, and reddish-brown or grey. Areas of haemorrhage and necrosis are frequently present, and there are often large or small cystic spaces. Both compact and cancellous bone in the region of the tumour is destroyed; the cortex is usually replaced by a thin shell of new periosteal bone. The more malignant giant cell tumours sometimes disrupt the periosteum and invade the adjacent soft tissues.

Histology

Histologically, the tumour consists of two characteristic components, the giant cells and the stroma-like spindle-celled tissue (Figs 37.92C and 37.92D). The latter includes occasional blood vessels and scanty collagen fibres. The giant cells show a morphological similarity to osteoclasts. They contain many nuclei, most of which are situated in the central part of the cell. It is thought that they are derived from the spindle-shaped cells.

The relative proportions of the two components vary in different tumours, and in different parts of the same tumour (Figs 37.92C and 37.92D). It is generally agreed that it is the appearance of the spindle-cell component that indicates the malignant potentialities of the tumour. A high degree of cellularity and the presence of large, hyperchromatic nuclei, or of numerous mitotic figures, are features indicative of malignancy. It must be stressed, however, that the absence of these histological features is no guarantee that, with the passage of time, the lesion in question will not behave as a malignant tumour.

Diagnosis

A presumptive clinical diagnosis of giant cell tumour should always be confirmed by biopsy. If any indication of the degree of malignancy of the lesion is sought, the biopsy specimen must be an adequately representative sample: aspiration biopsy is not satisfactory for this purpose.

Differential Diagnosis.—The giant cell tumour must be distinguished from other tumours that include

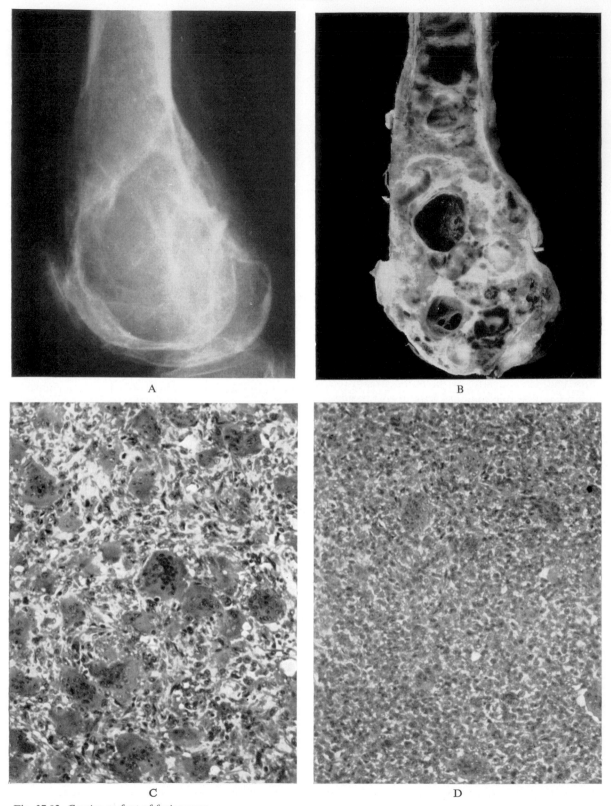

A

B

C

D

Fig. 37.92. *Caption at foot of facing page.*

osteoclast-like giant cells in their composition, such as the chondroblastoma (see page 2452), the chondromyxoid fibroma (see page 2455) and the non-ossifying fibroma (see page 2455). The distinction is indicated not only by the difference in histological appearance between the giant cell tumour and the benign bone tumours but also by the different age incidence and the different skeletal distribution of the growths. The uniformly good prognosis of the benign tumours is a further distinctive and important feature.

Occasional osteosarcomas contain a sufficient proportion of giant cells to lead to confusion with giant cell tumours, but they can be identified by the presence of bony differentiation.

The 'brown tumours' of bone in cases of hyperparathyroidism (see page 2431) have often been confused with giant cell tumour. They can be distinguished from it both by the presence of the biochemical changes of hyperparathyroidism and by their different behaviour. The histological similarity may in some cases be very close. The peculiar local condition termed *giant cell granuloma of the jaw bones* is also to be distinguished from giant cell tumour (see page 942, Volume 3).[444]

Various other lesions in which the presence of osteoclasts may create confusion include simple bone cyst (see page 2442), aneurysmal bone cyst (see page 2458) and fibrous dysplasia of bone (see page 2439).

Course and Prognosis

As already noted, true giant cell tumours may metastasize. Dissemination occurs by the blood stream, and secondary deposits develop in the lungs. The metastatic tumours usually retain the characteristic histological appearance of a giant cell tumour; occasionally, the primary and secondary growths lack the histological features that ordinarily indicate malignancy (see above).[445, 446]

Ewing's Tumour

In 1921, Ewing[447] briefly reported a series of obscure bone tumours that he described as 'endothelial myelomas'. Since then, most pathologists interested in the study of bone tumours have used the term *Ewing's tumour* to designate a group of non-osteogenic, round-celled tumours, usually involving a long bone in a young patient.[448–451] These tumours are highly malignant, but characteristically show a dramatic, but temporary, response to radiotherapy. In radiographs, the tumours usually appear as osteolytic lesions, but the destruction is sometimes associated with patchy reactive bone formation or diffuse periosteal bone formation.

Histology

Histological examination shows that the tumour consists of indistinctly outlined cells, with a large, round nucleus. There are many mitotic figures. Areas of haemorrhage and necrosis are common. The tumour cells sometimes show a 'perithelial' arrangement round blood vessels, and they may form indistinct rosettes. Ewing's tumour lacks the intercellular framework of reticulin fibres that is characteristic of true reticulum cell sarcomas. A feature of some cases of Ewing's tumour that may be of diagnostic help is the presence of glycogen within the tumour cells.[452]

Diagnosis

Willis[453] emphasized that a solitary metastatic deposit of an adrenal or sympathetic neuroblastoma can produce the appearances of Ewing's tumour. He suggested that most of the tumours that have been interpreted as instances of 'Ewing's tumour' have been either metastatic, or 'reticulum cell sarcomas', or poorly differentiated osteosarcomas. However, the term Ewing's tumour continues to be used, although the histological criteria for diagnosis remain somewhat vague: the diagnosis is consequently difficult, particularly in limited biopsy material. Some patients with metastatic neuroblastoma excrete an increased amount of catecholamines and their derivatives in the urine (see page 1959, Volume 4):[451] this is a useful diagnostic feature.

Fig. 37.92.§ Giant cell tumour: femur.

A.§ Radiograph showing expansion of lower end of the bone by an osteolytic lesion.

B.§ Longitudinally divided femur. The lower end of the bone is largely replaced by the tumour, the cut surface of which shows cysts and areas of haemorrhage.

C.§ Part of the tumour, composed of many giant cells separated by a small amount of stromal tissue. *Haematoxylin–eosin.* ×160.

D.§ Another field, showing more conspicuous stromal tissue and relatively few giant cells. *Haematoxylin–eosin.* ×160.

Course

Metastasis occurs early in the course of the disease, secondary tumours developing particularly in the lungs and liver. Quite often, the skeleton itself is the site of multiple tumours that are probably metastatic.

Myelomatosis[454-456]

Myelomatosis (multiple myeloma) is a neoplastic condition originating in the bone marrow and not from skeletal connective tissue (see page 448 in Volume 2). The tumour cells usually resemble plasma cells. The presence of abnormal plasma proteins is a feature characteristic of the condition.

Myelomatosis usually occurs in people above the age of 50 years; men are more frequently affected than women. Multiple bone lesions are usually present at the time of clinical presentation. They may appear as focal osteolytic lesions (Figs 37.93 and 37.94) or as areas of diffuse marrow replacement, with or without local bone destruction. Diffuse bony rarefaction may be the only radiographic indication of widespread myelomatosis. The bones that contain haemopoietic marrow

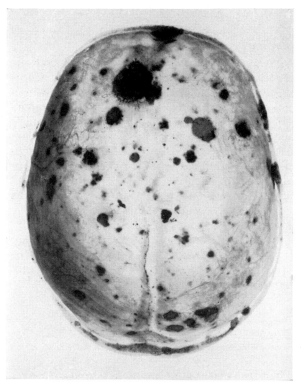

Fig. 37.93.§ Myelomatosis. Inner aspect of the vault of a skull, showing numerous focal osteolytic lesions.

(spine, pelvis, ribs, sternum and vault of the skull) are the common sites of the lesions, although other parts of the skeleton may be involved.

Occasionally, an apparently single osteolytic bone lesion is found to have the histological structure of myeloma. The term *solitary myeloma* is sometimes applied to such lesions. In most instances of these 'solitary' myelomas the typical picture of myelomatosis ultimately develops.[457] There are a very few cases on record in which prolonged follow-up, and even necropsy, failed to show involvement of other bones.[458-462]

Myelomatous tissue appears greyish white or brown on macroscopical examination. It often forms discrete nodules that are sharply defined from the cortical or cancellous bone that they have eroded. The larger lesions are frequently haemorrhagic, and predispose to fracture of the eroded or expanded bones. Collapse of involved vertebral bodies is not infrequent (Fig. 37.94), and may result in compression of the spinal cord and consequent paraplegia.

Histology

The microscopical appearances are characteristic, if somewhat variable. The tumour cells are small and rounded; their cytoplasm is clearly defined and their nucleus—which often is eccentric in position—usually shows clumping of chromatin toward its periphery, as in plasma cells (Fig. 37.95). There is usually very little supporting stromal tissue. In most cases, the histological structure is strikingly uniform, but occasionally some of the cells are larger and irregular, and have two or sometimes three hyperchromatic nuclei. It is unusual to see any reactive bone formation in or round myelomatous lesions. The mechanism of bone removal in myelomatosis has not been studied in detail, but it may be assumed to be brought about by osteoclasts.

Extra-Skeletal Involvement

Extraskeletal lesions are sometimes encountered in myelomatosis. They usually take the form of microscopical accumulations of myeloma cells in the spleen, liver and lymph nodes.[463] Occasionally, more massive nodular lesions have been encountered, particularly in the spleen.[464] Extensive marrow involvement by myelomatous tissue is usually accompanied by severe anaemia, which, in many cases, is of the leucoerythroblastic type.

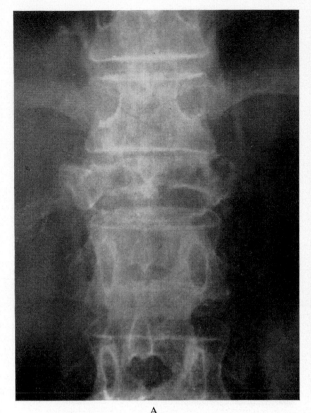
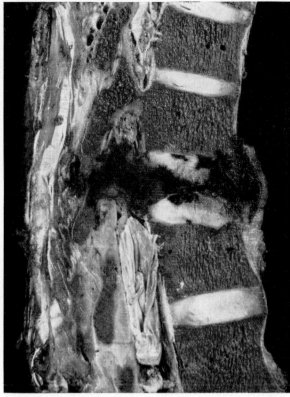

A   B

Fig. 37.94.§ Myelomatosis.

A.§ Radiograph of spine, showing a collapsed vertebral body.

B.§ Longitudinally divided vertebrae (same case as Fig. 37.94A): the body and pedicle of the collapsed vertebra are replaced by haemorrhagic myelomatous tissue; although the other vertebrae appear normal macroscopically, their marrow was found to be diffusely replaced by myelomatous tissue when sections were examined.

Occasionally, myeloma cells can be identified in the peripheral blood, and sometimes they are present in such numbers that the term *plasma cell leukaemia* may be applied.[465]

Biochemical Changes

Myelomatosis is often associated with abnormalities of plasma proteins.[466] The globulin content of the plasma is increased, and abnormal beta or gamma globulin fractions can be demonstrated by electrophoresis. A characteristic feature of the disease is the continuous or intermittent presence of a distinctive protein in the urine (Bence Jones proteinuria—see page 489 in Volume 2). It has been shown that the myeloma tissue contains abnormal globulins of the types that are present in the blood.[467, 468]

Hypercalcaemia may be present when bone destruction is particularly active.

Changes in the Kidneys

The kidneys frequently show certain characteristic changes; the picture is usually referred to as '*myeloma kidney*' (see page 1438 in Volume 4). The tubules are obstructed by protein casts, many of which are surrounded by multinucleate giant cells. The tubular obstruction can lead to renal failure.

Amyloidosis

Another complication of myelomatosis is amyloidosis.[469] It is present in about 10 per cent of cases studied at necropsy. The distribution of the amyloid material is that ordinarily associated with

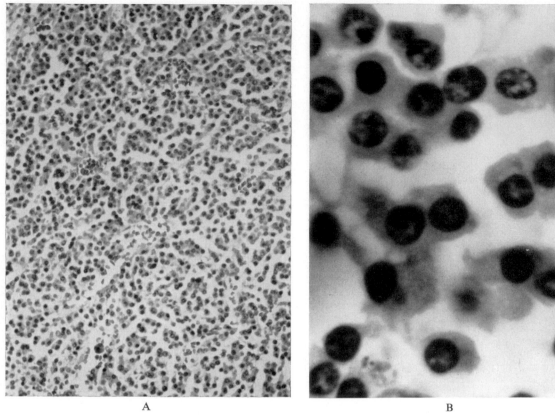

A   B

Fig. 37.95. Myelomatosis. *Haematoxylin–eosin.*

A. The uniform, diffusely cellular appearance of the tumour is characteristic. × 160.

B.§ Higher magnification of the same tumour, showing the resemblance of the myeloma cells to plasma cells. × 1400.

so-called primary ('pericollagenous') amyloidosis, with predominant involvement of the myocardium, skeletal muscle, blood vessels and gastrointestinal tract, rather than the liver, spleen and kidneys as in amyloidosis secondary to chronic sepsis and other predisposing diseases ('perireticular amyloidosis'). However, the clinical and pathological picture of amyloidosis complicating myelomatosis may be that of secondary amyloidosis.

Diagnosis

The diagnosis of myelomatosis is confirmed microscopically either by examination of sternal marrow or by biopsy of a bone lesion. Identification of the so-called 'myeloma protein' by electrophoresis is diagnostic, and is particularly important as a guide to the diagnosis when bone lesions are inconspicuous, or when they are confused with those of metastatic carcinoma.

Tumours of Lymphoreticular and Haemopoietic Tissue (Lymphomas and Leukaemia)[470–472]

Lymphomas

The skeleton is involved in a considerable proportion of cases of primary malignant disease of the lymphoreticular system (see pages 794 and 820 in Volume 2). Careful post-mortem examination in fatal cases of Hodgkin's disease and of other malignant lymphomas frequently reveals widespread replacement of haemopoietic bone marrow by tumour tissue: in perhaps 10 per cent of cases this is accompanied by localized alterations in bony structure. The vertebral column is a common site for such lesions; ribs, skull and pelvis are less frequently involved, and other bones only rarely. The lesions are usually osteolytic: this sometimes leads to pathological fracture.

In the majority of cases of lymphoma involving bone, it is clear that the bone lesions are metastatic or, oftener, a manifestation of the multicentric origin of the disease. Hodgkin's disease and lymphocytic lymphomas very rarely originate in bone. In contrast, immunoblastic lymphomas and tumours that have been described as reticulum cell sarcomas (reticulosarcomas) arising in bone form a recognized clinicopathological entity.[473-475] Men are affected more frequently than women; most of the patients are between 20 and 40 years of age. The long bones of the limbs are most commonly affected. The lesions are sometimes osteolytic, but often there is widespread infiltration without much alteration in bone structure and radiographic appearance. The tumour tissue is greyish-white or pink. Histologically, it has essentially the same characteristics as immunoblastic lymphomas or, more rarely, true reticulum cell sarcomas (histiocytic lymphomas) elsewhere (see pages 849 and 851 in Volume 2). Abundant reticulin fibres may be demonstrable in appropriately prepared sections, forming a delicate network round and between individual tumour cells.

Primary lymphomas of bone usually are less malignant than most other types of sarcoma arising in bone. It is sometimes difficult to distinguish between them and Ewing's tumour: the better prognosis of the lymphomas emphasizes the desirability of making the distinction.

Leukaemia

In cases of leukaemia in adults there is frequently the same diffuse replacement of the marrow and the same focal distribution of osteolytic bone lesions that are found when the skeleton is heavily involved in the course of dissemination of Hodgkin's disease and other lymphomas.

In childhood, leukaemia is frequently associated with diffuse bony rarefaction and areas of focal bone destruction, particularly in the metaphyses of rapidly growing long bones, such as the tibiae and femora. Reactive periosteal bone formation may also be a feature. The radiological appearances of the lesions, in association with pain and fever, occasionally simulate acute osteomyelitis.

Chordoma[476-480]

This is a relatively rare tumour. It occurs only in the axial skeleton and it is usually considered to take origin from remnants of notochordal tissue. Such remnants are occasionally encountered in normal individuals, particularly in the spheno-occipital region, where they take the form of small flattened masses of soft tissue attached—often by a narrow pedicle—to the inner surface of the dura. The term *ecchordosis* is often used to describe these notochordal remnants (see page 2230).

Despite their origin from developmental remnants, chordomas are not usually found before the age of 40 years and may present as late as the eighth decade. They are more frequent in men. Most occur in the sacral region, the next commonest site being the spheno-occipital region of the base of the skull; the intervening vertebrae are exceptionally rare sites of these growths. Sacral chordomas usually present as pelvic tumours; those of the spheno-occipital region produce the signs and symptoms of an intracranial tumour, with evidence of involvement of structures at the base of the skull (see page 2230). Cervical, thoracic and lumbar tumours may compress the spinal cord or nerve roots. By the time symptoms occur, chordomas are usually large and associated with considerable destruction of bone (Figs 37.96A and 37.96B): there is often infiltration of adjacent muscle and other soft tissues. The tumour tissue is gelatinous, and shows conspicuous lobulation; areas of necrosis and haemorrhage are frequent.

Histology

Histologically, chordomas have some resemblance to notochordal tissue. They are characterized by large amounts of mucoid intercellular material in which strands and masses of tumour cells are scattered (Figs 37.96C and 37.96D). The tumour cells themselves are conspicuously vacuolate ('physaliphorous' cells). Sometimes these features are less evident, and parts of the tumour present an undifferentiated, pleomorphic appearance. This may lead to problems of diagnosis in small biopsy specimens, but careful scrutiny of a representative sample should reveal characteristic features and enable the diagnosis to be established unequivocally.

Occasionally, the mucoid intercellular material of a chordoma may show a remarkably close resemblance to the degenerate intercellular matrix of a chondrosarcoma: the cells of the latter, however, are rounded, lie in definite spaces in the matrix, and fail to show the conspicuous vacuolation of chordoma cells. Diagnostic confusion between the two tumours should not arise.

Course

Chordomas grow slowly. They are locally malignant, infiltrating adjacent structures and recurring

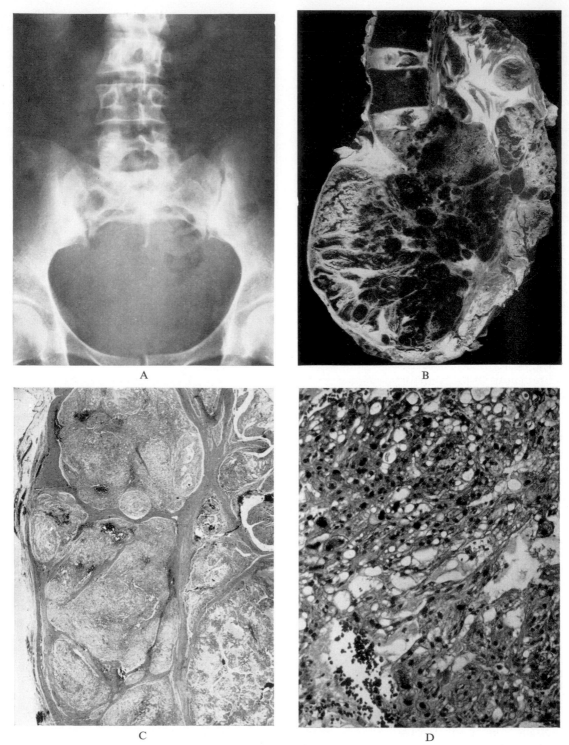

A

B

C

D

Fig. 37.96.§ Chordomas.

A.§ Radiograph showing destruction of the lower part of the sacrum by the tumour.

B.§ Longitudinally divided lumbosacral spine in another case of chordoma.

C.§ Low-power magnification of part of a chordoma to show the characteristic lobulation of the tumour tissue. *Haematoxylin–eosin.* ×8.

D.§ An area of tumour tissue showing conspicuous vacuolation of the cells ('physaliphorous cells'). *Haematoxylin–eosin.* ×130.

after local resection; they are almost invariably fatal. Metastasis occurs rarely.[481, 482]

'Adamantinoma' of Limb Bones[483–485]

The name 'adamantinoma' is applied to a rare tumour of limb bones that has a histological resemblance to the ameloblastoma (adamantinoma) of the jaws (see page 984 in Volume 3). There has been much discussion of its histogenesis. Generally, it has been regarded as an epithelial tumour, despite its site of origin, and the identification of tonofibrils and desmosomes in the tumour cells on electron microscopy supports this view, at least in the case of some specimens.[486] The development of a primary epithelial tumour within a long bone appears a paradox. An early suggestion was that the growth has its origin in epithelial tissue displaced into the underlying bone during embryonic development,[487] but there is no evidence that such displacement occurs. Traumatic displacement of epithelium during postnatal life has also been suggested,[488] again without direct evidence. Congenital abnormalities of the affected tibia, and sometimes of the other tibia also, have been present in some cases.[489] Some authorities have contested the epithelial nature of the tumours, regarding them as synovial[490, 491] or vascular ('malignant angioblastoma'[492]). In exceptional cases an adamantinoma has developed in a long bone in association with fibrous dysplasia;[493] the implications of such observations are not clear.

Fewer than 100 cases have been reported.[483–485] Most of the patients are adults. In almost every case the tumour is in a tibia. It takes the form of a circumscribed mass that expands the shaft of the bone (Figs 37.97A and 37.97B).

Histology (Fig. 37.97C)

Histologically, 'adamantinomas' of bone consist of groups or sheets of cells, separated by spindle-celled connective tissue that is presumed to be stromal in nature. In some instances the tumour cells have an alveolar arrangement, and the cells abutting on the 'stroma' are oriented into a more or less columnar layer that gives a distinctly epithelial aspect to the pattern. These features may effect a remarkable resemblance to the ameloblastoma of the jaws. Squamous transformation of the tumour cells is occasionally seen, and provides further evidence that the growth is epithelial.

Course and Prognosis

Adamantinomas of limb bones grow slowly. Local excision is commonly followed by recurrence in the same site. Metastasis to regional lymph nodes or to the lungs occurred in 8 of 25 cases in which the ultimate outcome of the disease was known.[492]

Other Primary Malignant Tumours

Malignant Vascular Tumours

Malignant vascular tumours are very rare in bone.[494] Their nomenclature is confused.

Angiosarcoma.—This is a highly malignant growth, characterized histologically by conspicuous vascular spaces lined by immature endothelial cells. It usually metastasizes rapidly to the lungs. Multiple angiosarcomas are sometimes found in the bones or in bones and soft tissues.

Haemangioendothelioma.—This name has been given to a group of less malignant tumours of vascular endothelium that are intermediate between the angiosarcomas and the benign haemangiomas both in structure and in behaviour.[495, 495a] The tumours of this group commonly recur after excision, but they rarely metastasize. They may be multiple.

Kaposi's Sarcoma.—Lesions were present in bone in 20 per cent of a series of 229 cases of Kaposi's sarcoma studied in South Africa.[495b] The disease is considered on page 711 in Volume 2 and in Chapter 39, Volume 6.

Liposarcoma and Tumours with Liposarcomatous Components

Liposarcoma.—Bone is a rare but well-recognized site of primary liposarcoma.[496, 497]

Malignant 'Mesenchymoma' of Bone.—Liposarcomatous tissue is associated with osteosarcomatous tissue in the exceptionally rare tumours of bone that have sometimes been described as *malignant mesenchymomas*,[498, 499] a term that gives a misleading indication of their histogenesis.[500]

Miscellaneous Unclassifiable Malignant Tumours

In any large series of bone tumours there are always some that cannot be put in any of the established groups. Most of these are undifferentiated malignant tumours, the histological structure

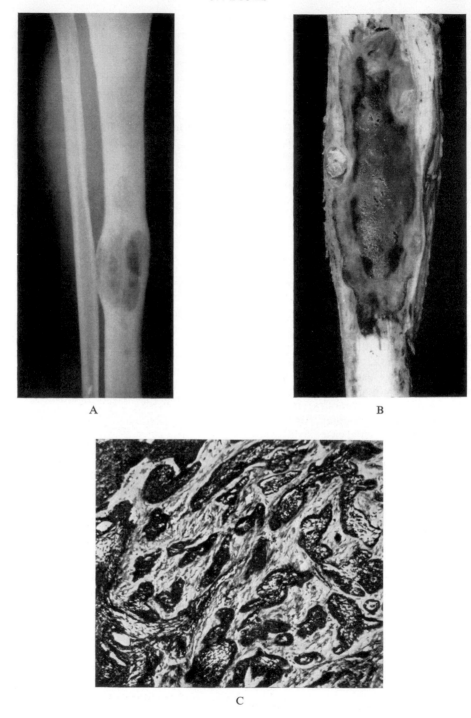

A   B

C

Fig. 37.97. A so-called 'adamantinoma' of tibia.

A.§ Radiograph showing an expanding osteolytic lesion in the middle part of the shaft.

B.§ Longitudinally divided specimen. Much of the tumour is necrotic, possibly as a result of X-irradiation.

C. Islands of darkly staining tumour cells are separated by stroma formed of spindle-shaped cells, presumably fibroblasts. *Haematoxylin–eosin.* × 65.

of which gives no indication of their histogenesis: they can be identified as primary bone tumours only when careful search has failed to demonstrate a primary tumour elsewhere. In bone, metastatic tumours are relatively much more frequent than primary tumours (see below). This must be borne in mind, particularly when investigating the nature of neoplasms in older patients: in the absence of definite evidence to the contrary, any obscure malignant tumour of the skeleton should be regarded as probably metastatic.

Secondary Tumours in Bone[501]

The skeleton is a frequent site for metastasis of many types of malignant epithelial tumour. In a series of 500 cases of carcinoma, studied at necropsy, metastasis to bone was found in 13·6 per cent:[501] only the lungs and liver were more frequently the site of metastatic deposits. In this series the examination of the skeleton, apart from the standard exposure of the thoracic cage, and of the cranial bones in the course of removing the brain, was usually confined to sawing a slice off the abdominal aspect of the lumbar vertebral bodies.[501a] In a larger series the incidence of secondary tumours in bone was 27 per cent.[502] In another series, comprising 575 necropsies in cases of carcinoma, the entire length of the spinal column was divided longitudinally: tumour deposits were found in the vertebrae in 33 per cent of the series as a whole and in 47·5 per cent of the cases in which there were secondary deposits in viscera apart from the organ in which the tumour had arisen.[502a]

Some types of primary tumour give rise to secondary deposits in bone with exceptional frequency, examples being carcinoma of breast and carcinoma of prostate, which are found to have metastasized to bone in from 50 to 70 per cent of fatal cases respectively. Deposits in bones are also very commonly found in cases of bronchial carcinoma. Next in frequency come carcinomas of colon, stomach and urinary bladder. A primary tumour responsible for secondary growths in bone may be clinically latent: carcinomas of the thyroid and of the kidneys have a special reputation in this connexion.

In children, adrenal neuroblastoma is the commonest source of secondary tumours in bone. The neuroblastomatous deposits are usually multiple; a solitary metastasis may simulate Ewing's tumour (see page 2471). The urinary excretion of catecholamines and their metabolites is sometimes increased in cases of neuroblastoma; this may aid the identification of these tumours and in particular enable them to be distinguished from Ewing's tumour.[451]

Sites and Routes of Metastasis

Metastatic bone tumours almost exclusively involve the haemopoietic bone marrow, which in the adult is normally present in the vertebral bodies, the pelvis, the calvarium, the ribs and sternum, and the proximal end of the femora and humeri. The tumour cells are blood borne, and it is clear that they usually reach the bone marrow as emboli in the systemic arterial system. The vertebral plexuses of veins have been suggested as a pathway for metastasis from the pelvic viscera, particularly the prostate, to the bodies of the lumbar vertebrae,[503] but its role is unproved.

Occasionally, bones may be directly invaded by an adjacent malignant tumour. Examples of this are the invasion of the subcutaneous part of the tibia by a carcinoma originating in an overlying varicose ulcer and invasion of the bone of the face

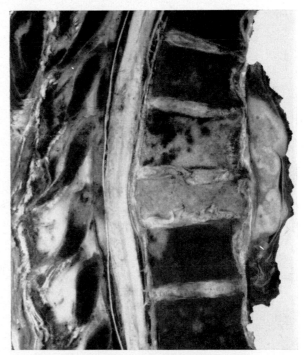

Fig. 37.98.§ Metastatic carcinoma in the spine. The primary growth was a renal carcinoma. An isolated metastatic deposit in a vertebral body has resulted in collapse of the vertebra and compression of the spinal cord. The tumour has invaded the adjoining soft tissues; it has also spread from the vertebral body first affected into that immediately above.

by a basal cell carcinoma of the skin. Sometimes a squamous carcinoma or, more rarely, a sarcoma arises in an old osteomyelitic sinus and has its origin close to, or even within, a bone (see page 2408).

Effects on Involved Bone

Secondary deposits in bone are usually multiple. When solitary, or apparently solitary, lesions are encountered they may simulate primary bone tumours. They may be circumscribed or diffuse (Figs 37.98 and 37.99). Most of them are associated with destruction of the involved bone tissue, and therefore are described as *osteolytic*. Some tumours, however, particularly those of prostatic origin, stimulate local bone formation (Figs 37.99 and 37.100) and produce lesions that appear dense on radiographic examination and therefore are termed *osteosclerotic*. Bone formation in metastatic tumours is due to osteoblastic activity (Fig. 37.100): bone destruction is usually regarded as being the

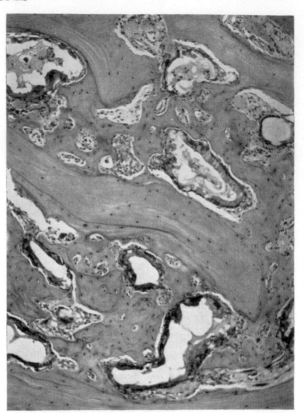

Fig. 37.100.§ Metastatic carcinoma. An osteosclerotic deposit from a prostatic carcinoma. Scattered adenocarcinomatous structures are separated by a close meshwork of bony tissue. A few of the original trabeculae of lamellar bone remain; the rest of the osseous tissue is non-lamellar, newly formed bone that has been produced in response to the presence of the tumour. *Haematoxylin–eosin.* × 70.

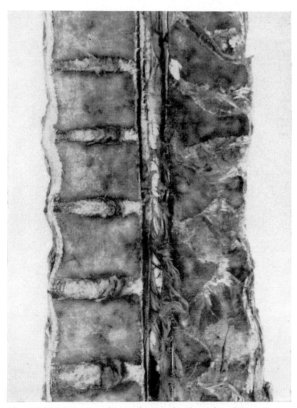

Fig. 37.99.§ Metastatic carcinoma in the spine. The primary growth was a prostatic carcinoma. The external contour of each vertebra is normal, but each is diffusely infiltrated by tumour tissue and has been converted into abnormally dense bone. See also Fig. 37.100.

result of osteoclastic activity, although it has been suggested[504] that it may sometimes be caused by the tumour cells themselves. Although the terms osteolytic and osteosclerotic are convenient ones, they denote differences of predominance, bone destruction and bone formation both being present in relation to most metastatic tumours. Secondary tumours in bone are not always associated with alteration of bony structure: very extensive, heavy invasion may be present in the absence of any demonstrable radiographic change.[505]

Biochemical Effects

Some metastatic bone tumours produce important chemical changes in the blood. Extensive deposits are often accompanied by elevation of the serum alkaline phosphatase: this is usually ascribed to the associated reactive osteoblastic response. In cases of metastasis of carcinoma of the prostate, there may also be a large rise in serum acid phosphatase, as this enzyme is secreted by the tumour cells.

Widespread bone destruction may result in hypercalcaemia, and this may be accompanied by mestastic calcification and renal damage.

REFERENCES

BONE STRUCTURE AND PHYSIOLOGY

1. McLean, F. C., Urist, M. R., *Bone—Fundamentals of the Physiology of Skeletal Tissue*, 3rd edn. Chicago, 1968.
2. *The Biochemistry and Physiology of Bone*, 2nd edn, edited by G. H. Bourne. New York, 1972.
3. Rodahl, K., Nicholson, J. T., Brown, E. M., *Bone as a Tissue*. New York, 1960.
4. Vaughan, J. M., *The Physiology of Bone*. Oxford, 1970.
5. Ham, A. W., *Histology*, 7th edn, chaps 14 and 15. Philadelphia and Toronto, 1974.
6. Hancox, N. M., *Biology of Bone*. Cambridge, 1972.
7. Cohen, J., Harris, W. H., *J. Bone Jt Surg.*, 1958, **40A**, 419.
7a. Göthlin, G., Ericsson, J. L. E., *Virchows Arch. Abt. B*, 1972, **12**, 318.
8. Robinson, R. A., Watson, M. L., *Ann. N.Y. Acad. Sci.*, 1955, **60**, 596.
9. Irving, J. T., *Arch. oral Biol.*, 1963, **8**, 735.
10. Matrajt, H., Hioco, D., *Stain Technol.*, 1966, **41**, 97.
11. Loe, H., *Acta odont. scand.*, 1959, **17**, suppl. 27.
12. Vincent, J., *Recherches sur la constitution de l'os adulte*. Brussels, 1955.
13. Vincent, J., *Rev. belge Path.*, 1957, **26**, 161.
14. Frost, H. M., Villanueva, A. R., Roth, H., *Henry Ford Hosp. Bull.*, 1960, **8**, 239.
15. Harris, W. H., *Nature (Lond.)*, 1960, **188**, 1038.
16. Lee, W. R., *J. Anat. (Lond.)*, 1964, **98**, 665.
17. Young, R. W., *Exp. Cell Res.*, 1962, **26**, 562.
18. Young, R. W., *J. Cell Biol.*, 1962, **14**, 357.
19. Owen, M., *Int. Rev. Cytol.*, 1970, **28**, 213.
20. Howship, J., *On the Natural and Diseased State of the Bones*. London, 1820.
20a. Baker, S. L., in *A Text-Book of X-Ray Diagnosis*, 3rd edn, edited by S. C. Shanks and P. J. Kerley, vol. 4, page 68. London, 1959.
21. Kölliker, A. von, *Die normale Resorption des Knochengewebes und ihre Bedeutung für die Entstehung der typischen Knochenformen*. Leipzig, 1873.
22. Weinmann, J. P., Sicher, H., *Bone and Bones*, 2nd edn, page 284. St Louis, 1955.
23. Bailie, J. M., Irving, J. H., *Acta med. scand.*, 1955, suppl. 306.
24. Scott, B. L., Pease, D. C., *Anat. Rec.*, 1956, **126**, 465.
25. Cameron, D. A., Paschall, H. A., Robinson, R. A., in *Bone Biodynamics*, edited by H. M. Frost, page 91. Boston, 1964.
26. Schenk, R. K., Müller, J., Zinkernagel, R., Willenegger, H., *Calcif. Tiss. Res.*, 1970, **4**, suppl., 110.
27. Cameron, D. A., in *The Biochemistry and Physiology of Bone*, 2nd edn, edited by G. H. Bourne, vol. 1, page 191. New York, 1972.
28. Baud, C. A., *Clin. Orthop.*, 1968, **56**, 227.
29. Bélanger, L. F., in *The Biochemistry and Physiology of Bone*, 2nd edn, edited by G. H. Bourne, vol. 3, page 239. New York, 1972.
30. Boyde, A., Hobdell, M., *Z. Zellforsch.*, 1969, **93**, 213.
31. Tomes, J., de Morgan, C., *Phil. Trans.*, 1853, **143**, 109.
32. Sissons, H. A., in *Bone as a Tissue*, edited by K. Rodahl, J. T. Nicholson and E. M. Brown, chap. 1. New York, 1960.
33. Amprino, R., Marotti, G., in *Bone and Tooth*, edited by H. J. J. Blackwood, page 21. Oxford, 1964.
34. Lee, W. R., Marshall, J. H., Sissons, H. A., *J. Bone Jt Surg.*, 1965, **47B**, 157.
35. Bauer, G. C. H., Carlsson, A., Lindquist, B., *Kgl. Fysiograf. Sällskap. Lund, Förh.*, 1955, **25**, 1.
36. Bauer, G. C. H., Ray, R. D., *J. Bone Jt Surg.*, 1958, **40A**, 171.
37. Heaney, R. P., Whedon, G. D., *J. clin. Endocr.*, 1958, **18**, 1246.
38. Marshall, J. H., in *Bone as a Tissue*, edited by K. Rodahl, J. T. Nicholson and E. M. Brown, chap. 8. New York, 1960.
39. McLean, F. C., Urist, M. R., *Bone—Fundamentals of the Physiology of Skeletal Tissue*, 3rd edn. Chicago, 1968.
40. Copp, D. H., Cameron, E. C., Cheney, B. A., Davidson, A. G. F., Henze, K. G., *Endocrinology*, 1962, **70**, 638.
41. Hirsch, P. F., Gauthier, G. F., Munson, P. L., *Endocrinology*, 1963, **73**, 244.
42. Foster, G. V., Baghdiantz, A., Kumar, M. A., Slack, E., Soliman, H. A., MacIntyre, I., *Nature (Lond.)*, 1964, **202**, 1303.
43. Parsons, J. A., Potts, J. T., Jr, *Clin. Endocr. Metab.*, 1972, **1**, 33.
44. Foster, G. V., Byfield, P. G. H., Gudmundsson, T. V., *Clin. Endocr. Metab.*, 1972, **1**, 93.
45. Friedman, J., Raisz, L. G., *Science*, 1965, **150**, 1465.
46. Aliapoulios, M. A., Goldhaber, P., Munson, P. L., *Science*, 1966, **151**, 330.
47. Milhaud, G., Pérault, A. M., Moukhtar, M. S., *C.R. Acad. Sci. (Paris)*, 1965, **261**, 813.
48. Martin, T. J., Robertson, C. J., MacIntyre, I., *Lancet*, 1966, **1**, 900.
49. Foster, G. V., Doyle, F. H., Bordier, P., Matrajt, H., *Lancet*, 1966, **2**, 1428.
50. Amprino, R., Engström, A., *Acta anat. (Basel)*, 1952, **15**, 1.
51. Amprino, R., *Arch. Putti Chir. Organi Mov.*, 1952, **2**, 173.
52. Vincent, J., *Recherches sur la constitution de l'os adulte*. Brussels, 1955.
53. Robinson, A. A., Elliott, S. R., *J. Bone Jt Surg.*, 1957, **39A**, 167.
54. Smith, J. W., *J. Bone Jt Surg.*, 1960, **42B**, 588.
55. Engfeldt, B., Engström, A., Zetterström, R., *Biochim. biophys. Acta (Amst.)*, 1952, **8**, 375.

56. Lacroix, P., in *Bone as a Tissue*, edited by K. Rodahl, J. T. Nicholson and E. M. Brown, chap. 12. New York, 1960.
57. Ponlot, R., *Le Radiocalcium dans l'étude de l'os*. Brussels, 1960.
58. Sissons, H. A., Holley, K. J., Heighway, J., in *L'Ostéomalacie*, edited by D. J. Hioco, page 19. Paris, 1967.
59. Dunnill, M. S., Anderson, J. A., Whitehead, R., *J. Path. Bact.*, 1967, **94**, 275.
60. Atkinson, P. J., *Calcif. Tiss. Res.*, 1967, **1**, 24.
61. Wakamatsu, E., Sissons, H. A., *Calcif. Tiss. Res.*, 1969, **4**, 147.
62. Ellis, H. A., Peart, K. M., *J. clin. Path.*, 1972, **25**, 277.
63. Trotter, M., Broman, G. E., Peterson, R. R., *J. Bone Jt Surg.*, 1960, **42A**, 50.
64. Barnett, E., Nordin, B. E. C., *Clin. Radiol.*, 1960, **11**, 166.
65. Bernard, J., Laval-Jeantet, M., *Presse méd.*, 1962, **70**, 889.
66. Exton-Smith, A. N., Millard, P. H., Payne, P. R., Wheeler, E., *Lancet*, 1969, **2**, 1153.
67. Dequeker, J., *Bone Loss in Normal and Pathological Conditions*. Leuven, 1972.
68. Anderson, J. B., Shimmis, J., Smith, D. A., *Brit. J. Radiol.*, 1966, **39**, 443.
69. Sorenson, J. A., Cameron, J. R., in *Symposium Ossium*, edited by A. M. Jelliffe and B. Strickland, page 155. Edinburgh and London, 1970.
70. Caldwell, R. A., Collins, D. H., *J. Bone Jt Surg.*, 1961, **43B**, 346.
71. Caldwell, R. A., *J. clin. Path.*, 1962, **15**, 421.
72. Lindahl, O., Lindgren, A. G. H., *Acta orthop. scand.*, 1962, **32**, 85.
73. Jowsey, J., *Clin. Orthop.*, 1960, **17**, 210.
74. Sissons, H. A., in *The Biochemistry and Physiology of Bone*, 2nd edn, edited by G. H. Bourne, vol. 3, page 145. New York, 1972.
75. Wilkins, L., *The Diagnosis and Treatment of Endocrine Disorders in Childhood and Adolescence*, 2nd edn. Oxford, 1957.
76. Harris, H. A., *Bone Growth in Health and Disease*. London, 1933.
77. Follis, R. H., Park, E. A., *Amer. J. Roentgenol.*, 1952, **68**, 709.
78. Trueta, J., *Bull. Hosp. Jt Dis. (N.Y.)*, 1953, **14**, 147.
79. Trueta, J., Amato, V. P., *J. Bone Jt Surg.*, 1960, **42B**, 571.
80. Howland, J., Kramer, B., *Mschr. Kinderheilk.*, 1923, **22**, 105.
81. Howland, J., *Harvey Lect.*, 1923, **18**, 189.
82. Robison, R., *Biochem. J.*, 1923, **17**, 286.
83. Glimcher, M. J., Hodge, A. J., Schmitt, F. O., *Proc. nat. Acad. Sci. (Wash.)*, 1957, **43**, 860.
84. Jackson, S. Fitton, *Proc. roy. Soc. B*, 1957, **146**, 270.
85. Sheldon, H., Robinson, R. A., *J. biophys. biochem. Cytol.*, 1957, **3**, 1011.
85a. Anderson, H. C., in *The Biochemistry and Physiology of Bone*, 2nd edn, edited by G. H. Bourne, vol. 4, page 135. New York, 1972.
86. Fleisch, H., Neuman, W. F., *Amer. J. Physiol.*, 1961, **200**, 1296.

DEVELOPMENTAL ABNORMALITIES

87. Werthemann, A., in *Handbuch der speziellen pathologischen Anatomie und Histologie*, edited by O. Lubarsch, F. Henke and R. Rössle, vol. 9, part 6, *Die Entwicklungsstörungen der Extremitäten*. Berlin, 1952.
87a. Smithells, R. W., *Brit. med. J.*, 1973, **1**, 269.
88. McKusick, V. A., *Heritable Disorders of Connective Tissue*, 4th edn. St Louis, 1972.
89. Roberts, J. A. Fraser, *An Introduction to Medical Genetics*, 6th edn, page 281. London, 1973.
90. Fairbank, H. A. T., *An Atlas of General Affections of the Skeleton*. Edinburgh and London, 1951.
91. Knaggs, R. L., *Brit. J. Surg.*, 1923–24, **11**, 737.
92. Seedorff, K. S., *Osteogenesis Imperfecta*. Copenhagen, 1949.
93. Engfeldt, B., Engström, A., Zetterström, R., *J. Bone Jt Surg.*, 1954, **36B**, 654.
94. Falvo, K. A., Bullough, P. G., *J. Bone Jt Surg.*, 1973, **55A**, 275.
95. Fairbank, H. A. T., Baker, S. L., *Brit. J. Surg.*, 1948–1949, **36**, 1.
96. Knaggs, R. L., *Brit. J. Surg.*, 1927–28, **15**, 10.
97. Mörch, E. T., *Chondrodystrophic Dwarfs in Denmark*. Copenhagen, 1949.
98. Murdoch, J. K., Walker, B. A., Hall, J. G., Smith, K. K., Abbey, H., McKusick, V. A., *Ann. hum. Genet.*, 1970, **33**, 227.
99. Zawisch, C., *Arch. Path. (Chic.)*, 1947, **43**, 55.
100. Cohen, J., *J. Bone Jt Surg.*, 1951, **33A**, 923.
101. Albers-Schönberg, H., *Münch. med. Wschr.*, 1904, **51**, 365.
102. Hanart, E., *Helv. paediat. Acta*, 1948, **3**, 113.
103. Ollier, L. X. E. L., *Bull. Soc. Chir. Lyon*, 1899–1900, **3**, 22.
104. Fairbank, H. A. T., *An Atlas of General Affections of the Skeleton*, page 69. Edinburgh and London, 1951.
105. Maffucci, A., *Mov. med.-chir.*, 1881, 2nd ser., **3**, 399.
106. Torri, O., *Clin. chir.*, 1902, **10**, 81.
107. Carleton, A., Elkington, J. St. G., Greenfield, J. G., Robb-Smith, A. H. T., *Quart. J. Med.*, 1942, N.S. **11**, 203.
108. Speiser, F., *Virchows Arch. path. Anat.*, 1925, **258**, 126.
109. Lichtenstein, L., Jaffe, H. L., *Amer. J. Path.*, 1943, **19**, 553.
110. Coley, B. L., Higinbotham, N. L., *Ann. Surg.*, 1954, **139**, 547.
111. Keith, A., *J. Anat. (Lond.)*, 1919–20, **54**, 101.
112. Stocks, P., Barrington, A., in *Treasury of Human Inheritance*, edited by Karl Pearson, vol. 3, page 1. Cambridge, 1925.
112a. Ollier, L. X. E. L., *Mém. C.R. Soc. Sci. méd. Lyon*, 1890, **29**, 2, 12.
113. Müller, E., *Beitr. path. Anat.*, 1913–14, **57**, 232.
114. Jaffe, H. L., *Arch. Path. (Chic.)*, 1943, **36**, 335.
115. Morquio, L., *Arch. Méd. Enf.*, 1929, **32**, 129.
116. Brailsford, J. F., *Amer. J. Surg.*, 1929, **7**, 404.
117. Camurati, M., *Chir. Organi Mov.*, 1922, **6**, 662.
118. Engelmann, G., *Fortschr. Röntgenstr.*, 1929, **39**, 1101.

REACTION TO TRAUMA

119. Ham, A. W., Harris, W. R., in *The Biochemistry and Physiology of Bone*, 2nd edn, edited by G. H. Bourne, vol. 3, page 337. New York, 1972.
120. Bast, T. H., Sullivan, W. E., Geist, F. D., *Anat. Rec.*, 1925, **31**, 255.
121. Blaisdell, F. E., Cowan, J. F., *Arch. Surg. (Chic.)*, 1926, **12**, 619.
122. Urist, M. R., McLean, F. C., *J. Bone Jt Surg.*, 1941, **23**, 1.

123. Pritchard, J. J., *J. Anat.* (*Lond.*), 1946, **80**, 55.
124. Urist, M. R., Johnson, R. W., *J. Bone Jt Surg.*, 1943, **25**, 375.
125. Cohen, J., *Lab. Invest.*, 1956, **5**, 53.
126. Charnley, J., Baker, S. L., *J. Bone Jt Surg.*, 1952, **34B**, 187.
127. Wolff, J., *Virchows Arch. path. Anat.*, 1899, **155**, 256.
128. Bauer, G. C. H., Wendeberg, B., *J. Bone Jt Surg.*, 1959, **41B**, 558.
129. Buhr, A. J., Cooke, A. M., *Lancet*, 1959, **1**, 531.
130. Gallie, W. E., Robertson, D. E., *Brit. J. Surg.*, 1919–1920, **7**, 211.
131. Chalmers, J., *J. Bone Jt Surg.*, 1959, **41B**, 160.
132. Huggins, C. B., *Arch. Surg.* (*Chic.*), 1931, **22**, 377.
133. Bertelsen, A., *Acta orthop. scand.*, 1944, **15**, 139.

VASCULAR DISTURBANCES

134. Gorham, L. W., Stout, A. P., *J. Bone Jt Surg.*, 1955, **37A**, 985.
135. Jaffe, H. L., Pomeranz, M. M., *Arch. Surg.* (*Chic.*), 1934, **29**, 566.
136. Sherman, M. S., Phemister, D. B., *J. Bone Jt Surg.*, 1947, **29**, 19.
137. Sevitt, S., *J. Bone Jt Surg.*, 1964, **46B**, 280.
138. Catto, M., *J. Bone Jt Surg.*, 1965, **47B**, 749.
139. Phemister, D. B., *J. Bone Jt Surg.*, 1930, **12**, 769.
140. Catto, M., *J. Bone Jt Surg.*, 1965, **47B**, 777.
141. Baker, S. L., in *A Text-Book of X-Ray Diagnosis*, 3rd edn, edited by S. C. Shanks and P. J. Kerley, vol. 4, page 83. London, 1959.
142. Sutro, C. J., Pomeranz, M. M., *Arch. Surg.*, 1937, **34**, 360.
143. Gall, E. A., Bennett, G. A., *Arch. Path.* (*Chic.*), 1942, **33**, 866.
144. Calvé, F., *Rev. Chir.* (*Paris*), 1910, **42**, 54.
145. Legg, A. T., *Boston med. surg. J.*, 1910, **162**, 202.
146. Perthes, G. C., *Dtsch. Z. Chir.*, 1910, **107**, 111.
147. Waldenström, H., *Z. orthop. Chir.*, 1909, **24**, 487.
148. Patterson, R. J., Bickel, W. H., Dahlin, D. C., *J. Bone Jt Surg.*, 1964, **46A**, 267.
149. Solomon, L., *J. Bone Jt. Surg*, 1973, **55B**, 246.
150. Kahlstrom, S. C., Burton, C. C., Phemister, D. B., *Surg. Gynec. Obstet.*, 1939, **68**, 129.
151. McCallum, R. I., Walder, D. N., Barnes, R., Catto, M. E., Davidson, J. K., Fryer, D. I., Golding, F. C., Paton, W. D. M., *J. Bone Jt Surg.*, 1966, **48B**, 207.
152. Amstutz, H. C., Carey, E. J., *J. Bone Jt Surg.*, 1966, **48A**, 670.
153. Reich, R. S., Rosenberg, N. J., *J. Bone Jt Surg.*, 1953, **35A**, 894.
154. Moseley, J. E., Manley, J. B., *Radiology*, 1953, **60**, 656.
155. Chung, S. M. K., Ralston, E. L., *J. Bone Jt Surg.*, 1969, **51A**, 33.
156. Axhausen, B., Bergmann, E., in *Handbuch der speziellen pathologischen Anatomie und Histologie*, edited by F. Henke, O. Lubarsch and R. Rössle, vol. 9, part 3, *Die Ernährungsunterbrechungen am Knochen*. Berlin, 1937.
157. Osgood, R. B., *Boston med. surg. J.*, 1903, **148**, 114.
158. Schlatter, C., *Bruns' Beitr. klin. Chir.*, 1903, **38**, 874.
159. Köhler, A., *Münch. med. Wschr.*, 1908, **55**, 1923.
160. Köhler, A., *Münch. med. Wschr.*, 1920, **67**, 1289.
161. Freiberg, A. H., *J. Bone Jt Surg.*, 1926, **8**, 257.
162. Kienböck, R., *Fortschr. Röntgenstr.*, 1910, **16**, 103.
163. Crump, C., *Virchows Arch. path. Anat.*, 1929, **271**, 467.

164. Gall, E. A., Bennett, G. A., Bauer, W., *Amer. J. Path.*, 1951, **27**, 349.
165. Marie, P., *Rev. Méd.* (*Paris*), 1890, **10**, 1.
166. Mendlowitz, M., *J. clin. Invest.*, 1941, **20**, 113.

IRRADIATION DAMAGE

167. Vaughan, J. M., *The Effects of Irradiation on the Skeleton*. Oxford, 1973.
168. Jaffe, H. L., *Tumors and Tumorous Conditions of the Bones and Joints*, page 479. Philadelphia, 1958.
169. Stephenson, W. H., Cohen, B., *J. Bone Jt Surg.*, 1956, **38B**, 830.
170. Leabhart, J. W., Bonfiglio, M., *J. Bone Jt Surg.*, 1961, **43A**, 1056.
171. Martland, H. S., *J. Amer. med. Ass.*, 1929, **92**, 466, 552.
172. Aub, J. C., Evans, R. D., Hempelmann, L. H., Martland, H. S., *Medicine* (*Baltimore*), 1952, **31**, 221.
173. Looney, W. B., *Amer. J. Roentgenol.*, 1956, **75**, 559.
174. Sissons, H. A., Duthie, R. B., *A Survey of the Biological Properties of Tumours of Bone*, in *Surgical Progress*, edited by E. Rock Carling and J. Paterson Ross, page 158. London, 1959.
175. Finkel, M. P., Biskis, B. O., *Acta Un. int. Cancr.*, 1959, **15**, 99.

INFLAMMATORY CONDITIONS

176. Knaggs, R. L., *Inflammatory and Toxic Diseases of Bone*. Bristol, 1926.
177. Marks, K. L., Turner, W. L., *Brit. J. Surg.*, 1950–51, **38**, 206.
178. Brodie, B. C., *Med.-chir. Trans.*, 1832, **17**, 239.
179. Zammit, F., *Brit. J. Radiol.*, 1958, **31**, 683.
179a. Kelly, P. J., Martin, W. J., Schirger, A., Weed, L. A., *J. Amer. med. Ass.*, 1960, **174**, 347.
180. Houston, T., Murdock, C. R., Symmers, W. St C., Withers, R. J. W., *unpublished observations* (*Belfast*), 1939-41.
181. Lowbeer, L., *Proc. Hillcrest mem. Hosp.* (*Tulsa*), 1949, **6**, 1.
182. Huckstep, R. L., *Typhoid Fever*, page 180. Edinburgh and London, 1962.
182a. Groll, A., Smith, J., *S. Afr. med. J.*, 1965, **39**, 417.
183. Hendrickse, R. G., Collard, P., *Lancet*, 1960, **1**, 80.
183a. Specht, E. E., *Clin. Orthop.*, 1971, **79**, 110.
184. Pott, P., *Remarks on That Kind of Palsy of the Lower Limbs, Which Is Frequently Found to Accompany a Curvature of the Spine*. London, 1779. [Reprinted in: *Med. Classics*, 1936, **1**, 281.]
185. David, J. P., *Dissertation sur les effets du mouvement et du repos dans les maladies chirurgicales*. Paris, 1779.
186. Griffiths, D. L., Seddon, H. J., Roaf, R., *Pott's Paraplegia*. London, 1956.
187. McLean, S., *Amer. J. Dis. Child*, 1931, **41**, 130, 363, 607, 887, 1128, 1411.
188. Schmidt, M. B., *Verh. dtsch. path. Ges.*, 1905, **2**, 223.
189. Virchow, R., *Derm. Z.*, 1896, **3**, 1.
190. Hackett, C. J., *Bone Lesions of Yaws in Uganda*. Oxford, 1951.
191. Baker, R. D., *Human Infection with Fungi, Actinomycetes and Algae*. New York, Heidelberg and Berlin, 1971.
191a. Conant, N. F., Smith, D. T., Baker, R. D., Callaway, J. L., *Manual of Clinical Mycology*, 3rd edn. Philadelphia, London and Toronto, 1971.
192. Symmers, W. St C., *Brit. med. J.*, 1973, **2**, 423.

193. Symmers, W. St C., *personal communication*, 1974.
193a. Cope, V. Z., *J. Bone Jt Surg.*, 1951, **33B**, 205.
194. Destombes, P., Camain, R., Nazimoff, O., *Bull. Soc. Path. exot.*, 1958, **51**, 863.
195. Destombes, P., *Proc. int. Congr. trop. Med. Malar.*, 1959, **4**, 570.
196. Osmond, J. D., Schweitzer, G., Dunbar, J. M., Villet, W., *S. Afr. med. J.*, 1971, **45**, 431.
197. Symmers, W. St C., *Brit. med. J.*, 1973, **4**, 460 [Case 4].
198. Cockshott, W. P., Lucas, A. O., *Quart. J. Med.*, 1964, N.S. **33**, 223.
199. Allcock, E. A., *J. Bone Jt Surg.*, 1961, **43B**, 71.
200. Pankovich, A. M., Jevtic, M. M., *J. Bone Jt Surg.*, 1973, **55A**, 1525.

METABOLIC AND ENDOCRINE DISORDERS
201. Ball, J., in *Recent Advances in Pathology*, edited by C. V. Harrison, 7th edn, chap. 9. London, 1960.
202. Fourman, P., Royer, P., *Calcium Metabolism and the Bone*, 2nd edn. Oxford, 1968.
202a. Rasmussen, H., Bordier, P., *The Physiological and Cellular Basis of Metabolic Bone Disease*. Baltimore, 1974.
203. Follis, R. H., *Deficiency Disease*. Springfield, Ill., 1958.
204. Wolbach, S. B., Howe, R. P., *Arch. Path. Lab. Med.*, 1926, **1**, 1.
205. Wolbach, S. B., *Amer. J. Path.*, 1933, **9**, 689.
206. Boyle, P. E., Wolbach, S. B., Bessey, O. A., *J. dent. Res.*, 1936, **15**, 331.
207. Follis, R. H., *Arch. Path. (Chic.)*, 1943, **35**, 579.
208. Follis, R. H., *Bull. Johns Hopk. Hosp.*, 1951, **89**, 9.
209. Boyle, P. E., Bessey, O. A., Howe, P. R., *Arch. Path. (Chic.)*, 1940, **30**, 90.
210. Park, E. A., *Harvey Lect.*, 1938–39, **34**, 157.
211. Pommer, G., *Untersuchungen über Osteomalacie und Rachitis*. Leipzig, 1885.
212. Howland, J., Kramer, B., *Amer. J. Dis. Child.*, 1921, **22**, 105.
213. Follis, R. H., *Amer. J. Path.*, 1955, **31**, 568.
214. Follis, R. H., *Amer. J. clin. Path.*, 1956, **26**, 400.
215. Crawford, J. D., Gribetz, D., Diner, W. C., Hurst, P., Castleman, B., *Endocrinology*, 1957, **61**, 59.
216. Dodds, G. S., Cameron, H. C., *Amer. J. Anat.*, 1934, **55**, 135.
217. Looser, E., *Zbl. Chir.*, 1920, **47**, 1470.
218. Kind, A., *Schweiz. Z. allg. Path.*, 1947, **10**, 143.
219. Meyer, P. C., *J. Path. Bact.*, 1956, **71**, 325.
220. Sissons, H. A., Aga, V., in *Symposium Ossium*, edited by A. M. Jelliffe and B. Strickland, page 285. Edinburgh and London, 1970.
221. Ball, J., *J. clin. Path.*, 1957, **10**, 281.
222. Ueckert, E., *Stain Technol.*, 1960, **35**, 261.
223. Dent, C. E., *Proc. roy. Soc. Med.*, 1970, **63**, 401.
224. Morgan, D. B., Paterson, C. R., Woods, C. G., Pulvertaft, C. N., Fourman, P., *Lancet*, 1965, **2**, 1085, 1089.
225. Rathbun, J. C., *Amer. J. Dis. Child.*, 1948, **75**, 822.
226. Fraser, D., *Amer. J. Med.*, 1957, **22**, 730.
227. Currarino, G., Neuhauser, E. B., Reyersbach, G. C., Sobel, E. H., *Amer. J. Roentgenol.*, 1957, **78**, 392.
228. Wolbach, S. B., Bessey, O. A., *Physiol. Rev.*, 1942, **22**, 233.
229. Mellanby, E., *A Story of Nutritional Research*. Baltimore, 1950.
230. Wolbach, S. B., Bessey, O. A., *Arch. Path. (Chic.)*, 1941, **32**, 689.

231. Maddock, C. L., Wolbach, S. B., Maddock, W., *J. Nutr.*, 1949, **39**, 117.
232. Fell, H. B., Mellanby, E., *J. Physiol. (Lond.)*, 1952, **116**, 320.
233. Allison, N., Brooks, B., *Surg. Gynec. Obstet.*, 1921, **33**, 250.
234. Sissons, H. A., *J. Bone Jt Surg.*, 1952, **34B**, 275.
235. Weidenreich, F., *Wilhelm Roux' Arch. Entwickl.-Mech. Org.*, 1922, **61**, 436.
236. Geiser, M., Trueta, J., *J. Bone Jt Surg.*, 1958, **40B**, 282.
237. Landry, M., Fleisch, H., *J. Bone Jt Surg.*, 1964, **46B**, 764.
238. Sudeck, P., *Arch. klin. Chir.*, 1900, **62**, 147.
239. Whedon, G. D., in *Bone as a Tissue*, edited by K. Rodahl, J. T. Nicholson and E. M. Brown, chap. 4. New York, 1960.
240. Albright, F., Burnett, C. H., Cope, O., Parson, W., *J. clin. Endocr.*, 1941, **1**, 711.
241. Reifenstein, E. C., Albright, F., *New Engl. J. Med.*, 1944, **231**, 343.
242. Lutwak, L., Whedon, G. D., Lachance, R. A., Reid, J. M., Lipscomb, H. S., *J. clin. Endocr.*, 1969, **29**, 1140.
243. Cooke, A. M., *Lancet*, 1955, **1**, 877, 929.
244. Barzel, U. S., *Osteoporosis*. New York, 1970.
245. Dequeker, J., *Bone Loss in Normal and Pathological Conditions*. Leuven, 1972.
246. Albright, F., Bloomberg, E., Smith, P. H., *Trans. Ass. Amer. Phycns*, 1940, **55**, 298.
247. Albright, F., *Harvey Lect.*, 1943, **38**, 123.
248. Reifenstein, E. C., *Clin. Orthop.*, 1957, **10**, 206.
249. Nordin, B. E. C., in *Bone as a Tissue*, edited by K. Rodahl, J. T. Nicholson and E. M. Brown, chap. 3. New York, 1960.
250. Nordin, B. E. C., *Clin. Orthop.*, 1960, **17**, 235.
251. Sissons, H. A., Holley, K. J., Heighway, J., in *L'Ostéomalacie*, edited by D. J. Hioco, page 19. Paris, 1967.
252. Exton-Smith, A. N., Millard, P. H., Payne, P. R., Wheeler, E. F., *Lancet*, 1969, **2**, 1154.
253. Goldsmith, N. F., Johnston, J. O., Picetti, G., Garcia, C., *J. Bone Jt Surg.*, 1973, **55A**, 1276.
254. Buhr, A. J., Cooke, A. M., *Lancet*, 1959, **1**, 531.
255. Heaney, R. P., Whedon, G. D., *J. clin. Endocr.*, 1958, **18**, 1246.
256. Jowsey, J., *Clin. Orthop.*, 1960, **17**, 210.
257. Cushing, H., *Bull. Johns Hopk. Hosp.*, 1932, **50**, 137.
258. De Martini, F. Groboest, A. W., Ragan, C., *J. Amer. med. Ass.*, 1952, **149**, 750.
259. Teicher, R., Nelson, R., *J. invest. Derm.*, 1952, **19**, 205.
260. Curtiss, P. H., Clark, W. S., Herndon, C. H., *J. Amer. med. Ass.*, 1954, **156**, 467.
261. Sissons, H. A., in *Bone as a Tissue*, edited by K. Rodahl, J. T. Nicholson, and E. M. Brown, chap. 1. New York, 1960.
262. Follis, R. H., *Proc. Soc. exp. Biol. (N.Y.)*, 1951, **76**, 722.
263. Sissons, H. A., Hadfield, G. J., *J. Anat. (Lond.)*, 1955, **89**, 69.
264. Blunt, J. W., Plotz, C. M., Lattes, R., Howes, E. L., Meyer, K., Ragan, G., *Proc. Soc. exp. Biol. (N.Y.)*, 1950, **73**, 678.
265. Sissons, H. A., Hadfield, G. J., *Brit. J. Surg.*, 1951–52, **39**, 172.
266. Storey, E., *J. Bone Jt Surg.*, 1958, **40B**, 558.
266a. Frankcom, G., Musgrave, J. H., *The Irish Giant*. London, 1976.
267. Keith, A., *Lancet*, 1911, **1**, 993.
268. Erdheim, J., *Virchows Arch. path. Anat.*, 1931, **281**, 197.

269. Waine, H., Bennett, G. A., Bauer, W., *Amer. J. med. Sci.*, 1945, **209**, 671.

270. Erdheim, J., *Beitr. path. Anat.*, 1916, **62**, 302.

271. Askanazy, M., Rutishauser, E., *Virchows Arch. path. Anat.*, 1933, **291**, 653.

272. Martos, J., *Beitr. path. Anat.*, 1938, **100**, 293.

273. Follis, R. H., *Bull. Johns Hopk. Hosp.*, 1953, **92**, 405.

274. Wilkins, L., *Amer. J. Dis. Child.*, 1941, **61**, 13.

275. Looser, E., *Verh. dtsch. path. Ges.*, 1929, **24**, 352.

276. Simpson, S., *Quart. J. exp. Physiol.*, 1924, **14**, 161.

277. Ray, R. D., Simpson, M. E., Li, C. H., Asling, C. W., Evans, H. M., *Amer. J. Anat.*, 1950, **86**, 479.

278. Lusted, L. B., Pickering, D. E., Fisher, D., Smyth, F. S., *Amer. J. Dis. Child.*, 1953, **86**, 426.

279. Silberberg, M., Silberberg, R., *Arch. Path.* (*Chic.*), 1943, **36**, 512.

280. Becks, H., Scow, R. O., Simpson, M. E., Asling, C. W., Li, C. H., Evans, H. M., *Anat. Rec.*, 1950, **197**, 299.

281. Albright, F., Reifenstein, E. C., Jr, *The Parathyroid Glands and Metabolic Bone Disease.* Baltimore, 1948.

282. Hunter, D., Turnbull, H. M., *Brit. J. Surg.*, 1931–32, **19**, 203.

283. Jaffe, H. L., *Arch. Path.* (*Chic.*), 1933, **16**, 63, 236.

284. Erdheim, J., *S.-B. Akad. Wiss. Wien, math.-nat. Kl.*, 1907, **116**, 311.

285. Erdheim J., *Denkschr. Akad. Wiss. Wien*, 1914, **30**, 363.

286. Liu, S. H., Ch'in, K. Y., Chu, H. I., Pai, H. C., *Chin. med. J.*, 1940, **58**, 141.

287. Ham, A. W., Littner, N., Drake, T. G. H., Robertson, E. C., Tisdall, F. E., *Amer. J. Path.*, 1940, **16**, 277.

287a. Barnicot, N. A., *J. Anat.* (*Lond.*), 1948, **82**, 233.

287b. Chang, H., *Anat. Rec.*, 1951, **111**, 23.

287c. Gaillard, P. J., in *The Parathyroids*, edited by R. O. Greep and R. V. Talmage, page 20. Springfield, Ill., 1961.

287d. Raisz, L. G., *Fed. Proc.*, 1962, **21**, 207.

288. Recklinghausen, F. von, in *Festschrift, Rudolf Virchow.* Berlin, 1891.

288a. Engel, G., *Ueber einen Fall von cystoider Entartung des ganzen Skelettes.* Giessen, 1864.

289. Erdheim, J., *Mitt. Grenzgeb. Med. Chir.*, 1906, **16**, 632.

290. Mandl, F., *Arch. klin. Chir.*, 1926, **143**, 245.

291. Pugh, D. G., *Amer. J. Roentgenol.*, 1951, **66**, 577.

292. Albright, F., Reifenstein, E. C., Jr, *The Parathyroid Glands and Metabolic Bone Disease*, page 57. Baltimore, 1948.

293. Byers, P. D., Smith, R., *Quart. J. Med.*, 1971, N.S. **40**, 471.

294. Jaffe, H. L., Bodansky, A., *J. exp. Med.*, 1930, **52**, 669.

294a. Bodansky, A., Jaffe, H. L., *J. exp. Med.*, 1931, **53**, 591.

295. Bronsky, D., Kushner, D. S., Dubin, A., Snapper, I., *Medicine* (*Baltimore*), 1958, **37**, 317.

296. Emerson, K., Walsh, F. B., Howard, J. E., *Ann. intern. Med.*, 1941, **14**, 1256.

297. Ginzler, A. M., Jaffe, H. L., *Amer. J. Path.*, 1941, **17**, 293.

298. Follis, R. H., Jackson, D. A., *Bull. Johns Hopk. Hosp.*, 1943, **72**, 232.

299. Gilmour, J. R., *The Parathyroid Glands and Skeleton in Renal Disease.* London, 1947.

300. Ellis, H. A., Peart, K. M., *J. clin. Path.*, 1973, **26**, 83.

301. Stanbury, S. W., *Brit. med. Bull.*, 1957, **13**, 57.

302. Pappenheimer, A. M., Wilens, S. L., *Amer. J. Path.*, 1935, **11**, 73.

303. Gilmour, J. B., Martin, W. J., *J. Path. Bact.*, 1937, **44**, 431.

304. Castleman, B., Mallory, T. B., *Amer. J. Path.*, 1937, **13**, 553.

305. Mach, R. S., Rutishauser, E., *Helv. med. Acta*, 1937, **4**, 423.

306. Claireaux, A. E., *J. Path. Bact.*, 1953, **65**, 291.

307. Herbert, F. K., Miller, H. G., Richardson, G. O., *J. Path. Bact.*, 1941, **53**, 161.

308. Dent, C. E., *J. Bone Jt Surg.*, 1952, **34B**, 266.

309. Winters, R. W., Graham, J. B., Williams, T. F., McFalls, V. W., Burnett, C. H., *Medicine* (*Baltimore*), 1958, **37**, 97.

310. Dent, C. E., Harris, H., *J. Bone Jt Surg.*, 1956, **38B**, 204.

311. De Toni, G., *Acta paediat.* (*Uppsala*), 1933, **16**, 479.

311a. Fanconi, G., *Helv. paediat. Acta*, 1946, **1**, 183.

311b Debré, R., Marie, J., Cléret, F., Messimy, *Arch. Méd. Enf.*, 1934, **37**, 597.

312. Darmady, E. M., Stranack, F., *Brit. med. Bull.*, 1957, **13**, 21.

313. Barr, H. S., Bickel, H., *Acta paediat.* (*Uppsala*), 1952, **42**, suppl. 90, 71.

313a. Dent, C. E., Stamp, T. C. B., *Quart. J. Med.*, 1971, N.S. **40**, 303.

313b. Wyman, A. L., Paradinas, F. J., Daly, J. R., *J. clin. Path.*, 1977, **30**, 328.

313c. Hosking, D. J., Chamberlain, M. J., Shortland-Webb, W. R., *Brit. J. Radiol.*, 1975, **48**, 451.

PAGET'S DISEASE OF BONE

314. Sissons, H. A., in *Bones and Joints*, edited by L. V. Ackerman, H. J. Spjut and M. R. Abell, chap. 10. Baltimore, 1976.

314a. Paget, J., *Med.-chir. Trans.*, 1877, **60**, 37.

315. Schmorl, G., *Virchows Arch. path. Anat.*, 1932, **283**, 694.

316. Jaffe, H. L., *Arch. Path.* (*Chic.*), 1933, **15**, 83.

317. Collins, D. H., *Lancet*, 1956, **2**, 51.

318. Choremis, C., Yannakos, D., Papadatos, C., Baroutsou, E., *Helv. paediat. Acta*, 1958, **13**, 185.

319. Fanconi, G., Moreira, G., Uehlinger, E., Giedon, A., *Helv. paediat. Acta*, 1964, **19**, 279.

320. Stemmermann, G. N., *Amer. J. Path.*, 1966, **48**, 641.

321. Woodhouse, N. J. Y., Fisher, M. T., Sigurdsson, G., Joplin, G. F., MacIntyre, I., *Brit. med. J.*, 1972, **4**, 267.

321a. Barker, D. J. P., Clough, P. W. L., Guyer, P. B., Gardner, M. J., *Brit. med. J.*, 1977, **2**, 1181.

321b. Luxton, R. W., *Lancet*, 1957, **1**, 441.

322. Schüller, H., *Brit. J. Radiol.*, 1926, **31**, 156.

323. Collins, D. H., Winn, J. M., *J. Path. Bact.*, 1955, **69**, 1.

324. Wycis, H. T., *J. Neurosurg.*, 1944, **1**, 299.

325. Edholm, O. G., Howarth, S., McMichael, J., *Clin. Sci.*, 1945, **5**, 249.

326. Storsteen, K. A., Janes, J. M., *J. Amer. med. Ass.*, 1954, **154**, 472.

327. Edholm, O. G., Howarth, S., *Clin. Sci.*, 1953, **12**, 277.

328. Sornberger, C. F., Smedal, M. I., *Circulation*, 1952, **6**, 711.

329. Howarth, S., *Clin. Sci.*, 1953, **12**, 271.

330. Heaney, R. P., Whedon, G. D., *J. clin. Endocr.*, 1958, **18**, 1246.

331. Bauer, G. C. H., Wendeberg, B., *J. Bone Jt Surg.*, 1959, **41B**, 558.

332. Deuxchaisnes, C. N. de, Krane, S. M., *Medicine* (*Baltimore*), 1964, **43**, 558.

333. Woodhouse, N. J. Y., *Clin. Endocr. Metab.*, 1972, **1**, 125.

334. Sissons, H. A., *Clin. Orthop.*, 1966, **45**, 73.

335. Jaffe, H. L., Selin, G., *Bull. N.Y. Acad. Med.*, 1951, **27**, 165.
336. Summey, T. J., Pressly, C. L., *Ann. Surg.*, 1946, **123**, 135.
337. Price, C. H. G., Goldie, W., *J. Bone Jt Surg.*, 1969, **51B**, 205.
338. Sissons, H. A., in *Cancer*, edited by R. W. Raven, vol. 2, chap. 17. London, 1958.

FIBROUS DYSPLASIA OF BONE

339. Lichtenstein, L., Jaffe, H. L., *Arch. Path. (Chic.)*, 1942, **33**, 777.
340. Pritchard, J. E., *Amer. J. med. Sci.*, 1951, **222**, 313.
341. Jaffe, H. L., *Tumors and Tumorous Conditions of the Bones and Joints*, page 117. Philadelphia, 1958.
342. Albright, F., Butler, A. M., Hampton, A. O., Smith, P., *New Engl. J. Med.*, 1937, **216**, 727.
343. Falconer, M. A., Cope, C. L., Robb-Smith, A. H. T., *Quart. J. Med.*, 1942, N.S. **11**, 121.
344. Hunter, D., Turnbull, H. M., *Brit. J. Surg.*, 1931–32, **19**, 203.
345. Lichtenstein, L., *Arch. Surg. (Chic.)*, 1938, **36**, 874.
346. Sissons, H. A., in *Cancer*, edited by R. W. Raven, vol. 2, chap. 17. London, 1958.
347. Phemister, D. B., Grimson, K. S., *Ann. Surg.*, 1937, **105**, 564.
348. Pugh, D. G., *Radiology*, 1945, **44**, 1945.

MISCELLANEOUS CONDITIONS

349. Jaffe, H. L., Lichtenstein, L., *Arch. Surg. (Chic.)*, 1942, **44**, 1004.
350. Woods, C. G., *J. Bone Jt Surg.*, 1961, **43B**, 758.
351. Sim, F. H., Dahlin, D. C., *Mayo Clin. Proc.*, 1974, **46**, 484.
352. Kambolis, C., Bullough, P. G., Jaffe, H. L., *J. Bone Jt Surg.*, 1973, **55A**, 496.
353. Thannhauser, S. J., *Lipidoses—Diseases of the Cellular Lipid Metabolism*, 3rd edn. New York, 1958.
354. Todd, R. McL., Keidan, S. E., *J. Bone Jt Surg.*, 1952, **34B**, 447.
355. Amstutz, H. C., Carey, E. J., *J. Bone Jt Surg.*, 1966, **48A**, 670.
356. Crocker, A. C., Farber, S., *Medicine (Baltimore)*, 1958, **37**, 1.
357. Holm, J. E., Teilum, G., Christensen, E., *Acta med. scand.*, 1944, **118**, 292.
358. Green, W. T., Farber, S., *J. Bone Jt Surg.*, 1942, **24**, 499.
359. Jaffe, H. L., Lichtenstein, L., *Arch. Path. (Chic.)*, 1944, **37**, 99.
360. Lichtenstein, L., *J. Bone Jt Surg.*, 1964, **46A**, 76.
361. Schajowicz, F., Slullitel, J., *J. Bone Jt Surg.*, 1973, **55B**, 545.
362. Grinnau, A. G., *Amer. J. Roentgenol.*, 1935, **34**, 297.
363. Caffey, J., *Amer. J. Roentgenol.*, 1937, **37**, 293.
364. Moseley, J. E., Manly, J. B., *Radiology*, 1953, **60**, 656.
365. Reich, R. S., Rosenberg, N. J., *J. Bone Jt Surg.*, 1953, **35A**, 894.
365a. Cockshott, P., in *Abnormal Haemoglobins in Africa*, edited by J. H. P. Jonxis, page 131. Oxford and Edinburgh, 1965.
366. Diggs, L. W., Pulliam, H. N., King, J. C., *Sth. med. J. (Bgham, Ala.)*, 1937, **30**, 249.
367. Sherman, M., *Sth. med. J. (Bgham, Ala.)*, 1959, **52**, 632.
368. Chung. S. M. K., Ralston, E. L., *J. Bone Jt Surg.*, 1969, **51A**, 33.

368a. Specht, E. E., *Clin. Orthop.*, 1971, **79**, 110.

TUMOURS OF BONE

369. Schajowicz, F., Ackerman, L. V., Sissons, H. A., Sobin, L. H., Torloni, H., *Histological Typing of Bone Tumours*. Geneva, 1972.
370. Jaffe, H. L., *Tumors and Tumorous Conditions of the Bones and Joints*. Philadelphia, 1958.
371. Dahlin, D. C., *Bone Tumors*, 2nd edn. Springfield, Illinois, 1967.
372. Spjut, H. J., Dorfman, H. D., Fechner, R. E., Ackerman, L. V., *Tumors of Bone and Cartilage* (Atlas of Tumor Pathology, 2nd series, fasc. 5). Washington, D.C., 1971.
373. Lichtenstein, L., *Bone Tumors*, 4th edn. St Louis, 1972.
374. Sissons, H. A., Duthie, R. B., in *Surgical Progress*, edited by E. Rock Carling and J. Paterson Ross, page 158. London, 1959.
375. Mackenzie, A., Doll, R., Court Brown, W. M., Sissons, H. A., *Brit. med. J.*, 1961, **1**, 1782.
376. Soehner, R. L., Dmochowski, L., *Nature (Lond.)*, 1969, **224**, 191.
377. Finkel, M. P., Reilly, C. A., Biskis, B. O., Greco, I. L., in *Bone—Certain Aspects of Neoplasia*, edited by C. H. G. Price and F. G. M. Ross, page 353. London, 1973.
378. Jaffe, H. L., *Arch. Surg. (Chic.)*, 1935, **31**, 709.
379. Lichtenstein, L., *Cancer (Philad.)*, 1956, **9**, 1044.
380. Jaffe, H. L., *Bull. Hosp. Jt Dis. (N.Y.)*, 1956, **17**, 141.
381. Dahlin, D. C., Johnson, E. W., *J. Bone Jt Surg.*, 1954, **36A**, 559.
382. Byers, P. D., *Cancer (Philad.)*, 1968, **22**, 43.
383. Schajowicz, F., Lemos, C., *Acta orthop. scand.*, 1970, **41**, 272.
384. Schajowicz, F., Gallardo, H., *J. Bone Jt Surg.*, 1970, **52B**, 205.
385. Ewing, J., *The Classification and Treatment of Bone Sarcoma*, in *Report of the International Conference on Cancer, London, 1928*, page 365. Bristol and London, 1928.
386. Codman, E. A., *Surg. Gynec. Obstet.*, 1931, **52**, 543.
387. Jaffe, H. L., Lichtenstein, L., *Amer. J. Path.*, 1942, **18**, 969.
388. Kahn, L. B., Wood, F. M., Ackerman, L. V., *Arch. Path.*, 1969, **88**, 371.
389. Riddell, R. J., Louis, C. J., Bromberger, N. A., *J. Bone Jt Surg.*, 1973, **55B**, 848.
390. Hatcher, C. H., Campbell, J. C., *Bull. Hosp. Jt Dis. (N.Y.)*, 1951, **12**, 411.
391. Dahlin, D. C., *Cancer (Philad.)*, 1956, **9**, 195.
392. Geschickter, C. F., Copeland, M. M., *Tumors of Bone*, 3rd edn, page 164. Philadelphia, 1949.
393. Jaffe, H. L., Lichtenstein, L., *Arch. Path. (Chic.)*, 1948, **45**, 541.
394. Schajowicz, F., Gallardo, H., *J. Bone Jt Surg.*, 1971, **53B**, 198.
395. Jaffe, H. L., Lichtenstein, L., *Amer. J. Path.*, 1942, **18**, 205.
396. Jaffe, H. L., *Tumors and Tumorous Conditions of the Bones and Joints*, page 83. Philadelphia, 1958.
397. Campbell, C. J., Harkness, J., *Surg. Gynec. Obstet.*, 1957, **104**, 392.
398. Jaffe, H. L., *Tumors and Tumorous Conditions of the Bones and Joints*, page 298. Philadelphia, 1958.
399. Rabhan, W. N., Rosai, J., *J. Bone Jt Surg.*, 1968, **50A**, 487.

400. Nilsonne, V., Göthlin, G., *Acta orthop. scand.*, 1969, **40**, 205.

401. Lattes, R., Bull, D. C., *Ann. Surg.*, 1948, **127**, 187.

402. Siegel, M. W., *Amer. J. Orthop.*, 1967, **9**, 68.

403. Junghanns, H., *Arch. klin. Chir.*, 1932, **169**, 204.

404. Perman, E., *Acta chir. scand.*, 1926, **61**, 91.

405. Macrycostas, K., *Virchows Arch. path. Anat.*, 1927, **265**, 259.

406. Ritchie, G., Zeier, F. G., *J. Bone Jt Surg.*, 1956, **38A**, 115.

407. Bickel, W. H., Broders, A. C., *J. Bone Jt Surg.*, 1947, **29**, 517.

408. Harris, R., Prandoni, A. G., *Ann. intern. Med.*, 1950, **33**, 1302.

409. Cohen, J., Craig, J. M., *J. Bone Jt Surg.*, 1955, **37A**, 585.

410. Besse, B. E., Dahlin, D. C., Bruwer, A., Svien, H. J., Ghormley, R. K., *Proc. Mayo Clin.*, 1953, **28**, 249.

411. Thompson, P. C., *J. Bone Jt Surg.*, 1954, **36A**, 281.

412. Barnes, R., *J. Bone Jt Surg.*, 1956, **38B**, 301.

413. Jaffe, H. L., *Bull. Hosp. Jt Dis. (N.Y.)*, 1950, **11**, 3.

414. Lichtenstein, L., *Cancer (Philad.)*, 1950, **3**, 279.

415. Hadders, H. N., Oterdoom, H. J., *J. Path. Bact.*, 1956, **71**, 193.

416. Biesecker, J. L., Marcove, R. C., Huvos, A. G., Mike, V., *Cancer (Philad.)*, 1970, **26**, 615.

417. Tillman, B. P., Dahlin, D. C., Lipscomb, P. R., Stewart, J. R., *Mayo Clin. Proc.*, 1968, **43**, 478.

418. Gorham, L. W., Stout, A. P., *J. Bone Jt Surg.*, 1955, **37A**, 985.

418a. Gorham, L. W., Wright, A. W., Shultz, H. H., Maxon, F. C., Jr, *Amer. J. Med.*, 1954, **17**, 674.

418b. [Jackson, J. B. S.] *Boston med. surg. J.*, 1838, **18**, 368.

419. Child, P. L., *Amer. J. clin. Path.*, 1955, **25**, 1050.

420. Smith, W. E., Fienberg, R., *Cancer (Philad.)*, 1957, **10**, 1151.

421. Peers, J. H., *Amer. J. Path.*, 1934, **10**, 811.

422. Gross, P., Bailey, F. R., Jacox, H. W., *Arch. Path. (Chic.)*, 1939, **28**, 716.

423. De Santo, D. A., Burgess, E., *Surg. Gynec. Obstet.*, 1940, **71**, 454.

424. Holt, J. F., Wright, E. M., *Radiology*, 1948, **51**, 647.

424a. Dahlin, D. C., Coventry, M. B., *J. Bone Jt Surg.*, 1967, **49A**, 101.

425. Jeffree, G. M., Price, C. H. G., *J. Bone Jt Surg.*, 1965, **47B**, 120.

426. Coley, B. L., Sharp, G. S., Ellis, E. B., *Amer. J. Surg.*, 1931, **13**, 215.

427. Ottolenghi, C. E., *J. Bone Jt Surg.*, 1955, **37A**, 443.

428. Schajowicz, F., *J. Bone Jt. Surg.*, 1955, **37A**, 465.

428a. Sweetnam, R., Knowelden, J., Seddon, H., *Brit. med. J.*, 1971, **2**, 363.

428b. Jeffree, G. M., Price, C. H. G., Sissons, H. A., *Brit. J. Cancer*, 1975, **32**, 87.

428c. Geschickter, C. F., Copeland, M. M., *Ann. Surg.*, 1951, **14**, 790.

428d. Jaffe, H. L., Selin, G., *Bull. N.Y. Acad. Med.*, 1951, **27**, 165.

429. Lichtenstein, L., Jaffe, H. L., *Amer. J. Path.*, 1943, **19**, 553.

429a. Barnes, R., Catto, M., *J. Bone Jt Surg.*, 1966, **48B**, 729.

430. Coley, B. L., Higinbotham, N. L., *Ann. Surg.*, 1954, **139**, 547.

431. O'Neal, L. W., Ackerman, L. V., *Cancer (Philad.)*, 1952, **5**, 551.

432. Thomson, A. D., Turner-Warwick, R. T., *J. Bone Jt Surg.*, 1955, **37B**, 266.

433. Henderson, E. D., Dahlin, D. C., *J. Bone Jt Surg.*, 1963, **45A**, 1450.

434. Lichtenstein, L., Bernstein, D., *Cancer (Philad.)*, 1959, **12**, 1142.

435. Dahlin, D. C., Henderson, E. D., *Cancer (Philad.)*, 1962, **15**, 410.

436. Dahlin, D. C., Ivins, J. C., *Cancer (Philad.)*, 1969, **23**, 35.

437. Eyre-Brook, A. L., Price, C. H. G., *J. Bone Jt Surg.*, 1969, **51B**, 20.

438. Spanier, S. S., Enneking, W. F., Enriquez, P., *Cancer (Philad.)*, 1975, **36**, 2084.

439. Jaffe, H. L., Lichtenstein, L., Portis, R. B., *Arch. Path. (Chic.)*, 1940, **30**, 993.

440. Jaffe, H. L., *Ann. roy. Coll. Surg. Engl.*, 1953, **13**, 343.

441. Hutter, R. V. P., Worcester, J. N., Francis, K. C., Foote, F. W., Stewart, F. W., *Cancer (Philad.)*, 1962, **15**, 653.

442. Dahlin, D. C., Cupps, R. E., Johnson, E. W., *Cancer (Philad.)*, 1970, **25**, 1061.

443. Schajowicz, F., *J. Bone Jt Surg.*, 1961, **43A**, 1.

444. Jaffe, H. L., *Oral Surg.*, 1953, **6**, 159.

445. Jewell, J. H., Bush, L. F., *J. Bone Jt Surg.*, 1964, **46A**, 848.

446. Pan, P., Dahlin, D. C., Lipscomb, P. R., Bernatz, P. E., *Mayo Clin. Proc.*, 1964, **39**, 344.

447. Ewing, J., *Proc. N.Y. path. Soc.*, 1921, **21**, 17, 24, 93.

448. Foote, F. W., Anderson, H. R., *Amer. J. Path.*, 1941, **17**, 497.

449. Stout, A. P., *Amer. J. Roentgenol.*, 1943, **50**, 334.

450. Dahlin, D. C., Coventry, M. B., Scanlon, P. W., *J. Bone Jt Surg.*, 1961, **43A**, 185.

451. Marsden, H. B., Steward, J. K., *J. clin. Path.*, 1964, **17**, 411.

452. Schajowicz, F., *J. Bone Jt Surg.*, 1959, **41A**, 349.

453. Willis, R. A., *Amer. J. Path.*, 1940, **16**, 317.

454. Jaffe, H. L., Lichtenstein, L., *Arch. Path. (Chic.)*, 1947, **44**, 207.

455. Lumb, G., *Ann. roy. Coll. Surg. Engl.*, 1952, **10**, 241.

456. Snapper, I., Turner, L. B., Moscovitz, H. L., *Multiple Myeloma*. New York, 1953.

457. Christopherson, W. M., Miller, A. J., *Cancer (Philad.)*, 1950, **3**, 240.

458. Stewart, M. J., Taylor, A. L., *J. Path. Bact.*, 1932, **35**, 541.

459. Rutishauser, E., *Zbl. allg. Path. path. Anat.*, 1933, **58**, 355.

460. Raven, R. W., Willis, R. A., *J. Bone Jt Surg.*, 1949, **31B**, 369.

461. Lumb, G., *Brit. J. Surg.*, 1948–49, **36**, 16.

462. Wright, C. J., *J. Bone Jt Surg.*, 1961, **43B**, 767.

463. Lowenhaupt, E., *Amer. J. Path.*, 1945, **21**, 171.

464. Churg, J., Gordon, A. J., *Arch. Path. (Chic.)*, 1942, **34**, 546.

465. Patek, A. J., Castle, W. B., *Amer. J. med. Sci.*, 1936, **191**, 788.

466. Rundles, R. W., Cooper, G. R., Willett, R., *J. clin. Invest.*, 1951, **30**, 1125.

467. Martin, N. H., *J. clin. Invest.*, 1947, **26**, 1189.

468. Miller, G. L., Brown, C. E., Miller, E. E., Eitelman, E. S., *Cancer Res.*, 1952, **12**, 716.

469. Bayrd, E. D., Bennett, W. A., *Med. Clin. N. Amer.*, 1950, **34**, 1151.

470. Jaffe, H. L., *Tumors and Tumorous Conditions of the Bones and Joints*, page 396. Philadelphia, 1958.

471. Thomas, L. B., Forkner, C. E., Frei, E., Besse, B. E., Stabenam, J. R., *Cancer (Philad.)*, 1961, **14**, 608.

472. Chabner, B. A., Haskell, C. M., Canellos, G. P., *Medicine (Baltimore)*, 1969, **48**, 401.

473. Parker, F., Jackson, H., *Surg. Gynec. Obstet.*, 1939, **68**, 45.

474. McCormack, L. J., Ivins, J. C., Dahlin, D. C., Johnson, E. W., *Cancer (Philad.)*, 1952, **5**, 1182.

475. Francis, K. C., Higinbotham, N. L., Coley, B. L., *Surg. Gynec. Obstet.*, 1954, **99**, 142.

476. Dahlin, D. C., McCarty, C. S., *Cancer (Philad.)*, 1952, **5**, 1170.

477. Willis, R. A., *The Pathology of Tumours*, 4th edn, page 937. London, 1967.

478. Sissons, H. A., in *Modern Trends in Diseases of the Vertebral Column*, edited by J. R. Nassim and H. J. Burrows, page 198. London, 1959.

479. Jaffe, H. L., *Tumors and Tumorous Conditions of the Bones and Joints*, page 451. Philadelphia, 1958.

480. Higinbotham, N. L., Phillips, R. F., Hollon, F. W., Hustu, H. O., *Cancer (Philad.).*, 1967, **20**, 1841.

481. Littman, L., *Ann. Surg.*, 1953, **137**, 80.

482. Chalmers, J., Coulson, W. F., *J Bone Jt Surg.*, 1960, **42B**, 556.

483. Baker, P. L., Dockerty, M. B., Coventry, M. B., *J. Bone Jt Surg.*, 1954, **36A**, 704.

484. Desaive, P., *Bull. Acad. roy. Méd. Belg.*, 1955, **20**, 105.

485. Moon, N. F., *Clin. Orthop.*, 1965, **43**, 189.

486. Rosai, J., *Amer. J. clin. Path.*, 1969, **51**, 786.

487. Fischer, B., *Frankfurt. Z. Path.*, 1913, **12**, 422.

488. Ryrie, B. J., *Brit. med. J.*, 1932, **2**, 1000.

489. Willis, R. A., *The Pathology of Tumours*, 4th edn, page 288. London, 1967.

490. Hicks, J. D., *J. Path. Bact.*, 1954, **67**, 151.

491. Lederer, H., Sinclair, A. J., *J. Path. Bact.*, 1954, **67**, 163.

492. Changus, G. W., Speed, J. S., Stewart, F. W., *Cancer (Philad.)*, 1957, **10**, 540.

493. Cohen, D. M., Dahlin, D. C., Pugh, D. G., *Cancer (Philad.)*, 1962, **15**, 515.

494. Jaffe, H. L., *Tumors and Tumorous Conditions of the Bones and Joints*, page 341. Philadelphia, 1958.

495. Otis, J., Hutter, R. V. P., Foote F. W., Marcove, R. C., Stewart, F. W., *Surg. Gynec. Obstet.*, 1968, **127**, 295.

495a. Unni, K. K., Ivins, J. C., Beabout, J. W., Dahlin, D. C., *Cancer (Philad.)*, 1971, **27**, 1403.

495b. Keen, P., in *Symposium on Kaposi's Sarcoma*, edited by L. V. Ackerman and J. F. Murray, pages 67–74 [page 69]. Basel and New York, 1963.

496. Catto, M., Stevens, J., *J. Path. Bact.*, 1963, **96**, 248.

497. Goldman, R. L., *Amer. J. clin. Path.*, 1964, **42**, 503.

498. Ross, O. F., Hadfield, G., *J. Bone Jt Surg.*, 1968, **50B**, 639.

499. Schajowicz, F., Cuevillas, A. R., Silberman, F. S., *Cancer (Philad.)*, 1966, **19**, 1423.

500. Symmers, W. St C., Nangle, E. J., *J. Path. Bact.*, 1951, **63**, 417.

501. Willis, R. A., *The Spread of Tumours in the Human Body*, 3rd edn, Chap. 24. London, 1973.

501a. Willis, R. A., *The Spread of Tumours in the Human Body*, 3rd edn, appendix [page 297]. London, 1973.

502. Abrams, H. L., *Radiology*, 1950, **55**, 534.

502a. Drury, R. A. B., Palmer, P. H., Highman, W. J., *J. clin. Path.*, 1964, **17**, 448.

503. Batson, O. V., *Ann. Surg.*, 1940, **112**, 138.

504. Milch, R. A., Changus, G. W., *Cancer (Philad.)*, 1956, **3**, 340.

505. Shackman, R., Harrison, C. V., *Brit. J. Surg.*, 1947–48, **35**, 385.

ACKNOWLEDGEMENTS FOR ILLUSTRATIONS

Figs 37.14, 48. Pathology Museum, University College Hospital Medical School, London; reproduced by permission of the Curator, Mr W. R. Merrington.

Figs 37.15, 37, 90. Pathology Museum, Royal Free Hospital Medical School, London; reproduced by permission of Professor G. B. D. Scott.

Figs 37.17A, 17B, 29A, 29B, 31B, 46A, 46B, 61A, 61B, 65A, 65B, 67A, 67B, 67C, 77A, 77B, 77C, 77D, 86A, 86B, 86C, 89A, 89B, 92A, 92B, 94A, 94B, 96A, 96B, 97A, 97B. Wellcome Museum, Institute of Orthopaedics, London.

Figs 37.19, 33. Pathology Museum, St Mary's Hospital Medical School, London; reproduced by permission of Professor K. A. Porter.

Figs 37.20, 21. Reproduced by permission of the editor of the journal from: Sissons, H. A., *J. Bone Jt Surg.*, 1956, **38B**, 418.

Fig. 37.30. Pathology Museum, King's College Hospital Medical School, London; reproduced by permission of Professor E. A. Wright.

Fig. 37.31A. Pathology Museum, St Bartholomew's Hospital Medical College, London; reproduced by permission of Professor W. G. Spector.

Figs 37.32, 72, 78, 99. Museum of London Hospital Medical College; reproduced by permission of the Curator, Mr E. C. B. Butler.

Figs 37.35A, 35B. Photograph and radiograph provided by Mr J. K. Oyston, Royal Halifax Infirmary, Halifax, Yorkshire; reproduced by permission of the editors from: Oyston, J. K., *J. Bone Jt Surg.*, 1961, **43B**, 259, *and* Symmers, W. St C., *Nurs. Mirror*, 1963 (Dec. 6), **117**, x.

Figs 37.35C, 35D. Specimen presented to the Pathology Museum, Charing Cross Hospital Medical School, London, by Professor G. D. Pegrum, Charing Cross Hospital Medical School, and Mr J. K. Oyston, Royal Halifax Infirmary, Halifax, Yorkshire; reproduced by permission of the Curator, Dr F. J. Paradinas, Photographs by Miss P, M. Turnbull, Charing Cross Hospital Medical School; Fig. 37.35C reproduced by permission of the editor from: Symmers, W. St C., *Nurs. Mirror*, 1963 (Dec. 6), **117**, x.

Figs 37.35E, 35F, 35G. Photomicrographs provided by W. St C. Symmers.

Fig. 37.36. Pathology Museum, St Thomas's Hospital Medical School, London; reproduced by permission of Professor H. Spencer.

Figs 37.43A, 43B. Reproduced by permission of the editor of the journal from: Sissons, H. A., *J. Bone Jt Surg.*, 1952, **34B**, 275.

Figs 37.47A, 47B. Reproduced by permission of the editors, Dr K. Rodahl, Dr J. R. Nicholson and Dr E. M. Brown, and publishers, Messrs McGraw-Hill, from: Sissons, H. A., in *Bone as a Tissue*, chap. 1; New York, 1960.

Fig. 37.60. Pathology Museum, Royal Postgraduate Medical School, London; reproduced by permission of Professor K. Weinbren.

Fig. 37.82. Pathology Museum, University of Cambridge; reproduced by permission of the Curator, Dr S. Thirunavuk-karasu, and Professor P. Wildy.

Figs 37.84A, 84B. Pathology Museum, University of Manchester Medical School; reproduced by permission of the Curator, Dr J. Davson.

Figs 37.85A, 85B, 85C. Reproduced by permission of the author, and of the editor of the journal, from: Barnes, R., *J. Bone Jt Surg.*, 1956, **38B**, 301.

Figs 37.88A, 89A, 89B, 91A, 91B, 92A, 92B, 92C, 92D. Reproduced by permission of the editor, Mr R. W. Raven, and publishers, Messrs Butterworth and Company, from: Sissons, H. A., in *Cancer*, vol. 2, chap. 17; London, 1958.

Fig. 37.93. Pathology Museum, Royal Marsden Hospital, London; reproduced by permission of Professor N. F. C. Gowing.

Figs 37.94A, 94B, 95B, 96A, 96B, 96C, 96D, 98, 99, 100. Reproduced by permission of the editors, Mr H. J. Burrows and Dr J. R. Nassim, and publishers, Messrs Butterworth and Company, from: Sissons, H. A., in *Modern Trends in Diseases of the Vertebral Column*; London, 1958.

Fig. 37.98. Pathology Museum, Royal College of Surgeons of England; reproduced by permission of the Conservator, Professor J. L. Turk.

38: *Diseases of Joints, Tendon Sheaths, Bursae and Other Soft Tissues*

by H. A. SISSONS

CONTENTS

38: *Diseases of Joints, Tendon Sheaths, Bursae and Other Soft Tissues*

by H. A. SISSONS

ANATOMY AND PHYSIOLOGY

Most joints are complex structures, consisting of articular cartilage, capsular tissues and synovial membrane. These components are specialized connective tissues: together with the adjacent bones they can all be involved in diseases of the joints. The normal histology,[1] ultrastructure[2] and physiology[3-5] of joints have been extensively studied.

Normal articular cartilage is a connective tissue in which the intercellular matrix contains large amounts of mucopolysaccharide (mucoprotein, proteoglycan). Most of the mucopolysaccharide is chondroitin 6-sulphate, which consists of sulphated *N*-acetylgalactosamine conjugated with hexuronic acid; there are smaller amounts of chondroitin 4-sulphate and keratan sulphate.[6, 7] The acidic glycosaminoglycans are responsible for the metachromatic staining of cartilage,[8, 9] while neutral glycosaminoglycans are thought to be responsible for the positive periodic-acid/Schiff reaction given by certain areas of cartilage, particularly those undergoing calcification. The high mucopolysaccharide content, together with the arcade arrangement of the collagen fibres,[10] is responsible for the strength and elasticity of articular cartilage. The articular surfaces themselves are smooth; they are lubricated by the synovial fluid present in the joint. Cartilage is a tissue that contains relatively few cells, and its overall rate of metabolism is low.[11] It is devoid of blood vessels, and the nutritional and respiratory requirements of its cells are met by diffusion from the synovial fluid and the blood vessels of the subchondral bone.

The synovial membrane covers all the intra-articular structures except the articular cartilages, and it is responsible for the formation of the synovial fluid. Histologically,[12, 13] it consists of an 'intima' formed of flattened connective tissue cells that are not always clearly distinguishable from those of the immediately adjoining tissue. In some situations the lining cells are closely applied to the fibrous capsule of the joint: in others they are separated from it by loose connective tissue, which is usually highly vascular and often contains local accumulations of fat. Some parts of the synovial surface are smooth: others present numerous villous projections.

Bursae and tendon sheaths are also lined by synovial membrane and can show pathological changes similar to those affecting joints. Synovial tissue can be formed from other types of connective tissue by metaplasia: this is the origin of the synovial lining of adventitious bursae and of pseudarthroses.

A normal joint contains a small amount of clear, viscous fluid. About 1 ml is present in a normal knee joint of an adult. This synovial fluid is a protein-containing dialysate of the blood plasma to which mucin (hyaluronic acid) is added as a secretion of the synovial cells.[3, 14, 15]

DEVELOPMENTAL ABNORMALITIES

Joints are, of course, involved in the developmental abnormalities of the skeleton (see page 2395). In some conditions, however, the abnormality affects predominantly the articular structures: *congenital dislocation of the hip* and *talipes equinovarus* are examples. A combination of genetical and environmental factors is thought to be concerned in the aetiology of these conditions.[16] For example, in congenital dislocation of the hip (Fig. 38.1) there is laxity of the ligamentous structures of the joint, and this is often associated with underdevelopment of the upper part of the articular surface of the acetabulum (the acetabular roof). The femoral head consequently becomes dislocated — particularly when walking commences—and a false joint forms

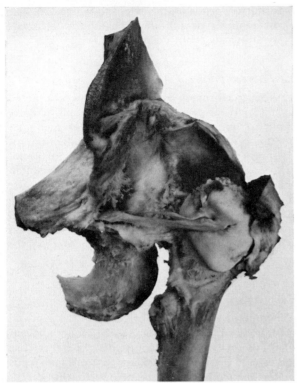

Fig. 38.1.§ Congenital dislocation of hip. Dissected specimen showing longstanding lesion. The femoral head is deformed and displaced, and there is a 'false acetabulum' above the normal position of the articular surface.

above the acetabulum. Somewhat similar joint deformities can occur as a result of muscle imbalance resulting from congenital or acquired paralysis, particularly as a manifestation of poliomyelitis.

TRAUMATIC LESIONS

A variety of effects may follow trauma to a joint. The synovial and capsular tissues may be stretched or lacerated. With greater violence, the joint may be dislocated or the bones fractured; sometimes the articular cartilage is detached from the bone. When the knee is injured its menisci may be torn or displaced (see page 2506).

Minor sprains or lacerations heal promptly, with no residual disability: in such cases, extravasated blood is usually rapidly absorbed from the joint space and it is only very occasionally that fibrous adhesions form. Detached fragments of articular cartilage often persist as loose bodies: the

§ See *Acknowledgements*, page 2522.

cartilage cells at the surface of these loose bodies are able to survive and even proliferate in the absence of any vascular attachment; the deeper—usually necrotic—parts of the detached cartilage undergo calcification.

Experimental studies[17] and observations in man[18] indicate that articular cartilage has little capacity for regeneration following injury. Repair of gaps in articular cartilage is usually brought about by cartilaginous metaplasia of adjacent connective tissue. Cartilaginous metaplasia also occurs in fracture callus (see page 2402); it is also responsible for the formation of the articular surfaces of a pseudarthrosis.

Non-Specific Synovial Reaction

Following injury, synovia shows histological changes that are usually referred to as the *non-specific synovial reaction*. The synovial tissues become hyperaemic and oedematous, and there are accumulations of neutrophils and mononuclear cells. If the synovial trauma is repeated, or if it is long continued, the cells that accumulate are chiefly lymphocytes and plasma cells; they may form conspicuous focal aggregates in the synovial tissues. Defects in the synovial membrane, in contrast to those in articular cartilage, are repaired rapidly;[19] proliferation of synovial cells and synovial metaplasia of other connective tissue cells are concerned in this process.

INFLAMMATORY CONDITIONS

The term *arthritis* is applied to a variety of conditions that affect joints, not all of which are inflammatory in nature: *osteoarthritis*, for example, is a degenerative process (see page 2501) and *gouty arthritis* is the reaction of joint tissues to deposited urates (see page 2505).

Most true inflammatory diseases of joints—such as *suppurative arthritis* and *tuberculous arthritis*—are caused by known infective agents. One major type—*rheumatoid arthritis*—is of uncertain aetiology.

Suppurative Arthritis

Bacteria usually reach the joints from the blood stream: they establish infection in the synovial tissues, and the resulting inflammatory changes involve the whole joint surface. The organisms concerned include *Staphylococcus aureus*, streptococci, pneumococci, meningococci and, less commonly, the gonococcus and various salmonellae. Suppurative arthritis usually occurs in childhood, and cases have been reported in the neonatal period. The hips, knees, elbows, shoulders and ankle joints are those most frequently involved.

In the typical case of staphylococcal or streptococcal arthritis, the inflamed synovial tissues are hyperaemic and oedematous, and there is an effusion of fluid into the joint. The fluid contains fibrin and neutrophils, and the synovial surface is covered with fibrinopurulent exudate. The articular cartilage is rapidly devitalized, and within a few days of the onset it has become thin and incomplete (Fig. 38.2). This rapid removal of cartilage may be effected either by proteolytic enzymes produced by the leucocytes in the purulent joint fluid[20] or by activation of the proteolytic enzymes of the blood.[21] In the untreated, but non-fatal, case of suppurative arthritis, repair is effected by the formation of granulation tissue, with subsequent fibrosis and ossification. Suppurative arthritis frequently becomes chronic, with the development of discharging sinuses. The degree of residual

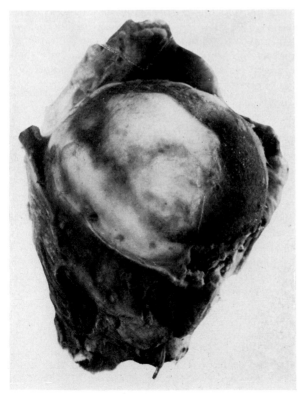

Fig. 38.2.§ Acute suppurative arthritis of shoulder. The articular surface of the head of the humerus shows destruction of cartilage (right).

deformity depends on the extent to which articular cartilage and synovial tissues have been damaged: bony ankylosis is not uncommon.

Less Severe Forms of Acute Infective Arthritis

Less severe forms of arthritis may be encountered in a variety of generalized infections, particularly those of gonococcal, pneumococcal or meningococcal origin.[22–24] Before the introduction of chemotherapy, 2 to 5 per cent of cases of gonorrhoea were complicated by acute arthritis, often involving several joints. Knees, ankles, wrists, fingers, clavicular joints, shoulders and toes are the sites most liable to be affected by this often relatively mild type of infective arthritis. The extent of the inflammatory changes within the joint and the degree of residual damage vary.

Tuberculous Arthritis

Tuberculous arthritis may originate in the synovial membrane or it may be consequent on an adjacent focus of tuberculous osteomyelitis. In either case the disease is usually secondary to a primary focus in the lungs:[25, 26] as in comparable instances of localized tuberculous lesions—for instance, in the genitourinary organs and in the brain—the pulmonary lesion has usually healed long before the distant focus becomes clinically evident. The hips and the knees are the joints most commonly affected by tuberculosis. The disease usually develops during childhood. Occasionally, several joints are involved.

The macroscopical changes depend on the duration and severity of the infection. The joint cavity rarely contains appreciable amounts of pus. The synovial surface appears congested and some areas may be covered by shaggy, fibrinous exudate. The synovial membrane becomes thickened and the capsular tissues are oedematous. A pannus of tuberculous granulation tissue may extend over the surface of the articular cartilage from its margin. Tuberculous tissue commonly extends into the marrow spaces of the cancellous bone underlying the articular cartilage. The cartilage is devitalized and appears dull and wrinkled: it becomes separated from the bone, exposing an uneven surface of bone and tuberculous tissue (Fig. 38.3). The juxta-articular bone is seldom involved to a depth of more than a few millimetres in any area. The bone trabeculae in the involved parts are necrotic, and may form small sequestra. More extensive bone involvement, with massive sequestra-

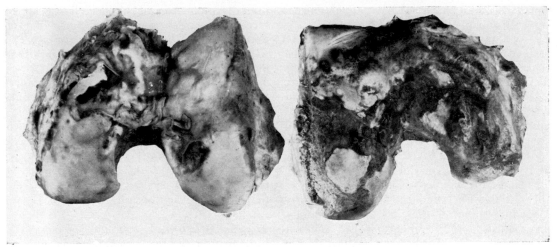

Fig. 38.3.§ Tuberculous arthritis of knee joint. Articular surfaces of femur (two different specimens) showing undermining and separation of cartilage.

tion, is rare. Local osteoporosis, secondary to the inflammatory lesion but extending much more widely than the tuberculous tissue, may contribute to the radiological changes. Generalized osteoporosis of the affected limb may result from disuse and immobilization.[27]

Histological sections of the synovial membrane usually show extensive caseous necrosis, bordered by areas of typical tuberculous tissue. In some cases tubercles are few, and much of the synovial surface shows only diffuse, non-specific inflammatory changes: a limited biopsy may then fail to establish that the lesion is tuberculous. Biopsy of the synovial membrane itself or of a regional lymph node is the accepted procedure for diagnosis: the biopsy material should be examined both histologically and by bacteriological methods.

Tuberculous arthritis may become arrested without extension beyond the synovial tissues; in such cases only a limited restriction of joint mobility may result. More frequently, however, other structures are involved and fibrous or bony ankylosis follows.

Syphilitic Arthritis

Syphilitic arthritis is uncommon, but can occur in both congenital and acquired syphilis.

The joint lesions of congenital syphilis were described by Clutton[28] in 1886, and are sometimes referred to as *Clutton's joints*. In most cases there is a chronic, painless effusion in both knees; occasionally, other joints are affected. The synovial tissues are thickened and oedematous, and usually show only non-specific inflammatory changes; miliary gummas are sometimes present.[29, 30]

Transient arthritis may develop during the secondary stage of syphilis. In some cases this manifestation of syphilitic arthritis may simulate rheumatoid arthritis.[31, 32] Gummatous lesions may develop in joints in the tertiary stage.

Neuropathic joint disease (see page 2504) may develop as a result of syphilitic involvement of the nervous system.

Other Forms of Infective Arthritis

Transient arthritis has been noted in the course of many other infective diseases, including salmonella infections, infections by *Brucella abortus*, *Brucella melitensis* and *Brucella suis*, and smallpox. In cases of brucella infection the spinal joints are particularly liable to involvement and the arthritis, in whatever part of the body, tends to be chronic.[33]

The term *Reiter's syndrome*[33a] is currently applied to the clinical triad of non-gonococcal urethritis, conjunctivitis and arthritis (see page 1540, Volume 4).[33b]

Rheumatoid Arthritis[34–37]

Rheumatoid arthritis is a systemic disease of unknown aetiology, usually involving joints, but also affecting with varying frequency the lymph nodes, spleen, bone marrow and other tissues. The possible role of a variety of infective agents, including mycoplasmas and viruses, has been much discussed[38] but without any more definite conclusion than that infective and immunological factors are probably concerned.

The widespread involvement of connective tissues and the presence of fibrinoid change in the lesions have led some authorities to add rheumatoid arthritis to the group of so-called *collagen diseases*, or systemic diseases of connective tissue, which include, for example, rheumatic fever, polyarteritis, systemic lupus erythematosus, dermatomyositis and systemic sclerosis; this view is coupled with the suggestion that some type of hypersensitivity reaction may be concerned in its pathogenesis, or that it may be the manifestation of autoimmunization against a tissue component. However, it clearly does not follow that all these diseases are aetiologically related.[39, 40] In about 80 per cent of cases of rheumatoid arthritis, the serum contains factors—apparently gammaglobulins of high molecular weight—with specific agglutinating properties: a number of systems, utilizing sensitized sheep red cells or latex particles, have been developed for the detection of these 'rheumatoid factors' and are often of use in diagnosis (see also Chapter 39, Volume 6).[41, 42]

Clinical Features.—Rheumatoid arthritis occurs more commonly in women than in men. It may develop at any age; in a fairly high proportion of cases in women the age at onset is between 40 and 60 years. There is evidence that the disease has a familial incidence in some cases. Joint involvement is usually multiple and often symmetrical: the knee joints and the joints of the hands and feet are affected most frequently. Early in its course there is pain, swelling and stiffness of the involved joints. The disease is progressive, but its course is characterized by remissions and exacerbations. The later stages are marked by deformity and ankylosis of the involved joints, and by atrophy of the related bones, muscles and skin.

Histopathology.—The initial change in the joints is an inflammatory reaction in the synovial tissues,[43] with hyperaemia and an accumulation of inflammatory cells. Most of the cells are lymphocytes and plasma cells, but neutrophils and macrophages, and—occasionally—multinucleate giant cells, are also found. Sometimes the cells are distributed diffusely throughout the synovial tissues (Figs 38.4A and 38.4B), but oftener they are arranged in focal collections: these may be conspicuous and bulky, and associated with marked villous change (Fig. 38.4C). There is usually effusion of fluid into the joint. A synovial reaction with focal accumula-

tions of lymphocytes and plasma cells was sometimes formerly regarded as pathognomonic of rheumatoid arthritis,[44] but it has been emphasized that such a reaction can result from a number of causes, including trauma, infection and osteoarthritis.[45] Nonetheless, the morphological appearances of the advanced synovial lesions of rheumatoid arthritis are distinctive, if only because of the bulk of the cellular infiltrate and the extent of the villous change associated with it. The microscopical picture may be greatly modified in cases treated with corticosteroids: the interpretation of biopsy findings must always be related to the treatment that the patient has been having.

Electron Microscopy and Immunofluorescence.—Investigation by these methods has shown that both type B lymphocytes and type T lymphocytes participate in the rheumatoid synovial reaction.[46, 46a] Immunofluorescent studies have demonstrated the presence of rheumatoid factor in the plasma cells in the lesions, thus confirming that an immunological process is concerned.[47, 48] Rheumatoid factor has been shown to be present in cells—particularly neutrophils—in the synovial fluid of affected joints:[49] the cytoplasm of these

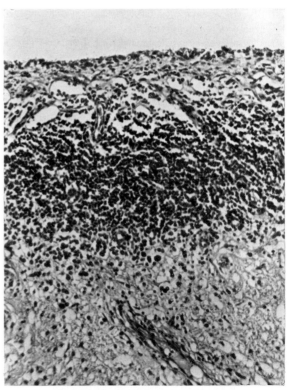

Fig. 38.4A. *Caption on opposite page.*

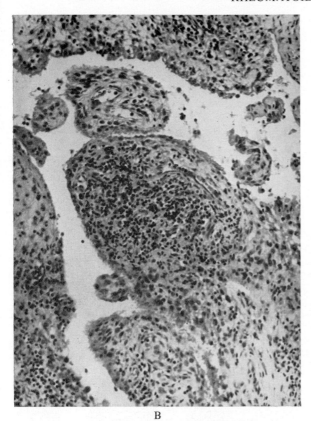

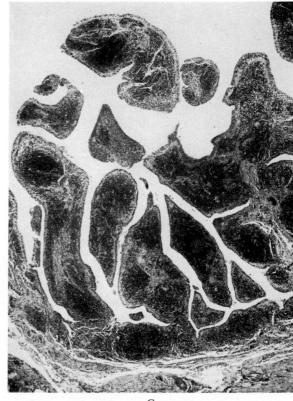

B   C

Fig. 38.4. Rheumatoid arthritis. Synovial membrane. *Haematoxylin–eosin.*

A. Dilated blood vessels, oedema, and diffuse infiltration by lymphocytes and plasma cells. × 140.

B. Diffuse infiltration by lymphocytes and plasma cells, and proliferation of surface synovial cells. × 140.

C.§ Conspicuous focal collections of inflammatory cells, with pronounced villous change of the synovial surface. × 25.

cells often contains granules that are regarded as immune complexes related to rheumatoid factor.

Progress.—As the synovial changes progress, a pannus of granulation tissue covers and replaces the surfaces of the articular cartilages, growing centripetally from their margins (Figs 38.5A and 38.5B). Fibrous adhesions form between the opposed joint surfaces, and the changes sometimes progress to complete destruction of articular cartilage and bony ankylosis. Disuse of the affected limb leads to atrophy of muscle and bone, and to contracture and deformity of joints. In some long-standing cases the inflammatory changes may disappear; the joint deformities persist.

Histological changes similar to those in the joints have been observed in the synovial tissues of tendon sheaths and of bursae in cases of rheumatoid arthritis. Focal accumulations of lymphocytes and plasma cells may be present in the muscles.

Rheumatoid Nodules.—Another lesion characteristic of rheumatoid arthritis is the subcutaneous rheumatoid nodule. Such nodules are present in about 20 per cent of cases. They are located over bony prominences, particularly along the subcutaneous border of the ulna. Their pathological appearances are characteristic.[50–53] They are firm and fibrous in consistency, and range from a few millimetres to a few centimetres in diameter. Histologically, they consist of fibrous tissue showing conspicuous foci of the so-called *fibrinoid necrosis* (Fig. 38.6). The zones of necrosis are sharply outlined, and are surrounded by radially oriented ('palisaded') connective tissue cells. The nature of the fibrinoid material has been much discussed.[53a] The original

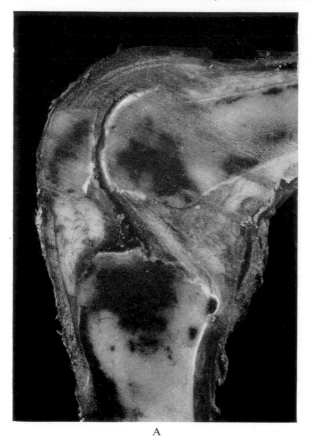

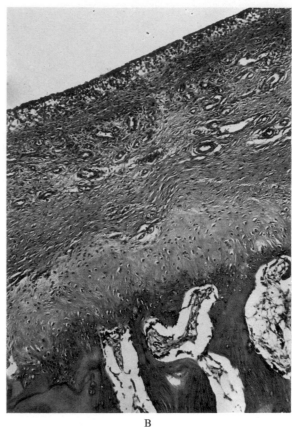

A   B

Fig. 38.5. Rheumatoid arthritis.

A.§ Sagitally divided knee-joint, showing destruction of articular cartilage and replacement by pannus.

B. Histological appearance of fibrous pannus replacing articular cartilage. *Haematoxylin–eosin.* × 80.

concept of the 'collagen diseases' implied that the fibrinoid material represented a degeneration of collagen, but more recent work suggests that accumulation of fibrin, or of material resembling fibrin, is more important. In particular, chemical[54, 55] and electron microscopical[56, 57] studies have failed to show any resemblance between fibrinoid and collagen. Fluorescent antibodies to human fibrin are selectively fixed by the fibrinoid material.[58]

Visceral lesions occur in a minority of cases of rheumatoid arthritis.[59–61] They include valvular and other lesions of the heart, somewhat similar to the lesions of rheumatic heart disease, arteritis,[62, 63] pulmonary lesions (page 370 in Volume 1), pleurisy, splenomegaly, renal changes (including a mild form of glomerulonephritis) (page 1429 in Volume 4), lymph node enlargement (page 690 in Volume 2), and inflammatory ocular lesions, particularly non-granulomatous non-suppurative uveitis (Chapter 40, Volume 6).[64] Amyloidosis is present in 10 to 20 per cent of cases at necropsy: the spleen, liver, kidneys and lymph nodes tend to be the organs most heavily involved.

The term *Still's disease*[65] is sometimes applied to juvenile rheumatoid arthritis, particularly when associated with splenomegaly and lymph node enlargement, and also to cases of rheumatoid arthritis with splenomegaly in adults (see page 690 in Volume 2). There is no real need to distinguish these two groups by a special name. The association of rheumatoid arthritis with splenomegaly and leucopenia is sometimes referred to as *Felty's syndrome,*[66] but again there is no justification for regarding such cases as representing another entity.

Arthritis Associated with Psoriasis[67, 68, 68a]

Rheumatoid arthritis is sometimes associated with psoriasis. This may represent the chance co-

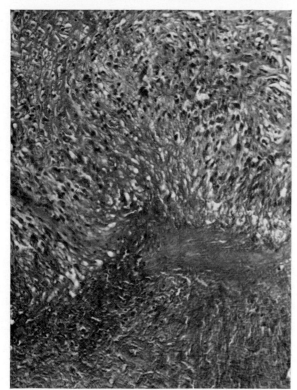

Fig. 38.6. Rheumatoid arthritis. Histological appearance of part of a subcutaneous nodule, showing extensive fibrinoid necrosis with palisading of adjacent connective tissue cells. See also Fig. 39.118 in Volume 6. *Haematoxylin–eosin.* × 110.

existence of two common, independent diseases. Alternatively, it has been considered that there is a specific psoriatic arthritis, or arthropathy, distinct from rheumatoid arthritis. The evidence for this is clinical and serological. The joints that are affected are characteristically the distal interphalangeal joints of the hands and feet; this may be associated with psoriasis of the nails (psoriasis unguium). Other joints are usually involved too, including any of the major and smaller joints of the limbs; there may be temporomandibular arthritis, sacroiliac arthritis and a widespread spinal arthritis that presents the picture of ankylosing spondylitis. Clinically, the polyarthritis may be indistinguishable from rheumatoid arthritis. However, rheumatoid factor is not demonstrable in the serum, rheumatoid nodules do not occur and there are no visceral lesions such as may accompany classic rheumatoid arthritis. It is particularly these features that have been considered to support the view that psoriatic arthritis is an entity distinct from rheumatoid arthritis. The pathological findings in the

joints do not differ from those that may be found in rheumatoid arthritis.[68b]

Whether 'psoriatic arthritis' is an entity or a variant of rheumatoid arthritis remains controversial. Confusion is caused by the occurrence of clinically typical rheumatoid arthritis, with rheumatoid factor, in patients with psoriasis or who subsequently develop psoriasis. This is generally regarded as a chance association by those who believe psoriatic arthritis to be an entity; correspondingly, they take the finding of rheumatoid factor or of a rheumatoid nodule in a case of arthritis accompanying psoriasis to exclude the diagnosis of psoriatic arthritis and to indicate coexistent but independently caused arthritis.

Ankylosing Spondylitis

Ankylosing spondylitis (Strümpell–Marie disease[69, 70]) is characterized by arthritis and bony ankylosis of the costovertebral joints, the joints of the vertebral arches and the sacroiliac joints, and by ossification of the spinal ligaments and of the margin of the intervertebral discs (the ossified structures at the margin of the discs are known as *syndesmophytes*). Involvement of peripheral joints, also leading to bony ankylosis, is frequent. A relationship to rheumatoid arthritis has been postulated, although the disease mainly occurs in men: the grounds for this view are the similarity of the histological picture of the synovial lesions in the peripheral and intervertebral joints in ankylosing spondylitis to that of rheumatoid arthritis.[71–73] The term *rheumatoid spondylitis* is sometimes used as a synonym of ankylosing spondylitis.

The arthritis results in bony ankylosis of all the vertebral joints, the spinal column becoming converted into a continuous bony structure (Fig. 38.7), usually with a pronounced dorsal kyphosis. The pelvis and the thoracic cage are usually involved. The hips (Fig. 38.8) and knees are frequently affected also. Histologically, the involved joints show progressive inflammatory changes in the synovial membrane, with focal collections of lymphocytes and plasma cells. The articular cartilage becomes covered by pannus, and is destroyed, with consequent fibrous and eventually bony ankylosis.

Ankylosis of the vertebral bodies results from ossification in the *anulus fibrosus*: the central part of the intervertebral discs usually remains unossified.

The changes in the vertebrae in ankylosing spondylitis differ from those associated with

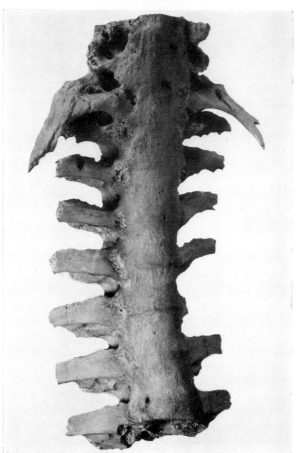

Fig. 38.7.§ Ankylosing spondylitis. Macerated specimen of thoracic spine, showing bony ankylosis of all vertebral articulations.

rheumatoid arthritis. In the latter, the cervical vertebrae are involved predominantly and the arthritis takes the form of a marginal synovitis of the posterior intervertebral joints, with secondary destruction of bone.[74]

Heart Disease.—Various reports have described the association of ankylosing spondylitis with cardiac lesions,[75, 76] including pericarditis and myocarditis, and a variety of valvular lesions, of which the most frequent is aortic insufficiency.

Human Leucocyte Antigen System and Ankylosing Spondylitis.—Ankylosing spondylitis is one of a number of diseases that have been found to occur significantly more frequently among people who have particular antigens of the HLA ('human leucocyte system A') antigen system than among those with

other HLA antigens.* The antigen associated with ankylosing spondylitis is B27 (also referred to as HLA-B27): it is present in a very large proportion both of the patients and of their close relatives.[76a, 76b] The detailed significance of this observation is uncertain, but it evidently indicates a genetic predisposition to the disease. The antigen B27 is also important in transplantation practice as it is one of the major histocompatibility antigens.

Arthritis in Rheumatic Fever

In addition to the characteristic cardiac lesions (see page 24 in Volume 1), rheumatic fever is

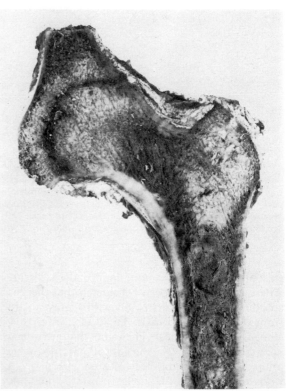

Fig. 38.8.§ Ankylosing spondylitis. Longitudinally divided femur and part of pelvis, showing bony ankylosis of hip joint.

* Other diseases that have been recognized to have an association with particular HLA antigens include Hodgkin's disease (Zervas, J. D., Delamore, I. W., Israëls, M. C. G., *Lancet*, 1970, **2**, 634), adult coeliac disease (idiopathic steatorrhoea) (Stokes, P. L., Asquith, P., Holmes, G. K. T., Macintosh, P., Cooke, W. T., *Lancet*, 1972, **2**, 162), psoriasis (Krulig, L., Farber, E. M., Grumet, F. C., Payne, R. O., *Arch. Derm.*, 1975, **111**, 857) and systemic lupus erythematosus (Waters, H., Konrad, P., Walford, R. L., *Tissue Antigens*, 1971, **1**, 68). In none of these is the association with particular HLA antigens so frequent as the association of ankylosing spondylitis with B27. See also: *The HLA System*, edited by W. F. Bodmer (*Brit. med. Bull.*, 1978, **34**, 213–316).

accompanied by transient arthritic involvement of various joints, particularly the ankles, knees and wrists. The synovial fluid contains many neutrophils. The synovial membrane is hyperaemic and infiltrated by inflammatory cells, particularly lymphocytes and plasma cells. The cellular infiltration is characteristically diffuse: the focal aggregates of cells that are typical of rheumatoid arthritis are not a feature of the synovitis of rheumatic fever. Foci of fibrinoid necrosis may be present in the synovia but are not a constant finding. The joint lesions of rheumatic fever usually subside without residual damage.

Rheumatic Nodules.—Subcutaneous nodules may develop in the course of rheumatic fever. Their histological appearance is somewhat similar to that of the subcutaneous nodules of rheumatoid arthritis (see page 2497), but the nodules of the two diseases can usually be distinguished.[53] Fibrinoid change is rather inconspicuous in the rheumatic nodule, and necrosis of the affected structures is rarely complete. The rheumatic nodule is less clearly demarcated from the surrounding tissues than is the rheumatoid nodule; it undergoes organization and replacement by fibrous tissue after a relatively short period.[50] Such morphological resemblance as there is between the lesions of rheumatic fever and those of rheumatoid arthritis does not indicate an aetiological relationship between the two conditions.[77]

OSTEOARTHRITIS[78-82]

Osteoarthritis is a common disease. The essential pathological change is degeneration of articular cartilage. Some degree of degenerative change is always present in the major joints of individuals over the age of 30 years, and these changes slowly progress with increasing age:[78, 79] the term osteoarthritis is applied to any exaggeration of this normal ageing process. Although some repair can occur in articular cartilage,[82a] it has been suggested that the development of osteoarthritis is related to the relatively limited reparative capacity of this tissue, representing a failure to respond to the wear and tear occasioned by the mechanical stresses to which joints are normally subjected. Genetical factors may play a part in predisposing to the disease. The influence of other general factors, at least in experimental animals, is illustrated by the demonstration that prolonged feeding of mice on a diet enriched with fat accelerates articular ageing and accentuates the development of osteoarthritis.[83]

Local factors that either increase the mechanical stresses and strains to which joints are subjected or interfere with the integrity of the articular surface often produce osteoarthritis: this is usually known as *secondary osteoarthritis*, and may be seen following a variety of disturbances, including trauma, developmental anomalies, osteochondritis, Paget's disease, infection of joints and rheumatoid arthritis.

The distinction between osteoarthritis and the condition that we now know as rheumatoid arthritis began to be defined toward the end of the nineteenth century. In 1909, Nichols and Richardson[84] clearly differentiated the two on morbid anatomical grounds, and recognized that osteoarthritis arises as a 'degeneration of joint cartilage'.

In primary osteoarthritis, one or several joints may be affected, the major weight-bearing joints (the hips, knees and spinal joints) being those usually involved. The parts of the articular surface that are most subject to mechanical stress are specially affected. In the hip, these are the upper surface of the femoral head and the apposed part of the acetabulum; in the knee, they are the patellar surface of the femur and the weight-bearing areas of the femoral and tibial condyles.

The initial degenerative change in osteoarthritis consists of a softening of the normally firm articular cartilage. Histological changes first appear in its superficial part (Fig. 38.9A). There is loss of the basiphile, metachromatic, mucopolysaccharide constituents of the cartilage matrix,[82] and the tissue becomes frayed by the development of numerous vertical clefts between groups of cartilage cells. This change is referred to as *fibrillation*, and is characteristic of osteoarthritis.[85] Despite the absence of effective regeneration of the articular cartilage, the 'degenerating' tissue appears to be in an active metabolic state. Biochemical investigation, including enzymatic studies, shows evidence of increased cellular activity—for instance, synthesis of deoxyribonucleic acid and of mucopolysaccharides—in areas where the overall loss of mucopolysaccharides has been greatest.[86] Lysosomal enzyme activity, possibly concerned in the breakdown of cartilage matrix,[87] is also increased.[88, 89]

Later, the affected articular cartilage becomes thinned because of the disorganization and fragmentation of the superficial tissue. The degenerative changes now extend to the deeper part of the cartilage (Fig. 38.9B). Ultimately, the subchondral bone is exposed (Fig. 38.11): it becomes denser and its surface becomes worn and polished, the process

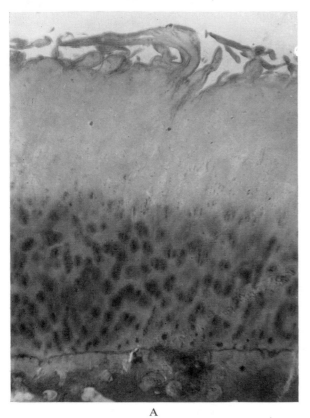
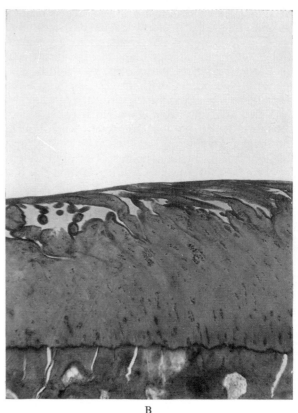

A   B

Fig. 38.9. Osteoarthritis. *Haematoxylin–eosin.* × 25.

A. Histological appearance of the articular surface of the femoral head, showing fibrillation and loss of basiphile staining of matrix in the superficial tissue.

B. A more severely affected zone of the same articular surface: the articular cartilage is thinned, and the fibrillation and loss of staining of the matrix have extended to the deep part. The fissures in the subchondral bone are artefacts.

that is known as *eburnation*. Small pseudocysts commonly occur in the bone deep to the eroded surfaces (Figs 38.10 to 38.13): they appear to be the result of degeneration in fibrous tissue that has come to occupy the marrow spaces of the subchondral bone. Patches of necrotic (acellular) bone are sometimes seen in the neighbourhood of such cysts (Figs 38.12 and 38.13). Elsewhere the sclerotic subchondral bone is not necrotic: indeed, injection studies show increased vascularity in this region.[90]

While these changes are occurring in the articular cartilage and the subchondral bone, a different process occurs at the margin of the articular surface, leading to the formation of outgrowths known as *marginal osteophytes*. The earliest change consists of reactivation of endochondral ossification in the deep part of the articular cartilage (Fig. 38.11). As ossification extends into the articular cartilage, the cartilage increases in size, either by proliferation of its own cells or by proliferation and metaplasia of adjacent fibrous tissue and fibrocartilage. The result is the formation, at the margin of the articular surface, of a 'lip' of bone, covered by a layer of cartilage or fibrocartilage continuous with the articular surface. This peripheral reshaping of the joint tissues, together with the erosion of the cartilage and bone in the central part of the articular surface, can result in marked alteration in the contour of the joint surface, often with restriction of mobility.

The ineffectiveness of regeneration or repair of articular cartilage means that the changes of osteoarthritis are progressive. Degeneration of articular cartilage leads to exposure of bony surfaces and to mechanical disorganization of the joint: this increases the mechanical stresses to which the remaining articular cartilage is subjected, and a vicious circle of change is established.

In the early stages of osteoarthritis the synovial membrane of an affected joint is substantially

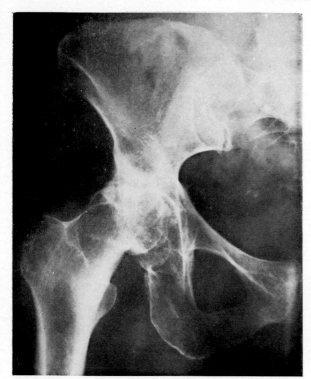

Fig. 38.10. Osteoarthritis. Radiograph of hip, showing moderately severe changes. The joint space is narrowed and the contour of the femoral head altered. The subchondral bone of the femoral head shows increased density and the presence of pseudocysts (see Figs 38.11A and 38.11B).

normal. Later, it may show a mild degree of non-specific synovial reaction (see page 2493), often accompanied by considerable fibrosis of the synovial and capsular tissues. When the subchondral bone is eroded, microscopical fragments of abraded bone may become embedded in the synovial membrane and contribute to the synovial changes.[91]

Osteoarthritis in Specific Sites

Hips.—The increasing frequency of surgical treatment of osteoarthritis of the hip by removing the diseased bone and inserting a prosthesis has stimulated interest in the anatomical changes in the head of the femur and in the acetabulum in this condition.[92–95] These studies have provided valuable information on various aspects that are of pathological importance also, such as the distribution of wear of the articular cartilage in the normal course of ageing and in relation to the congruity of the opposed joint surfaces.[95]

Patellae.—Osteoarthritis affecting the patella[95a] gives rise to the condition known as *chondro-*

malacia patellae, characterized by fibrillation of the articular cartilage. The changes may develop in a series of parallel vertical bands indicative of the sites of greatest friction of the patella on the femur. Eburnation of the exposed bone is often particularly marked. Osteophytes at the patellar margin may seriously interfere with the mobility of the knee.

First Metatarsophalangeal Joints.—The metatarsophalangeal joint of the great toe is frequently affected with osteoarthritis. In cases of *hallux rigidus* there is limitation of the movement of the joint by osteophytes or bony 'lipping' at the periphery of the articular surface. Most frequently the toe cannot be dorsiflexed (extended) but in

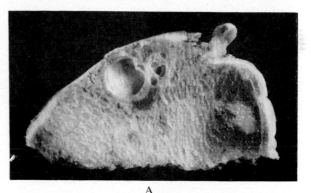

A

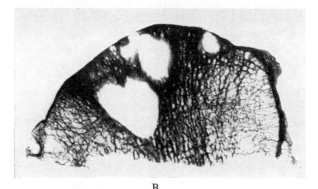

B

Fig. 38.11. Osteoarthritis.

A. The cut surface of part of the femoral head, from a case similar to that shown in Fig. 38.10. The articular cartilage is thinned and its central part is eroded: the subchondral bone contains a number of pseudocysts. At the right of the figure there is bone formation within the deep part of the articular cartilage.

B. Radiograph of a slab of bone from the same femoral head. The flattened surface of the eroded bone and the sclerosis surrounding the pseudocysts are evident. At the right of the figure the outline of the bone formation in the deep part of the articular cartilage is seen.

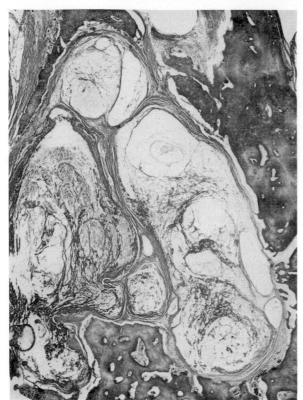

Fig. 38.12.§ Osteoarthritis. Histological appearance of tissue from 'cyst' in femoral head. The space in the bone is occupied by degenerate fibrous tissue. *Haematoxylin–eosin.* × 10.

some cases the limitation is in plantar flexion; occasionally all movement at the joint is restricted or prevented. The condition may follow injury, particularly neglected fracture of the base of the phalanx; often no cause is apparent.

Hallux valgus is a commoner condition. Its causation is uncertain. The osteoarthritic changes that frequently, but not invariably, accompany it are probably secondary. The basic abnormality is medial displacement of the head of the metatarsal bone: this, with a marginal osteophyte on the medial surface of the bone, produces the characteristic 'bunion'.

Finger Joints.—In the fingers, which are among the commonest sites of osteoarthritis, the marginal osteophytes—particularly those on the base of the *terminal phalanx*—are known as *Heberden's nodes.*[96]

Spine.—Osteoarthritis of the spine takes the form of changes in the articular cartilages of the joints of the vertebral arches.

A common abnormality, sometimes confused with true osteoarthritic change, is the formation of

marginal osteophytes on the vertebral bodies themselves, usually involving the anterior surface of the lumbar or cervical spine. This change, which is related to degeneration of intervertebral discs,[97, 98] should not be confused with osteoarthritis or with ankylosing spondylitis. It is sometimes known as *spinal osteophytosis* or *spondylitis deformans*. The latter term has been applied also to ankylosing spondylitis (see page 2499), a practice that may cause confusion. The osteophytes, particularly in the cervical region, may press on the spinal cord or obstruct its blood vessels (see page 2196).

Neuropathic Arthropathy ('Neuropathic Joints')

A particularly severe form of degenerative and destructive change may occur in certain joints in certain types of neurological disorder in which there is interference with sensory pathways. Tabes dorsalis and syringomyelia are the commonest conditions of this type, but similar joint changes can occur in leprosy and in a variety of other neurological disorders. The term *Charcot's joint*[99]

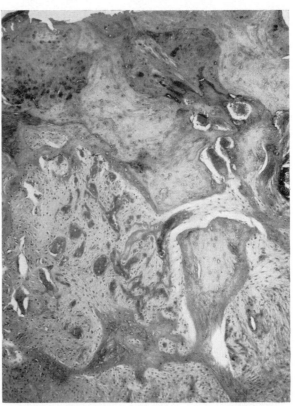

Fig. 38.13. Osteoarthritis. Another 'cystic' area from a femoral head, showing fibrous tissue. Note the patches of necrosis in parts of the subchondral bone. *Haematoxylin–eosin.* × 40.

is commonly applied to this condition. Apart from the severity of involvement, the changes are similar to those of osteoarthritis. There is often very severe destruction of cartilage and bone, with marked osteophyte formation. Dislocation and other displacements of the severely affected joints are frequently seen. The exceptional severity of the destructive changes is usually ascribed to the lessening or loss of sensibility to pain that is symptomatic of the associated neurological disease: this deprives the diseased joint of the protection that the need to avoid painful movements ordinarily gives, and articular damage is therefore severer, and rapider in development, than would otherwise be the case.

GOUT[100–102]

Gout is a disorder of purine metabolism in which sodium urate is deposited in a variety of tissues, and particularly in the tissues of the joints. About 90 per cent of affected individuals are men; there is often evidence of familial liability to the disease. The symptoms of gout usually develop after middle age.

Uric acid is derived chiefly from the degradation of nucleoproteins. It is present in the blood, and is excreted in the urine after filtration through the glomeruli and concentration by the renal tubules. The fasting serum urate concentration is less than 350 μmol/l (or 6 mg/dl) in 97 per cent of people who have not suffered from gout; it is above these figures in 98 per cent of gouty patients.[102a]

The deposition of urate crystals in the superficial part of the articular cartilage is the earliest change in the joints. Various joints may be affected, but particularly the metatarsophalangeal joint of the great toe. Other tissues in which urates may be deposited include the synovial membrane of joints and bursae, the juxta-articular tissues (including bone, tendons and ligaments), and the cartilage of the external ear. The larger gouty deposits are known as *tophi*, and consist of masses of urate crystals surrounded by fibrous tissue containing numerous 'foreign body' giant cells. The urate crystals are best preserved in alcohol-fixed material, and the deposits usually have an amorphous appearance in ordinary sections of formalin-fixed tissue (Fig. 38.14). Deposition of calcium salts sometimes occurs, and cholesterol is often present in older lesions.[103] The crystalline material in a gouty lesion can be identified as urate by the application of the murexide test.[104]

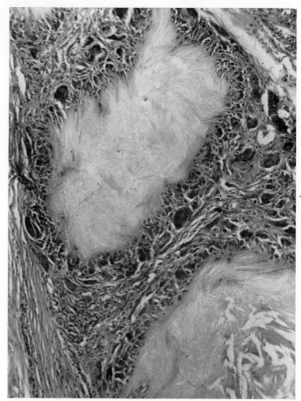

Fig. 38.14. Gout. Section of a tophus, showing deposits of urate surrounded by fibrous tissue containing numerous 'foreign body' giant cells. *Haematoxylin–eosin.* $\times 80$.

The joint lesions of gout are usually slowly progressive. The clinical course is marked by a series of acute attacks, characterized by general constitutional disturbance and by pain in the affected joint, which is very tender to touch. In an attack, the tissues that adjoin tophi appear acutely inflamed, and the synovial fluid of the joint contains many neutrophils. As the lesions become chronic, progressive destruction of the adjacent bone may occur, and secondary osteoarthritic changes frequently develop.

Bulky subcutaneous tophi can lead to ulceration of the covering skin, with sinus formation and secondary infection.

Renal Changes in Gout.—Urate deposits frequently form in the kidneys, and may ultimately lead to renal failure (see page 1430 in Volume 4).[100] The tubules contain urate crystals and casts, and there is a variable amount of interstitial fibrosis and inflammatory change. Uric acid calculi are sometimes found in the urinary tract; however, the presence of such stones is not in itself evidence of gout as they are frequently seen in patients who are not affected with the latter (see page 1458 in Volume 4).

Pseudogout[105]

In recent years a condition has been recognized in which calcified deposits, free from urates, develop in articular cartilage and in adjacent fibro-cartilaginous or ligamentous tissues. This condition is referred to as articular chondrocalcinosis, or 'pseudogout'.[105–108] Joint involvement is often multiple: the knees are the most commonly affected joints, followed by the wrists, elbows, hips and shoulders. As in gout, the condition is marked by intermittent pain and swelling of the involved joints. X-ray diffraction studies have established that the material deposited in the articular cartilage is not hydroxyapatite (see page 2384) but calcium pyrophosphate dihydrate.[108a]

The distinction between crystals of urate, characterizing gout, and those of calcium pyrophosphate dihydrate, characterizing pseudogout, can be made by comparison of their optical qualities under the polarizing microscope. This examination, applied to fluid aspirated from the affected joint, readily distinguishes the two conditions.[109]

Calcification of Joint Structures in Other Diseases

Calcification of articular cartilage occurs in other joint diseases also, including osteoarthritis, rheumatoid arthritis[110, 111] and neuropathic arthropathy.[111a] It may also be found in cases of hyperparathyroidism.[111b]

MISCELLANEOUS DISEASES

Synovial Chondromatosis[112, 113]

Synovial chondromatosis is a rare condition. There is doubt whether it is a neoplastic disease or an unusual manifestation of hyperplasia. It is characterized by the presence of numerous cartilaginous nodules that develop as a result of metaplasia of the synovial tissues. Most of the patients are adults. The lesions usually involve one or more large joints, such as the knees, hips and shoulders. The nodules of cartilage can be as large as a centimetre in diameter; they are visible in radiographs only when they have undergone calcification or ossification. Sometimes they are pedunculate, and they may then become separated as loose bodies; however, cartilaginous loose bodies in joints are

much more commonly a result of osteochondritis dissecans or of fragmentation of osteophytes in osteoarthritis.

Very rarely, a chondrosarcoma develops in a joint already affected by chondromatosis.[114] It may also be noted here that a chondrosarcoma may arise from synovia in the absence of chondromatosis.[115]

Lesions of the Menisci of the Knee Joints

The menisci or semilunar cartilages of the knee joints are wedge-shaped, fibrocartilaginous structures. They are attached by their outer margin to the joint capsule and their anterior and posterior horns are attached to the intercondylar region of the tibia. Their free edge projects into the joint between the marginal parts of the articular surfaces of the femur and tibia.

They are liable to be torn or avulsed in injuries to the knee, the medial meniscus being much more frequently involved than the lateral one. The medial meniscus is more securely attached to neighbouring structures than the lateral meniscus and this fixation renders it less capable of adaptation to sudden changes of position. The lateral meniscus is less firmly attached; moreover, it tends to be drawn backward by the popliteus muscle, part of the tendon of which is attached to the meniscus, and this may protect it from becoming trapped between the articular surfaces. Tears in the menisci are usually longitudinal, and the torn fragment, or the avulsed cartilage, can become displaced and cause 'locking' of the joint. Damage to a meniscus is usually accompanied by damage to the synovial membrane and capsular tissues. The fibrocartilage of a damaged meniscus usually fails to show any appreciable evidence of the reparative processes ordinarily seen following damage to connective tissue, and a major tear will persist indefinitely.

The surgical removal of a meniscus is followed by the slow regeneration of a new wedge-shaped structure.[116] In contrast to the original structure the regenerated meniscus usually consists of fibrous tissue and not of fibrocartilage.

The menisci may also be the site of *pseudocyst formation*, which can usually be ascribed to trauma or to degenerative change. The lateral meniscus is more commonly involved than the medial. The pseudocysts involve the outer part of the meniscus and the adjacent capsular tissue (Figs 38.15A and 38.15B); they are usually multilocular. Histologically, they are similar to a ganglion (see below),

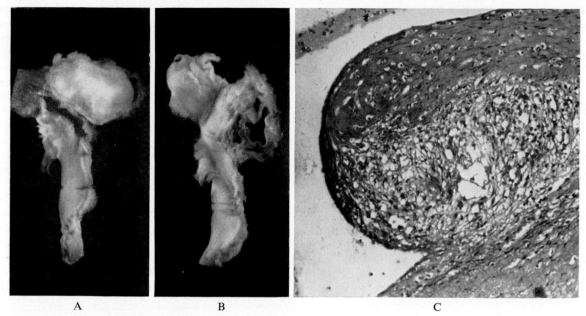

A   B   C

Fig. 38.15. Pseudocyst of lateral meniscus of a knee joint.

A,§ B.§ Two different specimens, showing the relationship of the pseudocysts to the meniscus and the adjacent capsular tissue.

C. Section of the wall of the pseudocyst illustrated in Fig. 38.15B, showing that it consists of fibrous tissue undergoing mucoid change. *Haematoxylin–eosin.* × 80.

their wall consisting of fibrous tissue, often with areas of mucoid degeneration (Fig. 38.15C).

Bursae

Some bursae have an obvious communication with a joint and are lined by typical synovial tissue. Others, known as *adventitious bursae*, form in connective tissue covering bony prominences or at other sites of abnormal tissue movement: they usually consist merely of fibrous tissue showing pronounced mucoid change, but a synovial lining is sometimes formed by metaplasia of cells abutting on the cavities that result.

Ganglia

Ganglia are small pseudocystic swellings that may develop on the dorsum of the wrists and hands, or near the ankles. They result from mucoid degeneration in the fibrous tissue of tendon sheaths, ligaments or aponeuroses. They seldom have a synovial lining.

Lesions of Intervertebral Discs[117, 118]

The normal intervertebral disc in the adult consists of the semifluid *nucleus pulposus* surrounded by the *anulus fibrosus*, which firmly unites the margins of adjacent vertebral bodies. Above and below, the nucleus pulposus is separated from the cancellous bone of the vertebral body by the *cartilaginous end-plate* of the vertebra. The nucleus pulposus consists of poorly cellular, chondroid material, while the structures bounding it are fibrous tissue and fibrocartilage. Our knowledge of the pathology of the intervertebral disc is due chiefly to the work of Schmorl and his colleagues.[117]

The most important abnormality of the intervertebral discs is prolapse. Normally, the nucleus pulposus is under pressure, and any weakening of the surrounding structures may result in outward displacement of its semifluid substance. Prolapse can occur vertically into the cancellous bone of the adjacent vertebral body or posteriorly into the spinal canal: the anterior longitudinal ligament prevents forward prolapse. Prolapse into the vertebral body produces a *Schmorl's node*—a rounded mass of disc tissue deep to the end-plate of the vertebral body. Schmorl's nodes are often demonstrable at necropsy, sometimes in many vertebrae; they do not cause symptoms. Posterior prolapse of disc tissue is also a frequent necropsy finding: sometimes, particularly in the lumbar and cervical regions, the prolapsed tissue produces compression or stretching of nerve roots, with consequent pain, paraesthesiae and muscle wasting.

The discs between the fourth and fifth lumbar vertebrae and between the fifth lumbar and first sacral vertebrae are the ones that most frequently prolapse. Prolapse of intervertebral discs is not infrequently responsible for the development of *spinal osteophytosis* (see page 2504).

Pigmented Villonodular Synovitis[119, 120]

The name pigmented villonodular synovitis was given by Jaffe and his colleagues[121] in 1941 to a group of lesions characterized by villous and nodular proliferation of the synovial tissues, with pigmentation of the hyperplastic tissue, and a histological structure of synovial cells, macrophages and osteoclast-like giant cells. Similar lesions occur in tendon sheaths and bursae, and also in fascial tissue. The nature of these lesions and their nomenclature have been much debated: terms such as xanthoma, giant cell tumour and benign synovioma have been used, with the implication that the lesions are neoplastic.[122–124] The nodularity of some of the lesions, their capacity for growth and their highly cellular histological appearance are features that favour this concept; in contrast, the diffuseness of the synovial involvement exhibited by the more villous lesions, and the reactive quality of the histological appearance, when it is considered in detail, seem to be out of keeping with this view. One point requiring emphasis is that these pigmented synovial lesions are benign: they are quite distinct from synovial sarcomas (see opposite), and there is no evidence to suggest that they ever undergo malignant change.

When it involves a major joint, pigmented villonodular synovitis appears as a brownish mass of villous or nodular projections from the synovial surface (Figs 38.16A and 38.16B). The involvement is usually diffuse, although localized lesions also occur. Most of the patients are young adults, and the knee is most commonly affected: there is usually

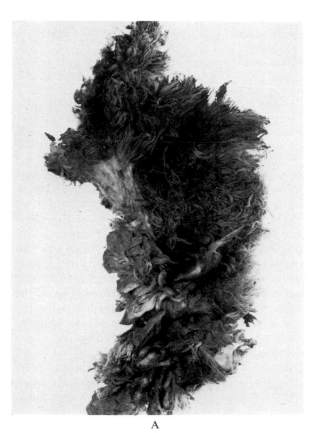
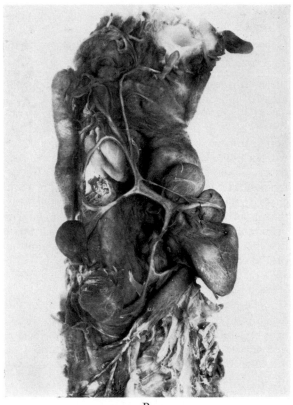

A   B

Fig. 38.16.§ Pigmented villonodular synovitis.

A.§ Synovectomy specimen from lesion of knee joint showing a predominantly villous, darkly pigmented lesion.

B.§ Another synovectomy specimen showing a more nodular lesion. Both the synovial surface and the deeper tissues are pigmented.

a history of pain and swelling of the involved joint, often with episodes of acute exacerbation. Aspiration yields dark brown or frankly bloody fluid.

As already noted, the gross appearance is variable: villi and nodules may be intermingled, and in some cases both types of structure become matted into a sponge-like mass. The synovial surface of the lesion is usually heavily pigmented, appearing reddish brown or tan; the cut surface of solid areas is a paler yellow-brown. Histologically, the villous tissue (Fig. 38.17A) consists of thin strands of vascular connective tissue covered by synovial cells and presenting a diffuse or focal accumulation of lymphocytes and plasma cells. Granules of haemosiderin are present in the superficial synovial cells, in many of the deeper cells, and lying free in the tissue spaces. Giant cells may be present. In nodular or solid areas (Figs 38.17B to 38.17D) the tissue is made up of rounded or spindle-shaped cells: variable amounts of haemosiderin are present, and there are many vacuolate macrophages containing lipid. Multinucleate giant cells are present in these areas, and are sometimes a very conspicuous feature: many of them resemble osteoclasts in size and appearance, their nuclei being located in the central part of the cell body. Some nodules are conspicuously fibrotic; others show a remarkably high degree of cellularity, with numerous cells in mitosis. In some cases the pigmented tissue extends into the interstices of the capsular tissue of the joint (Fig. 38.18), simulating invasion: it may even erode bone. Because of these sinister-looking histological features, which sometimes are misinterpreted as indicative of a sarcomatous process, it must be stressed that these lesions have never been reported to metastasize.

Localized Nodular Synovitis.—More localized lesions with a similar histological structure are frequently seen. These take the form of solitary, pedunculate masses, attached to the synovial surface.[124a] Localized nodular lesions of tendon sheaths are also quite common, and, because of the conspicuous multinucleate cells, are often referred to as *giant cell tumours of tendon sheaths.* They occur particularly in the fingers, generally appearing as lobulate nodules, 1 to 2 cm in diameter: they have a brownish colour, and they are often referred to by surgeons as 'brown tumours'. Histologically, they consist of rather fibrous tissue, containing round and spindle-shaped cells and scattered multinucleate giant cells. Haemosiderin and lipid material are present. Occasionally, such lesions show histological evidence of evolution from a

number of smaller nodules, or from villous structures, and the proponents of the concept of pigmented villonodular synovitis argue that this links them with the more diffuse, villonodular synovial lesions. It is for this reason that they are often described by the term *localized nodular synovitis*, in order to indicate that they are not tumours.

Aetiology.—If pigmented villonodular synovitis is to be regarded as a reactive condition rather than a neoplasm, it must be admitted that the cause of the reaction is obscure. Histological changes somewhat similar to those of pigmented villonodular synovitis occur as a sequel of repeated episodes of haemarthrosis (bleeding into the joint cavity) in haemophiliacs,[125, 126] and they have also been produced in dogs by the repeated intra-articular injection of blood.[127, 128] Although the lesions in haemophiliacs and those produced experimentally show marked villous change, pigmentation by haemosiderin and the presence of scattered giant cells and lipid-containing macrophages, they do not progress to form the bulky, proliferating, nodular lesions characteristic of the fully-developed picture of pigmented villonodular synovitis.

Reticulohistiocytic Granulomatosis

This uncommon disease of adults, usually women, in which a peculiar giant-celled and histiocytic granuloma occurs widely in the skin and in synovial membranes, is considered in Chapter 39, Volume 6.

SYNOVIAL TUMOURS

Primary tumours of joints, bursae and tendon sheaths are uncommon. The condition known as pigmented villonodular synovitis has been discussed above (see opposite): it has been noted that lesions of this type are regarded by some authorities as benign synoviomas.

Benign Tumours and Tumour-Like Lesions

Angiomas, lipomas and chondromas arising in joint tissues have been reported.[129]

Synovial Sarcoma

Synovial sarcoma,[129–132] or *malignant synovioma*, is the only variety of malignant tumour that requires particular discussion in relation to joints. Its

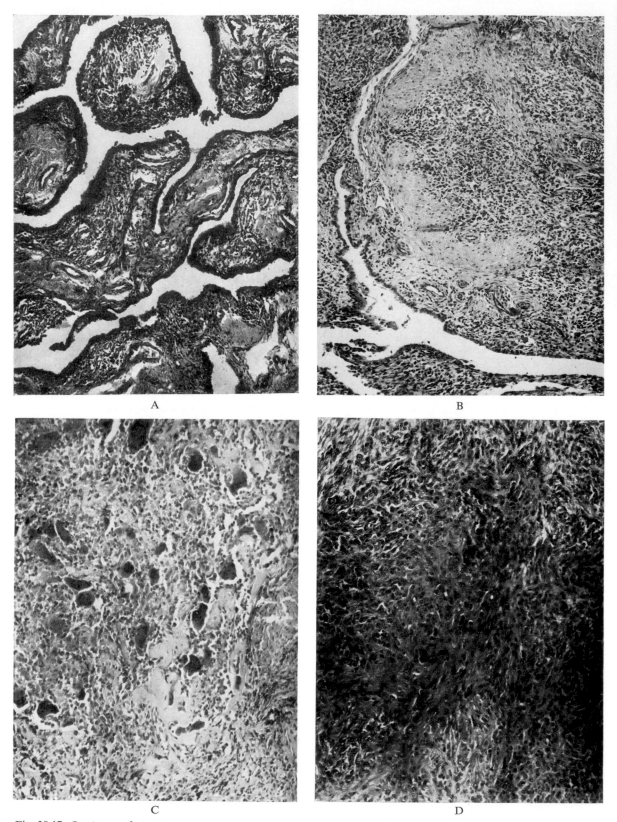

Fig. 38.17. *Captions on facing page*.

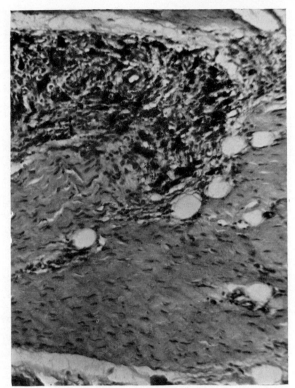

Fig. 38.18. Pigmented villonodular synovitis. Pigmented tissue extends between the fibrous bundles of the joint capsule. *Haematoxylin–eosin.* × 105.

pattern of histological differentiation shows a similarity to synovial tissue. It usually originates in the juxta-articular soft tissues rather than in the synovial membrane itself, and it not infrequently occurs in sites remote from pre-existing synovial structures.[130–132] It is only in recent years that synovial sarcomas have been clearly distinguished from other malignant soft tissue tumours and from benign pigmented synovial lesions (see above).

Synovial sarcoma is predominantly a tumour of young adults. There has been no particular sex difference among the reported cases. It usually arises in a limb: a leg, particularly the region of the knee, is the commonest site. In the upper limb the vicinity of the shoulder is the usual site. In some cases the tumour appears to originate in relation to one of the bursae in that region.

A synovial sarcoma usually appears as a rounded, apparently encapsulate mass of fleshy tissue (Fig. 38.19A). The cut surface may present areas of necrosis or haemorrhage. The nearby joint spaces, and less commonly the adjacent bones, may be invaded. Foci of calcification are occasionally present in the tumour and may be a conspicuous feature in radiographs.

The characteristic—indeed the definitive—histological feature of synovial sarcoma is the presence of synovial spaces in the tumour tissue. Careful search, however, may be required for the identification of these spaces, as the bulk of the tumour usually consists of undifferentiated spindle-celled tissue (Fig. 38.19B). The synovial spaces frequently show a resemblance to epithelial structures: they are usually lined by cuboidal or columnar cells and are arranged in simple or branching gland-like structures that contrast with the surrounding spindle-celled tissue (Figs 38.19C and 38.19D). The synovial spaces frequently contain mucinous fluid. Despite their resemblance to epithelial tissue, these gland-like structures are the neoplastic counterpart of normal synovial tissue, the cells of which, although not to be rigidly distinguished from other types of connective tissue cell, both form a surface covering for the synovial membranes and secrete the mucin of synovial fluid.

Synovial sarcomas are highly malignant tumours. In a series of 104 cases, only three patients were alive and apparently free from metastasis after five years.[130] The tumours metastasize by the blood stream, and also to the regional lymph nodes. The secondary deposits usually show the same morphological features as the primary tumour.

TUMOURS OF OTHER SOFT TISSUES

There are many different types of tumour of soft tissues:[133–135] they vary widely in clinical presentation, pathology and behaviour. A currently acceptable nomenclature and classification are set out in a World Health Organization publication.[133]

The term *soft tissue tumour* is applicable to growths arising in a range of connective tissues, including fibrous tissue, adipose tissue, muscle and synovia, and also blood and lymphatic vessels and

Fig. 38.17. Pigmented villonodular synovitis. *Haematoxylin–eosin.*

A. Histological appearance of a villous lesion. The dark superficial synovial cells contain haemosiderin. × 80.

B.§ A nodular lesion. A considerable amount of fibrous tissue is present, and many heavily pigmented cells are seen. × 85.

C. Another nodular lesion, showing scattered giant cells. × 125.

D. A highly cellular field in a nodular lesion. × 125.

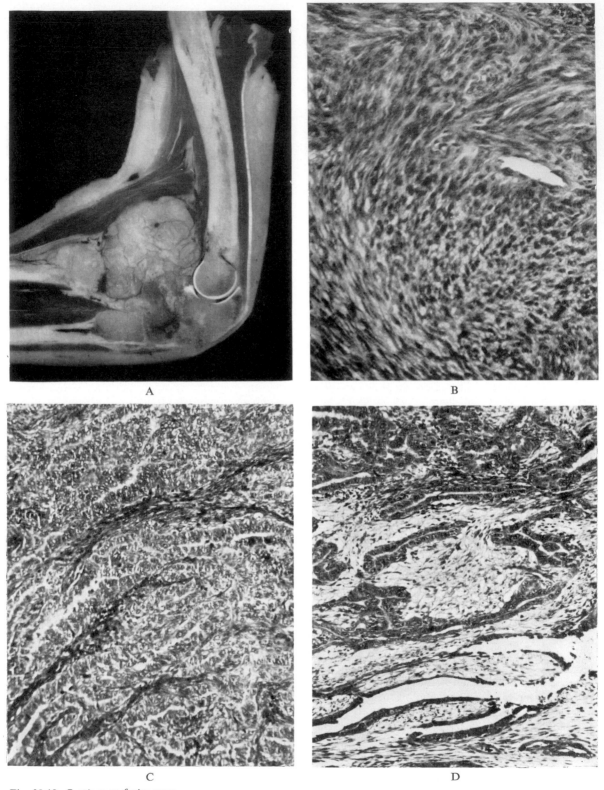

Fig. 38.19. *Captions on facing page.*

peripheral nerves. Tumours of sympathetic ganglia and of paraganglia (see page 1962, Volume 4) are sometimes also considered under this term, as are various tumours of disputed or uncertain histogenesis, particularly when they originate in the soft tissues of the limbs or in the subcutaneous tissue or musculature of other parts of the body.

The histological criteria for the specific identification of many varieties of soft tissue tumour, both benign and malignant, have changed with advancing knowledge in recent years. The exact pathological features and the behaviour of many supposed tumour entities are not yet established, and there is justification for the use of expressions such as '*benign soft tissue tumour (unspecified)*' and '*malignant soft tissue tumour (unspecified)*' when a specific diagnosis cannot be made.

The benign soft tissue tumours include familiar, relatively common, entities such as the *dermatofibroma* (dermal nodular fibrosis—Chapter 39, Volume 6), *lipoma*, *leiomyoma* (Chapter 39, Volume 6), *haemangioma* (Chapter 39, Volume 6), *glomus tumour* (Chapter 39, Volume 6) and *neurolemmoma* (page 2334). Each has a distinctive histological pattern that in each variety is based on a single type of cell. A leiomyoma, for example, is composed of smooth muscle cells that may be specifically identified by the presence of non-striate myofibrils in their cytoplasm; the tumour cells may have a particular relation to the muscle of blood vessels (Fig. 38.20). Similarly, a neurolemmoma is characterized by a distinctive histological structure, at least in part, with a more or less orderly arrangement of the nuclei in twisted rows or palisades: although this pattern may be mimicked in some leiomyomas, diagnostic confusion is unusual because the cells themselves have distinctive features (see page 2335).

The malignant soft tissue tumours include such well-defined entities as fibrosarcoma, liposarcoma, angiosarcoma, rhabdomyosarcoma and neurosarcoma, which are referred to in more detail below, and synovial sarcoma, which is considered on page 2509. It must be emphasized that, in contrast to these sarcomas of identifiable origin, a considerable number of malignant soft tissue tum-

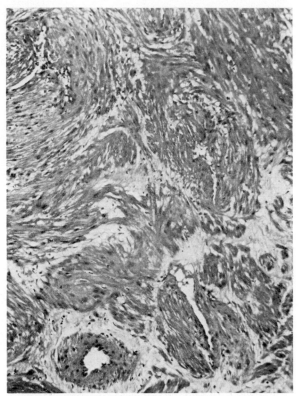

Fig. 38.20. Leiomyoma. In places the smooth muscle cells of the tumour are arranged round irregular spaces lined by endothelium: this relation to blood channels is a feature of leiomyomas of vascular origin. The tendency of the tumour cells to stream and twist in bundles through the tissues is characteristic of leiomyomas in general. *Haematoxylin–eosin.* × 110.

ours cannot be specifically identified because they fail to show a specific pattern of histological differentiation. In practice, this does not seriously limit prognostication, since most of these undifferentiated sarcomas are clearly malignant, and significant differences of behaviour have not yet been established between their possible subgroups.

All soft tissue sarcomas include parts that consist of spindle-shaped cells. Specific identification depends on the recognition of a distinctive cell type, such as a developing fat cell or striated muscle cell, or of a distinctive pattern of arrangement of the cells, or of a particular anatomical origin.

Fig. 38.19. Synovial sarcoma.

A.§ Longitudinally divided arm and forearm, showing tumour of the elbow region. The radius and ulna are invaded.

B. Histological appearance of an undifferentiated area from the tumour in Fig. 38.19A. No synovial structures are present. *Haematoxylin–eosin.* × 245.

C. Another field from the same tumour, showing conspicuous pseudoepithelial structures. *Haematoxylin–eosin.* × 115.

D. The histological appearance of another tumour of this type. Conspicuous pseudoepithelial structures are separated by spindle-celled connective tissue. *Haematoxylin–eosin.* × 115.

Fibrosarcoma[134, 136, 137]

The term fibrosarcoma is commonly applied to malignant tumours formed of spindle-shaped cells that produce reticulin and collagen (Fig. 38.21). Formerly, a large proportion of malignant soft tissue tumours were placed in this group: more careful study and greater knowledge of the histogenesis of the tumours now make it possible to allocate a substantial number of them to other groups. Similarly, the various members of the heterogeneous group of fibroblastic lesions that constitute the so-called fibromatoses (see page 2517) were usually misdiagnosed as fibrosarcomas.

Liposarcoma[138, 139]

The liposarcomas are identifiable histologically by the presence of fat-forming cells—lipoblasts—at various stages of differentiation (Fig. 38.22A). A number of types of liposarcoma may be distinguished; the three that are seen oftenest are the well-differentiated liposarcoma, the myxoid liposarcoma (see below) and the pleomorphic liposarcoma. These types differ considerably in

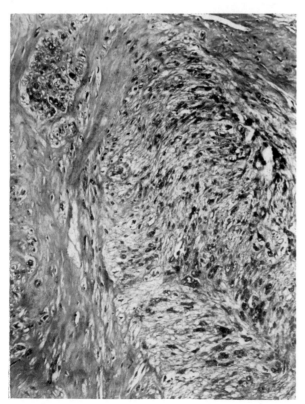

Fig. 38.21. Fibrosarcoma. A pleomorphic example with abundant intercellular collagen. *Haematoxylin–eosin.* × 110.

behaviour: metastasis occurs most frequently in cases of the pleomorphic tumours.

Myxoid Liposarcoma.—The myxoid liposarcomas may contain relatively little fat. They are characterized by the presence of abundant intercellular mucin and conspicuous fluid-filled spaces (Fig. 38.22B). Such tumours were formerly referred to as *myxomas* and *myxosarcomas* (the former term was also applied to fibromas and similar benign lesions that had undergone myxoid change). They commonly recur locally after excision; metastasis rarely takes place.

Angiosarcoma and Other Tumours of Vascular Origin[140–144]

A diversity of histological structures is seen among both benign and malignant tumours of vascular origin. The benign tumours include various types of haemangioma (capillary, cavernous and racemose), the benign haemangiopericytoma and the glomus tumour (see Chapter 39, Volume 6); the malignant tumours include the angiosarcomas and the malignant haemangiopericytoma. All these are characterized by the presence of vascular spaces as an integral part of the tumour. Although, in typical cases, each variety has its own distinctive histological features, there can be difficulty in making a specific identification of some specimens and even in distinguishing them from other tumours such as synovial sarcoma and mesothelioma.

Rhabdomyosarcoma[145–147]

The term rhabdomyosarcoma is applied to a group of highly malignant tumours that are characterized by the presence of cells that are regarded as tumour myoblasts because in a proportion of the tumours there are recognizable cross-striate myofibrils. The histological features vary greatly: embryonal, alveolar and pleomorphic types are distinguishable.

Embryonal Rhabdomyosarcoma.—The embryonal rhabdomyosarcomas are highly malignant tumours that occur almost exclusively in early childhood. They arise particularly in the uterine cervix (see page 1714*), the vagina (see page 1716*), the prostate (see page 1594*) and the urinary bladder (see page 1534*). They belong to the group of so-called 'botryoid sarcomas', the mixed mesodermal tumours: the latter name is the preferred term, particularly as a considerable proportion of the

* In Volume 4.

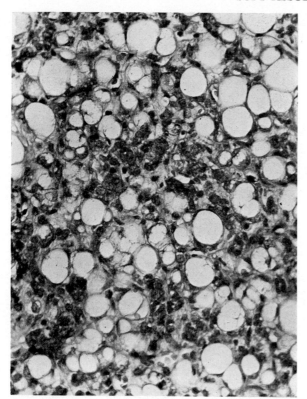

Fig. 38.22A. Pleomorphic liposarcoma. The tumour consists of lipoblasts of various degrees of differentiation. *Haematoxylin–eosin.* × 250.

tumours lack an identifiable muscle cell component.

Alveolar Rhabdomyosarcoma.—The alveolar rhabdomyosarcoma[148] (see Fig. 18.7 on page 1164, Volume 3) should not be confused with the somewhat similarly named alveolar soft-part sarcoma (see below): there is no histological resemblance between them, and no evidence that the latter is in any way derived from muscle. The alveolar rhabdomyosarcoma may be seen at any age; it is less rare in children and young adults than in older people.

Pleomorphic Rhabdomyosarcoma.—The pleomorphic rhabdomyosarcoma is characterized by the presence of bizarre, multinucleate giant cells (Fig. 38.23). A long search of many sections of many samples of a given tumour may be necessary before tumour cells are found that show unequivocal cross-striation of the cytoplasm under the light microscope. It can be very difficult to be sure that cross-striate cells in a sarcoma are not degenerating non-

neoplastic muscle fibres that have been surrounded by the tumour in the course of its growth. Electron microscopy may be invaluable, when practicable, as it enables myofibrils to be recognized in a proportion of unquestionably neoplastic cells.

It is of the greatest practical importance to remember that a diagnosis of rhabdomyosarcoma can be made mistakenly through misinterpretation of the often pleomorphic appearance of healing infarcts and traumatic lesions (tears and haematomas) of muscle. It must also be remembered that rhabdomyosarcomas arise in sites other than the skeletal muscles. The nasopharynx is one of the more frequent of these (see page 243, Volume 1).

Alveolar Soft-Part Sarcoma[149–151]

The tumour that has become known as the alveolar soft-part sarcoma is a rare and distinctive growth that is characterized by an 'organoid' or 'aggregated' arrangement of polygonal cells (Fig. 38.24) and by the presence of granular, intracellular material

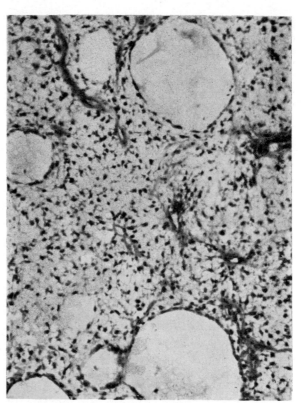

Fig. 38.22B. Myxoid liposarcoma. The characteristically mucoid intercellular material and conspicuous fluid-filled spaces are seen. *Haematoxylin–eosin.* × 135.

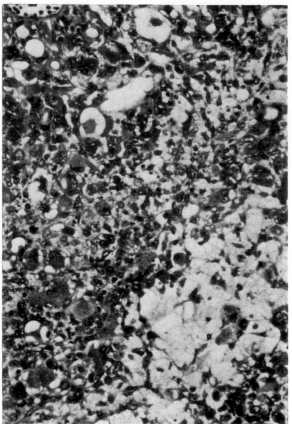

Fig. 38.23. Rhabdomyosarcoma. Pleomorphic type, with conspicuous giant cells. Cross-striate myofibrils were demonstrated in appropriately stained sections. *Haematoxylin–eosin.* × 165.

that gives a positive periodic-acid/Schiff reaction. Its histogenesis is unknown. Some of these tumours have been described as malignant granular cell myoblastomas (see Chapter 39, Volume 6), but they seem in fact to be quite distinct from the very rare, genuine examples of the latter. The alveolar soft-part sarcoma is sometimes mistaken for a metastatic carcinoma or for a non-chromaffin paraganglioma (see page 2342). Some authorities regard it as an example of the latter.[151a]

Other Malignant Tumours of the Soft Tissues

Malignant synoviomas are discussed on page 2509. Other well-defined but rare malignant tumours of soft tissues include neurosarcomas,[152] chondrosarcoma arising in soft tissues,[153, 154] osteosarcoma arising in soft tissues,[155] clear cell sarcoma of tendons and aponeuroses,[156] giant cell tumour of soft tissues,[157, 158] and the malignant fibrous

histiocytoma (malignant fibroxanthoma) (see page 2468).[159, 160] Mesotheliomas are considered on page 407 in Volume 1 and page 1193 in Volume 3.

MYOSITIS OSSIFICANS[161, 162]

At least two distinct conditions are known as myositis ossificans. The rarer, *generalized myositis ossificans*, is considered on page 2356. *Localized myositis ossificans* ('solitary myositis ossificans', or pseudomalignant osseous tumour of soft tissues) is of particular importance because its histological appearances are liable to be misinterpreted as sarcomatous: it is a benign condition, and probably not neoplastic. It is to be distinguished from so-called traumatic myositis ossificans (see page 2355). It takes the form of a circumscribed mass within a muscle or in the intermuscular tissue of a limb, and it is quite separate from the skeleton; there is usually no history of trauma.

The most peripheral part of the lesion of localized myositis ossificans consists of a spongework of relatively mature bone trabeculae (Fig. 38.25A).

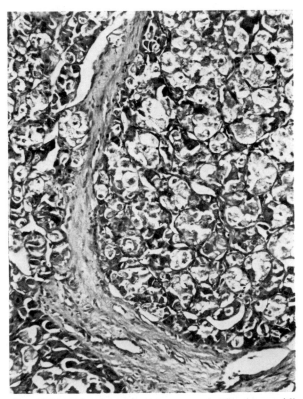

Fig. 38.24. 'Alveolar soft-part sarcoma'. The 'organoid' appearance is characteristic. *Haematoxylin–eosin.* × 100.

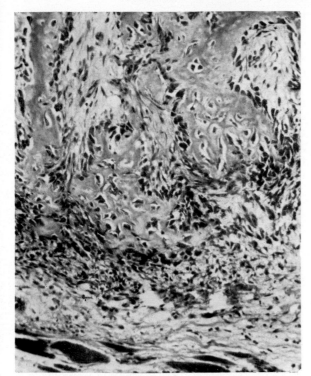

Fig. 38.25A. *Caption at foot of adjoining column.*

The deeper part is usually without bone formation and consists of more or less pleomorphic spindle-shaped cells. It is this central, cellular tissue that is sometimes misinterpreted as sarcomatous (Fig. 38.25B), particularly as mitotic figures may be numerous.

FASCIAL 'FIBROMATOSES'[163, 163a, 164]

Various relatively benign, proliferative fibroblastic lesions of uncertain aetiology have been grouped under the term 'fibromatosis'. They include reactive processes like keloid (see Chapter 39, Volume 6), slowly-growing lesions like Dupuytren's contracture and plantar fibromatosis (see below) and more aggressive lesions that may be confused with sarcomas of soft tissues. Some forms of 'fibromatosis' occur in infants and young children, others in adults; some involve particular areas of the body, others have a less specific distribution.

Dupuytren's Contracture[165–167]

This is one of the commonest of the proliferative fibrous tissue lesions under consideration. The palmar fascia and the overlying subcutaneous tissue

are the site of small, firm, nodular masses. The lesions are formed of spindle-celled and highly collagenous fibrous tissue that merges at its margin with the normal fibrous tissue of the palmar fascia (Figs 38.26A and 38.26B). It is the collagenous tissue that is eventually responsible for the characteristic contracture, which causes puckering of the overlying skin, limitation of extension of the involved fingers and, ultimately, fixed flexion deformity. The condition is infrequent under the age of 40 years; its incidence increases with age, and as many as 40 per cent of octogenarians are found to show some degree of the change. Men are more commonly affected than women, and there is an increased incidence among those suffering from epilepsy and certain other diseases.[166, 167] Trauma does not appear to be a factor. Multiple, often bilateral, lesions are common. There is a family history in some cases. The condition may be associated with other types of fibrous tissue

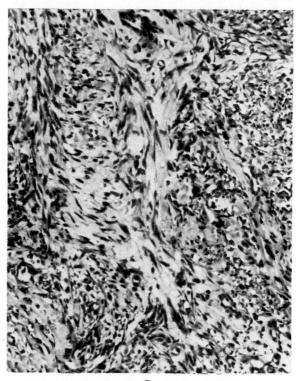

B

Fig. 38.25. Solitary form of 'myositis ossificans'. *Haematoxylin–eosin.* × 130.

A. This field is from the peripheral part of the lesion, which consists of mature bone trabeculae.

B. In this field, from the central part of the lesion, the very cellular nature of the tissue in this region is seen; the cells are predominantly spindle-shaped.

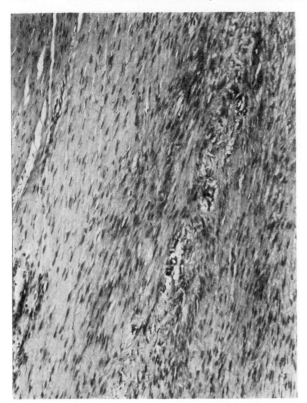

Fig. 38.26A. *Caption at foot of adjoining column.*

proliferation, including lesions of the soles of the feet (plantar 'fibromatosis'—see below), of the penis (Peyronie's disease—see page 1548 in Volume 4) and of the extensor surface of the proximal interphalangeal joints of the hand.

It is important that the spindle-celled tissue of the Dupuytren lesion, which may be very cellular, should not be mistaken for a malignant tumour.

Plantar 'Fibromatosis'[168]

'Fibromatosis' of the plantar fascia of a foot, or of both feet, is much less frequent than Dupuytren's contracture and tends to occur in younger patients. It presents as single or multiple nodules; these have been known to reach a diameter of 10 cm. As in Dupuytren's contracture, the lesion is made up of spindle-celled fibrous tissue: histological distinction from a slowly growing fibrosarcoma can be difficult.

Other 'Fibromatoses'

In recent years it has been established that a number of diffuse proliferative fibrous tissue lesions previously regarded as sarcomatous are, in fact, benign. The characteristics of many of these lesions

have not been studied in detail. Although there is not yet agreement on the names by which they should be known, the terms 'fasciitis',[169] 'nodular fasciitis',[170] 'juvenile fibromatosis',[171] 'diffuse infantile fibromatosis'[164] and 'juvenile aponeurotic fibroma'[172, 173] are coming into use. The lesions arise particularly in the superficial fasciae or subcutaneous tissues, particularly in the limbs. All are relatively rare; most varieties occur predominantly in children or in infants. Distinction from soft tissue tumours (fibrosarcoma, so-called desmoid tumours and dermatofibrosarcoma protuberans—see Chapter 39, Volume 6) is sometimes difficult. The microscopical picture is usually characterized by relatively mature fibrous tissue (Fig. 38.27A), sometimes in a pattern of interlacing fibres and cells. Some examples show a considerable degree of cellularity and mitotic activity. Involvement of the adjoining tissue is not uncommon and may give

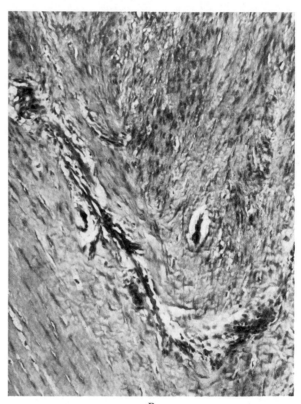

B

Figs 38.26. Dupuytren's contracture. *Haematoxylin–eosin.* ×110.

A. Cellular tissue characteristic of the lesion.

B. Margin of the lesion, showing the abnormal tissue (above) merging with the normal fibrous tissue of the palmar fascia (below): the lesion is more cellular than the normal tissue and its cells are more conspicuous.

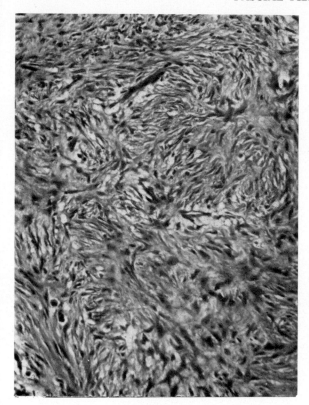
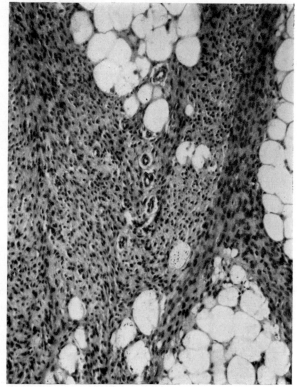

A   B

Fig 38.27. 'Fibromatosis'. *Haematoxylin–eosin.* × 165.

A. Relatively mature fibrous tissue, consisting of interlacing bundles of cells and fibres.

B. Intrusion of the abnormal tissue into subcutaneous fat at the margin of the lesion.

an appearance that suggests infiltration by a malignant tumour (Fig. 38.27B), although the condition is benign.

Some cases of retroperitoneal fibrosis are probably of the same nature as the fascial 'fibromatoses' (see page 1185, Volume 3).

REFERENCES

ANATOMY AND PHYSIOLOGY

1. Ham, A. W., *Histology*, 7th edn, chap. 16. Philadelphia and Toronto, 1974.
2. Ghadially, F. N., Roy, S., *Ultrastructure of Synovial Joints in Health and Disease.* London, 1969.
3. Bauer, W., Ropes, M. W., Waine, H., *Physiol. Rev.*, 1940, **20**, 272.
4. Davies, D. V., *Ann. rheum. Dis.*, 1945, **5**, 29.
5. Freeman, M. A. R., *Adult Articular Cartilage.* London, 1973.
6. McDevitt, C. A., *Ann. rheum. Dis.*, 1973, **32**, 364.
7. Serafini-Fracassini, A., Smith, J. W., *The Structure and Biochemistry of Cartilage.* Edinburgh and London, 1974.
8. Hooghwinkel, G. J., Smits, G., *J. Histochem. Cytochem.*, 1957, **5**, 120.
9. Stockwell, R. A., Scott, J. E., *Nature* (*Lond.*), 1967, **215**, 1376.
10. Benninghoff, A., *Z. Zellforsch.*, 1925, **2**, 783.
11. Bywaters, E. G. L., *J. Path. Bact.*, 1937, **44**, 247.

12. Collins, D. H., *The Pathology of Articular and Spinal Diseases*, page 24. London, 1949.
13. Shaw, N. E., Martin, B. F., *J. Anat.* (*Lond.*), 1962, **96**, 359.
14. Vaubel, E., *J. exp. Med.*, 1933, **58**, 85.
15. Blau, S., Janis, R., Hamerman, D., Sanderson, J., *Science*, 1965, **150**, 353.

DEVELOPMENTAL ABNORMALITIES

16. Carter, C., *J. Bone Jt Surg.*, 1957, **39B**, 778.

TRAUMATIC LESIONS

17. Bennett, G. A., Bauer, W., Maddock, S. J., *Amer. J. Path.*, 1932, **8**, 499.
18. Landells, J. W., *J. Bone Jt Surg.*, 1957, **39B**, 548.
19. Key, J. A., *J. Bone Jt Surg.*, 1925, **23**, 793.

INFLAMMATORY CONDITIONS

20. Phemister, D. B., *Ann. Surg.*, 1924, **80**, 481.
21. Lack, C. H., *J. Bone Jt Surg.*, 1959, **41B**, 384.

22. Copeman, W. S. C., *Brit. med. J.*, 1942, **1**, 760.
23. Keefer, C. S., Parker, P., Myers, W. K., *Arch. Path. (Chic.)*, 1934, **18**, 199.
24. Boger, W. P., *J. Amer. med. Ass.*, 1944, **126**, 1062.
25. Rosencrantz, E., Piscitelli, A., Bost, F. C., *J. Bone Jt Surg.*, 1941, **23**, 628.
26. Mann, K. J., *Lancet*, 1946, **2**, 744.
27. Sissons, H. A., *J. Bone Jt. Surg.*, 1952, **34B**, 275.
28. Clutton, H. H., *Lancet*, 1886, **1**, 391.
29. Kling, D. H., *Amer. J. med. Sci.*, 1932, **183**, 538.
30. Klauder, J. V., Robertson, H. F., *J. Amer. med. Ass.*, 1934, **103**, 236.
31. Chesney, A. M., Kemp, J. E., Resnik, W. H., *Bull. Johns Hopk. Hosp.*, 1924, **35**, 235.
32. Chesney, A. M., Kemp, J. E., Baetjer, F. H., *J. clin. Invest.*, 1926, **3**, 131.
33. Dalrymple–Champneys, W., *Brucella Infection and Undulant Fever in Man*, page 72. London, New York and Toronto, 1960.
33a Reiter, H., *Dtsch. med. Wschr.*, 1916, **42**, 1535.
33b.Weinberger, H. J., Bauer, W., *Med. Clin. N. Amer.*, 1955, **39**, 587.
34. Collins, D. H., *The Pathology of Articular and Spinal Diseases*, page 169. London, 1949.
35. Short, C. L., Bauer, W., Reynolds, W. E., *Rheumatoid Arthritis*. Cambridge, Mass., 1957.
36. Gardner, D. L., *The Pathology of Rheumatoid Arthritis*. London, 1972.
37. Sokoloff, L., in *Arthritis and Allied Conditions*, 7th edn, edited by J. L. Hollander, page 187. Philadelphia, 1966.
38. Duthie, J. J. R., in *Modern Trends in Rheumatology*, edited by A. G. S. Hill, vol. 2, page 78. London, 1971.
39. Klemperer, P., *Ann. intern. Med.*, 1948, **28**, 1.
40. Klemperer, P., *Harvey Lect.*, 1953–54, **49**, 100.
41. Ragan, C., in *Progress in Arthritis*, edited by J. H. Talbot and L. M. Lockie, page 22. New York, 1958.
42. Waller, M., *Ann. N.Y. Acad. Sci.*, 1969, **168**, 5.
43. Kulka, J. P., Bocking, D., Ropes, M. W., Bauer, W., *A.M.A. Arch. Path.*, 1955, **59**, 129.
44. Allison, N., Ghormley, R. K., *Diagnosis in Joint Diseases*. Baltimore, 1931.
45. Sherman, M. S., *Bull. Hosp. Jt Dis. (N.Y.)*, 1951, **12**, 110.
46. Kobayshi, I., Ziff, M., *Arthr. and Rheum.*, 1973, **16**, 471.
46a. Bankhurst, A. D., Husby, G., Williams, R. C., *Arthr. and Rheum.*, 1976, **19**, 555.
47. Mellors, R. C., Nowoslawski, A., Korngold, L., Sengson, B. C., *J. exp. Med.*, 1961, **113**, 475.
48. Kaplan, M. H., *Arthr. and Rheum.*, 1963, **6**, 475.
49. Hollander, J. L., McCarty, D. J., Astorga, G., Casto-Murillo, E., *Ann. intern. Med.*, 1965, **62**, 271.
50. Bennett, G. A., Zeller, J. W., Bauer, W., *Arch. Path. (Chic.)*, 1940, **30**, 70.
51. Collins, D. H., *The Pathology of Articular and Spinal Diseases*, page 191. London, 1949.
52. Sokoloff, L., McCluskey, R. T., Bunin, J. J., *A.M.A. Arch. Path.*, 1953, **55**, 475.
53. Bywaters, E. G. L., Glynn, L. E., Zeldis, A., *Ann. rheum. Dis.*, 1958, **17**, 278.
53a. Howell, D. S., in *Progress in Arthritis*, edited by J. H. Talbot and L. M. Lockie, page 1. New York, 1958.
54. Kantor, T., Sokoloff, L., Smith, A., Ziff, M., *Ann. rheum. Dis.*, 1951, **10**, 471.
55. Ziff, M., Kantor, T., Bien, E., Smith, A., *J. clin. Invest.*, 1953, **32**, 1253.
56. Kellgren, J. H., Ball, J., Astbury, W. T., Reed, R., Beighton, E., *Nature (Lond.)*, 1951, **168**, 493.
57. Gale, J. C., *Amer. J. Path.*, 1951, **27**, 455.
58. Gitlin, D., Craig, J. M., Janeway, C. A., *Amer. J. Path.*, 1957, **33**, 55.
59. Baggenstoss, A. H., Rosenberg, E. F., *Arch. Path. (Chic.)*, 1943, **35**, 503.
60. Rosenberg, E. F., Baggenstoss, A. H., Hench, P. S., *Ann. intern. Med.*, 1944, **20**, 903.
61. Sinclair, R. J. G., Cruickshank, B., *Quart. J. Med.*, 1956, N.S. **25**, 313.
62. Sokoloff, L., Bunin, J. J., *J. chron. Dis.*, 1957, **5**, 668.
63. Kulka, J. P., in *Modern Trends in Rheumatology*, edited by A. G. S. Hill, vol. 1, page 49. London, 1966.
64. Sorsby, A., Gormag, A., *Brit. med. J.*, 1946, **1**, 597.
65. Still, G. F., *Med.-chir. Trans.*, 1897, **80**, 47.
66. Felty, A. R., *Bull. Johns Hopk. Hosp.*, 1924, **35**, 16.
67. Jaffe, H. L., *Metabolic, Degenerative, and Inflammatory Diseases of Bones and Joints*, page 817. Philadelphia, 1972.
68. Bauer, W., Bennett, G. A., Zeller, J. W., *Trans. Ass. Amer. Phycns*, 1941, **56**, 349.
68a. Wassermann, K., *Ann. rheum. Dis.*, 1949, **8**, 70.
68b. Sherman, M. S., *J. Bone Jt Surg.*, 1952, **34A**, 831.
69. Strümpell, A., *Dtsch. Z. Nervenheilk.*, 1897, **11**, 338.
70. Marie, P., *Rev. Méd. (Paris)*, 1898, **18**, 285.
71. Tyson, T. L., *Med. Clin. N. Amer.*, 1937, **21**, 1755.
72. Collins, D. H., *The Pathology of Articular and Spinal Diseases*, page 313. London, 1949.
73. Cruikshank, B., *Bull. rheum. Dis.*, 1960, **10**, 211.
74. Ball, J., Sharp, J., in *Modern Trends in Rheumatology*, edited by A. G. S. Hill, vol. 2, page 117. London, 1971.
75. Bernstein, L., *Rheumatism*, 1951, **7**, 18.
76. Toone, E. C., Pierce, E. L., Hennigar, G., in *Progress in Arthritis*, edited by J. H. Talbott and L. M. Lockie, page 154. New York, 1958.
76a. Schlosstein, L., Terasaki, P. I., Bluestone, R., Pearson, C. M., *New Engl. J. Med.*, 1973, **288**, 14, 704.
76b. Brewerton, D. A., Caffrey, M., Hart, F. D., James, D. C. O., Nicholls, A., Sturrock, R. D., *Lancet*, 1973, **1**, 904.
77. Bennett, G. A., *Ann. intern. Med.*, 1943, **19**, 11.

OSTEOARTHRITIS

78. Heine, J., *Virchows Arch. path. Anat.*, 1926, **260**, 521.
79. Bennett, G. A., Waine, H., Bauer, W., *Changes in the Knee Joint at Various Ages with Particular Reference to the Nature and Development of Degenerative Joint Disease*. New York, 1942.
80. Collins, D. H., *The Pathology of Spinal and Articular Diseases*, page 74. London, 1949.
81. Sokoloff, L., *The Biology of Degenerative Joint Disease*. Chicago, 1969.
82. Muir, H., *Ann. rheum. Dis.*, 1977, **36**, 199.
82a. Meachim, G., Osborn, G. V., *J. Path.*, 1970, **102**, 1.
83. Silberberg, M., Silberberg, R., *Arch. Path. (Chic.)*, 1950, **50**, 828.
84. Nichols, E. H., Richardson, F. L., *J. med. Res.*, 1909, **21**, 149.
85. Meachim, G., *Ann. rheum. Dis.*, 1972, **31**, 457.
86. Mankin, H. J., Dorfman, H., Lippiello, L., Zarins, A., *J. Bone Jt Surg.*, 1971, **53A**, 523.
87. Dingle, J. T., *J. Bone Jt Surg.*, 1973, **55B**, 87.
88. Ehrlich, M. G., Mankin, H. J., Treadwell, B. V., *J. Bone Jt Surg.*, 1973, **55A**, 1068.

89. Ali, S. Y., Bayliss, M. T., in *Normal and Osteoarthrotic Articular Cartilage*, edited by S. Y. Ali, M. W. Elves and D. H. Leaback, page 189. London, 1974.

90. Harrison, M. H. M., Schajowicz, F., Trueta, J., *J. Bone Jt Surg.*, 1953, **35B**, 598.

91. Lloyd-Roberts, G. C., *J. Bone Jt Surg.*, 1955, **37B**, 8.

92. Byers, P. D., Contepomi, C. A., Farkas, T. A., *Ann. rheum. Dis.*, 1970, **29**, 15.

93. Byers, P. D., Contepomi, C. A., Farkas, T. A., *Ann. rheum. Dis.*, 1976, **35**, 114.

94. Meachim, G., *J. Path.*, 1972, **107**, 199.

95. Bullough, P., Goodfellow, J., O'Connor, J., *J. Bone Jt Surg.*, 1973, **55B**, 746.

95a. Hirsch, C., *Acta chir. scand.*, 1954, suppl. 83.

96. Heberden, G. [W.], *Commentarii de morborum historia*, page 130. London, 1802.

97. Collins, D. H., *The Pathology of Articular and Spinal Diseases*, chap.14. London, 1949.

98. Vernon-Roberts, B., Pirie, C. J., Trenwith, V., *Ann. rheum. Dis.*, 1974, **33**, 281.

99. Charcot, J. M., *Arch. Physiol. norm. path.*, 1868, **1**, 161.

GOUT

100. Talbott, J. H., *Gout*, 2nd edn. New York, 1964.

101. Wyngaarden, J. B., Kelley, W. N., *Gout and Hyperuricemia*. New York, San Francisco and London, 1976.

102. Lichtenstein, L., Scott, H. W., Levin, M. H., *Amer. J. Path.*, 1956, **32**, 871.

102a. Jacobson, B. M., *Ann. intern. Med.*, 1938, **11**, 1277.

103. Sherman, M. S., *Arch. Path. (Chic.)*, 1946, **42**, 557.

104. Collins, D. H., *The Pathology of Articular and Spinal Diseases*, page 119, London, 1949.

105. McCarty, D. J., Jr, in *Arthritis and Allied Conditions— A Textbook of Rheumatology*, 8th edn, edited by J. L. Hollander and D. J. McCarty, Jr, page 1140. Philadelphia, 1972.

106. McCarty, D. J., Jr, Kohn, N. N., Faires, J. S., *Ann. intern. Med.*, 1962, **56**, 711.

107. Bundens, W. D., Brighton, C. T., Weitzman, G., *J. Bone Jt Surg.*, 1965, **47A**, 111.

108. McCarty, D. J., Jr, Hogan, J. M., Gatter, R. A., Grossman, M., *J. Bone Jt Surg.*, 1966, **48A**, 309.

108a. Kohn, N. N., Hughes, R. E., McCarty, D. J., Jr, Faires, J. S., *Ann. intern. Med.*, 1962, **56**, 738.

109. Currey, H. L. F., *Proc. roy. Soc. Med.*, 1968, **61**, 969.

110. Moskowitz, R. W., Katz, D., *Arch. intern. Med.*, 1965, **115**, 680.

111. McCarty, D. J., Hogan, J. M., Gatter, R. A., Grossman, M., *J. Bone Jt Surg.*, 1966, **48A**, 309.

111a. Jacobelli, S., McCarty, D. J., Silcox, D. C., Mall, J. C., *Ann. intern. Med.*, 1973, **79**, 340.

111b. Bywaters, E. G. L., Dixon, A. St J., Scott, J. T., *Ann. rheum. Dis.*, 1963, **22**, 171.

MISCELLANEOUS DISEASES

112. Freund, E., *Arch. Surg. (Chic.)*, 1937, **34**, 670.

113. Murphy, F. P., Dahlin, D. C., Sullivan, R., *J. Bone Jt Surg.*, 1962, **44A**, 77.

114. Mullins, F., Benard, C. W., Eisenberg, S. H., *Cancer (Philad.)*, 1965, **18**, 1180.

115. Goldman, R. L., Lichtenstein, L., *Cancer (Philad.)*, 1964, **17**, 1233.

116. Bruce, J., Walmsley, R., *Brit. J. Surg.*, 1937–38, **25**, 17.

117. Schmorl, G., Junghanns, H., *Die gesunde und kranke Wirbelsäule im Röntgenbild*. Leipzig, 1932.

118. Beadle, O. A., *Spec. Rep. Ser. med. Res. Coun. (Lond.)*, No. 161, 1931.

119. Jaffe, H. L., *Tumors and Tumorous Conditions of the Bones and Joints*, page 532. Philadelphia, 1958.

120. Byers, P. D., Cotton, R. E., Deacon, O. W., Lowy, M., Newman, P. H., Sissons, H. A., Thomson, A. D., *J. Bone Jt Surg.*, 1968, **50B**, 290.

121. Jaffe, H. L., Lichtenstein, L., Sutro, C. J., *Arch. Path. (Chic.)*, 1941, **31**, 731.

122. De Santo, D. A., Wilson, P. D., *J. Bone Jt Surg.*, 1939, **21**, 531.

123. Stewart, M. J., *J. Bone Jt Surg.*, 1948, **30B**, 522.

124. Wright, C. J. E., *Brit. J. Surg.*, 1950–51, **38**, 257.

124a. Fraire, A. E., Fechner, R. E., *Arch. Path.*, 1972, **93**, 473.

125. Key, J. A., *Ann. Surg.*, 1932, **95**, 198.

126. De Palma, A. F., Cotler, J., *Clin. Orthop.*, 1956, **8**, 163.

127. Young, J. M., Hudacek, A. G., *Amer. J. Path.*, 1954, **30**, 799.

128. Hoaglund, F. T., *J. Bone Jt Surg.*, 1967, **49A**, 285.

SYNOVIAL TUMOURS

129. Jaffe, H. L., *Tumors and Tumorous Conditions of the Bones and Joints*, page 576. Philadelphia, 1958.

130. Haagensen, C. D., Stout, A. P., *Ann. Surg.*, 1944, **120**, 826.

131. Bennett, G. A., *J. Bone Jt Surg.*, 1947, **29**, 259.

132. Cadman, N. L., Soule, E. H., Kelly, P. J., *Cancer (Philad.)*, 1965, **18**, 613.

TUMOURS OF OTHER SOFT TISSUES

133. Enzinger, F. M., Lattes, R., Torloni, H., *Histological Typing of Soft Tissue Tumours*. Geneva, 1969.

134. Stout, A. P., Lattes, R., *Tumors of the Soft Tissues* (Atlas of Tumor Pathology, 2nd ser., fasc. 1). Washington, D.C., 1967.

135. Mackenzie, D. H., *Differential Diagnosis of Fibroblastic Disorders*. Oxford, 1970.

136. Stout, A. P., *Cancer (Philad.)*, 1948, **1**, 30.

137. Mackenzie, D. H., *Brit. J. Surg.*, 1964, **51**, 607.

138. Stout, A. P., *Ann. Surg.*, 1944, **119**, 86.

139. Enzinger, F. M., Winslow, D. J., *Virchows Arch. path. Anat.*, 1962, **335**, 367.

140. Murray, M. R., Stout, A. P., *Amer. J. Path.*, 1942, **18**, 183.

141. Stout, A. P., *Cancer (Philad.)*, 1949, **2**, 1027.

142. Kauffman, S. L., Stout, A. P., *Cancer (Philad.)*, 1960, **13**, 695.

143. Steingaszner, L. C., Enzinger, F. M., Taylor, H. B., *Cancer (Philad.)*, 1965, **18**, 352.

144. Ramsey, H. J., *Cancer (Philad.)*, 1966, **19**, 2005.

145. Patton, R. B., Horn, R. C., *Surgery*, 1962, **52**, 572.

146. Lawrence, W., Jegge, G., Foote, F. W., *Cancer (Philad.)*, 1964 **17**, 361.

147. Kauffman, S. L., Stout, A. P., *Cancer (Philad.)*, 1965, **18**, 460.

148. Enzinger, F. M., Shiraki, M., *Cancer (Philad.)*, 1969, **24**, 18.

149. Christopherson, W. M., Foote, F. W., Stewart, F. W., *Cancer (Philad.)*, 1952, **5**, 100.

150. Fisher, E. R., *Amer. J. Path.*, 1956, **32**, 721.

151. Stein, A. H., *J. Bone Jt Surg.*, 1956, **38A**, 1126.

151a. Ashley, D. J. B., *Evans' Histological Appearances of Tumours*, 3rd edn, page 96. Edinburgh, London and New York, 1978.

152. Stewart, F. W., Copeland, M. M., *Amer. J. Cancer*, 1931, **15**, 1235.
153. Stout, A. P., Verner, E. W., *Cancer (Philad.)*, 1953, **6**, 581.
154. Lichtenstein, L., Goldman, R. L., *Cancer (Philad.)*, 1964, **17**, 1203.
155. Fine, G., Stout, A. P., *Cancer (Philad.)*, 1956, **9**, 1027.
156. Enzinger, F. M., *Cancer (Philad.)*, 1965, **18**, 1163.
157. Guccion, J. G., Enzinger, F. M., *Cancer (Philad.)*, 1972, **29**, 1518.
158. Salm, R., Sissons, H. A., *J. Path.*, 1972, **27**, 107.
159. Kempson, R. L., Kyriakos, M., *Cancer (Philad.)*, 1972, **29**, 961.
160. Soule, E. H., Enriquez, P., *Cancer (Philad.)*, 1972, **30**, 128.

'MYOSITIS OSSIFICANS'
161. Ackerman, L. V., *J. Bone Jt Surg.*, 1958, **40A**, 279.
162. Jaffe, H. L., *Tumors and Tumorous Conditions of the Bones and Joints*, page 526. Philadelphia, 1958.

FASCIAL 'FIBROMATOSES'
163. Mackenzie, D. H., *The Differential Diagnosis of Fibroblastic Disorders*. Oxford and Edinburgh, 1970.
163a. Mackenzie, D. H., *Brit. med. J.*, 1972, **4**, 277.
164. Enzinger, F. M., in *Tumors of Bone and Soft Tissue*, page 375. Chicago, 1965.
165. Dupuytren, G., *J. univ. hebd. Méd. Chir. prat.*, 1831, sér. 2, **5**, 352.
166. Hueston, J. T., *Dupuytren's Contracture*. Edinburgh and London, 1963.
167. Skoog, T., *Acta chir. scand.*, 1948, **96**, suppl. 139.
168. Pickren, J. W., Smith, A. G., Stevenson, T. W., Stout, A. P., *Cancer (Philad.)*, 1951, **4**, 846.
169. Hutter, R. V. P., Stewart, F. W., Foote, F. W., *Cancer (Philad.)*, 1962, **15**, 999.
170. Konwaler, B. E., Keasby, L., Kaplan, L., *Amer. J. clin. Path.*, 1955, **25**, 241.
171. Stout, A. P., *Cancer (Philad.)*, 1954, **7**, 953.
172. Keasby, L. E., *Cancer (Philad.)*, 1953, **6**, 338.
173. Allen, P. W., Enzinger, F. M., *Cancer (Philad.)*, 1970 **26**, 857.

ACKNOWLEDGEMENTS FOR ILLUSTRATIONS

Figs 38.1, 7. Pathology Museum, St Bartholomew's Hospital Medical College, London; reproduced by permission of Professor W. G. Spector.

Figs 38.2, 3. Pathology Museum, King's College Hospital Medical School, London; reproduced by permission of Professor E. A. Wright.

Figs 38.4C, 12, 17B. Photomicrographs of the author's specimens by Mr R. S. Barnett, Department of Histopathology, Charing Cross Hospital Medical School, London.

Figs 38.5A, 15A, 15B, 19A. Wellcome Museum, Institute of Orthopaedics, London.

Fig. 38.8. Museum of London Hospital Medical College, London; reproduced by permission of the Curator, Mr E. C. B. Butler.

Figs 38.16A, 16B. Pathology Museum, Royal College of Surgeons of England, London; reproduced by permission of the Conservator, Professor J. L. Turk.

Index to Volume 5

prepared by the editor and Jean N. Symmers

Some entries include a cross-reference to another part of the index where the subject is covered in more detail or under a preferred synonym, or where a related condition is cited. To lessen the possible inconvenience of this practice, if there is a major account of the topic its page is indicated in parentheses: for example—

avitaminosis B_1 2317, *and see* thiamin deficiency
neurosyphilis, *see* syphilis, CNS (2118)

Multiple Page Entries. When more than one page reference is given in an entry, bold type is used to indicate a main account of the topic, if appropriate.

Illustrations and Tables. Reference to an illustration or table is indicated by noting its number in parentheses after the number of the page on which it appears. In general, illustrations and tables are not included in the index as they are referred to in the part of the text to which the relevant subject entries relate.

Footnotes. Reference to a footnote is indicated by the appropriate symbol (asterisk [*], dagger [†] or double dagger [‡]) after the page number.

Cases. Reference to a particular case of a disease is indicated by the word *case* in parentheses after the text of the entry.

Alternative Spellings. Terms that in American usage are generally spelt more simply than is usual in Britain, such as celiac disease (coeliac disease), edema (oedema), hemangioblastoma (haemangioblastoma) and nevus (naevus), should be looked for in the spelling that accords with British practice (shown in parentheses in the examples noted).

The spellings catabolic, leucodystrophy, leucoviruses and the like are used in this book rather than katabolic, leukodystrophy and leukoviruses. It is also in accordance with current practice in Britain that the spelling leukaemia is used.

Abbreviations. CNS: central nervous system. Other abbreviations that appear in the index refer to abbreviations used—and explained—in the text of the book: the terms for which these abbreviations stand are also indexed, in their appropriate alphabetical place.

Index to Volume 5

D